The Clinical Practice of
Critical Care Neurology

THE
CLINICAL PRACTICE
OF
CRITICAL CARE
NEUROLOGY
SECOND EDITION

Eelco F. M. Wijdicks, M.D., Ph.D., F.A.C.P.

Consultant, Department of Neurology
Mayo Clinic and Mayo Foundation
Professor of Neurology, Mayo Medical School
Medical Director, Neurological/Neurosurgical
Intensive Care Unit, Saint Marys Hospital
Rochester, Minnesota

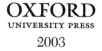

OXFORD
UNIVERSITY PRESS
2003

OXFORD
UNIVERSITY PRESS

Oxford   New York
Auckland   Bangkok   Buenos Aires   Cape Town   Chennai
Dar es Salaam   Delhi   Hong Kong   Istanbul   Karachi   Kolkata
Kuala Lumpur   Madrid   Melbourne   Mexico City   Mumbai
Nairobi   São Paulo   Shanghai   Singapore   Taipei   Tokyo   Toronto

© 2003 Mayo Foundation for Medical Education and Research.

Published by Oxford University Press, Inc.
198 Madison Avenue, New York, New York, 10016
http://www.oup-usa.org

Oxford is a registered trademark of Oxford University Press.

Library of Congress Cataloging-in-Publication Data
Wijdicks, Eelco F. M., 1954–
The clinical practice of critical care neurology / Eelco F.M. Wijdicks—2nd ed.
p. ; cm. Includes bibliographical references and index.
ISBN 0-19-515729-X (cloth)
1. Neurological intensive care.   I. Title.
[DNLM: 1. Nervous System Diseases.   2. Critical Care.   3. Emergencies.
4. Intensive Care Units—organizations & administration.
WL 100 W662c 2003]
RC350.N49 W549 2003
616.8'0428—dc   2002030775

Nothing in this publication implies that Mayo Foundation endorses any of the products mentioned in this book. Care has been taken to confirm the accuracy of the information presented and to describe generally accepted practices. However, the authors, editors, and publisher are not responsible for errors or omissions or for any consequences from application of the information in this book and make no warranty, express or implied, with respect to the contents of the publication.

The authors, editors, and publisher have exerted every effort to ensure that drug selection and dosage set forth in this text are in accordance with current recommendations and practice at the time of publication. However, in view of ongoing research, changes in government regulations, and the constant flow of information relating to drug therapy and drug reactions, the reader is urged to check the package insert for each drug for any change in indications and dosage and for added warnings and precautions. This is particularly important when the recommended agent is a new or infrequently employed drug.

Some drugs and medical devices presented in this publication have U.S. Food and Drug Administration (FDA) clearance for limited use in restricted research settings. It is the responsibility of health care providers to ascertain the FDA status of each drug or device planned for use in their clinical practice.

2 4 6 8 9 7 5 3 1

Printed in the United States of America
on acid-free paper.

For Barbara-Jane,
Coen,
and Marilou,
always

Preface to the Second Edition

This second edition follows soon after the first edition for the very obvious reason that the field is moving rather quickly and because I have a few more words to say. I have kept the layout and organization but have expanded the book with five new chapters. One of these is on the organization of intensive care units, including options for different types and models that can be used in intensive care units all over the world. In some hospitals, the closed unit form fits nicely; in others, the logistics or funding may not allow for such a model, but care of the patient can still be superb. A chapter on acute spinal cord disorders has been added because occasionally patients with this type of disorder have rapid deterioration and are admitted to the neurologic intensive care unit. I felt a discussion was needed in this edition to assist in evaluation and management, albeit in most circumstances to bridge neurosurgical intervention. I have added a two-chapter part on management of common postoperative neurosurgical complications. Critical care neurologists are often involved in postoperative complications and should have at least a working knowledge of these complications. These chapters are abbreviated to match the scope of neurologists. The book closes with the sensitive subject of ethical and legal decisions. Many families are shaken by the aftermath of a neurologic catastrophe and feel that care is futile, and some are angry. This chapter highlights some of the current ethical controversies and legal risks. Also new to this edition are algorithms on outcome prediction in the specific disorders. The branches of the trees in these algorithms have been carefully chosen and may guide the practitioner in discussions with family members. The decision trees are based on the best available medical knowledge, but the user of this book should acknowledge their limitations.

I have tried to maintain a practical format, to keep the language clear and succinct, and to remove gross generalizations and efforts to force-feed the reader with strong opinions. I rewrote, corrected, and improved paragraphs that I did not get right the first time and revised some of my conclusions. Multiple new sections have filtered into this second edition. The booklet with tables and figures that accompanied the first edition was well received but wore out quickly. I have added new tables and algorithms, and the quality of the cover and paper has been improved.

It is easy to overreach in a second edition, but the book should be condensed enough for neurologists of all stripes, adequately transparent for the junior residents, and sufficiently specific to be useful to my peers. It tries to paint a broad canvas incorporating all topics needed in daily practice. Thus it is intended not only for beginning neurointensivists but also for anyone who demands a full treatment of the complexity of acute neurologic disorders. I hope that it will be accepted as a responsible work on the subject of neurologic critical care and acute neurology.

Eelco F. M. Wijdicks

Acknowledgments

I much appreciate the invaluable and continuing assistance of the Mayo Clinic Section of Scientific Publications. I specifically thank Sharon L. Wadleigh, who has been involved with my book projects since the beginning and has always been ahead of me. John L. Prickman's astute editing of the text is greatfully acknowledged. David A. Factor is a peerless illustrator whose wonderful halftone drawings are again interspersed throughout the book. Roberta J. Schwartz coordinated the entire effort with much resolve and made timely submission possible. I am very pleased to be connected with Oxford University Press (Leslie Anglin) and greatly value their commitment to publish my work.

Contents

PART I

GENERAL PRINCIPLES OF MANAGEMENT OF CRITICALLY ILL NEUROLOGIC PATIENTS

1

Organization of the Neurologic Critical Care Unit

The essence of neurologic critical care lies in the acute decision making and management of emergency neurologic conditions. Surely, new skills, support structures, and attitudes are necessary to practice neurologic critical care—or acute neurology, for that matter. Avatars in critical care medicine contend that you need driven, primed neurologists, a team, and colleagues who understand the distinctive features of neurologic critical illness and belaud the presence of a service and a location. At the risk of oversimplification, the neurologic critical care unit is a better place from the perspective of the patient and is the locus in quo of critical care neurologists. Usually, this unit is a combined neurologic and neurosurgical intensive care unit, but some have remained largely neurosurgical or specifically designated trauma units. Most of these units are labeled *neurologic intensive care unit* (NICU), but some institutions have embroidered the designation: *neurosciences intensive care unit.*

Neurologic critical care is an appealing subspecialty of neurology, providing considerable job satisfaction. Although at times the patient's clinical course is hopeless, many days are filled with accomplishments resulting in patients with intact or nondisabling neurologic function.

This chapter introduces the complexity and hustle and bustle of daily practice and the ever more visible role of a director overseeing the clinical activity. Its focus is on management and types of administrative structure. Microeco-

nomics is beyond the scope of this book, but excellent monographs on policymaking are available.[2,12]

STAFFING

The physicians, nurses, and ancillary staff who determine care in the NICU may include but are not limited to the medical or surgical director (responsible for clinical affairs), the neurointensivist (primary and overseeing care) (Table 1–1), neurosurgeons, anesthesiologists, neurologic intensive care fellows in training, senior neurology or neurosurgery residents, the nurse manager (responsible for nursing affairs), neuroscience intensive care nurses, and nurses in training. Respiratory therapists have become crucial in the management of critically ill patients, and efficient strategies have been developed. Physician assistants in critical care units have become a reality and provide excellent practice. Other teams consist of nutritional consultants, infectious disease consultants, and acute code responders. Physical therapists are indispensable in the NICU (Chapter 3).

The major task of the neurointensivist is to orchestrate a cohesive policy and to prevent fractionation of care.[5] Fundamentally, on any given day in the NICU, a certain mission or code of conduct is required. Significant challenges to some of these principles may occur, such as limited resources and capacity, nursing

Table 1–1. The Neurointensivist

Is trained in medical management of critically ill patients
  with neurologic or neurosurgical disease
Has clinical credibility
Makes daily rounds
Develops novel research and publishes widely
Implements collaborative practices
Spends 30% to 50% of professional time in practice

Table 1–2. Code of Conduct for the Neurointensivist

Make the care of patients your first concern
Be sure that communication with family is the next
  concern
Do not let personal beliefs prejudice the provision of
  care
Maintain veracity
Respect all laws and uphold the honor of the profession
Obtain consultation from other experts when the need is
  clear
Accept any patient in need of intensive care
Be academic, teach, and publish new observations

staff shortage, and excessive expense. The mission or code of conduct of the neurointensivist (a neurologist but also in some institutions a neurosurgeon or neuroanesthesiologist) is shown in Table 1–2.

DESIGN

As a rule, the NICU is close to other intensive care units, the emergency department, and the radiology department. The typical floor plan includes single-patient rooms, nursing station, support storage and utility areas, pharmacy, conference rooms, and family waiting rooms (Fig. 1–1). A large space should be allowed for family members, and sleep facilities should be offered to them in times of crisis. Multiple hand-washing facilities, decreased crowding, and efficient airflow may reduce nosocomial infections. Current NICUs accommodate multiple computer workstations for immediate access to patient data and radiologic studies. In the patient area are a universal bed, a power column, equipment space, and, preferably, mobile monitoring devices. Our NICU room is depicted in Figure 1–2.

Driven by regulations and the need for cost-effectiveness, NICUs have evolved through several models of organization. The main models are open, transitional (semiopen or hybrid), and closed units (Table 1–3). The main feature of the transitional model is a more active role for the neurointensivist. There has been a major push toward a closed unit in which the neu-

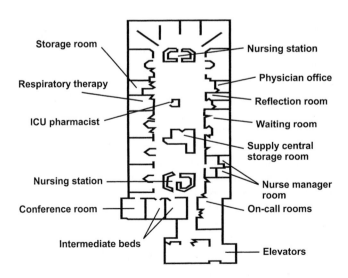

Figure 1–1. Floor plan of the neurologic-neurosurgical intensive care unit (ICU) at the Mayo Clinic.

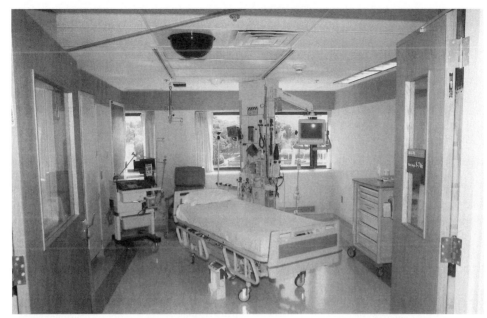

A

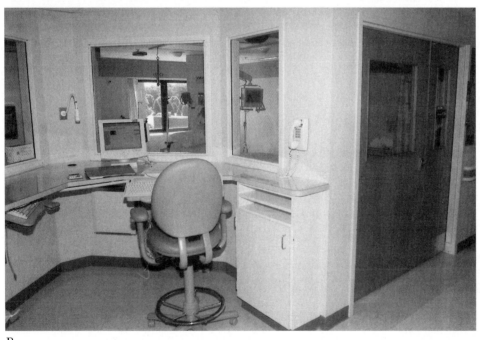

B

Figure 1–2. (*A*) Neurologic intensive care unit room with power column and monitors. Note video monitor (for continuous electroencephalographic video monitoring), attached to ceiling. Patient rooms in the unit should be at least 225 square feet, and an anteroom (not in our unit) for washing hands and applying gowns should be at least 20 square feet. Natural illumination is important to maintain day and night orientation. Monitors should display electrocardiogram, intracranial pressure, cerebral perfusion pressure, and cardiac and respiratory data. Tracings of Swan–Ganz catheters are continuously displayed when used.[6] (*B*) A computer workstation provides electronic medical records and laboratory tests. Most neuroradiologic studies are readily available on-line.

Table 1–3. Neurologic-Neurosurgical Intensive Care Unit Models

Key Features	MODEL		
	Open	*Transitional*	*Closed*
Hospital type	Nonteaching	Teaching	Referral center
Triage approval	Any neurologist or neurosurgeon	Neurointensivist or unit director	Neurointensivist
Patient care	Any neurologist or neurosurgeon	Neurointensivist	Neurointensivist
Rounds and orders	Each physician separate	Neurointensivist on selected patients	Neurointensivist on all patients
Advantages	Continuity of neurosurgical care	Collaborative practice Nurse satisfaction	Neurointensivist is the responsible person Protocols facilitated Improved efficiency and reduced resources Nurse satisfaction
Disadvantages	Increased subspecialty consultation No team leader	Role of neurointensivist brittle House staff not always present	Physician conflict and alienation Less continuity of care

rointensivist becomes the team leader with significant administrative powers but also makes rounds on every patient, manages the day-to-day care, and forges a collaborative practice.[4,11] Transitional models may be very workable in other hospitals where there is in-house angst to relegate care to one person. Studies in other intensive care units suggest that closed units reduce complications and mortality,[1] but these data are not available from NICUs.

ROUNDS

Initial daily rounds are needed to integrate findings at the bedside with laboratory test results, current therapies, and technologic support into a "plan for the day." Intermittent visits to the bedside are frequent, but care is facilitated if responsible team members meet in the morning and late afternoon. Morning rounds may or may not include the respiratory therapist and pharmacist, but the charge nurse, responsible assigned nurse, senior resident, fellow, and consultant should be present. The attending physician is briefed by the residents or fellow. After a general overview of the neurologic condition is provided, specific problems

are discussed. These include careful review of systems (cardiac, pulmonary, gastrointestinal, bladder, skin), intercurrent infections, prophylactic medication, and recent institution of drugs. Rates of adverse drug events may be substantially lower when the pharmacist participates.[10] The necessity of procedural interventions (arterial line, pulmonary artery catheter, nasogastric tube, ventriculostomy) should be addressed. Neuroimaging studies should be reviewed and, when appropriate, compared.

Major emphasis is placed on causes of deterioration, which require discussion. Orders that trigger calls to the resident should be written, and the rationale should be explained. Overt laboratory abnormalities are important, but trends also need attention and management. The results of recent discussions with the patient or family members should be communicated. A plan of management should be clear before the next patient is approached.

Morning rounds are a fertile ground for teaching and to channel certain ideas for research to interested residents or fellows. The late afternoon round can be truncated and should typically involve only follow-up of earlier plans and reiteration of potential nighttime problems. It is ill advised to use afternoon rounds to dismiss patients, but patients can be identified when such a need arises. Sufficient observation requires at least 24 hours, and transfer of patients from 6 P.M. to 6 A.M. is not good practice. Early communication with the neurosurgical resident or staff is important and may prevent conflicting opinions when triage is needed to accommodate a new patient in greater need of critical care.

MORALE

A budding neurointensivist may constantly need to be two steps ahead while developing credibility and respect, which come at a considerable personal cost. Overworking has to be balanced with slack time, but the critical care unit invites a psychologic phenomenon called *burnout* among the staff.

The term *burnout* has been coined to describe physical and emotional exhaustion typified by negative self-concept, negative job attitude, and a loss of concern and feeling for patients.[8,9] Most worrisome is a feeling of "just going through the motions."[7] Other signs of burnout are a run-down feeling, disillusionment, sarcasm and rigidity, and fading enthusiasm. Burnout may largely depend on the individual. Being "on call" 24 hours a day, 7 days a week; facing high mortality and, more significantly, damaging morbidity in patients, knowing what will happen to a person; experiencing overwhelming tragedies, constant exposure to grieving family reactions, and sleep deprivation; and resolving conflicts between physicians and nursing staff are common triggers for burnout.[7,9] Very few studies of intensive care unit physicians are available. One study in pediatric critical care medicine (probably comparable to neurology intensive care because of frequent family interaction and sudden loss) found 50% at risk.[3] A study in Australia suggested a possible link between excessive workload (using a creative definition of occupancy per shift and peak occupancy) and mortality in the intensive care unit.[13]

Protection against these stressors may include restriction to 2-week shifts, a total of three rotating attending neurointensivists, no clinic responsibilities, protected downtime, regular exercise, few administrative meetings, and time to write.

LEGITIMACY

Most academically affiliated medical centers have some area of critical care dedicated to neurologic and neurosurgical patients. There has been significant growth in the number of neurointensivists in the United States and Europe. Generally, neurointensivists are not anesthesiologists, pulmonologists, or cardiologists but are neurologists with formal training in neurologic intensive care. Fellowship programs are available throughout the United States and in some countries in Europe (e.g., Germany and Austria). Neurointensivists may have earlier been pulmonologists or anesthesiologists, but most have not fully completed critical care training. Complex preconceptions are the result, and beginning neurointensivists with lack of authority find themselves in the wild blue yonder. Critical care physicians may point out that neurointensivists are not board-certified in critical care medicine, do not understand the ventilator, and cannot take care of "really sick" patients. Some consider it an assault on their autonomy and prestige. Neurosurgeons may argue that neurosurgical emergencies should not be managed by neurologists and justly feel threatened losing responsibility after many hours in the operating room. Moreover, perioperative care is a core requirement for training of residents and fellows. Others would degrade the neurointensivist's work to a mere custodial function ("baby-sitting") or ask for prognostication only. Other subspecialists with overlapping interests may be even more disdainful and may believe that neurointensivists are an "endangered species," are much too aggressive, and think there is nothing they cannot do and that a paradigm shift is not justified. All of the above is understandable but such a position is not excusable.

As this book shows, neurologic critical care is complex and neurologists in the field have training in neurosurgical issues, appreciate the impact of cardiopulmonary manipulation on central nervous system function, understand secondary deterioration in major catastrophes, integrate systemic illness with neurologic illness, and can fully manage acute disorders of the nervous system but also have core skills in neuroimaging interpretation and critical care. To compare neurologic intensive care with medical or surgical intensive care is to measure incommensurables with the same ruler. Neurointensivists should rise to the challenge and build bridges, foster collaborative relationships,[14] convince skeptics of their complementary expertise, share clinical responsibility, and create opportunity for mutual research. We share the NICU directorship with neurosurgery

and have a visible role of critical care anesthesiologists.

Within an environment of trust, patient care and education should improve tremendously. Neurointensivists should try to find the best model in their institution, comply with the requirements of the Joint Commission on the Accreditation of Health Organizations, and negotiate management strategies. The impact of neurointensivists has not been rigorously evaluated, but future studies could potentially demonstrate reduced mortality, shortened stays in the NICU, shorter duration of mechanical ventilation, fewer consultations, reduction in both readmissions to the NICU and inappropriate early dismissals, and, finally, reduced NICU costs.

CONCLUSIONS

- NICU practice is collaborative, but several models exist. A closed model is ideal.
- Practice in the NICU is totally different from that in other intensive care units.
- Daily rounds are best standardized to address specific problems and should incorporate other health care workers.

REFERENCES

1. Carson SS, Stocking C, Podsadecki T, et al: Effects of organizational change in the medical intensive care unit of a teaching hospital: a comparison of 'open' and 'closed' formats. *JAMA* 276:322–328, 1996.
2. Felstein PJ: *Health Care Economics*. 5th ed. Albany, NY, Delmar Publishers, 1999.
3. Fields AI, Cuerdon TT, Brasseux CO, et al: Physician burnout in pediatric critical care medicine. *Crit Care Med* 23:1425–1429, 1995.
4. Ghorra S, Reinert SE, Cioffi W, et al: Analysis of the effect of conversion from open to closed surgical intensive care unit. *Ann Surg* 229:163–171, 1999.
5. Guidelines Committee, Society of Critical Care Medicine: Guidelines for the definition of an intensivist and the practice of critical care medicine. Retrieved July 2, 2001, from the World Wide Web: www.sccm.org/accm/guidelines/guide_body_g11.html.
6. Guidelines/Practice Parameters Committee of the American College of Critical Care Medicine, Society of Critical Care Medicine: Guidelines for intensive care unit design. *Crit Care Med* 23:582–588, 1995.
7. Gundersen L: Physician burnout. *Ann Intern Med* 135:145–148, 2001.

8. Hoff T, Whitcomb WF, Nelson JR: Thriving and surviving in a new medical career: the case of hospitalist physicians. *J Health Soc Behav* 43:72–91, 2002.
9. Keidel GC: Burnout and compassion fatigue among hospice caregivers. *Am J Hosp Palliat Care* 19:200–205, 2002.
10. Leape LL, Cullen DJ, Clapp MD, et al: Pharmacist participation on physician rounds and adverse drug events in the intensive care unit. *JAMA* 282:267–270, 1999.
11. Multz AS, Chalfin DB, Samson IM, et al: A "closed" medical intensive care unit (MICU) improves resource utilization when compared with an "open" MICU. *Am J Respir Crit Care Med* 157:1468–1473, 1998.
12. Phelps CE: *Health Economics*. 3rd ed. Reading, Mass: Addison-Wesley, 2002.
13. Tarnow-Mordi WO, Hau C, Warden A, et al: Hospital mortality in relation to staff workload: a 4-year study in an adult intensive-care unit. *Lancet* 356:185–189, 2000.
14. Zimmerman JE, Shortell SM, Rousseau DM, et al: Improving intensive care: observations based on organizational case studies in nine intensive care units: a prospective, multicenter study. *Crit Care Med* 21:1443–1451, 1993.

2

Admission Criteria

By its nature, the NICU is utilized for medical and surgical management of critical neurologic disorders and postoperative care of neurosurgical patients, but it may also be used for patients with extensive spinal operations performed by orthopedic surgeons and neurosurgeons and for monitoring patients after epilepsy surgery. Characteristically, severe physiologic derangements, increased intracranial pressure, neuromuscular respiratory failure, refractory seizures, and any rapid neurologic deterioration without identified cause are admission criteria. Uniform criteria for admission are difficult to identify, and some ambiguity remains. Trauma triage rules have been recently validated and emphasize the need for admission with a Glasgow Coma Scale score less than 8, systolic blood pressure less than 90 mm Hg, and presence of gunshot wounds.[9] ICU case mix may differ between countries and may involve differences in utilization by age.[7] Although the economic pressures on hospital stay are substantial, they have not had an impact on intensive care units.[5] It is an unchallenged dictum that any patient with a craniotomy goes to the NICU, but whether fast-track programs apply is unknown. These truncated programs, currently in place in a few intensive care units in the United States but more prevalent in Europe, involve early extubation, reduced use of postoperative sedation, and preauthorized implementation of intensive care unit transfer orders.[1,6]

Admission to the NICU requires excellent rapport with the nurse manager and charge nurse, because criteria for admission are arbitrary and therefore should be flexible. For instance, in some patients, sedation for marked agitation or monitoring of the airway alone may justify admission. On the other hand, medical suitability may be very limited in any patient with a high probability of hospital mortality or severe disability, do-not-resuscitate orders, and no response to interventions, all suggesting an unsalvageable condition. Some of these patients on the verge of brain death, however, are admitted to activate a possible organ procurement protocol.

The admission criteria for each of the neurologic disorders discussed in Part III of this book are summarized in Table 2–1 for easy reference. This set of guidelines may facilitate communication and also possibly reduce the length of stay and thus costs. Any admission to the NICU should be democratic and free of cultural or religious bias.

Dismissal from the NICU is typically more haphazard and sometimes a result of pressure for beds. Inappropriate early dismissal may lead to readmission ("bounce back") or fatality on the ward.[2,4,8] Possibly, patients released at night fare worse than patients dismissed during the day.[3] The reason may be an insufficient number of staff at night.

Without audits and surveys in NICUs, only crude recommendations of transfer out of the NICU can be made. These include more than 24 hours of extubation, good gas exchange, no cardiac arrhythmias or recent discontinuation of pressors or antiarrhythmic agents, and no seizures over 48 hours and therapeutic levels of antiepileptic drugs or, at the other extreme, an order not to intubate or resuscitate.

Table 2–1. Proposed Criteria for Admission to the Neurologic Intensive Care Unit

Aneurysmal subarachnoid hemorrhage
  Drowsiness, stupor, or coma
  Any neurologic deterioration
  Seizures
  Neurogenic pulmonary edema
  Aspiration pneumonia
  Cardiac arrhythmias
  Abnormal electrocardiogram
  S/P coil placement
  S/P clipping of aneurysm
Ganglionic or lobar hemorrhage
  Drowsiness, stupor, or coma
  CT evidence of brain shift
  Hypertensive surges
  Recurrent seizures
  Coagulopathy
  Mechanical ventilation
  S/P ventriculostomy
  S/P craniotomy
Cerebellum or brain stem ICH
  Drowsiness, stupor, or coma
  CT or clinical signs of brain stem compression
  Cardiac arrhythmia
  Mechanical ventilation
  S/P ventriculostomy
  S/P craniotomy
Cerebral venous thrombosis
  Drowsiness, stupor, or coma
  CT evidence of hemorrhagic infarct
  Seizures
  Suspected pulmonary embolus
  S/P thrombolysis
Hemispheric stroke
  Drowsiness, stupor, or coma
  CT scan evidence of early swelling or hemorrhagic
    conversion
  Seizures
  Cardiac failure
  S/P craniotomy
Basilar artery occlusion
  Drowsiness, stupor, or coma
  Mechanical ventilation
  S/P thrombolysis
Cerebellar infarct
  Drowsiness, stupor, or coma
  CT or clinical evidence of brain stem compression
  Cardiac arrhythmias
  S/P ventriculostomy
  S/P craniotomy

Acute bacterial meningitis
  Drowsiness, stupor, or coma
  CT scan evidence of edema
  Any neurologic deterioration despite antibiotics
  Seizures
  Shock
  Pulmonary infiltrates
Brain abscess
  Drowsiness, stupor, or coma
  CT scan evidence of multiple locations
  Seizures
  S/P drainage
  S/P stereotactic puncture
Viral encephalitis
  Drowsiness, stupor, or coma
  CT scan evidence of swelling
  Seizures
  S/P brain biopsy
Acute spinal cord disorder
  Cervical lesion
  Ascending paralysis
  Suspicion of associated traumatic brain injury
  Aspiration
  Dysautonomia, bladder dysfunction
  Surgical intervention anticipated
Closed head injury
  Drowsiness, stupor, or coma
  CT scan evidence of ICH, axonal injury
  Seizures
  Evidence of multitrauma
  S/P craniotomy
Status epilepticus
  Drowsiness, stupor, or coma
  Mechanical ventilation or intubation
  Recurrence after intravenous phenytoin loading
  Agitation
Guillain-Barré syndrome
  VC < 20 mL/kg or 30% decrease
  Aspiration
  Rapid clinical progression
  Hypotension during physical examination
  Pneumonia, sepsis
Myasthenia gravis
  Cholinergic crisis
  Myasthenic crisis with neuromuscular failure
    (VC < 20 mL/kg or 30% decrease)
  Bulbar weakness

CSF, cerebrospinal fluid; CT, computed tomography; ICH, intracranial hemorrhage; SAH, subarachnoid hemorrhage; S/P, status post; VC, vital capacity.

CONCLUSIONS

- Admission and transfer criteria should be defined by disorder but with some flexibility maintained.
- Fast-track programs may not apply to the NICU.
- Admission may not be warranted for patients in unsalvageable condition or with do-not-resuscitate orders.

REFERENCES

1. Daly K, Beale R, Chang RW: Reduction in mortality after inappropriate early discharge from intensive care unit: logistic regression triage model. *BMJ* 322:1274–1276, 2001.
2. Franklin C, Jackson D: Discharge decision-making in a medical ICU: characteristics of unexpected readmissions. *Crit Care Med* 11:61–66, 1983.
3. Goldfrad C, Rowan K: Consequences of discharges from intensive care at night. *Lancet* 355:1138–1142, 2000.
4. Rosenberg AL, Hofer TP, Hayward RA, et al: Who bounces back? Physiologic and other predictors of intensive care unit readmission. *Crit Care Med* 29:511–518, 2001.
5. Rosenberg AL, Zimmerman FE, Alzola C, et al: Intensive care unit length of stay: recent changes and future challenges. *Crit Care Med* 28:3465–3473, 2000.
6. Sirio CA, Martich GD: Who goes to the ICU postoperatively? *Chest* 115 Suppl:125S–129S, 1999.
7. Sirio CA, Tajimi K, Taenaka N, et al: A cross-cultural comparison of critical care delivery: Japan and United States. *Chest* 121:539–548, 2002.
8. Snow N, Bergin KT, Horrigan TP: Readmission of patients to the surgical intensive care unit: patient profiles and possibilities for prevention. *Crit Care Med* 13:961–964, 1985.
9. Tinkoff GH, O'Connor RE: Validation of new trauma triage rules for trauma attending response to the emergency department. *J Trauma* 52:1153–1159, 2002.

3

General Perspectives on Care

Amid the multiple neurologic and medical complexities of care, neurologists may perhaps tend to take general daily matters of care for granted. Attending physicians in the NICU should be anticipatory to the many vexing needs of the critically ill neurologic patient. It is conventional wisdom that the daily care of patients with acute neurologic disorders is multifaceted. Its scope includes nursing care, physical therapy, infection precautions, and other prophylactic measures. Inattention to any of these may potentially result in a less favorable outcome. This chapter reviews the principles of nursing care and physical therapy. Communication with family members receives special attention because one should be prepared to engage with intricate sentimentalities.

GENERAL NURSING CARE AND PHYSICAL THERAPY

Patients admitted to the NICU have extensive nursing requirements. The nursing staff routinely evaluate patients every hour to measure the level of alertness, detect new neurologic signs, and recognize seizures, agitation, and pain. They are well aware that changes in neurologic condition may be subtle, and in many instances no exact physiologic measurement is available to confirm a change in neurologic status.

Nursing care of patients with neurologic illness is complex and outside the scope of this book, but several important facets must be familiar to anyone who manages critically ill neu-

rologic patients. Important categories of nursing care are attention to mouth, eye, and skin care; checking of Foley catheters, nasogastric tubes, and intravascular catheters; dressing changes for monitoring devices; and, most importantly, adequate body positioning and respiratory care. Equally important in intensive care is optimization of comfort and, if possible, sleep.

Skin care has a high priority in immobilized patients.[5] Decubital ulcers or, more often, patches of demarcated painful erythema indicative of developing ulcers may appear, even with meticulous care. Pressure ulcers appear in stages, commonly progressing from pressure-produced erythematous blanching to abrasions, shallow ulcers, or full-thickness skin loss. Sores occur mostly over the sacrum, greater trochanter, and heels (Fig. 3–1). Heavy smokers, patients older than 85 years, and patients with dry skin or hypoalbuminemia are at particularly high risk.[2,20,29] The risk for ischemic damage over the sacral skin area is most prominent in the supine position and less in the 45° position.[44] Low body mass, high degree of skin exposure to moisture, and limited sensory perception contribute considerably to pressure ulcer formation. In a recent study in the NICU, two-thirds of the patients with pressure sores acquired them within the first week of admission.[14] Frequent turning in bed, lanolin creams, and dry patting of the skin are essential. Use of air-fluidized mattresses is critical when prolonged immobilization from coma or quadriplegia (e.g., spinal cord injury or Guil-

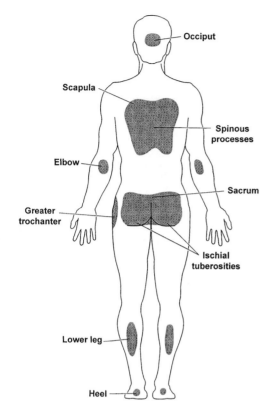

Figure 3–1. Common areas of pressure ulceration in the supine position. (Modified from Reuler JB, Cooney TG: The pressure sore: pathophysiology and principles of management. *Ann Intern Med* 94:661–666, 1981. By permission of the American College of Physicians–American Society of Internal Medicine.)

lain-Barré syndrome [GBS]) is expected.[21] On daily rounds, the skin should be inspected carefully at pressure points. Repositioning is performed every 2 hours but must be more frequent if erythema occurs. Medical management of pressure sores includes topical treatment with hydrocolloid occlusive dressing and polyurethane film dressings, but topical antibiotics such as neomycin and metronidazole may also be needed.[37] Without prospective trials, the benefits of medical treatments or even prophylaxis are not known, and as alluded to, pressure sores may occur very quickly, within days of admission.[10]

Skin breakdown may also occur from endotracheal tube contact. This can be minimized by adhesive tape and a combination of nystatin and tolnaftate (DuoDerm). Protective adhesive tape may reduce pressure on the patient's nares when nasogastric tubes are in place, and these tubes should never be positioned in upward flexion.

Eye care is important in comatose patients, and daily application of methylcellulose drops with taping of the eyelids is important to reduce corneal abrasions. In mechanically ventilated susceptible patients, positive pressure ventilation may cause severe conjunctival edema, resulting in inability to close the eyes.[27] Continuous sedation and muscle relaxation are risk factors for ocular surface disorders, but hypoxemia or hypercapnia may dilate conjunctival vessels (Fig. 3–2). Conjunctival edema is self-limited but can put patients at risk for

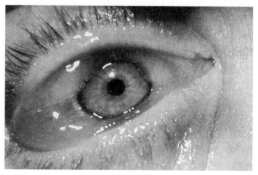

A

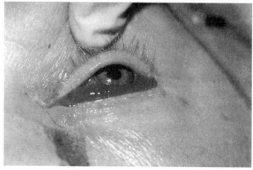

B

Figure 3–2. Chemosis due to accumulation of transudate causes conjunctiva to bulge over the cornea (*A*) or protrude between eyelids (*B*).

corneal exposure and corneal drying. Guibor eye bubbles, temporary tarsorrhaphy, or aggressive lubrication may prevent keratopathy.[23]

Mouth care includes use of lip balm and moistening of the gingiva and mouth. Oral candidiasis, recognized as creamy white patches on the pharynx or tongue, should be anticipated in patients receiving broad-spectrum antibiotics, corticosteroids, or total parenteral nutrition, but the probability is increased in any preceding debilitating state. Fluconazole, 100 mg orally per day, may treat this infection rapidly before it becomes invasive.

Positioning of comatose patients in an appropriate manner may reduce contractures.[11] Irrespective of whether the patient needs to have the head elevated (e.g., increased intracranial pressure [Chapter 9]) or to lie flat (e.g., acute basilar artery occlusion [Chapter 17]), a neutral or side-lying position should be adopted, with a pillow between the legs to prevent internal rotation, adduction, and inversion of the upper leg. Patients with a flaccid paralysis should have footboards, splinting to prevent contractures, and trochanter towel rolls to prevent entrapment neuropathy of the peroneal nerve. In addition, it is important to avoid compression at the elbows to protect the ulnar nerve. Nonetheless, comatose patients with marked extensor posturing are difficult to position. Footboards and splints in these patients are not useful, because they apply stretch and potentially further increase the tone of the hypertonic muscles. Unfortunately, despite long-term care, contractures are often observed in patients in a permanent vegetative state when they are reexamined months after the catastrophe.

In the properly aligned patient in a dorsal position, the head is in neutral position in line with the spine in the anteroposterior plane, the arms are flexed at the elbow with the hands resting at the side of the abdomen (pillows may be needed to support this position), and the fingers are extended over the edge of the pillow. (Inserting a rolled towel may create normal arching of the fingers.) The knees are extended or are slightly flexed, with trochanter rolls folded under the greater trochanter hip

joint area to distally reduce pressure on the peroneal nerve at the fibula head caused by external rotation at the hip joint. The feet are ideally at 70° to 90° to the legs, with the toes pointing upward (Fig. 3–3A). The lateral position places the patient on either side without twisting the head. The head is supported by a pillow, and a second pillow is placed between the legs (Fig. 3–3B).

Positioning of patients with hemiplegia is different. The head and neck should be in midline or, in patients with considerable hemibody neglect, preferably turned to the affected side. A pillow is placed in the axilla to counter the tendency of the arm to adduct and rotate internally. The paralyzed arm is supported on a pillow with the elbow partially flexed. The leg is placed in a neutral position supported by a trochanter roll. In the lateral position, patients should be turned on the unaffected side without flexion of the trunk and spine. Conventionally, the arm is positioned so that each joint is higher than the preceding one. Generally, extension, adduction, and internal rotation of the shoulder should be avoided. In patients with acute stroke who are lying on the unaffected side, the lower limb should be flexed. It may be beneficial to lift the affected hip forward while the limb is supported by a pillow.

Patients with flaccid quadriplegia favor the froglike position (a modification of Fowler's sitting position). The shoulders are supported with several pillows in the axilla and under the knees, and the hips are slightly abducted (Fig. 3–3C). In patients with virtually complete flaccid quadriplegia, splinting of the hands and use of footboards or sneakers are essential in preventing contractures.

Most NICUs have specially assigned physical therapy teams to assist in the care of critically ill patients. Physical therapy should begin virtually immediately; next to appropriate positioning, it includes passive range of motion and chest physiotherapy for postural drainage.

Initially, range-of-motion exercises are passive, consisting of abduction, adduction, flexion, and extension motions. Passive movements of the limbs are focused on the proximal limb

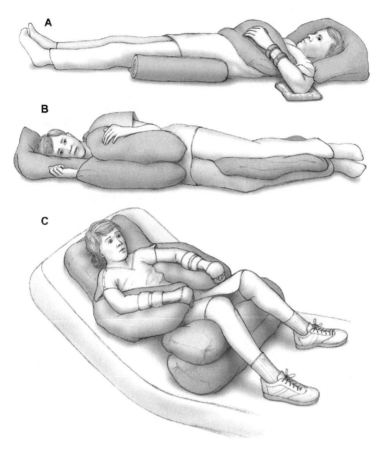

Figure 3–3. Properly aligned bed-bound patient. (*A*) Supine and (*B*) side-lying positions. Trochanter roll decreases compression on the peroneal nerve, and soft towel or sheepskin reduces pressure at the level of the ulnar nerve. (*C*) Froglike position in quadriplegic patient. Splints reduce contractures. (Sneakers can be used for splinting of feet.)

muscles, with flexion and extension of the knee while the hip is extended and the foot is held in dorsiflexion. Mild stretching after heat application may be added, but this causes additional discomfort for patients with muscle pain from GBS.

Range-of-motion exercises should be done daily and later can be performed by the patient actively. Active exercises should be done gradually, because prolonged bed rest leads to deconditioning, characterized by orthostatic hypotension and loss of muscle mass and contractile strength. Vigorous active range-of-motion exercises may cause oxygen desaturation or precipitate chest pain if a patient cannot meet the demands of low-level exercises.

Atelectasis with stagnant secretions is commonly developing in the left lower lobe because of poor drainage and compression by the heart in prolonged supine positions. Kinetic beds may be considered for comatose patients at high risk, but the costs are considerable despite clear benefit above physical therapy alone.[39] If hypoxemia occurs, bronchoscopy is required.

Use of routine physiotherapy remains a contentious issue.[12,31] Physiotherapy is likely to improve atelectasis and may have a short-lived beneficial effect on respiratory function. But whether routine physiotherapy in the NICU (or any other intensive care unit) reduces the chance of nosocomial pneumonia is questionable, and a study that used twice-daily physiotherapy suggested no effect.[32] In addition, no evidence exists that any of the other techniques (despite the empirical fact of efficacy) avoid atelectasis or decrease the incidence of pulmonary complications.[31,49] Nonetheless, chest physiotherapy is considered important in patients with neurologic critical illness. It involves positioning for postural drainage, suctioning, and, in cooperative patients, breathing exercises and forced expiratory techniques.

Many physical therapists briefly put the patient in a flat position before tracheal suctioning to assess the effect of position change on intracranial pressure. If intracranial pressure does not return to baseline value after a mild increase from change into a flat position, brief hyperventilation through a manual resuscitation bag is necessary. Marked intracranial pressure surges or plateau waves can be muted by an intravenous bolus of lidocaine (1 mg/kg) and, equally important, by simply limiting the number of tracheal passages. Percussion and vibration are additionally effective in mobilizing retained secretions. However, although the techniques of percussion and vibration reduce atelectasis, they may potentially increase intracranial pressure in susceptible patients with poor brain compliance.[16] Chest percussion generally should not increase intracranial pressure.

Coughing must be stimulated in alert patients with an acute neuromuscular disorder. Huffing (large inspiration followed by short expiratory blasts) may stimulate coughing, and gentle touch of the oropharynx with an oral suction tube may be helpful as well. The basic requirements for chest physical therapy are summarized in Table 3–1.

Table 3–1. Essentials of Chest Physiotherapy

Percussion and vibration
Coughing exercises (huffing techniques, oropharyngeal stimulation)
Suctioning (preceded by hyperoxygenation, FIO_2 1.0, for 15 seconds)
Mucolytic agents, bronchodilators, and nebulizers for humidification

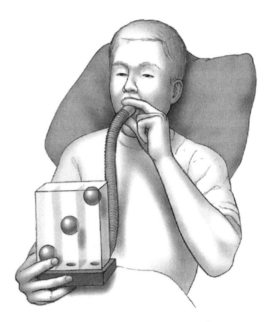

Figure 3–4. Incentive spirometry. The patient is encouraged to take a profound inspiratory breath, aiming at elevation of all three balls.

Incentive spirometry (Fig. 3–4) could be important in patients with neuromuscular respiratory failure and after craniotomy who have a proclivity for closure of the alveoli in the dependent lung zones. Obviously it requires alertness for coaching. A reasonable technique is to take 10 maximal inspirations every 2 hours between 8 A.M. and 8 P.M. to allow for a good night's rest. The use of incentive spirometry reduced the postoperative incidence of atelectasis in critically ill patients in some studies, but treatment benefit may be much less than claimed.[36] Systematic studies in patients with neurologic illness are not available. It is not expected that aggressive incentive spirometry may prevent mechanical ventilation in patients with GBS (Chapter 25) and myasthenia gravis (Chapter 26) and marginal respiratory function. Deterioration is too rapid to be averted with this simple measure.

Among the daily responsibilities of nursing care is safe in-hospital transfer.[3,19,42,50,52] Patients often need to be moved from the NICU to the radiology suite for neuroimaging. In-hospital transport results in a period in which patients are outside a critical care area and monitoring is potentially jeopardized.

Adverse events that have been noted during transport of acutely ill patients and that tentatively may lead to secondary insults to the brain are arterial oxygen saturation of less than 90%, hypoventilation in mechanically ventilated patients, severe hypocapnia by too-frequent manual bagging, cardiovascular changes induced by sudden alteration in the mode of ventilation, and surges of intracranial pressure, all of which may escape detection.[3,46] Catheters and tubes may be pulled, most often during transfer of patients to different beds. The consequences of dislodgment of intravascular catheters are particularly important if patients are receiving inotropic agents or drugs to control cardiac arrhythmias. For selected patients, it is effective to have mannitol and antiepileptic drugs prepared. The precautions are listed in Table 3–2. It is important to assess possible change in vital signs after several minutes of manual bagging. This precaution is useful because some patients do not even tolerate this brief intermission. The personnel transferring the patient should include the responsible neurologic critical care nurse most familiar with recent vital signs and should be further accompanied by a respiratory therapist or physician.

Table 3–2. Precautions before In-hospital Transport

Miminum of two persons (at least one assigned neurologic critical care nurse)
Stable vital signs for 1 hour
Tracheal suctioning before transport
Patency of intravenous sites checked (and flushed if needed)
Stable vital signs after manual bagging of the patient for several minutes
$SaO_2 \geq 90\%$
No recent seizures
Mannitol infusion prepared if needed
When indicated, supplies such as antiepileptic drugs (lorazepam, 4 mg), albumin 5% solution
Sufficient supply of administered fluids and drips
Monitor connected for arterial blood pressure tracings and electrocardiography
Pulse oximeter connected
Defibrillator

ISOLATION AND INFECTION PRECAUTIONS

Strict hand-washing between visits to patients, limitation of the use and duration of devices, proper isolation of infected patients, and aseptic techniques reduce nosocomial infections.[13,18] Identification of patients with antimicrobial-resistant strains (e.g., methicillin- and vancomycin-resistant *Staphylococcus aureus*) may control spread.[53] Risk factors are patients admitted from other hospitals, patients staying 4 days or more in the hospital, or prophylactic use of one or more antibiotics for more than one day after severe trauma.[51] These patients should be part of the screening of clinical specimens.[17]

The Centers for Disease Control and Prevention have defined categories of isolation: strict isolation, contact isolation, respiratory isolation, tuberculosis isolation, and several other disease-specific isolation precautions.[15] The isolation categories are shown in Table 3–3.

Body substance isolation has been proposed.[28] Body substance isolation implies that gloves should be worn for anticipated contact with blood, secretions, and any moist body substances. Gloves should be changed before another patient contact. Gowns, plastic aprons, masks, and goggles should be worn when secretions, blood, or body fluid is likely to soil or splash on clothing, skin, or face. Soiled reusable items should be contained. Needles should be placed in rigid containers without recapping.

Hand washing has been well recognized as the most effective method to prevent the spread of infectious agents.[1,40] Surprisingly, however, one study found virtually no relationship between hand washing rates and infection rates when two intensive care units were surveyed.[45] The type of soap or disinfectant probably is less important than the technique of hand washing. Adequate hand washing should ideally last 20 seconds, and a large volume of soap should be used. The faucet should be closed with a piece of paper towel if a lever is not available. Warning labels on me-

Table 3–3. Isolation Categories and Examples of Infectious Diseases in Each Category

Category	Requirements
Strict isolation	Private room
Rabies	Negative-pressure ventilation
Varicella	Masks, gowns, and gloves at all times
Hemorrhagic fever	Hand washing after glove removal
Contact isolation	Private room
Adenovirus	Mask when close to patient
Herpes simplex (disseminated)	Gowns if soiling likely
Major staphylococcal infections	Gloves for touching infectious material
	Hand washing after glove removal
Respiratory isolation	Private room
Infectious mononucleosis	Mask when close to patient
	Hand washing
Enteric precautions	Gowns if soiling likely
Enterovirus	Gloves for touching infectious material
Hepatitis A, E	Hand washing after glove removal
Salmonella	
Shigella	
Campylobacter	
Giardia	
Rotavirus	
Drainage and secretion precautions	Gowns if soiling likely
Herpes simplex (local)	Gloves for touching infectious material
Localized herpes zoster	Hand washing after glove removal
Blood and body fluid precautions	Fluid-resistant gowns
Arbovirus	Gloves for touching infectious material
Cytomegalovirus	Mask and glasses with side shields, goggles,
Hepatitis B, C, D	or face shield
Human immunodeficiency virus	Care with needles and sharp instruments

chanical ventilators (wash hands, use gloves) improved hand washing in one study, but others found no measurable effect.[7,24,34] In addition, irritant dermatitis (dry, flaky skin with multiple cracks) may occur with solutions containing chlorhexidine and therefore may discourage hand washing. Many intensive care units now use alcohol-based hand-rubs for "waterless" hand disinfection.[22] Care should be taken not to use over-the-counter hand lotions, which may neutralize the antiseptic effect. A prospective, randomized trial proved better tolerance and better disinfection with alcohol-based hand washing, but reduction in nosocomial infection was not established.[9,26]

Another important aspect of infection precaution is the protection of patients from infections transmitted by blood or blood products. The most frequent serious transfusion complication is the transmission of hepatitis and human immunodeficiency virus-1, but the risks are very low. In patients with critical neurologic illness, albumin is often used, but it is a product of Cohn ethanol fractionation of plasma pools. With this method, all infectious viral particles should be inactivated after pasteurization at 60°C for 10 hours.

Many nosocomial infections are associated with specific devices (Chapter 33), but advice on how to prevent them changes frequently. Current recommendations are (1) maintenance of a sterile urinary closed drainage system and no breaking in to obtain urinary samples or to irrigate the bladder, (2) replacement of intravenous catheters every 2 or 3 days, (3) replacement of central lines every 7 days, and (4) proper handling of condensate in respiratory tubing, dispensing and storage of nebulized solutions, and changing of the tubing (but no more often than every 1 to 2 weeks).

THE PATIENT'S FAMILY

More than in any other type of medical or surgical intensive care unit, the family represents the patient's interests,[6] because patients with acute brain injury may not be able to communicate or comprehend adequately.

Neurologists involved in the care of patients with an unexpected acute neurologic condition should foster a very close physician–family relationship. The needs of family members are substantial and rather specific. A recently completed survey involving different intensive care units found important predictors of patient family satisfaction.[4] These were knowledge of the specific role of the caregiver, avoidance of contradictory information, and involvement of the family doctor in addition to adequate time to meet with the attending physician.

Neurologists should allow families to insert their tragedies into their lives, and it is important to establish positive rapport immediately. The main goals are (1) clarification and explanation of the acute neurologic disorder, (2) discussion of the level of responsiveness of the patient, (3) estimation of the expected progression or improvement in the first 3 days, (4) review of possible long-term outcome and expected level of functioning in broad categories of dependence and independence, and (5) establishment of the level of care. Of course, the coping of family members of patients with acute neurologic disorders varies from family to family and, more importantly, may vary within a particular family.

In most instances, the contacts with families are pleasant and cordial, leading to decisions by consensus. However, the sudden presentation of a very sick family member with a high likelihood of permanent intellectual disability may lead to rapid disintegration of an otherwise very caring family. Acute neurologic catastrophes may bring an acute stress reaction to some family members. Dissociative symptoms are often seen, characterized by depersonalization, a dazed look, crippling panic, and amnesia, which may be accompanied by sleeplessness and restlessness. Parental stress in young persons, particularly with change in appearance, is considerable. Watching resuscitation efforts, placement of lines, and physicians rushing in is wrenching enough for most families and causes bewilderment. This may become even more apparent if a poor prognosis leads to fatalistic answers. Some families may think that "somebody has to be doing something wrong" and continue to display an oppositional mentality. Some families remain opaque in their understanding and display eccentricities in cultural beliefs, so that communication remains unsettling. Other family members remain quiet all the time only to explode suddenly in anger and mistrust.

Discussion with family members may become convoluted when religious positions are voiced in such terms as "Only He who gave life has the right to take life," "We will hope and pray for the best," and "God may work a miracle if that is His will." Withholding care is permitted in some religions (Christianity) but not in others (Islam). Religious beliefs of physicians usually do not conflict with family beliefs, but if they do, the desire of physicians to treat patients fully may be affected.[41] Transfer of care to other hospitals may be considered if conflicts cannot be resolved with the intervention of an ethics committee, but the move is logistically difficult.

Family members who do not participate must be identified soon and integrated into the discussions. Families evolve as they try to cope with a sudden devastating illness, but the evolution of behavior is not well known. (Most likely, the stages are very different from the stages of coping with terminal illness outlined by Kübler-Ross.[25])

Very important patients and their families pose a particularly demanding problem.[43] A very important person (VIP) can be arbitrarily defined as a celebrity, a major political figure, or, closer to home, a department member or board member of a large institution. With a VIP comes the *VIP syndrome*,[54] loosely defined as unusual medical care and unconventional reactions by the attending physician. It is commonplace in tertiary referral hospitals.

The syndrome may be marked by extensive testing for borderline abnormalities or the withholding of necessary procedures that may cause additional discomfort or have potentially major adverse effects.[8] In some neurologists, complete paralysis of action may occur.

Families of VIPs may respond differently and have a tendency to raise questions about care more frequently. Colleagues who are friends of the family member may call, and some may even suggest changes in care, often well-meant. Friends who are simply curious nevertheless interfere with daily rounds and may potentially reduce the time spent with other patients and families. It is crucial to limit visits of persons not directly related to the patient, to restrict and concentrate communication with family members to certain time slots (morning and afternoon rounds), and to inform the family and patient (when alert) that care will be similar: "I will treat him (or her) as I would any other patient." Often this simple statement is very relieving.[47] However, the responsibility of the attending neurologist should be clear and not be diffused by multiple consultations.

The clinical condition of the patient must be presented to the family in an unambiguous manner. It is important to ascertain whether the most significant family members are present. When appropriate, family members should be encouraged to travel, if necessary, to meet with the clinical staff. The nursing staff who will care for the patient should ideally be present and become actively involved in the discussion. The presentation of the clinical neurologic situation should be lucid, and often actually showing the lesion on computed tomography scan may help clarify the gravity of the situation. It is important to discuss the level of coma, experience of pain, reasons for bucking the ventilator, meaning of twitching in the face or limbs, and cause of agitation.

Early in the discussion with the family, one should talk about the actual prospects for recovery. It is important to take time in discussing these matters and to make them painfully clear. One must realize that despite hard evidence to the contrary, the family's assessment of prognosis can be more optimistic than the physician's

initially.[33] It is ill-advised to use platitudes or to express a sense of hope and optimism in the first 24 hours when the family is recovering from an overwhelming impact. The following day, the significance of change (or no change) in neurologic condition must be openly discussed.

When no improvement in the neurologic deficit is seen and the outlook for a meaningful recovery is remote, withdrawal of treatment and withdrawal of support must be discussed with the family. It may be effective to say, "I wish we could do more to turn things around, and I wish it had been otherwise."[38] One should be aware of each person's right to refuse medical treatment, and some may have legally formalized this right in a so-called advance directive. It is imperative to follow these instructions to the fullest extent possible, and one should ask family members whether a directive is in effect. Of a number of advance directives, the two most common are (1) a living will, which gives specific directions about types of treatment and may appoint a proxy to make decisions on the patient's behalf when a terminal illness exists, and (2) a durable power of attorney, which authorizes another person to make decisions on the patient's behalf even though the patient is not terminally ill.

An advance directive, however, becomes effective only when patients cannot make and communicate their own decisions. In addition, these declarations do not override reasonable medical practice, such as care to provide comfort, to control pain, and to give food and water by mouth when a patient accepts them. The laws regulating advance directives may vary by state, and out-of-state directives may not comply with the laws of the state where the patient is admitted.

The decision of families to withdraw care in a patient who has not clearly expressed any wishes in an advance directive or in passing is very difficult, and the responsibility of family members is enormous. Guilt plays an important role; nonetheless, reiteration of hopelessness, if applicable, may overcome this feeling. Some families remain reluctant to accept a grim prognosis, voice distrust, and rationalize the continuation of therapy by recalling examples of acquaintances who "unexpectedly recovered" after long intervals. One should discourage the use of terms such as "miracles can happen" and be frank in prognostication. Opening of eyes, blinking, grimacing, grinding of teeth, and sleep–wake cycles could be part of a developing vegetative state and must be explained as unpurposeful.[30]

When withdrawal is considered, a plan should be discussed with the family.[35,56] It is useful to state a certain time period in which the next decision is to be made (e.g., no major improvement in 2 days, do not resuscitate). There are several levels of withdrawal of support. Withdrawal of treatment may proceed through several levels, from withdrawal from high technology support (e.g., mechanical ventilation, dialysis, pacemakers, Swan-Ganz catheters, cardiopulmonary resuscitation) to withdrawal of medication (e.g., antibiotics, vasopressors, insulin, antiarrhythmia agents) and withdrawal of hydration and nutrition. In some situations, families are immediately assured of the hopeless situation and make the decision early to pursue comfort care only.

The decision can be made not to intubate and resuscitate in patients with severe neurologic disability. The neurologist must state that resuscitation is likely to bring more suffering than benefit. Very often, one must make clear that this measure also includes transfer out of the intensive care unit and no invasive measures. The next level of withdrawal of support is treatment of infection. Pneumonia and urinary tract infections that develop in many patients can be treated easily and often when treated are not life-threatening. It should be decided whether sepsis or sepsis syndrome is to be treated, also because management requires additional hemodynamic monitoring and readmission to the intensive care unit. Withdrawal of support is discussed in Chapter 35.

Explaining a locked-in syndrome to family members is particularly difficult. Family members should be made aware that communication is possible only through "yes" and "no" replies conveyed by blinking or vertical eye movements. A simple code, such as one blink for "yes" and three blinks for "no," is helpful and should be posted at the bedside, although

responsiveness may wax and wane during the day. The patient and family may want to continue maximal support, including tracheostomy and gastrostomy, but often significant pneumonias intervene, resulting in early death.

Discussion of a patient who fulfills the clinical criteria of brain death is a common task of the neurointensivist (Chapter 34). Neurologists should be crystal clear and not procrastinate. The family should be told in unequivocal terms that brain function has ceased and the patient is no longer here, having passed away, and that there is 100% certainty. Mechanical ventilation and pharmaceutical support are continued in the event the family agrees to donation of organs and tissue. The initial discussion of organ donation with family members is necessary but potentially threatening, and occasionally the perception of family members is that the physician is rushing from one decision to another. It is helpful if the opportunity exists to frequently visit the family briefly before organ donation is discussed. Indeed, surveys of family members after the patient's death show that frequent communication is appreciated.[33] The family should understand that asking for donation so soon after the ordeal is also stressful for neurologists. An apologetic tone may create a closer relationship with the family members, so that they can better understand the enormous benefits of organ and tissue donation. Organ donation saves many lives or dramatically improves the quality of life (e.g., no more long-term dialysis). Comprehensive discussion of organ donation is done by organ-procurement officers, and their intervention is legally required in the United States. During these meetings, the procedure of organ procurement is described to emphasize that no additional medical costs will be incurred. The charges are the responsibility of the organ procurement agency, which reclaims them from the insurance carrier of the recipients. A follow-up letter on the outcome of donation is sent. The recipients remain anonymous, but occasionally family members have sought contact with them (and the meeting has been comforting).

Family members play an important role in the decision to forgo organ donation, because the patient's preference generally is not known. A recent telephone poll found that only 30% of respondents had decided to donate and that 38% had made their wishes known to family members.[48] Once a patient has given valid consent, it cannot be overridden (Uniform Anatomical Gift Act). It is exceedingly rare for family members to disagree with donation if signed consent by the patient is available (usually on a driver's license). Nonetheless, if this situation occurs, it is ill-advised to proceed with organ donation. In all U.S. states, transplant surgeons require the next of kin's permission before removing any organ.

Refusal of donation removes the rationale for further support. Most families understand this concept very well. The family must be given adequate time to visit the patient to pay their last respects. It is questionable whether family should be present during discontinuation of ventilation support, because some patients have agonal breathing that suggests discomfort or have reflex movements. Although these signs are uncommon, considerable effort is required to explain to observing family members that these are reflex movements originating in the spinal cord.

After a decision to donate organs has been made, family members need to visit before organ retrieval. Only a minority of families ask to see the patient after organ retrieval, but if they do, they need to be offered this chance to see their loved one after organ donation.

Infrequently, family members want continuation of mechanical ventilation and pharmacologic support because the concept of brain death is not understood. Repeated communication to family members explaining that brain death equates to loss of life is not always helpful and could even result in more distrust. Transfer to another hospital is the best (but least feasible) option, but cardiac arrest usually emerges. In New Jersey and New York, religious exemptions have been added to official statutes, creating possible liability if the mechanical ventilator is disconnected. The important ethical issues surrounding these complex situations have been discussed in a monograph.[55] Hospital ethics committee members may be consulted when this delicate problem occurs.

CONCLUSIONS

- Alignment of the body is monitored daily: arms flexed, hands on pillows, and trochanter rolls in place. Compression points are monitored for development of erythema or early decubital ulcers.
- Incentive spirometry (every 2 hours; 6 trials during the day) is begun in patients with neuromuscular respiratory failure and after craniotomy.
- The number of passages during bronchial suctioning must be limited. Evidence of further increase in intracranial pressure should be followed by muting of the response with lidocaine intravenously (1 mg/kg).
- Requirements for intrahospital transport are stable vital signs for 1 hour, adequate oxygen saturation, and absence of recent seizures. For patients at risk, albumin 5%, mannitol infusion, and anticonvulsants are prepared for possible use during transport.
- Categories of isolation (Centers for Disease Control and Prevention) are strict control, contact isolation, respiratory isolation, tuberculosis isolation, and specific disease isolation precautions (hepatitis, acquired immunodeficiency syndrome).
- Time is taken for daily compassionate communication with the family. Dissociative symptoms in family members should be recognized. Expectations for outcome should be explained early, and level of care should be clear.
- Organ donation should be discussed for every patient who fulfills the criteria for brain death.

REFERENCES

1. Albert RK, Condie F: Hand-washing patterns in medical intensive-care units. *N Engl J Med* 304:1465–1466, 1981.
2. Andersen KE, Jensen O, Kvorning SA, et al: Prevention of pressure sores by identifying patients at risk. *Br Med J* 284:1370–1371, 1982.
3. Andrews PJ, Piper IR, Dearden NM, et al: Secondary insults during intrahospital transport of head-injured patients. *Lancet* 335:327–330, 1990.
4. Azoulay E, Pochard F, Chevret S, et al: Meeting the needs of intensive care unit patient families: a multicenter study. *Am J Respir Crit Care Med* 163:135–139, 2001.
5. Bates-Jensen BM: Pressure ulcers: pathophysiology and prevention. In Sussman C, Bates-Jensen BM (eds): *Wound Care: A Collaborative Practice Manual for Physical Therapists and Nurses.* Gaithersburg, MD, Aspen Publishers, 1998, pp 235–270.
6. Bernstein LP: Family-centered care of the critically ill neurologic patient. *Crit Care Nurs Clin North Am* 2:41–50, 1990.
7. Bischoff WE, Reynolds TM, Sessler CN, et al: Hand-washing compliance by health care workers: the impact of introducing an accessible, alcohol-based hand antiseptic. *Arch Intern Med* 160:1017–1021, 2000.
8. Block AJ: Beware of the VIP syndrome (editorial). *Chest* 104:989, 1993.
9. Boyce JM, Kelliher S, Vallande N: Skin irritation and dryness associated with two hand-hygiene regimens: soap-and-water hand washing versus hand antisepsis with an alcoholic hand gel. *Infect Control Hosp Epidemiol* 21:442–448, 2000.
10. Carlson EV, Kemp MG, Shott S: Predicting the risk of pressure ulcers in critically ill patients. *Am J Crit Care* 8:262–269, 1999.
11. Carr EK, Kenney FD: Positioning of the stroke patient: a review of the literature. *Int J Nurs Stud* 29:355–369, 1992.
12. Ciesla ND: Chest physical therapy for patients in the intensive care unit. *Phys Ther* 76:609–625, 1996.
13. Dubbert PM, Dolce J, Richter W, et al: Increasing ICU staff handwashing: effects of education and group feedback. *Infect Control Hosp Epidemiol* 11:191–193, 1990.
14. Fife C, Otto G, Capsuto EG, et al: Incidence of pressure ulcers in a neurologic intensive care unit. *Crit Care Med* 29:283–290, 2001.
15. Garner JS: Guideline for isolation precautions in hospitals. The Hospital Infection Control Practices Advisory Committee. *Infect Control Hosp Epidemiol* 17:55–80, 1996.
16. Garradu J, Bullock M: The effect of respiratory therapy on intracranial pressure in ventilated neurosurgical patients. *Aust J Physiol* 32:107–111, 1986.
17. Girou E, Pujade G, Legrand P, et al: Selective screening of carriers for control of methicillin-resistant *Staphylococcus aureus* (MRSA) in high-risk hospital areas with a high level of endemic MRSA. *Clin Infect Dis* 27:543–550, 1998.
18. Graham M: Frequency and duration of handwashing in an intensive care unit. *Am J Infect Control* 18:77–81, 1990.
19. Guidelines for the transfer of critically ill patients. Retrieved October 19, 2001, from the World Wide Web: http://www.sccm.org.
20. Guralnik JM, Harris TB, White LR, et al: Occurrence and predictors of pressure sores in the National Health and Nutrition Examination survey follow-up. *J Am Geriatr Soc* 36:807–812, 1988.
21. Hofman A, Geelkerken RH, Wille J, et al: Pressure sores and pressure-decreasing mattresses: controlled clinical trial. *Lancet* 343:568–571, 1994.
22. Hugonnet S, Perneger TV, Pittet D: Alcohol-based hand-rub improves compliance with hand hygiene in intensive care units. *Arch Intern Med* 162:1037–1043, 2002.
23. Imanaka H, Taenaka N, Nakamura J, et al: Ocular surface disorders in the critically ill. *Anesth Analg* 85:343–346, 1997.
24. Khatib M, Jamaleddine G, Abdallah A, et al: Hand washing and use of gloves while managing patients receiving mechanical ventilation in the ICU. *Chest* 116:172–175, 1999.
25. Kübler-Ross E: *Death: The Final Stage of Growth.* Englewood Cliffs, New Jersey: Prentice-Hall, 1975.
26. Larson EL, Aiello AE, Bastyr J, et al: Assessment of two hand hygiene regimens for intensive care unit personnel. *Crit Care Med* 29:944–951, 2001.
27. Lee TS, Schrader MW, Wright BD: Subconjunctival emphysema as a complication of PEEP. *Ann Ophthalmol* 12:1080–1081, 1980.
28. Lynch P, Cummings MJ, Roberts PL, et al: Implementing and evaluating a system of generic infection precautions: body substance isolation. *Am J Infect Control* 18:1–12, 1990.
29. Margolis DJ, Bilker W, Knauss J, et al: The incidence and prevalence of pressure ulcers among elderly patients in general medical practice. *Ann Epidemiol* 12:321–325, 2002.
30. The Multi-society Task Force on PVS: Medical aspects of the persistent vegetative state (parts 1 and 2). *N Engl J Med* 330:1499–1508; 1572–1579, 1994.
31. Norrenberg M, Vincent J-L, with the collaboration of the European Society of Intensive Care Medicine: A profile of European intensive care unit physiotherapists. *Intensive Care Med* 26:988–994, 2000.
32. Ntoumenopoulos G, Gild A, Cooper DJ: The effect of manual lung hyperinflation and postural drainage on pulmonary complications in mechanically ventilated trauma patients. *Anaesth Intensive Care* 26:492–496, 1998.
33. O'Callahan JG, Fink C, Pitts LH, et al: Withholding and withdrawing of life support from patients with severe head injury. *Crit Care Med* 23:1567–1575, 1995.
34. O'Donnell A: Handwashing. *Lancet* 355:156, 2000.
35. O'Toole EE, Youngner SJ, Juknialis BW, et al: Evaluation of a treatment limitation policy with a specific

treatment-limiting order page. *Arch Intern Med* 154: 425–432, 1994.

36. Overend TJ, Anderson CM, Lucy SD, et al: The effect of incentive spirometry on postoperative pulmonary complications: a systematic review. *Chest* 120:971–978, 2001.

37. Peerless JR, Davies A, Klein D, et al: Skin complications in the intensive care unit. *Clin Chest Med* 20:453–467, 1999.

38. Quill TE, Arnold RM, Platt F: "I wish things were different": expressing wishes in response to loss, futility, and unrealistic hopes. *Ann Intern Med* 135:551–555, 2001.

39. Raoof S, Chowdhrey N, Raoof S, et al: Effect of combined kinetic therapy and percussion therapy on the resolution of atelectasis in critically ill patients. *Chest* 115:1658–1666, 1999.

40. Reybrouck G: Handwashing and hand disinfection. *J Hosp Infect* 8:5–23, 1986.

41. Rubin SB (ed): *When Doctors Say No: the Battleground of Medical Futility*. Bloomington, Indiana University Press, 1998.

42. Sarnaik AP, Lieh-Lai MW: Transporting the neurologically compromised child. *Pediatr Clin North Am* 40:337–354, 1993.

43. Schneck SA: "Doctoring" doctors and their families. *JAMA* 280:2039–2042, 1998.

44. Schubert V, Heraud J: The effects of pressure and shear on skin microcirculation in elderly stroke patients lying in supine or semi-recumbent positions. *Age Ageing* 23:405–410, 1994.

45. Simmons B, Bryant J, Neiman K, et al: The role of handwashing in prevention of endemic intensive care unit infections. *Infect Control Hosp Epidemiol* 11:589–594, 1990.

46. Smith I, Fleming S, Cernaianu A: Mishaps during transport from the intensive care unit. *Crit Care Med* 18:278–281, 1990.

47. Smith MS, Shesser RF: The emergency care of the VIP patient. *N Engl J Med* 319:1421–1423, 1988.

48. Spital A: Mandated choice. A plan to increase public commitment to organ donation. *JAMA* 273:504–506, 1995.

49. Stiller K: Physiotherapy in intensive care: towards an evidence-based practice. *Chest* 118:1801–1813, 2000.

50. Tompkins JM: Intrahospital transport of seriously ill or injured children. *Pediatr Nurs* 16:51–53, 1990.

51. Velmahos GC, Toutouzas KG, Sarkisyan G, et al: Severe trauma is not an excuse for prolonged antibiotic prophylaxis. *Arch Surg* 137:537–541, 2002.

52. Vernon DD, Woodward GA, Skjonsberg AK: Management of the patient with head injury during transport. *Crit Care Clin* 8:619–631, 1992.

53. Warren DK, Fraser VJ: Infection control measures to limit antimicrobial resistance. *Crit Care Med* 29 Suppl:N128–N134, 2001.

54. Weintraub W: "The VIP syndrome": a clinical study in hospital psychiatry. *J Nerv Ment Dis* 138:181–193, 1964.

55. Wijdicks EFM (ed): *Brain Death*. Philadelphia, Lippincott Williams & Wilkins, 2001.

56. Zimmerman JE, Knaus WA, Sharpe SM, et al: The use of implications of do not resuscitate orders in intensive care units. *JAMA* 255:351–356, 1986.

4

Agitation and Pain

Rapid administration of a sedative may seem appropriate in patients with an acute neurologic illness who are agitated and uncomfortable. It may not only provide proper anxiolysis but may also reduce oxygen consumption and mute the hyperdynamic stress response. In addition, pulling of intravascular and bladder catheters and endotracheal and nasogastric tubes, a danger to the patient, may be prevented.

Traditionally, neurologists have bitterly opposed the use of any form of sedation to counter agitation, particularly when administered in an uncertain neurologic condition that has the propensity to worsen. However, this reluctance can be overcome when recovery after discontinuation of sedation is rapid, interaction with other drugs is minimal, or sedation can be reversed with an appropriate antidote. Current examples are propofol and midazolam, both of which have some of these attributes. In addition, patients are benefited greatly by the additional amnestic properties of most newer agents. Postoperative sedation and pain control, which also attenuate cardiovascular responses to endotracheal intubation, may be achieved by a promising new agent, dexmedetomidine[67] (Chapter 28).

Effective pain management is limited by the poor safety profile of most currently used analgesic agents. Narcotics do not have amnestic or anxiolytic qualities. Furthermore, morphine or fentanyl has a perceptible risk of respiratory depression, an unacceptable situation in patients with neuromuscular respiratory failure

and in patients with poor brain compliance, who may not tolerate a relative increase in P_{CO_2} from hypoventilation. Newer nonsteroidal anti-inflammatory drugs may circumvent these concerns but may increase bleeding time and are obviously less suitable, if not contraindicated, for patients with intracranial hemorrhage.

This chapter discusses the assessment and management of agitation and pain and the pharmacologic choices currently available in the NICU.

CAUSES OF AGITATION

Extreme restlessness with a mixture of shouting, combative behavior, and disorganized thinking poses difficulties not only in neurologic assessment but also in management. Harm to patients should be anticipated as a result of self-extubation and pulling out of central venous access. It has been established that in one-third of patients with self-extubation, a potentially life-threatening event may occur.[20] Fairly typical neurologic causes for profound agitation and acute confusional state are bifrontal cerebral infarcts or hematomas in aneurysmal subarachnoid hemorrhage, infarction of the basal ganglia, large infarcts of the middle cerebral artery territory,[46] and involvement of the thalamus, such as that in basilar artery occlusion (Chapter 17).

The primary central nervous system injury can be implicated in many agitated patients, but other causes should be sought. Occasionally, a florid delirium is the basis of acute confusion. Delirium is typically seen first at night and should be suspected when clinical features such as restlessness, short attention span, persecutory delusions, and perceptual distortions or vivid hallucinations are present.[38,39] Substance withdrawal remains a very important possibility in acute delirium (Table 4–1). Therefore, neurologists should be aware that agitation in any recently hospitalized patient may point to possible substance addiction.[16] In patients with head injuries, ethanol withdrawal is one of the strongest contenders. Alcoholic delirium may be manifested by a generalized tonic-clonic seizure and is a psychiatric emergency. As early as 6 to 8 hours after stopping drinking, and usually on the day of admission, these patients manifest marked restlessness, disordered perception, shouting at hallucinated objects with lucidity between hallucinations, profound diaphoresis, generalized tremor, sustained tachycardia, respiratory alkalosis, and, often, a significant increase in blood pressure. Electrocardiographic abnormalities associated with chest pain may be seen in patients with underlying coronary artery disease. The prevalence of extreme manifestations or fatal cases is low, possibly because of increasing use of benzodiazepines for detoxification.

Table 4–1. Causes of Delirium in the Neurologic Intensive Care Unit

Withdrawal syndromes
  Benzodiazepines
  Barbiturates
  Opioids
  Central nervous system stimulants
Drug-induced
  Antibiotics
  Antiarrhythmic agents
  Anticholinergic agents
  Antihistamines
  β-blockers
  Opioids
Metabolic derangements
  Hyponatremia
  Hyperosmolar hyperglycemia
  Endocrine crises

Alcohol-related seizures are often from withdrawal despite a history of trauma. The time to the first seizure from withdrawal varies greatly (Fig. 4–1). More than 50% of patients have multiple seizures, but it may be an isolated manifestation because only one-third ultimately have delirium tremens. When seizures occur, it may be prudent to repeat CT scan of the brain. However, in a prospective study, the majority of 259 patients with alcohol-withdrawal seizures had normal computed tomography scan findings or cerebral atrophy. In 6%

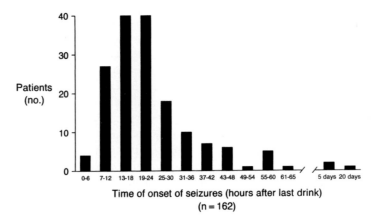

Figure 4–1. Time delay before seizures after alcohol withdrawal. (From Victor M, Brausch C: The role of abstinence in the genesis of alcoholic epilepsy. *Epilepsia* 8:1–20, 1967. By permission of the International League Against Epilepsy.)

of the patients, a structural lesion was found after the first alcohol-withdrawal seizure, with a potential neurosurgical lesion in half of the cases.[25] Particularly in alcoholic patients when initial CT is normal, cerebrospinal fluid examination is mandatory to exclude bacterial meningitis. Other considerations in a restless, agitated alcoholic patient are concomitant use of drugs such as cocaine, sepsis, and acute hepatic failure.

Agitation or delirium may be triggered by a toxic response to medication and, less commonly, by acute metabolic derangement. These possibilities, listed in Table 4–1, are not so well defined in the NICU but must be seriously considered in a delirious patient.

Postictal confusion after a seizure or nonconvulsive status epilepticus should come to mind. However, nonconvulsive status epilepticus produces a fluctuating twilight state more often than significant combativeness.

Agitation may also have its origin in marginal ventilation and gas exchange. Patients with aspiration pneumonitis or early adult respiratory distress syndrome may become significantly tachypneic and agitated, and oxygenation rapidly becomes insufficient. Mechanical ventilation is often only possible with some degree of sedation (intravenous infusion with lorazepam) and occasionally with use of neuromuscular junction blocking agents. Sedation alone allows positive end-expiratory pressure ventilation and improves gas exchange.

An uncommon cause is an adverse effect from a contrast agent after cerebral angiography. Acute combativeness, cortical blindness,[29] seizures, nonconvulsive status epilepticus,[68] and even anomic aphasia may occur but resolve within 24 hours in most patients. This rather dramatic side effect can be managed with mannitol 20% (1 g/kg) to osmotically draw the contrast material out and dexamethasone (10 mg bolus intravenously followed by 4 mg every 6 hours) to stabilize the blood–brain barrier. Sedation by repeated boluses of lorazepam (2–4 mg IV) or low doses of propofol per infusion (0.1 mg/kg per hour) is often required.

PHARMACEUTICAL AGENTS FOR SEDATION

Time-honored methods such as company, touch, and a comforting voice may not be effective in the NICU, and pharmacologic intervention is usually warranted.

The marked autonomic features of delirium warrant immediate treatment. The key steps in the treatment of alcohol withdrawal are rehydration, cooling, and prevention of self-harm and harm to others.[30] The use of chlordiazepoxide is possibly problematic because of marked, often persistent sedation. Therefore, lorazepam or haloperidol may be a better choice in neurologic patients. However, haloperidol may reduce the seizure threshold and is a less desirable choice in susceptible patients. Most experts treat alcohol withdrawal syndrome with intravenous or intramuscular administration of lorazepam, 1 to 2 mg every 4 hours, avoid phenothiazines and other benzodiazepines, but consider repeated doses of chlordiazepoxide, 50 to 100 mg IV or IM (up to 300 mg per day).[42] Recurrent seizures are markedly reduced with use of lorazepam in alcohol withdrawal syndrome.[23] Patients with severe tachycardia, diaphoresis, and hypertension may specifically benefit from oral clonidine (0.2 mg initially, then 0.2 mg three times a day for 2 days, and 0.2 mg on day 4).[7] Alcohol-related seizures may be associated with hypomagnesemia. Although this alleged association has been questioned, hypomagnesemia but also confounding derangements such as hypoglycemia or hypocalcemia must be corrected. Prophylactic antiepileptic medication is not needed, and treatment with phenytoin is indicated only for recurrent seizures or patients with prior seizures.

Management of the most common substance withdrawal syndromes is summarized in Table 4–2. A comprehensive account can be found in a seminal monograph.[16]

Although sedation in an evolving central nervous system disorder seems unacceptable, important improvements have been made by the development of extremely short-acting sedat-

Table 4–2. Substance Withdrawal Syndromes

Class	Common Symptoms and Signs	Treatment
Alcohol	Tachycardia, hypertension, diaphoresis, tremor, fever, respiratory alkalosis	Lorazepam, 2 mg IV Chlordiazepoxide, 50–100 mg IV or IM (up to 300 mg/day) q2h Clonidine, 0.1 mg p.o. b.i.d. (0.2 mg t.i.d. for 2 days; 0.2 mg on day 4) Haloperidol, 2–5 mg IM q4h Thiamine, 100 mg IM followed by 50 mg daily
Opioids (heroin, hydromorphone, oxycodone, methadone, meperidine)	Dilated pupils, sweating, goose flesh, rhinorrhea, lacrimation, mild hypertension, tachycardia, muscle twitching	Methadone, 40 mg single dose followed by 10 mg p.o. q4h Clonidine, 0.1 mg p.o. b.i.d.
Sedative-hypnotics (benzodiazepines, barbiturates, methaqualone, meprobamate)	Anxiety, irritability, myalgias, seizures, tachycardia, myoclonus, hyperreflexia	Consider phenobarbital, 200 mg p.o. (if drug or dosage is not known). Repeat dose to max 600 mg Restart medication and gradually taper
Stimulants (cocaine, amphetamine)	Disturbed sleep, dreaming, depression (suicidal), auditory hallucinations, headache, sweating, talkativeness, seizures	Haloperidol, 2–5 mg IM q4h, or lorazepam, 1–4 mg IV Antidepressants (if suicidal) Supportive therapy

Data from Hyman SE, Tesar GE (eds): *Manual of Psychiatric Emergencies*, 3rd ed. Boston, Little, Brown and Company, 1994.

ing agents and antagonists. Tolerance is excellent in most patients, and side effects are minimal. Propofol may become the preferred drug for treatment of agitated neurologic patients. Dexmedetomidine was recently introduced and may become a preferred agent after craniotomy; its use is discussed in Chapter 28. Currently available studies in intensive care units are insufficient to recommend one agent over another.[51] Continuous infusion of midazolam or propofol may be needed, but daily interruptions, if tolerated, are important to monitor the neurologic examination. An added benefit is shortened length of mechanical ventilation and stay in the intensive care unit. The aim is to have the patient awake at least 50% of the day.[34]

Another concern is common use of a rating scale that does not have a defined ideal level.[51] Many scales have been developed, but the surprisingly crude Ramsay scale (Table 4–3) remains the most widely used and has excellent inter-rater agreement. The sedation-agitation scale (SAS) grades patients in three severity levels and has excellent agreement among intensive care nurses, even without much training[12,63] (Table 4–4). A general but quite arbitrary rec-

ommendation found in anesthesiology texts is to achieve a Ramsay goal of level 2 to 3 (Table 4–3).[61] Monitoring in the intensive care unit with more objective tools, such as bispectral analysis of the electroencephalogram, could be useful, but early experience in the ICU suggests a poor correlation with depth of sedation.[26]

Propofol

Propofol (2,6-diisopropylphenol) is an anesthetic agent with pharmacologic properties and chemical structure unrelated to those of any other sedating drug.[31,35] The pharmacokinetics of this drug seem ideal, and rapid crossing

Table 4–3. Ramsay Scale

Level	Clinical Description
1	Anxious and agitated
2	Cooperative, oriented, tranquil
3	Responds only to verbal commands
4	Asleep with brisk response to light stimulation (glabellar tap)
5	Asleep without response to light stimulation (glabellar tap)
6	Nonresponsive, unarousable

Table 4–4. Sedation-Agitation Scale

Level	Label	Clinical Description
7	Dangerous agitation	Pulls at endotracheal tube, tries to remove catheters, climbs over bedrail, strikes at staff, thrashes side-to-side
6	Very agitated	Does not calm down despite frequent verbal reminding of limits, requires physical restraints, bites endotracheal tube
5	Agitated	Anxious or mildly agitated, attempts to sit up, calms down to verbal instructions
4	Calm and cooperative	Calm, awakens easily, follows commands
3	Sedated	Difficult to arouse, awakens to verbal stimuli or gentle shaking but drifts off again, follows simple commands
2	Very sedated	Arouses to physical stimuli but does not communicate or follow commands, may move spontaneously
1	Unarousable	Minimal or no response to noxious stimuli, does not communicate or follow commands

Source: From Riker RR, Fraser GL, Simmons LE, et al: Validating the Sedation-Agitation Scale with the Bispectral Index and Visual Analog Scale in adult ICU patients after cardiac surgery. *Intensive Care Med* 27:853–858, 2001. By permission of Springer-Verlag.

of the blood–brain barrier produces a marked hypnotic effect.[2,4] The major distinguishing feature of propofol is the rate of recovery, within minutes in almost all patients when incidentally used. Additionally, clearance of propofol is not altered by hepatic or renal failure, which is a well-recognized limitation to the use of benzodiazepines and opiates. Even after high-dose propofol infusion for almost a full day, awakening after discontinuation is comparatively rapid (longest time to following specific commands was 105 minutes for propofol).[1,33] In our experience, full awakening is markedly prolonged with high doses and infusion lasting several days (hours rather than minutes). Increased fat body mass may also contribute.[5] Antagonists for propofol are not available.

Nonetheless, brain stem reflexes may become abolished and only pupil size and light response may remain preserved. The corollary is that this agent is contraindicated in rapidly evolving neurologic catastrophes because infusion of the drug may cause serious difficulties in neurologic assessment.

Propofol for sedation of agitated patients is given as an intravenous infusion at a low-dose rate of 0.1 mg/kg per hour, with incremental doses at 5-minute intervals until reasonable sedation is achieved. Although the response may vary, continuous sedation can be achieved with a dose of 0.3 to 0.6 mg/kg per hour. In two comparative studies with midazolam, propofol was superior for sedation of critically ill patients.

Propofol may have a place in the management of increased intracranial pressure.[32,70] In a randomized, controlled trial, the intensity of intracranial pressure therapy was less[32] (see Chapter 9). Its emerging role as a second-line antiepileptic drug for status epilepticus is discussed in Chapter 24.[19]

Propofol has a safe pharmacologic profile in adults. However, with bolus doses it reduces blood pressure by reducing systemic vascular resistance, cardiac contractility, and preload. Hypotension with a low dose of propofol often indicates hypovolemia. Propofol increases serum triglycerides, and in fact concentrations of triglycerides can be monitored daily to judge the development of a propofol overdose. The 2% emulsion has reduced the lipid load by 50%. Caloric overload (1 mL = 1 kcal) and possible reactive airway disease in patients sensitive to sulfites are known side effects. Anaphylaxis may occur, predominantly in patients with a history of anaphylaxis to muscle relaxants.[37] When anaphylaxis occurs, it produces the typical symptoms of facial swelling, widespread urticaria, and life-threatening bronchospasm. Anaphylaxis should be managed by immediate intravenous administration of epinephrine (usually 1 mL of 1:1000 solution) or diphenhydramine hydrochloride, 25 to 50 mg intravenously, and volume resuscitation with 5% albumin. In more severe cases, aminophylline (6 mg/kg infused in 30 minutes) and hydrocortisone (100 mg intravenously) are needed. Propofol may reduce blood pressure through multiple mechanisms, but this unwanted effect can be minimized by careful titration. Other short-term side effects of propofol are pain at the site of injection (with use of peripheral veins), bacterial contamination (bottle open for more than 12 hours may lead to serious bacteremia), occasional clonic activity, involuntary movements such as choreoathetosis and opisthotonos (may mimic seizures).[43,69] Infusion of propofol in a 2% emulsion at extreme rates higher than 5 mg/kg per hour has been linked to cardiac failure and cardiac arrest, but the findings require confirmation.[21]

Major side effects of propofol have been reported only in children.[22,54] They consist of progressive myocardial failure, bradyarrhythmia, and, occasionally, metabolic acidosis with a fatal course. Its use in children therefore is not recommended.

Midazolam

The relative convenience of midazolam is best illustrated by the availability of an antidote and its distinctive amnestic quality, both of which are conspicuously absent with propofol.[73]

Midazolam is a short-acting benzodiazepine with mostly inactive metabolites.[66,72] Clearance occurs largely through the liver. Its elimination is rapid, but lipid and active metabolic accumulation may occur after 3 days of continuous intravenous infusion. Tolerance may occur, leading to increasing doses to achieve sedation. A study in critically ill patients, which included patients with multitrauma and respiratory failure, found that in those with renal failure, the mean time to awakening after midazolam administration was stopped was 44 hours.[58] The clearance of midazolam is reduced even more significantly with concomitant hepatic or renal failure, but both factors are in most instances not relevant in acutely ill patients with neurologic disorders. Thus, regardless of its short half-life, midazolam may result in sedation for days in some patients.[3,58] Sedation with midazolam is initiated with a bo-

lus of 0.2 mg/kg and is followed by infusion at a rate of 0.02 to 0.1 mg/kg per hour, but this low maintenance dose should be titrated to the response in the individual patient and may be adjusted up to 50% of the initial infusion rate.

Midazolam can be rapidly reversed with the imidazobenzodiazepine flumazenil.[11,14,52,59,65] Flumazenil has a half-life of 60 minutes and antagonizes any benzodiazepine through its specific action on central benzodiazepine receptors that are part of the γ-aminobutyric acid (GABA) A receptor complex. A dose of 0.2 to 0.4 mg of flumazenil intravenously over 15 seconds restores consciousness immediately, but resedation may occur, depending largely on the previous dose of benzodiazepines and the dose of flumazenil. Repeat doses of 0.5 mg at 1-minute intervals up to 3 mg may be needed for the maximal effect.

Side effects of flumazenil are minor, but seizures have been reported. Seizures occurred almost invariably in patients with preexisting epilepsy, in patients who regularly used benzodiazepines, and in patients using tricyclic antidepressants.[41] In predisposed patients, sudden withdrawal of benzodiazepines may also produce a nonconvulsive status epilepticus. Midazolam may produce withdrawal symptoms after 2 to 3 weeks of continuous use, but the actual risks are small.

Lorazepam

Lorazepam,[44] often used in critical care units for transient sedation, has almost no measurable effect on blood pressure and tidal volume. Nonetheless, patients with chronic obstructive pulmonary disease may be more at risk for hypoventilation. Lorazepam has a long-lasting effect after a single bolus injection and is very suitable in the elderly patient.[24] Its reliable absorption after intramuscular injection is another advantage. Administered with haloperidol, lorazepam has a synergistic effect that may be particularly useful if high doses of haloperidol are not sufficiently effective in the treatment of delirium. The comparatively long half-life of lorazepam (15 hours) makes it less suitable for patients with acute neurologic illness in whom the potential for rapid deterioration is great. Emergence from sedation is much more delayed with lorazepam than with midazolam infusion.[6] Lorazepam is cleared through the liver and excreted by the kidneys. An advantage over midazolam infusion is considerably less cost when several days of infusion are anticipated.[17] Lorazepam is usually given intravenously as a single dose of 2 mg. Others have reported a favorable response in extremely agitated patients with an infusion of lorazepam titrated to clinical response. A major side effect is severe arterial spasm causing gangrene if lorazepam is accidentally deposited intra-arterially.

Haloperidol

Haloperidol is the drug of choice in psychotic patients with acute disruptive behavior.[74] Approximately 20 minutes after intramuscular injection, a tranquil state can be achieved. The drug undergoes hepatic metabolism and has a half-life of 6 to 20 hours. Haloperidol may produce marked rigidity. Within days of oral treatment, haloperidol may lead to impressive side effects, such as akathisia (irresistible urge to move about and a feeling that something is crawling under the skin), which may, in fact, suggest ineffective treatment to the novice. This neuroleptic-induced movement disorder of almost continuous symptoms of restlessness responds to an anticholinergic agent such as benztropine, propranolol, or amantadine. Haloperidol can cause QT prolongation on electrocardiograms. Extremely high doses of haloperidol have been associated with oculogyral crises, torticollis, trismus, and a neuroleptic malignant syndrome, but these side effects should not occur with the typical low-dose schedules used in the NICU. There is a strong claim in the pharmacologic literature that extrapyramidal symptoms are much less common when the drug is given intravenously, but this mode of administration is not yet approved by the Food and Drug Administration.

Current recommendations for use of haloperidol are a starting dose of 2 to 5 mg intramuscularly followed by a similar dose 20 minutes later. Agitation can be further controlled by additional doses of 5 mg every 30 minutes until perceptional disturbances subside completely and the patient becomes calm and cooperative.

Miscellaneous Pharmacologic Choices for Management of Agitation

For patients in whom use of neuroleptic agents must be minimized, perphenazine (5 to 10 mg intramuscularly every 6 hours) or thioridazine (100 mg orally three times a day up to 800 mg/day) can be given but at the expense of moderate sedation and an increased risk of seizures. Diazepam has been the definitive drug for sedation in agitated patients for years and should not be easily dismissed as obsolete. In intubated patients, a low dose of 5 to 10 mg results in extremely rapid onset of sedation and can still be given randomly. However, accumulation (half-life, 35 to 100 hours) is substantial with advancing age and liver disease. This agent, therefore, is far less useful than the newer benzodiazepines.

A new generation of so-called atypical antipsychotics—risperidone (0.5 mg b.i.d. orally up to 3 mg daily), olanzapine (5–10 mg daily orally), and quetiapine (25 mg b.i.d., up to 300 mg daily)—developed for schizoaffective disorders, may also become useful in the management of agitation or delirium in patients with prior dementia and Parkinson's disease, but the side effects of sedation and reduced coughing are of concern. Dose adjustment is required in renal disease (risperidone) and liver disease (quetiapine). Clozapine, an alternative agent, can be given orally in a low dose, 6.25 to 50 mg/day (a fraction of the usual dose).[28,55]

The treatment of extremely agitated patients is summarized in Table 4–5.

PAIN MANAGEMENT

Pain is highly prevalent in patients with acute neurologic disorders and has widespread consequences. Disturbance of sleep from pain is

Table 4–5. Treatment of the Extremely
Agitated Patient

Lorazepam, 1–2 mg slowly IV every 4 hours
Haloperidol, 5 mg IM q2–4h
Chlordiazepoxide, 50–100 mg (up to 300 mg/day) IV or
    IM b.i.d.
Midazolam, IV infusion of 0.02–0.1 mg/kg per hour
Propofol, IV infusion of 0.1 mg/kg/hr (range, 0.3–0.6
    mg/kg per hour)

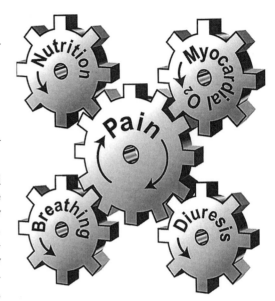

Figure 4–2. Pain has profound effects on physiologic well-being. Increasing pain causes low tidal volumes, decreased ventilation, gastric stasis, nausea and vomiting, poor nutritional intake, hypertension, and tachycardia and thus increased myocardial oxygen requirements and water and sodium retention due to an increase in antidiuretic hormone.

detrimental in fatigued patients with increased work of breathing from diaphragmatic failure due to acute neuromuscular disorders and may prematurely lead to endotracheal intubation. Excruciating head pain in patients with intracranial hemorrhage or after craniotomy may lead to hypertension as part of a complex neuroendocrine response and, more importantly, may result in myocardial ischemia in patients with underlying coronary artery disease.

Pain is signaled not only by moaning, crying, grimacing, and extreme restlessness but also by profuse sweating, sustained tachycardia, blood pressure fluctuations, and dilated pupils. However, one should be sensitive to the fact that lack of expression of pain does not mean lack of pain.

Pain that is insufficiently treated adversely impacts on many physiologic systems (Fig. 4–2); basic humanitarian principles require us to treat it. Immediate relief of pain not only results in visible comfort but also may considerably mute these potentially threatening physiologic responses.

Nursing personnel specifically trained in neurologic intensive care have a pivotal role in recognition and management of pain in various neurologic emergencies. In medical or surgical intensive care units, it has been well appreciated that most patients wait until pain becomes unbearable before they signal for analgesics, but more disturbing (at least in one survey in Australia), approximately only one-third of nursing personnel honor requests when they are made.[53]

The decision to pursue pain medication depends greatly on whether simple nursing measures (e.g., adequate positioning, catheterization) or use of distraction techniques (music, television, family visits) can reduce pain. When no other obvious cause is apparent, analgesics should be administered. The severity of pain is hard to quantify, but increased agitation with any type of stimulation and change in physiologic functions (e.g., tachycardia, blood pressure surges) are at times helpful indications. Patients who are alert can be asked to rate the pain on a scale of 0 to 10 (0, no pain; 10, excruciating and unbearable pain), but the reliability of this semiquantitative scoring is not known.

Adequate pain control has a high priority in the management of Guillain-Barré syndrome (GBS). Pain in GBS may appear in several forms, including hyperalgesia, sciatica, muscle pain and cramps, and joint stiffness (Chapter 25). Typical is the nocturnal aggravation of pain that keeps patients from rest and sleep. Positioning, splinting, and use of bed cages, gloves, or cotton socks may reduce burning, needle-like pain and a feeling of skin tightening. Hot or cold packs may be useful as well. Pain is generally managed with opioid analgesics, such as oxycodone, which should be administered ad libitum in patients with GBS and severe pain.[57,64] When large doses of opiates are needed to control pain, elective endotracheal intubation should be strongly considered in patients with marginal pulmonary function.

Treatment of pain in GBS can be notoriously difficult and frustrating and may in certain patients lead to administration of narcotics into the epidural space, a well-accepted treatment of postoperative pain in patients with thoracotomy.[27,40,47] A very good alternative is tramadol (150 mg followed by 400 mg/day),[10] and our anecdotal experience in a few cases has been impressive. A parenteral formulation is not available in the U.S.

Other effective drugs for pain associated with GBS are prednisone, 60 mg intramuscularly, and mexiletine, 200 mg/8 hours (mexiletine is contraindicated in patients with GBS and dysautonomia, e.g., with first-degree atrioventricular block). Success has also been claimed with capsaicin, specifically for superficial burning pain,[45] quinine sulfate (300 mg at bedtime) for nocturnal cramping and stiffness,[49] and carbamazepine[71] (400 mg before sleep) for sciatica. All these therapeutic measures have often unsuspectedly resulted in instant relief after trial and error with other drugs, but they have not been studied in series of patients.

Opioid analgesics remain the mainstay of pain management in patients with critical neurologic illness.

PHARMACEUTICAL AGENTS FOR PAIN

The choice of pain medication depends on the underlying neurologic condition, the possible interaction with other medication, and the type of pain as much as on the severity of the pain.[48]

Opiates

Opiates are invariably effective.[8,9] Fear of addiction after prolonged hospital use is vastly exaggerated. A survey of 11,882 consecutive patients identified 4 patients with new opiate dependency, only 1 of whom had major dependency.[60] Morphine is the prototype narcotic. Intravenous administration is preferred for acute pain management because transdermal patches delay the analgesic effect. Patient-controlled analgesia (by pump) has not yet found its way into NICUs because it requires patients to be awake and fully cooperative, but we have occasionally used it in patients with GBS whose distal muscle power is still preserved.

Fentanyl, although commonly used for postoperative pain control in other intensive care units, is not preferred because of a risk of seizures, an increase in intracranial pressure, and sedation. Alternative (but weaker) narcotic analgesics are codeine and meperidine. They may have less severe potential side effects (in particular, less sedation). They must be reserved for patients who cannot tolerate morphine or have mild to moderate pain and must be used preferentially in patients with acute central nervous system injury in whom seda-

Table 4–6. Opiates for Pain Management in the Neurologic Intensive Care Unit

Agent	Route	Starting dose (mg)	Peak effect (hour)	Duration (hour)
Codeine	IM	120	0.5–1	4–6
	p.o.	30–60	1.5–2	3–4
Morphine	IM	10	0.5–1	3–5
	p.o.	30	1.5–2	4
Meperidine	IM	75	0.5–1	2–3
	p.o.	200	1–2	2–3

tion is unacceptable. Codeine is the agent of choice for relief of severe pain in acute central nervous system disorders. The variety of narcotic drugs that can be used in the NICU is summarized in Table 4–6.

Side effects of opiates are considerable (Table 4–7). Nausea and vomiting occur in 30% of patients treated with repetitive doses of narcotics but these are rapidly reversible. Opioids are also known to cause water retention from suppression of antidiuretic hormone and combined with excessive vomiting potentially may lead to profound hyponatremia. Respiratory depression (detected by relative hypercapnia from hypoventilation) occurs in susceptible patients but is dose-dependent and usually appears with the initial doses. This important side effect abates with continuing doses, but hypoventilation remains in some patients. Constipation and potential for ileus, urinary retention, and itching are equally important side effects. Inability to temporarily overcome them with measures such as stool softeners and catheterization probably should prompt discontinuation. Meperidine has been linked to seizures, particularly in patients with decreased renal function.

Naloxone reverses opioid toxicity but, like all competitive antagonists, does not produce a long-lasting effect. Repeated intravenous doses

Table 4–7. Adverse Effects of Opiates

Respiratory depression
Hypotension (morphine)
Bronchospasm (morphine)
Euphoria (morphine)
Bradycardia (fentanyl)
Muscle rigidity
Ileus, impaired gastrointestinal motility
Seizures (meperidine)
Nausea and vomiting
Urinary retention
Pruritus
Possible withdrawal
Delayed emergence with prolonged infusions or with
    liver–kidney disease

of 0.2 mg every 3 minutes (up to 10 mg) are needed to obtain an effect. In addition, naloxone may have side effects of its own. Hypertensive crises, cardiac arrhythmias, and unexplained fatigue 24 hours after administration have been reported.

Nonsteroidal Anti-inflammatory Agents

Nonsteroidal anti-inflammatory drugs (NSAIDs) are linked together by their mode of action, not by their chemical structure. They are used increasingly in surgical intensive care units. One of the most recently introduced drugs, ketorolac, is as potent as morphine, and its parenteral form produces faster onset of analgesia, less sedation, and no depressant effect on the ventilatory response to carbon dioxide.[13,15,62] Ketorolac is metabolized by the liver and excreted by the kidneys.

Nonsteroidal anti-inflammatory agents are promising in patients with acute neurologic illness and severe headaches because they have a minimal effect on the level of consciousness.

Use of NSAIDs is associated potentially with major side effects. Gastropathy is noticeable in long-term use, typically including mucosal damage, gastrointestinal bleeding, and perforation, but these side effects are less common with brief exposure. Cimetidine and sucralfate are ineffective in protection against gastric ulcers from NSAIDs.[36] The major disadvantage is risk of hemorrhage or coagulopathy. Therefore, they are contraindicated in patients with intracranial hemorrhage.

Intramuscular administration of 30 mg of ketorolac is comparable to 10 mg of morphine and may be used to complement morphine and to reduce opioid requirements.[50,56] Ketorolac may cause renal vasoconstriction and renal failure through an effect on prostaglandin synthesis. Another agent, parecoxib, a new parenteral specific inhibitor of cyclo-oxygenase-2,[18] could become a good analgesic agent for postoperative pain control. A single dose of 40 mg/kg is well tolerated, and gastric ulceration may be less than with ketorolac.

CONCLUSIONS

- Agitation in a patient with an acute neurologic disorder may be from drug or alcohol withdrawal delirium.
- Alcohol-related delirium is best initially treated orally with chlordiazepoxide, 50 to 100 mg, up to 300 mg per day, or intravenously with lorazepam, 2 mg.
- Extremely agitated patients are best treated with lorazepam, 1–2 mg given slowly intravenously; haloperidol, 5 mg intramuscularly; midazolam, 0.02 to 0.1 mg/kg per hour; or propofol, 0.1 to 0.6 mg/kg per hour.
- Pain relief has a high priority in neurologic intensive care, and opiates are invariably effective. The preferred agent in acute central nervous system disorders is codeine.
- Pain relief in Guillain-Barré syndrome is crucial in management. The preferred agents are oxycodone or morphine. Tramadol may become a preferred treatment.

REFERENCES

1. Aitkenhead AR, Pepperman ML, Willatts SM, et al: Comparison of propofol and midazolam for sedation in critically ill patients. *Lancet* 2:704–709, 1989.
2. Albanese J, Martin C, Lacarelle B, et al: Pharmacokinetics of long-term propofol infusion used for sedation in ICU patients. *Anesthesiology* 73:214–217, 1990.
3. Ariano RE, Kassum DA, Aronson KJ: Comparison of sedative recovery time after midazolam versus diazepam administration. *Crit Care Med* 22:1492–1496, 1994.
4. Bailie GR, Cockshott ID, Douglas EJ, et al: Pharmacokinetics of propofol during and after long-term continuous infusion for maintenance of sedation in ICU patients. *Br J Anaesth* 68:486–491, 1992.
5. Barr J, Egan TD, Sandoval NF, et al: Propofol dosing regimens for ICU sedation based upon an integrated pharmacokinetic-pharmacodynamic model. *Anesthesiology* 95:324–333, 2001.
6. Barr J, Zomorodi K, Bertaccini EJ, et al: A double-blind, randomized comparison of i.v. lorazepam versus midazolam for sedation of ICU patients via a pharmacologic model. *Anesthesiology* 95:281–282, 2001.
7. Baumgartner GR, Rowen RC: Clonidine vs chlordiazepoxide in the management of acute alcohol withdrawal syndrome. *Arch Intern Med* 147:1223–1226, 1987.
8. Bernauer EA, Yeager MP: Optimal pain control in the intensive care unit. *Int Anesthesiol Clin* 31:201–221, 1993.
9. Black AMS, Alexander JI: Analgesia for postoperative pain. In Atkinson RS, Adams AP (eds): *Recent Advances in Anaesthesia and Analgesia 17.* Edinburgh, Churchill Livingstone, 1992.
10. Bloch MB, Dyer RA, Heijke SA, et al: Tramadol infusion for postthoracotomy pain relief: a placebo-controlled comparison with epidural morphine. *Anesth Analg* 94:523–528, 2002.
11. Bodenham A, Park GR: Reversal of prolonged sedation using flumazenil in critically ill patients. *Anaesthesia* 44:603–605, 1989.
12. Brandl KM, Langley KA, Riker RR, et al: Confirming the reliability of the sedation-agitation scale administered by ICU nurses without experience in its use. *Pharmacotherapy* 21:431–436, 2001.
13. Bravo LJ, Mattie H, Spierdijk J, et al: The effects on ventilation of ketorolac in comparison with morphine. *Eur J Clin Pharmacol* 35:491–494, 1988.
14. Breheny FX: Reversal of midazolam sedation with flumazenil. *Crit Care Med* 20:736–739, 1992.
15. Brown CR, Moodie JE, Wild VM, et al: Comparison of intravenous ketorolac tromethamine and morphine sulfate in the treatment of postoperative pain. *Pharmacotherapy* 10:116S–121S, 1990.
16. Brust JCM: *Neurological Aspects of Substance Abuse.* Boston, Butterworth-Heinemann, 1993.
17. Cernaianu AC, Delrossi AJ, Flum DR, et al: Lorazepam and midazolam in the intensive care unit: a randomized, prospective, multicenter study of hemodynamics, oxygen transport, efficacy, and cost. *Crit Care Med* 24:222–228, 1996.
18. Cheer SM, Goa KL: Parecoxib (parecoxib sodium). *Drugs* 61:1133–1141, 2001.
19. Claassen J, Hirsch LJ, Emerson RG, et al: Treatment of refractory status epilepticus with pentobarbital, propofol, or midazolam: systematic review. *Epilepsia* 43:146–153, 2002.
20. Coppolo DP, May JJ: Self-extubations. A 12-month experience. *Chest* 98:165–169, 1990.
21. Cremer OL, Moons KG, Bouman EA, et al: Long-term propofol infusion and cardiac failure in adult head-injured patients (letter to the editor). *Lancet* 357:117–118, 2001.
22. Deer TR, Rich GF: Propofol tolerance in a pediatric patient. *Anesthesiology* 77:828–829, 1992.
23. D'Onofrio G, Rathlev NK, Ulrich AS, et al: Lorazepam for the prevention of recurrent seizures related to alcohol. *N Engl J Med* 340:915–919, 1999.
24. Druckenbrod RW, Rosen J, Cluxton RJ Jr: As-needed

dosing of antipsychotic drugs: limitations and guidelines for use in the elderly agitated patient. *Ann Pharmacother* 27:645–648, 1993.

25. Earnest MP, Feldman H, Marx JA, et al: Intracranial lesions shown by CT scans in 259 cases of first alcohol-related seizures. *Neurology* 38:1561–1565, 1988.

26. Frenzel D, Greim CA, Sommer C, et al: Is the bispectral index appropriate for monitoring the sedation level of mechanically ventilated surgical ICU patients? *Intensive Care Med* 28:178–183, 2002.

27. Genis D, Busquets C, Manubens E, et al: Epidural morphine analgesia in Guillain-Barré syndrome. *J Neurol Neurosurg Psychiatry* 52:999–1001, 1989.

28. Glick ID, Murray SR, Vasudevan P, et al: Treatment with atypical antipsychotics: new indications and new populations. *J Psychiatr Res* 35:187–191, 2001.

29. Helsley JD: Cortical blindness following cerebral angiography. *W V Med J* 91:324, 1995.

30. Johnson JC: Delirium in the elderly. *Emerg Med Clin North Am* 8:255–265, 1990.

31. Kanto J, Gepts E: Pharmacokinetic implications for the clinical use of propofol. *Clin Pharmacokinet* 17:308–326, 1989.

32. Kelly DF, Goodale DB, Williams J, et al: Propofol in the treatment of moderate and severe head injury: a randomized, prospective double-blinded pilot trial. *J Neurosurg* 90:1042–1052, 1999.

33. Kress JP, O'Connor MF, Pohlman AS, et al: Sedation of critically ill patients during mechanical ventilation: a comparison of propofol and midazolam. *Am J Respir Crit Care Med* 153:1012–1018, 1996.

34. Kress JP, Pohlman AS, O'Connor MF, et al: Daily interruption of sedative infusions in critically ill patients undergoing mechanical ventilation. *N Engl J Med* 342:1471–1477, 2000.

35. Langley MS, Heel RC: Propofol. A review of its pharmacodynamic and pharmacokinetic properties and use as an intravenous anaesthetic. *Drugs* 35:334–372, 1988.

36. Lanza F, Peace K, Gustitus L, et al: A blinded endoscopic comparative study of misoprostol versus sucralfate and placebo in the prevention of aspirin-induced gastric and duodenal ulceration. *Am J Gastroenterol* 83:143–146, 1988.

37. Laxenaire MC, Mata-Bermejo E, Moneret-Vautrin DA, et al: Life-threatening anaphylactoid reactions to propofol (Diprivan). *Anesthesiology* 77:275–280, 1992.

38. Lipowski ZJ: Delirium (acute confusional states). *JAMA* 258:1789–1792, 1987.

39. Lipowski ZJ: Delirium in the elderly patient. *N Engl J Med* 320:578–582, 1989.

40. Longobardi JJ, Comens R, Jacobs AM: Epidural morphine as an adjuvant to the treatment of pain in a patient with acute inflammatory polyradiculopathy secondary to Guillain-Barré syndrome. *J Foot Surg* 30:267–268, 1991.

41. Marchant B, Wray R, Leach A, et al: Flumazenil causing convulsions and ventricular tachycardia. *BMJ* 299:860, 1989.

42. Mayo-Smith MF: Pharmacological management of al-

cohol withdrawal. A meta-analysis and evidence-based practice guideline. American Society of Addiction Medicine Working Group on Pharmacological Management of Alcohol Withdrawal. *JAMA* 278:144–151, 1997.

43. Mirenda J, Broyles G: Propofol as used for sedation in the ICU. *Chest* 108:539–548, 1995.

44. Modell JG: Further experience and observations with lorazepam in the management of behavioral agitation (letter to the editor). *J Clin Psychopharmacol* 6:385–387, 1986.

45. Morgenlander JC, Hurwitz BJ, Massey EW: Capsaicin for the treatment of pain in Guillain-Barré syndrome (letter to the editor). *Ann Neurol* 28:199, 1990.

46. Mori E, Yamadori A: Acute confusional state and acute agitated delirium. Occurrence after infarction in the right middle cerebral artery territory. *Arch Neurol* 44:1139–1143, 1987.

47. Moulin DE, Hagen N, Feasby TE, et al: Pain in Guillain-Barré syndrome. *Neurology* 48:328–331, 1997.

48. Murray MJ: Pain problems in the ICU. *Crit Care Clin* 6:235–253, 1990.

49. Nixon RA: Quinine sulfate for pain in the Guillain-Barré syndrome (letter to the editor). *Ann Neurol* 4:386–387, 1978.

50. O'Hara DA, Fragen RJ, Kinzer M, et al: Ketorolac tromethamine as compared with morphine sulfate for treatment of postoperative pain. *Clin Pharmacol Ther* 41:556–561, 1987.

51. Ostermann ME, Keenan SP, Seiferling RA, et al: Sedation in the intensive care unit: a systematic review. *JAMA* 283:1451–1459, 2000.

52. O'Sullivan GF, Wade DN: Flumazenil in the management of acute drug overdosage with benzodiazepines and other agents. *Clin Pharmacol Ther* 42:254–259, 1987.

53. Owen H, McMillan V, Rogowski D: Postoperative pain therapy: a survey of patients' expectations and their experiences. *Pain* 41:303–307, 1990.

54. Parke TJ, Stevens JE, Rice AS, et al: Metabolic acidosis and fatal myocardial failure after propofol infusion in children: five case reports. *BMJ* 305:613–616, 1992.

55. The Parkinson Study Group: Low-dose clozapine for the treatment of drug-induced psychosis in Parkinson's disease. *N Engl J Med* 340:757–763, 1999.

56. Peirce RJ, Fragen RJ, Pemberton DM: Intravenous ketorolac tromethamine versus morphine sulfate in the treatment of immediate postoperative pain. *Pharmacotherapy* 10:111S–115S, 1990.

57. Pentland B, Donald SM: Pain in the Guillain-Barré syndrome: a clinical review. *Pain* 59:159–164, 1994.

58. Pohlman AS, Simpson KP, Hall JB: Continuous intravenous infusions of lorazepam versus midazolam for sedation during mechanical ventilatory support: a prospective, randomized study. *Crit Care Med* 22:1241–1247, 1994.

59. Pollard BJ, Masters AP, Bunting P: The use of flumazenil (Anexate, Ro 15–1788) in the management of drug overdose. *Anaesthesia* 44:137–138, 1989.

60. Porter J, Jick H: Addiction rare in patients treated with narcotics (letter to the editor). *N Engl J Med* 302:123, 1980.

61. Ramsay MA, Savege TM, Simpson BR, et al: Controlled sedation with alphaxalone-alphadolone. *Br Med J* 2:656–659, 1974.

62. Rice AS, Lloyd J, Miller CG, et al: A double-blind study of the speed of onset of analgesia following intramuscular administration of ketorolac tromethamine in comparison to intramuscular morphine and placebo. *Anaesthesia* 46:541–544, 1991.

63. Riker RR, Picard JT, Fraser GL: Prospective evaluation of the sedation-agitation scale for adult critically ill patients. *Crit Care Med* 27:1325–1329, 1999.

64. Ropper AH, Wijdicks EFM, Truax BT: *Guillain-Barré Syndrome*. Philadelphia, FA Davis Company, 1991.

65. Sage DJ: Reversal of sedation with flumazenil in regional anaesthesia: a review. *Eur J Anaesthesiol* Suppl 2:201–207, 1988.

66. Shelly MP, Sultan MA, Bodenham A, et al: Midazolam infusions in critically ill patients. *Eur J Anaesthesiol* 8:21–27, 1991.

67. Venn RM, Karol MD, Grounds RM: Pharmacokinetics of dexmedetomide infusions for sedation of postoperative patients requiring intensive care. *Br J Anaesth* 88:669–675, 2002.

68. Vickrey BG, Bahls FH: Nonconvulsive status epilepticus following cerebral angiography. *Ann Neurol* 25:199–201, 1989.

69. Walder B, Tramer MR, Seeck M: Seizure-like phenomena and propofol: a systematic review. *Neurology* 58:1327–1332, 2002.

70. Wijdicks EFM, Nyberg SL: Propofol to control intracranial pressure in fulminant hepatic failure. *Transplant Proc* 34:1220–1222, 2002.

71. Winspur I: Tegretol for pain in the Guillain-Barré syndrome (letter to the editor). *Lancet* 1:85, 1970.

72. Wright SW, Chudnofsky CR, Dronen SC, et al: Comparison of midazolam and diazepam for conscious sedation in the emergency department. *Ann Emerg Med* 22:201–205, 1993.

73. Young C, Knudsen N, Hilton A, et al: Sedation in the intensive care unit. *Crit Care Med* 28:854–866, 2000.

74. Ziehm SR: Intravenous haloperidol for tranquilization in critical care patients: a review and critique. *AACN Clin Issues Crit Care Nurs* 2:765–777, 1991.

5

Airway and Mechanical Ventilation

Maintenance of a patent, unobstructed airway and normal gas exchange are two priorities and although each depends on the other, they are separate concerns. The tongue significantly contributes to airway obstruction when the oropharyngeal muscles lose their tone in impaired consciousness. Besides respiratory drive, ventilation depends on normal mechanics of the rib cage and includes a coordinated effort by respiratory muscles. Interruption of the neuronal control of breathing can occur at any level, inhibiting input to the medullary central pattern generator. Abnormal respiratory muscle function is most frequently seen in Guillain-Barré syndrome (GBS) and myasthenia gravis. Mechanical support is required, but respiratory function is completely reversible after therapeutic intervention. In addition, parenchymal lung disease due to aspiration may rapidly consolidate or collapse large areas in which an intrapulmonary shunt causes hypoxemia.

Neurologists have traditionally asked pulmonologists or anesthesiologists to take charge of the mechanical ventilator. With a new generation of neurologic intensive care specialists, the responsibilities have shifted. This change does not imply, however, that neurologists should routinely intubate or set ventilators. In many major institutions, mechanically ventilated patients are seen hourly by respiratory therapists under the supervision of anesthesiologists. However, neurologists with expertise in neurologic critical care should have a decisive role in airway management, establishing the need for mechanical ventilation, determining indications for tracheostomy, setting

the degree of respiratory alkalosis in induced hyperventilation, changing the mode of ventilation, and knowing when weaning is appropriate.

Management of the airway and mechanical ventilator is different in neurologic critical illness for several reasons. First, many patients in the neurologic intensive care unit (NICU) have normal baseline pulmonary function, unlike patients with exacerbation of obstructive respiratory disease or newly acquired serious pulmonary parenchymal disease typically found in medical intensive care units. Second, mode of ventilation in acutely ill neurologic patients is often intermittent mandatory or assisted control and, much less often, pressure control, inverse ratio, or permissive hypercapnia is used. Third, ventilator dependency is less common, and except for those with cervical spinal cord transection or end-stage amyotrophic lateral sclerosis, most acutely ill neurologic patients can later be successfully weaned from the ventilator.

The immense subject of mechanical ventilation[54] cannot be captured in a single chapter, and therefore the discussion is limited to the clinical applications of airway management and the basic principles of mechanical ventilation specifically focused on our patient population.

AIRWAY MANAGEMENT AND ENDOTRACHEAL INTUBATION

Inappropriate securing of the airway may rapidly result in hypoxemia. The risks of hypoxemia are considerable, even in controlled hospital settings such as emergency rooms and intensive care units. It is reasonable to assume that improper airway management in patients with a neurologic catastrophe may influence outcome. The most telling example of these subtle hazards in critically ill patients with neurologic disorders was recorded in an important survey of patients with head injury in whom a high frequency of a significant period of hypoxemia and hypercapnia was demonstrated.[3] If ignored, these events may potentially contribute to the initial insult and lead to a worse outcome than otherwise would be expected.

The physician can use the head-tilt maneuver to secure the airway by standing behind the patient, placing the thumb and index finger on the mask and the other fingers behind the vertical part of the mandible, and gently lifting the jaw upward to open the collapsed airway[18] (Fig. 5–1). Both thumb and index finger compress the ventilating mask to the face (the thumb presses the mask against the nasal bridge; the index finger presses the base of the mask against the chin). The other hand is free to operate the resuscitation bag, which should

be connected to an oxygen source (most resuscitation bags accommodate an oxygen flow rate of 10 to 15 L/minute).

The mask is pressed to the face just enough to create a seal. In a patient with a poorly fitting mask, particularly edentulous patients, two persons are needed, one to secure the maximal fit by pulling the cheeks to the rim of the mask and another to operate the resuscitation bag. The manual skills of airway management—bag and mask ventilation without intubation—are fairly easily acquired, can maintain the airway for at least 1 hour, and are of critical importance when one's intubation skills are in doubt or when intubation is expected to be difficult.

An oropharyngeal airway is inserted in many patients. This has the added advantage of protecting the tongue from biting in patients subject to seizures. The proper length of the tube can be estimated by holding one end to the corner of the mouth and the other to the ear. An airway that is too long pushes the epiglottis down and compresses the larynx, reducing the capacity to ventilate and, worse, increasing the risk of gastric insufflation. Too short an airway

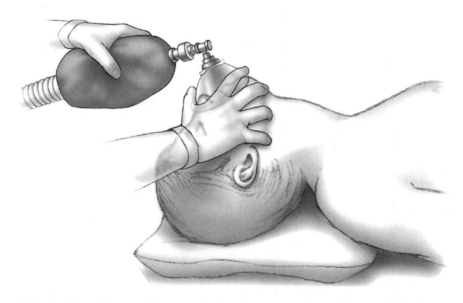

Figure 5–1. Position of resuscitation mask that fits over bridge of the nose, cheeks, and chin. An airtight seal is established by having two fingers hold the mask and three fingers lift the mandible.

pushes the tongue posteriorly, aggravating the obstruction. It is convenient to use a tongue depressor, which simplifies oral airway insertion and is followed by advancement of the device with the tip pointing at the palate and finally gradual turning of the tip toward the base of the tongue.

An adequate supply of oxygen can be provided through a large selection of delivery systems. Most commonly, nasal prongs or plastic face masks are used. Nasal prongs (flow rate of oxygen of 1 to 5 L/minute) may not deliver sufficient supplemental oxygen,[35] and a face mask with a flow rate of 6 to 12 L/minute and up to 60% oxygen should be considered.

Endotracheal intubation should follow in patients who cannot protect the airway, in those who may have aspirated gastric contents, and certainly in those with decreased alertness during which a brief unguarded moment may lead to airway obstruction. In addition, intubation is needed in patients with hypoventilation and hypoxia from neuromuscular disease.

The technique of intubation can be mastered by any physician. Elective intubation may be done by an experienced physician and supervisor, which may include neurologists, but probably should be done by experienced anesthesia teams. One may argue that neurologists with training in neurologic intensive care must learn how to manage an airway rather than force themselves to maintain the skill of endotracheal intubation. Generally, 70 to 100 intubations are needed for competency.

The choice of the intubation route is important. Nasal intubation has several advantages, including improved patient comfort, significantly tighter tube fixation, reduced laryngeal damage, and the possibility for proper mouth care. However, in patients with head injury and potential cerebrospinal fluid leak, nasal intubation may lead to contamination. Moreover, it has been well appreciated that nasal intubation produces a transient bacteremia. The infectious risks of prolonged nasotracheal intubation (more than 5 days) from purulent paranasal sinusitis are considerable, and patients with diabetes mellitus or corticosteroid coverage are at increased risk.[15,31] It may also lead to nasal septal necrosis and perforation of the nasal palate. Associated possible cervical spine injury should not necessarily sway the decision toward a nasal route for intubation, because if time allows, fiberoptic intubation more likely minimizes displacement of the unstable cervical spinal column.

The technique of endotracheal intubation begins with recognition of the difficult airway.[46] When a difficult endotracheal intubation is expected (only 8% incidence in critically ill patients)[49] and time allows elective intubation, a physician with daily expertise in endotracheal intubation should supervise or, more likely, perform the procedure. Important cues for a difficult intubation include inability to visualize oral structures—such as soft palate, tonsillar fossa, and uvula—when the mouth is wide open, significant facial trauma, cervical spine fracture, mandibular hypoplasia, history of rheumatoid arthritis, spondylitic ankylosis, morbid obesity, and short, muscular, thick neck.

Samsoon and Young[46] modified Mallampati's classification of a difficult airway, which is based on the visibility of the pharyngeal structures due to variation in tongue base. Class I is full exposure of soft palate, uvula, and tonsillar pillars; class II, exposure of the soft palate and base of the uvula with only a portion of the posterior pharyngeal wall visible; class III, visibility of soft palate only; and class IV, no visualization of pharyngeal structures except the hard palate. Its predictive value for a difficult intubation remains limited, and the classification should be incorporated with other physical signs.

Physical examination should at least include assessment of the temporomandibular joint, length of the mandible, and, most importantly, extension of the cervical spine. Important bedside estimates are the abilities to insert three fingers in the oral cavity (Fig. 5–2A) and to place three fingers between the thyroid bone and the mandible when the head is extended (Fig. 5–2B). Patients with long-standing insulin-dependent diabetes mellitus have a major limitation in cervical spine mobility. Difficulty in closing the palms and bowing at the

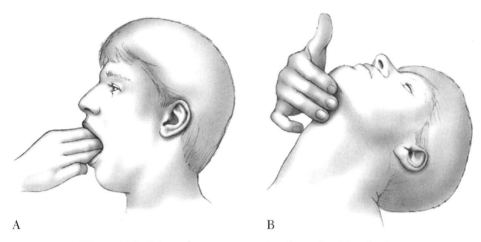

Figure 5–2. Manual assessment of endotracheal intubation.

interphalangeal area, creating a "prayer sign," also seem to be correlated with limitation in neck extension.[43]

Elective intubation can proceed if the patient has not taken food for at least 6 hours. The procedure of endotracheal intubation must be accompanied by cricoid pressure (Sel-

lick maneuver). Movement of this circle of cartilage posteriorly occludes the esophagus and may significantly prevent regurgitation (Fig. 5–3). The maneuver should be routine in any patient intubated in the NICU.

The technique of intubation is depicted in Figure 5–4. Stepwise performance is usually

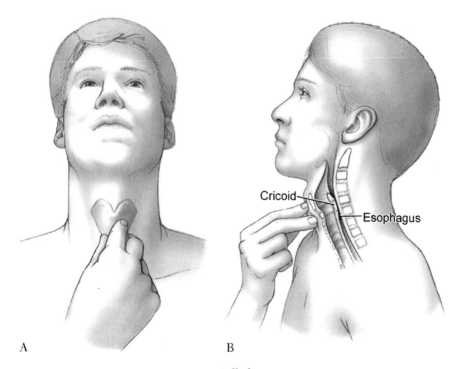

Figure 5–3. Sellick maneuver.

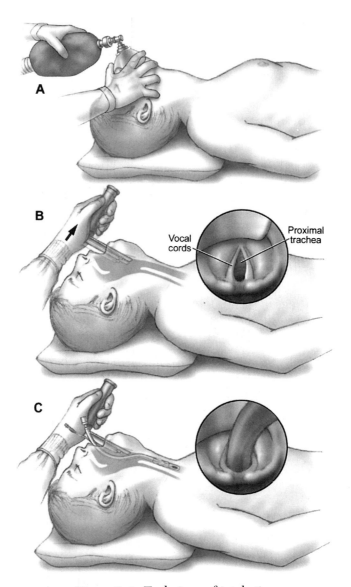

Figure 5–4. Technique of intubation.

successful. The patient is placed in the "sniffing position" (achieved by tilting the head backward) (Fig. 5–4A) and given 100% oxygen through ventilation with a bag and mask. To begin the laryngoscopy, the physician extends the patient's head and carefully introduces the laryngoscope into the patient's mouth with the left hand. The physician must be careful not to injure the patient's teeth and lips.

During the laryngoscopy, the base of the tongue is seen first. As the laryngoscope is ad-

vanced, the epiglottis appears. If the Miller blade is used, the tip is placed under the epiglottis to lift it up and out of the way. At this point, the laryngoscope is lifted in the direction of its handle. Pivoting the instrument back onto the upper incisor will injure the patient's teeth.

Lifting the laryngoscope brings the arytenoids, at the most posterior part of the larynx, into view. Further lifting exposes the cords (Fig. 5–4B). External pressure on the thyroid cartilage or cricoid cartilage by an assistant might help bring the laryngeal structures into view. As the endotracheal tube is advanced, it passes between the cords (Fig. 5–4C). After the cuff has passed the cords, advancement of only 3 cm is needed for proper placement. The endotracheal tube is shown in Figure 5–5.

The cuff is inflated up to 10–15 cm H_2O or more when a leak is still heard. The physician must auscultate over both lungs to ensure the presence of bilateral breath sounds. The gastric area is also auscultated to rule out esophageal ventilation. A secure method to confirm proper tube placement is use of a disposable capnometer that changes to yellow when exposed to carbon dioxide. The location must be confirmed by a routine chest radiograph, which identifies the tip of the endotracheal tube 5 to 7 cm above the carina or at the T-6 level.

Alternatively, a laryngeal mask airway has been used, particularly by emergency medical services in the field and nonanesthesiologists, in patients with difficult airways. The mask has been modified to facilitate tracheal intubation with a tracheal tube. The major incentives for its use are obscured vision of the larynx by blood and secretions and the potential for spinal cord damage when neck injuries are not yet known. Minimal training is required. Tracheal intubation is as successful as fiber-optic intubation, but oxygen saturation and bleeding complications are less frequent.[23,42] This may be a useful bridging device to a more traditional use of a cuffed tracheal tube in acute trauma care, but it is not particularly useful in the NICU.

INDICATIONS FOR MECHANICAL VENTILATION

The indications for mechanical ventilation in the heterogeneous NICU population can be most effectively discussed in reference to the hemispheres and brain stem (regulation of respiratory drive), peripheral effector organ (the mechanics of the respiratory system), and primary pulmonary causes of inadequate ventilation (intrinsic pulmonary disease).

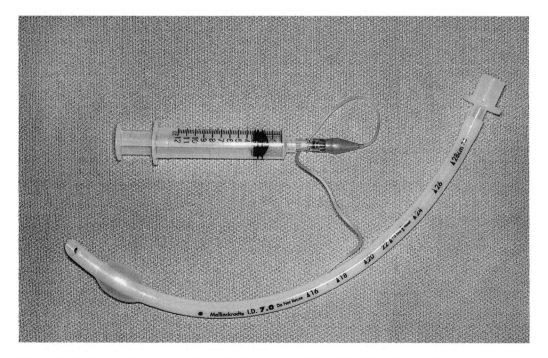

Figure 5–5. Soft endotracheal tube with inflated cuff (usually 10 to 12 cc of air in the syringe is sufficent).

Central Nervous System Dysfunction

Changes in respiratory drive may result from acute lesions in the hemispheres or brain stem. Many patients, particularly in the first hour, have marked spontaneous hyperventilation. There is a tendency to assume that the most prominent factor in hyperventilation is sustained resetting of the feedback loops in the respiratory centers, but in daily practice, some patients hyperventilate merely to compensate for considerable hypoxia. Rather than remaining in a marginal situation that without appropriate intervention results in ventilatory muscle fatigue, patients with prolonged hyperventilation are probably better served by assisted ventilation with mild sedation. In other patients, tachypnea compensates for metabolic acidosis, which needs correction first.[37] Sudden tachypnea in acute stroke may indicate pulmonary embolism,[36] and patients may not be able to signal pleuritic pain (see Chapter 29). Hyperventilation in a patient with an acute mass more centrally located may signal development of diencephalic herniation, and pathologic flexion or extension may emerge. Pupils usually remain in midposition and become fixed to light.

Depression of level of consciousness is not an absolute indication for mechanical ventilation. Intubated patients with an acute central nervous system event are generally well able to maintain efficient gas exchange that can be monitored by pulse oximeter and repeated blood gas determinations. Also, there is no rationale to prophylactically intubate patients to produce hypocapnia and respiratory alkalosis when there is a risk of brain swelling. However, patients with abnormal breathing patterns that result in inadequate oxygen delivery and hypercapnia need to be mechanically ventilated.

Archetypal breathing patterns are ataxic and cluster breathing, mostly in patients with acute brain stem syndromes.[38] Apneustic breathing characterized by prolonged end-expiratory pauses could be due to lesions in the rostral pons. Recurrent apnea in acute basilar artery occlusion may indicate a very poor outcome with a high probability of progression to loss of all brain stem reflexes.[60] Cheyne-Stokes respiration is recognized by an oscillating cycle (up to $1\frac{1}{2}$ minutes each) of hyperpnea separated by apnea. Touching the patient in an apneic period can easily start the crescendo hyperventilation phase. Cheyne-Stokes breathing is relatively frequent in patients in the NICU but should be left alone. A study found that 50% of patients had Cheyne-Stokes breathing after an acute ischemic stroke, but occasionally this occurred in association with oxygen desaturation below 90 mm Hg. Oxygen delivery through a nasal tube, or possibly theophylline, 250 mg intravenously,[32] probably is sufficient to circumvent this problem.

In our series of patients with hemispheric ischemic stroke who needed mechanical ventilation, we found that many had pulmonary edema from congestive heart failure.[61] In other patients, vigorous treatment with antiepileptic drugs to counter focal or generalized seizures resulted in hypoventilation and a need for airway protection and mechanical ventilation. Nonetheless, brain swelling with further impairment of consciousness remains the most common reason for intubation and mechanical ventilation in ischemic stroke.

Mechanical ventilation is often instituted for aneurysmal subarachnoid hemorrhage, particularly in patients who have had a rerupture, which often is associated with apnea. Within hours it should become clear whether apnea persists or if triggering of the ventilator occurs. Recovering patients need emergency clipping of the aneurysm, and it is prudent to continue mechanical ventilation until surgery (Chapter 12).

Neuromuscular Respiratory Failure

Before clinical features are discussed, it is useful to review the normal and pathologic state of respiratory muscles.[13] The muscles of inspiration are the diaphragm, intercostal muscles, and scalene muscles. Expiration is largely due to recoil of the lungs, but abdominal muscles contribute. When ventilatory demand is increased, accessory muscles (such as the sternocleidomastoid, pectoralis major and minor, latissimus dorsi) do service. The diaphragm has a central noncontractile tendon (dome) from which muscle fibers radiate to insert to the xiphoid in the front to the lower ribs and to the first two or three lumbar vertebral bodies. When the diaphragm contracts, the dome remains normal in shape but descends in a piston-like action. The rib cage expands with a much more complex vector. The lower ribs are lifted because the abdominal viscera counter the descent of the diaphragmatic dome and due to shortening of the costal part of the diaphragmatic fibers. The remaining rib cage expands as a result of synchronized contractile force of the parasternal intercostal muscles that run caudally and laterally between the ribs. Inspiration thus results in an outward movement of chest and abdomen (Fig. 5–6B). Expiration does involve relaxation of the diaphragm and recoil of the lungs. The abdominal muscles lengthen the diaphragm fibers and assist in the next inspiratory cycle but, most importantly, produce an increase in intra-abdominal pressure. Their function also involves coughing and clearing of secretions.

When respiratory weakness occurs, particularly within a brief period, the pulmonary mechanics change; but many other factors play a

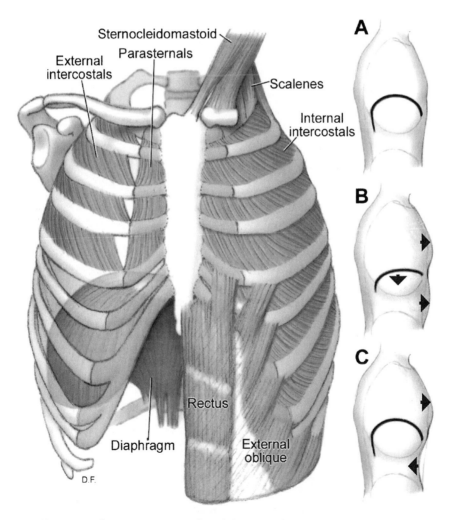

Figure 5–6. Drawing of respiratory muscles. (*A*) Normal position. (*B*) Normal breathing. (*C*) Paradoxical breathing. (See text for details.)

decisive role. Ineffective diaphragm contraction will result in pulling up of the rib cage by other inspiratory muscles, resulting in decrease of the intra-abdominal pressure, which will lead to inward movement of the anterior abdomen. This is called the respiratory paradox (Fig. 5–6C). In addition, the scalene and sternocleidomastoid muscles are recruited. The contraction of these muscles, which can be palpated, has been called the respiratory pulse ("pouls respiratoire").

Not only is pump failure a major concern but also lung function becomes impaired. This is partly due to the inability to cough, which results in atelectasis, shunting, and hypoxemia. However, when respiratory muscle weakness occurs, tidal volumes are reduced and this might reduce surfactant. Surfactant allows O_2 and CO_2 to diffuse freely across the alveolar membrane. It reduces the work of breathing, allows opening of collapsed lung regions with minimal inspiratory pressures, and prevents atelectasis. Therefore, in patients with neuromuscular respiratory failure, tachypnea in association with smaller lung volumes may decrease surfactant and cause decreased pulmonary compliance.

The clinical features that should alert one to the possibility of neuromuscular respiratory failure are listed in Table 5–1. The first signs are subtle and are typically not detected by bedside measurements of respiratory mechanics or by pulse oximeter.[17]

Patients with signs of diaphragmatic failure invariably have tachycardia and tachypnea. These clinical warning signs are usually associated with some sense of discomfort and anx-

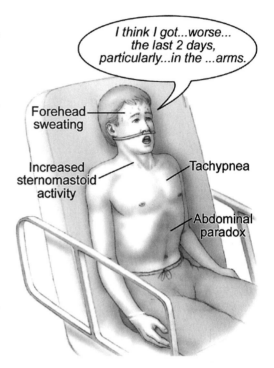

Figure 5–7. Bedside assessment of neuromuscular respiratory failure and imminent arrest: abdominal retraction, sternocleidomastoid contraction, sweating, and staccato speech (*balloon*). (Nasal flaring and sternal retraction may be seen as well.)

iety.[34] Many patients have staccato speech and a need to pause after a few words. Sweat is often found at the hairline or has collected in the eyebrows as a sign of the increased work of breathing. Restlessness may be apparent, but other patients are quiet and nod "yes" when asked if they are short of breath (Fig. 5–7). Vital capacity can be estimated by asking patients to take a deep breath and count to 20 (one number per second). Inability to perform this simple bedside test is associated with a markedly decreased vital capacity, but a comparative study is not available.

Use of accessory muscles is not always recognized well with the naked eye, and, as mentioned above, palpation of the sternocleidomastoid muscles may disclose muscle contractions during breathing. Contraction of the

Table 5–1. Clinical Features of Imminent Neuromuscular Respiratory Failure

Dyspnea at low levels of work
Restlessness
Tachycardia (rate > 100/minute)
Tachypnea (respiratory rate > 20/minute)
Use of sternocleidomastoid, scalene muscles (by palpation alone)
Forehead sweating
Staccato speech
Asynchronous (paradoxical) breathing

sternocleidomastoid muscles can be palpated long before florid paradoxical breathing becomes obvious clinically. At night, relaxation of these muscles may result in increased demand for diaphragmatic performance and thus hypoventilation and hypercapnia. Frequent nocturnal awakening may signal respiratory dysfunction that is not yet evident during daytime. Nonetheless, the clinical hallmark of diaphragmatic fatigue is dyssynchronous movement of the chest cage and abdomen. Dyspnea is much more significant when the patient is supine rather than sitting upright, and this also explains the tendency to worsen overnight.

Laboratory measurements are very useful, but they must be viewed together with the clinical manifestations of respiratory failure. All these tests are effort-dependent and require some training. The test results are not infrequently spuriously low from inadequate mouth closure, particularly in patients with bilateral facial palsy. In other patients, the Valsalva maneuver replaces exhalation. However, forced vital capacity remains a very useful bedside test. The vital capacity is defined as the volume of air that can be exhaled by force from the lungs after a full inhalation. The range in normal adults is approximately 3 to 5 L, and the critical value is approximately 15 mL/kg.

The maximum inspiratory pressure (PImax) and the maximum expiratory pressure (PEmax) are clinically useful for monitoring respiratory muscles in patients with possible neuromuscular failure. The investigation is done with the patient upright to increase efficiency. After placement of a nose clip and a scuba-type mouthpiece, the patient is instructed to exhale all residual volume and then to draw in as hard and quickly as possible for 2 to 5 seconds. The maneuver must be repeated at least three times, and only recorded values that vary not more than 20% from one another are reliable. For consistency, the best of the three measurements is recorded. The PImax is the true measure of respiratory muscle function, particularly the diaphragm. For PEmax measurements, the sequence is reversed (Fig. 5–8). The maximum respiratory pressures measure the ability of the patient to clear secretions and to

maintain a satisfactory airway. Effective coughing becomes severely compromised if PEmax values are below 40 cm H_2O.

When poor effort is suspected, one may measure intraesophageal pressure by inserting a balloon in the esophagus. The pressure is recorded during a cough or sniff, and a significant increase is a good indication of poor effort. In addition, several pulmonary conditions,

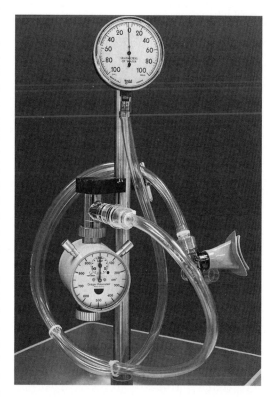

Figure 5–8. Bedside device for measurement of maximal inspiratory pressure and vital capacity. *Upper meter* measures pressure in cm H_2O. Sucking in gives a negative reading, and the needle moves to the left (normal, 100 cm H_2O). Blowing out gives a positive reading, and the needle moves to the right. *Lower meter* (Dräger Volumeter) shows the tidal volume (spontaneous breathing) or vital capacity (maximum exhalation). Normal tidal volume should be 7 to 9 mL/kg of ideal body weight. Normal vital capacity is approximately 70 mL/kg.

such as emphysema and chest wall deformities, can decrease PImax. Whether the positive predictive value of PImax for intubation is better than vital capacity is not exactly known, but vital capacity begins to decrease when these pressures approach -20 cm H_2O; above this value, vital capacities usually remain in the normal range.

In GBS, mechanical ventilation is indicated when clinical deterioration is associated with a vital capacity of 20 mL/kg or less and the PImax is less than -30 cm H_2O or the PEmax is less than 40 cm H_2O ("20–30–40" rule) (Table 5–2). A study found that when vital capacity is monitored three times a day, patients with GBS probably need mechanical ventilation within 36 hours if vital capacity decreases 50% from the initial value, even when vital capacity is within the normal range.[8]

A frequent harbinger of respiratory failure is transient oxygen desaturation (70s to 80s) during monitoring with a pulse oximeter. Hypercapnia is a late manifestation of acute neuromuscular respiratory failure and corresponds with vital capacities of less than 5 mL/kg, a life-threatening situation that mandates immediate intubation and mechanical ventilation.

Many patients readily accept endotracheal intubation followed by mechanical ventilation in the intermittent mandatory ventilation mode with pressure support to relieve the work of breathing and to unload the ventilatory muscles.

Primary Pulmonary Disease

Frequently, a primary pulmonary cause that leads to intubation is aspiration pneumonitis. It occurs, for example, in patients with acute oropharyngeal dysfunction, in patients who had seizures, and in vomiting patients with a diminished response of the pharyngeal reflex caused by drowsiness. Aspiration is rarely witnessed, but usually after an interval of 6 to 12 hours, the patient becomes breathless, with a productive cough.

Physical examination should include palpating the rib cage (place hands on chest and thumbs toward midline below ribs) and noting expansion after a deep breath. Percussion of the chest wall may differentiate pleural effusion or atelectasis (dull tone) from pneumothorax (tympanic tone). The characteristic tone of tympany can be simulated by tapping on one's own blown-out cheek. Auscultation may uncover late inspiratory crackles at the base of the lung (e.g., early congestive heart failure), wheeze at expiration (e.g., bronchial obstruction), stridor or wheeze at expiration (e.g., obstruction of the larynx or trachea), or pleural rub at both phases of respiration (e.g., pulmonary embolus). Vibration from the vocal cord after instructing the patient to make a sound with the mouth closed (the tactile fremitus) may increase (fluid-filled lung) or decrease (obstructed airway) on palpation.

Chest radiography may show abnormalities in the most dependent part of the lungs, typically including the superior parts of the lower lobes and the posterior segment of the right upper lobe (see Chapter 29). Mechanical ventilation should be considered if profound hypoxemia develops, but bronchoscopy must be performed when a segmental atelectasis is observed. Bronchoscopy may locate a large particle that can be removed without major effort.

Neurogenic pulmonary edema, commonly described in acute central nervous system

Table 5–2. Laboratory Values in Monitoring Respiratory Failure

Parameter	Normal Value	Critical Value
Vital capacity	40–70 mL/kg	20 mL/kg
Maximum inspiratory pressure	Male, > -100 cm H_2O	-30 cm H_2O
	Female, > -70 cm H_2O	
Maximum expiratory pressure	Male, > 200 cm H_2O	40 cm H_2O
	Female, > 140 cm H_2O	

catastrophes, is rare in clinical practice. Its clinical presentation is similar to that of adult respiratory distress syndrome, and mechanical ventilation with positive end-expiratory pressure (PEEP) is invariably indicated (Chapter 29).

In patients with trauma, pulmonary injuries should be strongly considered. Pulmonary contusions become apparent on chest radiographs, usually within the first hours of admission. Patients with associated flail chest (multiple rib fractures that result in paradoxical chest wall motion during respiration) are at considerable risk for hypoxemia and are best served by stabilization from mechanical ventilation (see Chapter 29). However, in some cases, incentive spirometry with adequate pain medication in patients with a pulmonary contusion may prevent intubation and mechanical ventilation.

In occasional patients, underlying pulmonary disease, such as asthma or emphysema, worsens at the time of an acute brain injury. Inability to cough frequently results in mucus plugs that may cause significant oxygen desaturation. Bronchodilators, sufficient rest, and mild sedation are often needed. In some patients, mechanical ventilation lasting several days is indicated.

Generally, mechanical ventilation is indicated when refractory hypoxemia exists irrespective of the pulmonary insult. Usually, a markedly widened alveolar-arterial oxygen gradient with a maximal F_{IO_2} of 1.0 or a P_{O_2} of less than 50 mm Hg despite 100% oxygen prompts ventilatory support (Chapter 29).

PHYSIOLOGIC PRINCIPLES AND STANDARD MODES OF MECHANICAL VENTILATION

This section contains common guidelines for setting the ventilator in acutely ill neurologic patients. (A position paper can be consulted as well.[51])

Many intensive care units are equipped with pneumatically driven ventilators. Typical examples are the Siemens Servo ventilator, the Puritan-Bennett ventilator, and the Hamilton Veolar ventilator, and they appear to currently dominate the market.[1] Recently introduced ventilators with digital touch screens are the Nellcor-Puritan-Bennett and the Esprit. It makes good sense to purchase only a few machines and become familiar with them. The control panels and typical settings for each of these ventilators are shown and described in Figures 5–9 through 5–13.

Settings of the Ventilator

The initial tidal volume delivered by the ventilator is usually set to be relatively large, ranging from 12 to 15 mL/kg[21] (based on ideal, not actual, body weight). A tidal volume of more than 15 mL/kg may significantly increase the risk of barotrauma. Patients with underlying pulmonary disease may need smaller tidal volumes (9 to 10 mL/kg). In some ventilators (e.g., Hamilton Veolar), the tidal volume is controlled by an independent adjustable knob. In others (e.g., Siemens Servo), the minute volume is dialed in. (The minute volume is determined by respiratory rate times tidal volume.) The respiratory rate usually ranges from 8 to 12 breaths/minute. The respiratory rate must be chosen at the lowest possible setting to reduce the phenomenon of intrinsic PEEP or gas trapping. When rapid rates are set, intrinsic PEEP is created when the time for expiration is diminished. This phenomenon is deleterious because it increases the work of breathing, increases the proximal airway pressures, and may cause hypotension.

Flow rate is set by the inspiratory time in most ventilators, usually through selection by the ratio of inspiration to expiration. This ratio is determined by inspiratory time, pause time, and expiratory time and is expressed in percentages of the total ventilatory cycle. Commonly, the inspiratory time is set for 20% and the pause time for 5%, with the remaining 75% allowed for expiration (inspiration:expiration ratio, 1:3).

An important setting is the fraction of inspired oxygen (F_{IO_2}), which is based on the arterial P_{O_2}. High F_{IO_2} values, those exceeding 0.8 for at least 2 days, are considered toxic (they

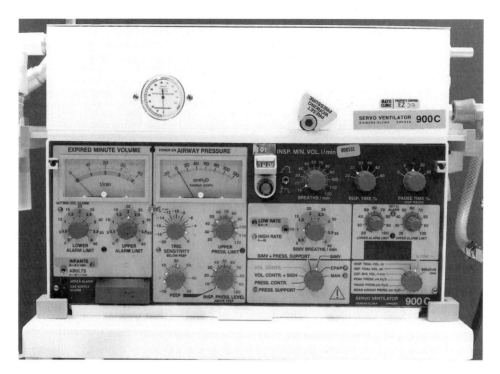

Figure 5–9. Servo Ventilator 900 C (Siemens). From left to right:

- *Expired minute volume* control section. The meter has two ranges—adult, 0–40 L/minute, and infant, 0–4 L/minute—and shows the minute volume with each breath (*0* in photograph). Typically, the lower alarm limit is set at *3 L/minute* and the upper alarm limit at *20 L/minute* (as shown).

- *Airway pressure* control section. The meter shows a peak airway pressure with each breath (*0* in photograph). The trigger sensitivity (below PEEP [positive end-expiratory pressure]) is set at −2 cm H_2O. This control sets the pressure at which the patient's effort can start an inspiratory phase. The upper pressure limit limits peak airway pressure. When high pressure is reached, the inspiratory valve shuts down and the expiratory valve opens. It is a pressure-release mechanism. Usually the limit is set at *50 cm H_2O* (as shown). The PEEP control is set at 5 cm H_2O. The inspiratory pressure level (above PEEP) is used in the pressure control or pressure support position and therefore is here set at *0 cm H_2O*.

- *Inspiratory minute volume* control section. In this section, four knobs are dialed in. The minute volume is set at *7.0 L/minute*, as shown. The breaths/minute is set at *10 breaths/minute* (the tidal volume, therefore, is 700 mL and is *not* dialed in). The inspiratory time is set at *25%* (inspiration:expiration ratio, 1:3). The pause time is set at *10%*. (This produces a volume hold by keeping the expiratory valve closed for a set portion [%] of the total ventilatory cycle.) The flow pattern is entered by a small switch moved to *square wave* (shown) for synchronized intermittent mandatory ventilation (SIMV) modes or decelerating taper in the pressure control mode.

- *SIMV breaths/minute* control section. This mode is used only for SIMV without pressure support. Here it is set at *10 breaths/minute*. The amount of time within one mandatory breath and the number of spontaneous breaths that can occur are determined by this control. In this setting of 10 breaths/minute, one breath is given every 6 seconds (SIMV rate of 10 divided into 60 seconds). The patient can breathe between the SIMV breaths.

- *Modes of operation* control section. *SIMV* (as set), volume control (= assist control), volume control + sigh (sigh automatic every 100 breaths), pressure control (often used in adult respiratory distress syndrome), pressure support, SIMV + pressure support, CPAP (continuous positive airway pressure), and manual (only in anesthesia).

- *O_2 alarm* control section. Lower alarm limit (FIO_2) is set at *50%*, and upper alarm limit is set at *70%*. Below the alarm knobs is a digital display of several selections (dial is set at O_2 concentration).

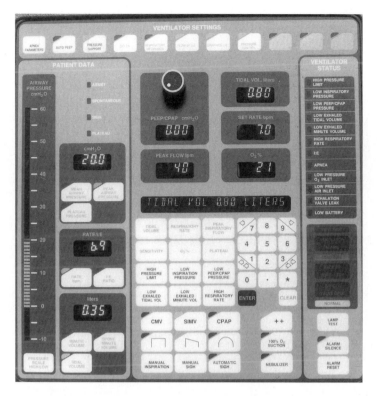

Figure 5–10. Puritan-Bennett (7200 Series). The control panel is divided into three sections: ventilator settings, patient data, and ventilator status.

- *Ventilator settings* control section. Three major modes of ventilation are set by pressing CMV (continuous mechanical ventilation) (= assisted control), *SIMV* (synchronized intermittent mandatory ventilation) (as shown), and CPAP (continuous positive airway pressure) (the settings are entered only when the ENTER command is used; the CPAP mode is also set by the rotating knob designated PEEP [positive end-expiratory pressure]/CPAP). Three inspiratory flow patterns can be chosen: constant, *decelerating* (as shown), and sinusoidal. (The airway pressure and inspiratory time increase when the decelerating mode is used.) Three different selections show manual inspiration, manual sigh, and automatic sigh (this key generally provides a 1.5 × set tidal volume sigh per 100 breaths). Tidal volume, respiratory rate, and peak inspiratory flow are set by pressing the numerical keypads; entries here are tidal volume, *0.8 L/minute*; respiratory rate, *7 set rate breaths/minute*; peak flow, *40 L/minute*; sensitivity (not shown; typically at −1 to −2 cm H_2O); O_2, 21%, and plateau, *0.0 to 2.0 seconds*, with 0.1-second increments (0.0 setting cancels plateau). Note that the inspiration:expiration ratio is not dialed in but is determined by tidal volume, rate, peak flow, and plateau settings. A set of six buttons identifies alarms: high-pressure limit (usually set at *50 cm H_2O*), low inspiration pressure (usually set at *5 cm H_2O*), low PEEP/CPAP pressure (usually set at *3 cm H_2O*), low exhaled tidal volume (usually set at *600 mL* in the assist-control mode, *100 to 200 mL* in the intermittent mandatory ventilation mode), low exhaled minute volume (usually set at *3 L/minute*), and high respiratory rate (usually set at *40 breaths/minute*). All alarms can be silenced or reset (two buttons in lower right corner). The ventilator settings (e.g., auto PEEP, pressure support, and flow-by) can be upgraded by the strip of buttons at the top. Flow-by provides a continuous background flow and decreases the patient's effort to obtain gas. With pressure control, all breaths become pressure-limited.
- *Patient Data*. Airway pressure shows a peak pressure of *20 cm H_2O* and a digital display of mean airway pressure, *peak airway pressure*, and plateau pressure; a digital display of *rate* and I:E (inspiration:expiration) ratio, and a digital display of minute volume, spontaneous minute volume, and *tidal volume*.
- *Ventilator status*. This section mostly involves specific alarm indicators.

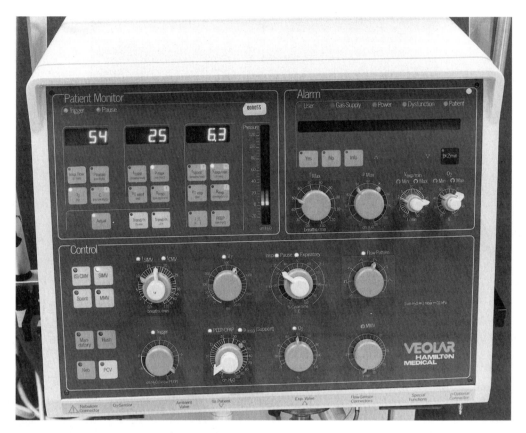

Figure 5–11. Hamilton Veolar. The display panel is divided into three sections: patient monitor, alarm, and control.

- *Control.* (S) CMV (continuous mechanical ventilation), SIMV (synchronized intermittent mandatory ventilation), Spont (spontaneous), and MMV (mandatory minute ventilation). The MMV mode is used for spontaneous breathing with pressure support. Dual knobs are used to set the SIMV mode (dark knob; *10 breaths/minute*) and the CMV (assist-control) mode (light knob). Tidal volume (V_T) is set at *700 mL*. I:E (inspiration:expiration) ratio is set at *1:2 and no pause* (pause is introduced by setting the inspiration and expiration time knobs apart, e.g., 10%). Flow pattern is set at the *deceleration* notch. Trigger sensitivity is set at *−2 cm H_2O*. Positive end-expiratory pressure (PEEP) is at *5 cm H_2O*. The pressure support level is set by activating the MMV, spontaneous, or SIMV mode and dialing in a pressure 0 to 40 cm H_2O above PEEP. Fraction of inspired O_2 is at *60%*. The MMV knob is infrequently used.
- *Alarm.* Breaths/min maximal is set at *50 breaths/minute*. Phase (peak airway pressure) is set at *50 cm H_2O*. Expiratory volume (V_{exp}/min) minimum is at *2 L/minute* and maximum at *20 L/minute*. The O_2 minimum is at *45%*, maximum at *70%*.
- *Patient Monitor.* Three separate controls show (*1*) *oxygen* (options are inspiratory flow, mean airway pressure, and compliance), (*2*) *peak airway pressure* with additional display (options are total frequency of breaths, inspired tidal volume, and respiratory resistance), and (*3*) *minute ventilation* in liters per minute (options are exhaled tidal volume, expiration resistance, I:E ratio, and PEEP). The indicator gives an *actual* reading but may show a trend.

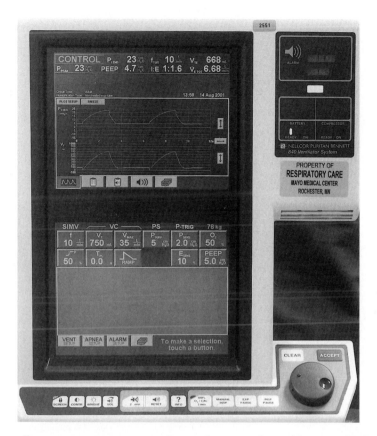

Figure 5–12. Nellcor-Puritan-Bennett ventilator. The control panel has two displays (any of the on-screen symbols can be pushed in the ventilator control squares). Turning the knob to the left digitally adjusts the required modes, which are entered when the ACCEPT button is pushed. The upper display (CONTROL) shows the actual patient settings. $P_{I\ END}$ is end inspiratory pressure; f_{TOT}, total rate of breathing; V_{TE}, end tidal volume; P_{PEAK}, peak pressure; *PEEP*, positive end-expiratory pressure; *I:E*, inspiratory:expiratory ratio; and $\dot{V}_{ETOT}$, total expiratory flow. The screen shows respiratory, pressure, and volume waveforms. The lower display shows the ventilator control settings. The settings for this patient are *f10*, frequency of 10/minute; V_T (tidal volume), *750 mL*; $\dot{V}_{MAX}$, maximum flow at *35 L/minute*; P_{SUPP}, support of *5 cm H_2O*; P_{SENS}, trigger of inspiration at *2.0 cm H_2O*; O_2, 50%; $\sqrt{P}$, working force of 50%; T_{PL}, plateau time of 0%; *RAMP, waveform*; E_{SENS}, expiratory sensitivity of 10%; and *PEEP*, 5 cm H_2O.

increased the chance of lung injury in animal experiments).[6,58] There should be a continuous incentive to decrease F_{IO_2} in patients receiving mechanical ventilation. However, if reduction of F_{IO_2} is not tolerated, adequate gas exchange can also be achieved with increasing PEEP. Positive end-expiratory pressure implies a setting that increases the end-expiratory pressure to produce a larger functional residual capacity. It maintains alveolar patency throughout respiration, recruits previously collapsed alveoli, and improves ventilation-perfusion matching. Most often, PEEP is indicated when the P_{O_2} remains less than 60 mm Hg despite an F_{IO_2} of 0.8. As indicated in cardiogenic pulmonary edema, adult respiratory distress syndrome, and diffuse bilateral pneumonia, PEEP is often added to ventilation.

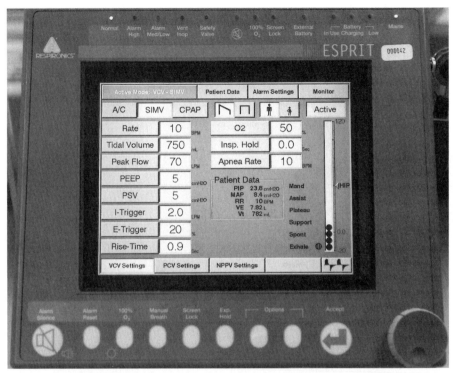

A

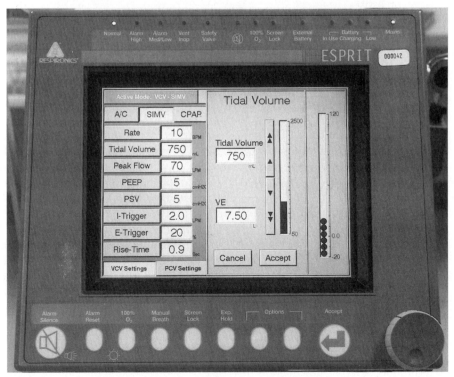

B

54

Figure 5–13. Esprit ventilator. The touch-screen display has additional displays when symbols are pushed. (*A*) Front panel control. (*B*) Display of tidal volume. Turning the knob adjusts the mode, and pushing the *Accept* key enters the data. In this example, SIMV (synchronized intermittent mandatory ventilation) is entered (button lights up if active). The *Rate* is *10 BPM* (breaths per minute); *Tidal Volume*, *750 mL*; *Peak Flow*, *70 L/minute*; *PEEP* (positive end-expiratory pressure), *5 cm H₂O*; *PSV* (pressure support), *5 cm H₂O*; *I-Trigger* (inspiratory sensitivity), *2.0 L/minute*; *E-Trigger* (percent of peak flow when the ventilator cycles from inspiration to exhalation), *20%*; and *Rise-Time* (amount of time the ventilator needs to reach a set level of pressure support), *0.9 second*. The bottom bar is at VCV settings (volume-controlled). Other options are PCV (pressure-controlled) and NPPV (bilevel positive airway pressure) settings.

Most mechanical ventilators have the capability of producing a breath of large volume (sigh) in an attempt to prevent alveolar collapse, but whether this function should be used routinely is unresolved. A typical ventilation order in a critically ill neurologic patient is shown in Table 5–3.

Modes of Ventilation

The most frequently used modes in critically ill neurologic patients are controlled mechanical ventilation or assist-control and synchronized intermittent mandatory ventilation, with or without pressure support. In a controlled mode, the ventilator takes over all the work in giving each breath. In a synchronized intermittent mandatory ventilation mode, the patient can add breaths spontaneously by triggering the ventilator. Pressure support may be added to reduce the work of breathing on each spontaneous breath. The most common modes are shown in Figure 5–14.

Many of the newer ventilators provide graphic display of pressure volume and flow

(see Fig. 5–14 for display of normal curves). The volume waveform should be scrutinized for possible leaks in the system, which may be caused by an inadequate endotracheal cuff. When such a leak exists, the expired limb of the waveform does not return to baseline (Fig. 5–15). The shape of the pressure waveform may indicate flow dyssynchrony. The work of breathing is increased if patient demand exceeds set flow. The pressure waveform becomes scalloped when the patient's demand exceeds the ventilator output. This anomaly is detected when an assisted patient-triggered breath is compared with an unassisted breath (Fig. 5–16).

Controlled Mechanical Ventilation

Controlled mode ventilation should be used in patients with no breathing drive. Some of these clinical situations are acute basilar artery occlusion, rebleeding after subarachnoid hemorrhage, pontine-medulla stage of herniation, severed high cervical cord, and treatment with barbiturates for status epilepticus, therapy-refractory increased intracranial pressure, or brain death. More often, it is used in mechanically ventilated combative patients treated with neuromuscular blockade, particularly in patients with multitrauma and significant respiratory distress. Its principle is a preset tidal volume with a dialed-in frequency without any necessary effort by the patient. The timing mechanism determines the delivery of breaths, and the patient is completely dependent on the ventilator.

Controlled mechanical ventilation has many disadvantages, largely related to use of seda-

Table 5–3. Typical Ventilation Order in the Critically Ill Neurologic Patient

Mode	IMV
FiO₂	0.4–0.9
Respiratory rate	8–12 breaths/minute
Tidal volume	10–15 mL/kg
PEEP	2–5 cm H₂O
I:E ratio	1:3

E, expiration; I, inspiration; IMV, intermittent mandatory ventilation; PEEP, positive end-expiratory pressure.

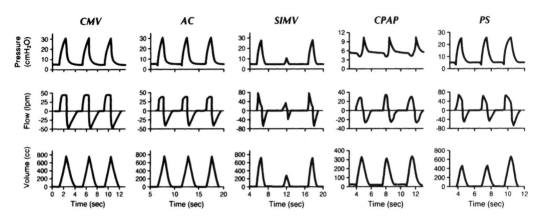

Figure 5–14. Modes of mechanical ventilation: three breaths with pressure curves and accompanying flow and volume waveforms illustrate the most commonly used selections.

- *CMV* (continuous mechanical ventilation). All breaths are machine-generated, and a positive end-expiratory pressure of 5 cm H_2O is evident.
- *AC* (assist-control). The first two breaths are patient-triggered, as evidenced by a brief negative deflection in airway pressure followed by a machine-triggered breath.
- *SIMV* (synchronized intermittent mandatory ventilation). Two machine-triggered breaths have a spontaneous breath in between.
- *CPAP* (continuous positive airway pressure). All breaths are patient-initiated.
- *PS* (pressure support). All breaths are patient-initiated. The waveforms of the volume and flow may vary with each breath but have a common rectangular shape.

tion and neuromuscular blockade. Important risks are disconnection from the machine and the inability to perform any spontaneous breathing. In addition, prolonged controlled mechanical ventilation may cause disuse atrophy and asynchrony of respiratory muscles, creating problems with weaning.[39]

Assist-Control Ventilation

Assist-control ventilation is a frequent initial mode of ventilation in patients with acute neurologic catastrophes. In this mode, the patient is dominant and the machine takes over if the patient fails to trigger the ventilator. Patients trigger the ventilator by creating a pressure drop in the system, which in turn starts an in-

spiration. (The trigger sensitivity is manually set and is referenced to the PEEP level.)

This ventilatory mode is often poorly tolerated by patients who are awake and acutely confused and may lead to patient–ventilator dyssynchrony that can be overcome only by additional sedation. Excessive work by the patient, certainly if ventilatory drive is increased, may result in inadequate peak flow or sensitivity settings. The most common side effect of this mode of ventilation is respiratory alkalosis.

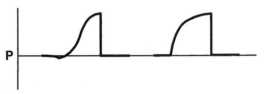

Figure 5–16. Dyssynchrony. *P*, pressure (cm H_2O).

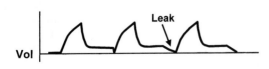

Figure 5–15. Cuff leak. *Vol*, volume (mL).

Intermittent Mandatory Ventilation

This mode is a combination of machine-initiated breathing at a fixed rate and spontaneous ventilation. Intermittent mandatory ventilation (IMV) is the mode chosen for most patients in the NICU after initial stabilization.[27] Again, a preset number of positive pressure breaths are available for the patient, but they are interrupted by spontaneous breaths. The major shortcoming of positive pressure ventilation—that ventilator breaths are out of phase with spontaneously generated breaths (*stacking*)—has been eliminated by synchronizing, which is standard in most ventilators on the market.

This mode has become widely used for weaning, but comparative studies with other regimens (e.g., increasing T-piece circuit intervals) are not available in the literature on critical care neurology. The major theoretical disadvantage is that because spontaneous breaths are not assisted, the mode is not responsive to the patient's needs and therefore may rapidly lead to inadequate ventilation.

Pressure Support Ventilation

This mode supplies a pressurized breath during spontaneous breathing. The patient generates each breath by triggering the ventilator, again by opening the valve that delivers the breath through creating a negative pressure similar to that in the IMV mode, but with the important difference of cutoff at a certain flow threshold. This mode essentially decreases the work of breathing, but the tidal volume and respiration cycle remain controlled by the effort of the patient. Inspiration is terminated when a certain flow threshold is reached.[28,29] This mode is often used to overcome the resistance of the endotracheal tube[50] and in combination with the IMV mode.

Continuous Positive Airway Pressure

This mode assists in spontaneous breathing and may improve oxygenation remarkably. The continuous positive airway pressure mode is often used in patients with sleep apnea, but in the medical intensive care unit, its major goal is to prevent mechanical ventilation. The range of continuous positive airway pressure varies from 0 to 30 cm H_2O.

Pressure Control Ventilation

This mode of ventilation is essentially the same as controlled mechanical ventilation, but instead of volume limits, a target inspiratory pressure is set. The flow wave characteristics are fairly similar. This mode is often combined with inverse ratio ventilation, and there is a strong claim of better oxygenation at lower PEEP and peak inspiratory pressure. Many, if not all, patients need additional sedation. Typical indications in the NICU are aspiration pneumonitis and early adult respiratory distress syndrome.[30]

Noninvasive Ventilation

Noninvasive bilevel positive pressure airway ventilation (BiPAP) has become an established alternative mode of mechanical ventilation in medical intensive care units[2,7] (Figs. 5–17 and 5–18). Its major objective is to maintain adequate gas exchange by avoiding intubation. In the intensive care unit, the procedure is typically used in patients with brief exacerbations of chronic obstructive pulmonary disease and in immunosuppressed patients with acute respiratory failure.[20] It may have a role in patients with acute neuromuscular disease. Its place in chronic neuromuscular disease, such as amyotrophic lateral sclerosis or muscular dystrophy, has been established. Experience in GBS and myasthenia gravis remains limited. We have not been successful in its use in deteriorating GBS, probably because of upper airway collapse and difficulty with secretions, but we have found it useful in myasthenia gravis and as a weaning device (Chapter 26). Experience with the noninvasive procedure in spinal cord injury is emerging.[57] Major limitations include discomfort from the close-fitting mask, failure to rest and sleep, leaks, and gastric distention.[62] Patients can be considered only if they do not require vasopressors, are alert and cooperative, can protect the airway, and have hypoxemia of < 60 mm Hg with FIO_2 > 50% or hypercapnia of < 50 mm Hg.

Many devices are available, but most experience has been gained with the bilevel positive

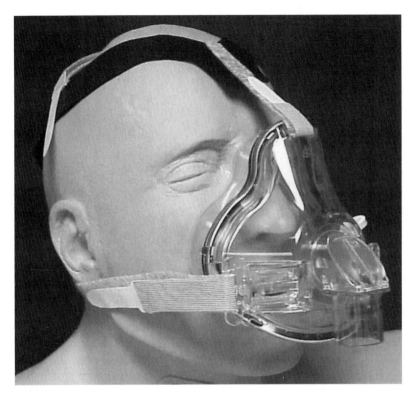

Figure 5–17. Noninvasive ventilation. Bilevel positive airway pressure (BiPAP) involves a special mask (shown here). Different sizes are available.

airway pressure ventilator from Respironics (Pittsburgh, PA) (Fig. 5–18). A full-face mask should fit from near the top of the bridge of the nose to just beneath the lower lip. The initial settings are 8 cm H_2O of inspiratory positive airway pressure and 4 cm H_2O of expiratory positive airway pressure, with oxygen flow of 6 L/minute and further adjustments for arterial blood gas and comfort. The maximal generating pressure is 22 cm H_2O. Whether the device can prevent intubation or assist in weaning in pulmonary disease remains unclear, and some studies suggest it does not.[12,22] A trial of 30 minutes should be sufficient to decide whether intubation can be deferred.[40]

TRACHEOSTOMY

Early tracheostomy should be considered when prolonged mechanical ventilation is anticipated (Fig. 5–19), but the timing of tracheostomy placement is controversial. It is self-evident that the potential serious complications and cosmetic disfiguration of tracheostomy should strongly influence this decision. Major complications of tracheostomy are massive hemorrhage manifested by hemoptysis and tracheal stenosis at the stoma site, but they are very rare when studied prospectively.[52] The central issues in the decision to proceed with early tracheostomy are the comfort of the patient, more effective tracheal suctioning, and the considerable risk of tracheolaryngeal stenosis from prolonged intubation that is difficult to repair. The prevalence of tracheal stenosis is nearly 10% within 2 weeks after endotracheal intubation. It is not known whether use of high residual volume and low-pressure cuffs (pressures < 25 cm H_2O) decreases this very distressing complication. Other techniques are to accept a slight leak (minimal leak technique), to use just enough volume to seal the airway

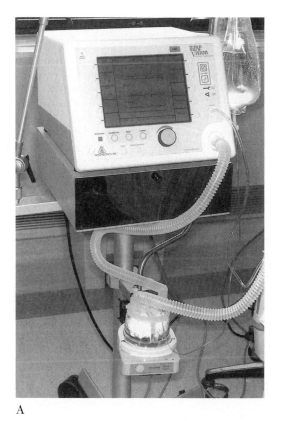

A

B

Figure 5–18. Bilevel positive airway pressure noninvasive ventilator. (*A*) Setup of the ventilator. The display and humidifier are shown. (*B*) Typical setting for the ventilatory support system. *IPAP* (inspiratory positive airway pressure), *10 cm H₂O* (range, 5 to 25 cm H₂O); *EPAP* (expiratory positive airway pressure), *5 cm H₂O* (range, 0 to 30 cm H₂O); and *Rate* (of breathing), *21 BPM* (breaths per minute). The display shows pressure (*P*), volume (*Vol*), and flow (*Flow*) curves. The percentage of *O₂* administered is *40*. When the round keypads at the right are touched, turning the knob at the bottom adjusts the display.

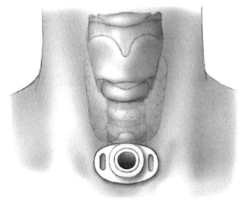

A

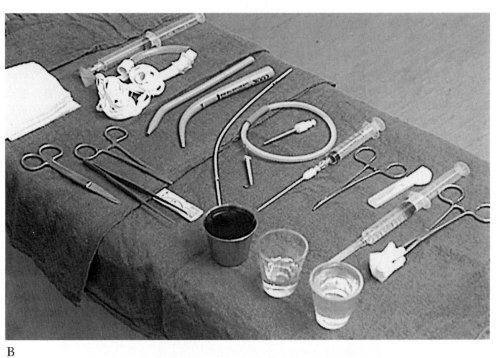

B

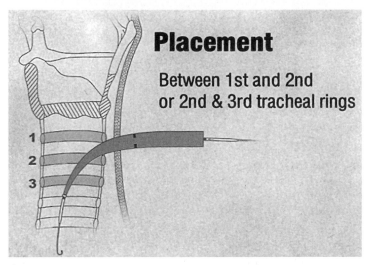

C

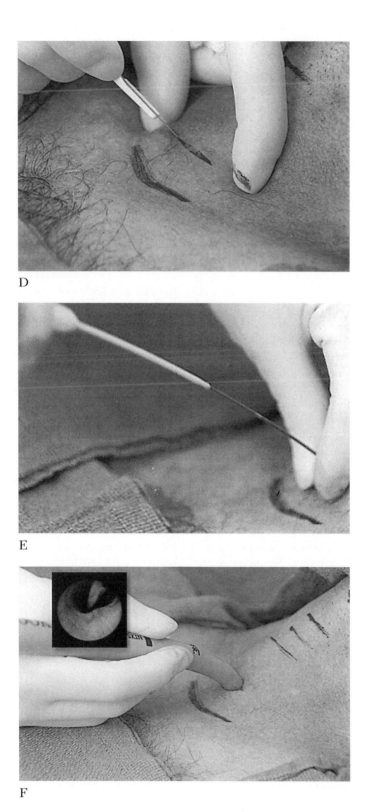

D

E

F

Figure 5–19. (A) Traditional surgical tracheostomy and (B–F) percutaneous dilatory tracheostomy. (B from Cook Ciaglia Blue Rhino Percutaneous Tracheostomy Introducer Set. Retrieved December 4, 2001, from the World Wide Web: http://www.cook-inc.com/cook_critical_care/education/slides/bluerhino/index.html. By permission.)

(minimal occluding volume technique), and to periodically deflate the cuff, but none has been tested to determine whether it is effective in preventing tracheal stenosis or increases the incidence of aspiration.

Indications for tracheostomy clearly depend on the clinical course of the acute neurologic illness. A general guideline is to wait 3 weeks to assess the need for tracheostomy but to proceed with tracheostomy earlier in patients who may significantly benefit from the increased comfort. Tracheostomy should probably be considered earlier for comatose patients with head injury who have facial trauma and swelling,[24,25] because inadvertent extubation may cause significant difficulties with reintubation. Early tracheostomy is also reasonable in patients with severe GBS characterized by severe quadriplegia and progressively abnormal results of electrophysiologic studies (inexcitable motor nerves, profuse fibrillations with no voluntary activity). In these unfortunate patients with GBS, prolonged mechanical ventilation is very likely, certainly when no response to plasma exchange or intravenous immune gamma globulin has been observed.

Many patients with ischemic or hemorrhagic stroke are weaned from the mechanical ventilator within 2 to 3 weeks (with the possible exception of patients with pontine hemorrhages or acute basilar artery occlusion), and tracheostomy should be postponed. The need for tracheostomy reflects the need for long-term mechanical ventilation, and outcome would seem very poor in these patients.

Our study in 97 patients[41] refuted the idea that prolonged ventilatory assistance leaves only crippled survivors. Tracheostomy reduced pulmonary complications and provided easier access for pulmonary toilet. In surviving patients, more than a fourth of those with a stroke who required a tracheostomy regained functional independence, and early tracheostomy shortened ICU stay.

Traditional tracheostomy involves a standard elective surgical procedure under general anesthesia (Fig. 5–18A). The procedure is usually event-free but may cause bleeding and loss of airway. Another technique is Ciaglia's percutaneous dilatational tracheostomy.[4,10,48] It is per-

formed by general surgeons and continues to be criticized by some otolaryngologists who see no reason to replace traditional tracheostomy. The major benefits of this procedure are use of the smallest possible skin incision, which may reduce scarring. As an illustration, our follow-up of 18 patients with surgical tracheostomy documented a satisfactory cosmetic result in only 4, and 1 patient lost a singing voice. Types of tracheostomy scars are shown in Figure 5–20.[59]

Percutaneous dilatational tracheostomy may be preferred in patients with GBS and myasthenia gravis when only comparatively brief periods of ventilation are anticipated. The technique may include fiberoptic bronchoscopy after the endotracheal tube is deflated and involves needle and Seldinger wire insertion and serial dilatation (Fig. 5–19B–F). Insertion is between the second and third tracheal cartilages. Elimination of operating room facilities and reduction of personnel contribute to lower costs.[16,19]

Complications of percutaneous dilatational tracheostomy are inadvertent endotracheal cuff rupture, subcutaneous emphysema, hemorrhage, false passage, pneumothorax, and tracheal stenosis,[5] all with incidences of less than 4%. Modification of the original technique may cause problems, too.[9] Contraindications to percutaneous dilatational tracheostomy are obscure anatomical landmarks (goiter, obesity, prior trauma), requirement of FIO_2 greater than 0.6 to ensure oxygen saturation, and abnormal coagulation. A randomized study in 100 patients documented a much lower surgical complication rate (2%) than that with traditional tracheostomy (25%).[33] However, a meta-analysis suggested that perioperative death and serious cardiorespiratory events were more common, albeit very rare (< 0.5%).[14] Systematic studies in critically ill neurologic patients are desirable.

WEANING FROM THE VENTILATOR

Discontinuation from the mechanical ventilator is a major focus of clinical studies, all in an attempt to define variables or indices that pre-

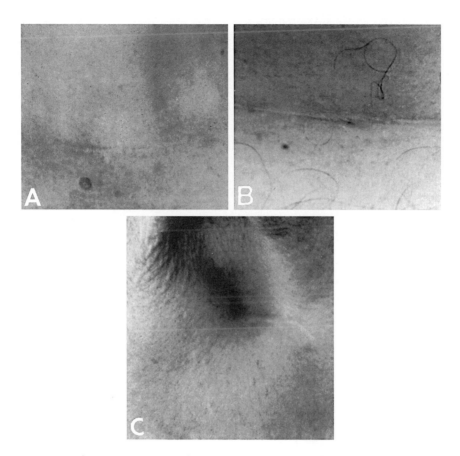

Figure 5–20. Tracheostomy scars in three patients. (*A*) A tracheostomy scar after two repairs. (*B*) Slightly hypertrophic scar, although clearly visible, was interpreted by the patient as satisfactory. (*C*) Unsatisfactory scar and retractive pit. The patient could bury a fingertip in the surgical area. (From Wijdicks et al.[59] By permission of Steinkopff Verlag.)

dict success.[34,47,55] Studies of weaning criteria in patients with central nervous system injury and neuromuscular weakness are virtually not available, and the published determinants in critically ill patients with prolonged mechanical ventilation may not apply to the vast majority of patients with acute brain injury.

The practice of weaning may differ, but no method should be entertained unless several clinical and laboratory criteria are fulfilled.[45] These criteria can be easily assessed at the bedside (Table 5–4). In addition, weaning should not be entertained in patients who still require PEEP for adequate oxygenation and patients who have significant chest X-ray abnormalities that do not show considerable remission (com-plete clearing on the chest radiograph is ideal but not required in the first attempt at weaning). Weaning should not be started if general anesthesia is planned within 1 or 2 days, the neurologic condition is deteriorating, or active therapy for intracranial pressure is administered. Reduced level of consciousness per se is not a contraindication.[11] Weaning from the ventilator also includes important adjunctive measures, such as correction of electrolyte imbalance, adequate hydration and nutrition, patient in upright position, proper care of secretions, and, perhaps most importantly, adequate sleep. It is critical that during weaning efforts, patients have effective rest at night. Weaning should be gradual, because a sudden transition may be

Table 5–4. General Laboratory Weaning Criteria

Measurement	Requirement
PaO$_2$	> 60 mm Hg
Tidal volume	> 5 mL/kg
Vital capacity	> 15 mL/kg
Minute ventilation	< 10 L/kg
Negative inspiratory pressure	> −30 mm Hg

stressful to patients with underlying cardiovascular disease.

We recently devised a pulmonary function ratio (PFR) based on the sum of pulmonary function test results in GBS:

$$PFR = \frac{PFint}{PF2w}$$

in which PF is vital capacity plus PImax plus PEmax, int is the value at intubation, and 2w is the value at the second week. Failure of this ratio to improve (< 1) predicted weaning failure and directed the timing of tracheostomy. The potential usefulness of this ratio in GBS implies that pulmonary function tests should continue during ventilation and may indicate trends in improvement that may set off an attempt at weaning.

In most patients with acute central nervous system lesions who have been intubated for a short time, weaning can be accomplished by gradual T-tube weaning.[56] Before the weaning effort is started, it is important to observe the patient for 5 minutes after placing a T piece. Next to looking for obvious signs of discomfort, one should specifically watch for an increase in respiratory rate (> 25 breaths/minute), a decrease in tidal volume (not below 300 mL), a change in blood pressure (either way), an increase in heart rate (increase of more than 20 beats/minute), or development of premature ventricular contractions or bigeminy. A T piece can remain in place for 30 minutes, with incremental increases in duration twice a day. Arterial blood gas values are determined regularly. Common practice is to begin with a trial of 30 minutes; if this is successful, the duration can be rapidly increased to 1 to 2 hours. Extu-

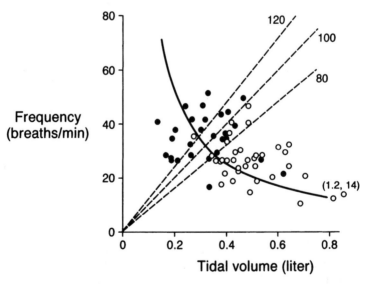

Figure 5–21. Rapid shallow breathing index. Weaning success (*open circles*), weaning failure (*solid circles*). Patients to the left of the threshold isopleth value of 100 for ratio of frequency to tidal volume had a 95% likelihood of weaning failure. For comparison, the hyperbola represents a minute ventilation of 10 L/minute, indicating poor predictive value (minute ventilation of 10 L/minute is a frequently used weaning criterion. See Table 5–4). (From Yang and Tobin.[64] By permission of the Massachusetts Medical Society.)

bation is performed when the arterial blood gas values remain satisfactory and no rapid shallow breathing is observed. If the T-tube trial fails, the patient is given at least 24 hours of rest with full ventilation, and then another attempt is made.[53]

Another approach is to change the settings of the IMV mode. The frequency is reduced in gradual steps. Arterial blood gas determinations are used to recognize potential trends to respiratory acidosis. Intermittent mandatory ventilation weaning is fairly simple, consisting of gradual reduction with 3 breaths/minute starting three times a day. It is prudent to add pressure support at low levels (5 to 10 cm H_2O) for further comfort. Pressure support weaning may be preferred to other weaning regimens and may increase synchronicity. Pressure support is set at a level that is comfortable for the patient, usually 15 to 40 cm H_2O, followed by decrements of 3 cm H_2O. When the pressure support level of 5 cm H_2O is tolerated (pressure just enough to overcome the resistance of the tubing) and the laboratory criteria are fulfilled, extubation can be undertaken.

It has been suggested that rapid shallow breathing diagnosed by the ratio of respiratory frequency to tidal volume accurately predicts weaning failure. Patients with a frequency-volume ratio of more than 100 had a 95% likelihood of failure in a weaning trial. Patients with a frequency-volume ratio of less than 100 had an 80% likelihood of successful weaning[63,64] (Fig. 5–21). A prospective study showed a less optimistic prognostic value (sensitivity, 72%; specificity, 11%).[26] Nonetheless, the use of the frequency-volume ratio may be very helpful as a clinical guide after extubation.

Extubation should be well tolerated, but inspiratory stridor may develop virtually immediately to 1 hour after extubation. Most patients have transient hoarseness alone. Topical epinephrine into the hypopharynx is a reasonable option, but reintubation is often necessary. Laryngospasm, however, is less common but life-threatening. It is much more common in children and young adults. Typically, the crowing sound of stridor is absent and strenuous efforts are seen, with significant desaturation.[44] Succinylcholine (0.1 mg/kg intravenously) usually effectively treats the spasm rapidly. Lidocaine, 2 mg/kg intravenously, may also significantly reduce laryngospasm if used several minutes before extubation in susceptible individuals.

CONCLUSIONS

- Appropriate airway management can be achieved for hours. This includes mask ventilation with oxygen (10 to 15 L/minute flow) after the jaw is lifted upward to open the airway. An oropharyngeal airway may facilitate mask ventilation.
- Intubation is needed in patients with acute brain injury who cannot protect their airway, as shown by frequent hypoxic episodes; in patients with tachycardia and tachypnea associated with neuromuscular failure (GBS, myasthenia gravis); and in patients with primary pulmonary disease (pulmonary edema or progressive aspiration pneumonitis).
- Clinical features of imminent respiratory failure in patients with neuromuscular failure are restlessness, staccato speech, asynchronous breathing, use of sternocleidomastoid muscles, and forehead sweating. Laboratory criteria are important but less reliable; the critical values are vital capacity, 20 mL/kg; maximum inspiratory pressure, −30 cm H_2O; and maximum expiratory pressure, 40 cm H_2O.
- A typical order for mechanical ventilation in a stable neurologic patient is IMV, 8 to 12; FIO_2, 0.4 to 0.9; tidal volume, 10 to 15 mL/kg; PEEP, 2 to 5 cm H_2O; and inspiration:expiration ratio, 1:3.
- Tracheostomy should be postponed 2 to 3 weeks except in patients with marked facial trauma, axonal type of GBS, or survivors with massive stroke.

REFERENCES

1. American Association for Respiratory Care: Consensus statement on the essentials of mechanical ventilators—1992. *Respir Care* 37:1000–1008, 1992.
2. American Thoracic Society, the European Respiratory Society, the European Society of Intensive Care Medicine, and the Society de Reanimation de Langue Française: International Consensus Conferences in Intensive Care Medicine: noninvasive positive pressure ventilation in acute respiratory failure. *Am J Respir Crit Care Med* 163:283–291, 2001.
3. Andrews PJ, Piper IR, Dearden NM, et al: Secondary insults during intrahospital transport of head-injured patients. *Lancet* 335:327–330, 1990.
4. Bewsher MS, Adams AM, Clarke CW, et al: Evaluation of a new percutaneous dilatational tracheostomy set apparatus. *Anaesthesia* 56:859–864, 2001.
5. Briche T, Le Manach Y, Pats B: Complications of percutaneous tracheostomy. *Chest* 119:1282–1283, 2001.
6. Bryan CL, Jenkinson SG: Oxygen toxicity. *Clin Chest Med* 9:141–152, 1988.
7. Carlucci A, Richard JC, Wysocki M, et al: Noninvasive versus conventional mechanical ventilation. An epidemiologic survey. *Am J Respir Crit Care Med* 163: 874–880, 2001.
8. Chevrolet JC, Deleamont P: Repeated vital capacity measurements as predictive parameters for mechanical ventilation need and weaning success in the Guillain-Barré syndrome. *Am Rev Respir Dis* 144:814–818, 1991.
9. Ciaglia P: Technique, complications, and improvements in percutaneous dilatational tracheostomy. *Chest* 115:1383–1389, 1999.
10. Ciaglia P, Firsching R, Syniec C: Elective percutaneous dilatational tracheostomy. A new simple bedside procedure; preliminary report. *Chest* 87:715–719, 1985.
11. Coplin WM, Pierson DJ, Cooley KD, et al: Implications of extubation delay in brain-injured patients meeting standard weaning criteria. *Am J Respir Crit Care Med* 161:1530–1536, 2000.
12. Delclaux C, L'Her E, Alberti C, et al: Treatment of acute hypoxemic nonhypercapnic respiratory insufficiency with continuous positive airway pressure delivered by a face mask: a randomized controlled trial. *JAMA* 284:2352–2360, 2000.
13. de Troyer A, Estenne M: The respiratory system in neuromuscular disorders. *Lung Biol Health Dis* 85 Part C:2177–2212, 1995.
14. Dulguerov P, Gysin C, Perneger TV, et al: Percutaneous or surgical tracheostomy: a meta-analysis. *Crit Care Med* 27:1617–1625, 1999.
15. Fassoulaki A, Pamouktsoglou P: Prolonged nasotracheal intubation and its association with inflammation of paranasal sinuses. *Anesth Analg* 69:50–52, 1989.
16. Freeman BD, Isabella K, Cobb JP, et al: A prospective, randomized study comparing percutaneous with surgical tracheostomy in critically ill patients. *Crit Care Med* 29:926–930, 2001.

17. Gibson GJ, Pride NB, Davis JN, et al: Pulmonary mechanics in patients with respiratory muscle weakness. *Am Rev Respir Dis* 115:389–395, 1977.
18. Heffner JE: Airway management in the critically ill patient. *Crit Care Clin* 6:533–550, 1990.
19. Heikkinen M, Aarnio P, Hannukainen J: Percutaneous dilational tracheostomy or conventional surgical tracheostomy? *Crit Care Med* 28:1399–1402, 2000.
20. Hilbert G, Gruson D, Vargas F, et al: Noninvasive ventilation in immunosuppressed patients with pulmonary infiltrates, fever, and acute respiratory failure. *N Engl J Med* 344:481–487, 2001.
21. Kacmarek RM, Venegas J: Mechanical ventilatory rates and tidal volumes. *Respir Care* 32:466–475, 1987.
22. Keenan SP, Powers C, McCormack DG, et al: Noninvasive positive-pressure ventilation for postextubation respiratory distress. A randomized controlled trial. *JAMA* 287:3238–3244, 2002.
23. Langeron O, Semjen F, Bourgain JL, et al: Comparison of the intubating laryngeal mask airway with the fiberoptic intubation in anticipated difficult airway management. *Anesthesiology* 94:968–972, 2001.
24. Lanza DC, Koltai PJ, Parnes SM, et al: Predictive value of the Glasgow Coma Scale for tracheotomy in head-injured patients. *Ann Otol Rhinol Laryngol* 99:38–41, 1990.
25. Lanza DC, Parnes SM, Koltai PJ, et al: Early complications of airway management in head-injured patients. *Laryngoscope* 100:958–961, 1990.
26. Lee KH, Hui KP, Chan TB, et al: Rapid shallow breathing (frequency-tidal volume ratio) did not predict extubation outcome. *Chest* 105:540–543, 1994.
27. Luce JM, Pierson DJ, Hudson LD: Intermittent mandatory ventilation. *Chest* 79:678–685, 1981.
28. MacIntyre NR: Respiratory function during pressure support ventilation. *Chest* 89:677–683, 1986.
29. MacIntyre NR, Ho LI: Effects of initial flow rate and breath termination criteria on pressure support ventilation. *Chest* 99:134–138, 1991.
30. Marini JJ: New approaches to the ventilatory management of the adult respiratory distress syndrome. *J Crit Care* 7:256–267, 1992.
31. Michelson A, Schuster B, Kamp HD: Paranasal sinusitis associated with nasotracheal and orotracheal long-term intubation. *Arch Otolaryngol Head Neck Surg* 118:937–939, 1992.
32. Nachtmann A, Siebler M, Rose G, et al: Cheyne-Stokes respiration in ischemic stroke. *Neurology* 45:820–821, 1995.
33. Nates NL, Cooper DJ, Myles PS, et al: Percutaneous tracheostomy in critically ill patients: a prospective, randomized comparison of two techniques. *Crit Care Med* 28:3734–3739, 2000.
34. O'Donohue WJ Jr, Baker JP, Bell GM, et al: Respiratory failure in neuromuscular disease: management in a respiratory intensive care unit. *JAMA* 235:733–735, 1976.
35. Ooi R, Joshi P, Soni N: An evaluation of oxygen delivery using nasal prongs. *Anaesthesia* 47:591–593, 1992.

36. Oppenheimer S, Hachinski V: Complications of acute stroke. *Lancet* 339:721–724, 1992.
37. Plum F: Hyperpnea, hyperventilation, and brain dysfunction (editorial). *Ann Intern Med* 76:328, 1972.
38. Plum F, Posner JB: *The Diagnosis of Stupor and Coma*, 3rd ed. Philadelphia, FA Davis Company, 1980.
39. Pontoppidan H, Geffin B, Lowenstein E: Acute respiratory failure in the adult. 2. *N Engl J Med* 287:743–752, 1972.
40. Poponick JM, Renston JP, Bennett RP, et al: Use of a ventilatory support system (BiPAP) for acute respiratory failure in the emergency department. *Chest* 116:166–171, 1999.
41. Rabinstein A, Wijdicks EFM: Outcome after prolonged ventilatory assistance and tracheostomy in survivors of acute stroke. (Submitted for publication.)
42. Reardon RF, Martel M: The intubating laryngeal mask airway: suggestions for use in the emergency department. *Acad Emerg Med* 8:833–838, 2001.
43. Reissell E, Orko R, Maunuksela EL, et al: Predictability of difficult laryngoscopy in patients with long-term diabetes mellitus. *Anaesthesia* 45:1024–1027, 1990.
44. Roy WL, Lerman J: Laryngospasm in paediatric anaesthesia. *Can J Anaesth* 35:93–98, 1988.
45. Sahn SA, Lakshminarayan S: Bedside criteria for discontinuation of mechanical ventilation. *Chest* 63:1002–1005, 1973.
46. Samsoon GL, Young JR: Difficult tracheal intubation: a retrospective study. *Anaesthesia* 42:487–490, 1987.
47. Scheinhorn DJ, Artinian BM, Catlin JL: Weaning from prolonged mechanical ventilation. The experience at a regional weaning center. *Chest* 105:534–539, 1994.
48. Schwann NM: Percutaneous dilational tracheostomy: anesthetic considerations for a growing trend. *Anesth Analg* 84:907–911, 1997.
49. Schwartz DE, Matthay MA, Cohen NH: Death and other complications of emergency airway management in critically ill adults. A prospective investigation of 297 tracheal intubations. *Anesthesiology* 82:367–376, 1995.
50. Shapiro M, Wilson RK, Casar G, et al: Work of breathing through different sized endotracheal tubes. *Crit Care Med* 14:1028–1031, 1986.
51. Slutsky AS: Mechanical ventilation. American College of Chest Physicians Consensus Conference. *Chest* 104:1833–1859, 1993.
52. Stock MC, Woodward CG, Shapiro BA, et al: Perioperative complications of elective tracheostomy in critically ill patients. *Crit Care Med* 14:861–863, 1986.
53. Tobin MJ: Advances in mechanical ventilation. *N Engl J Med* 344:1986–1996, 2001.
54. Tobin MJ (ed): *Principles and Practice of Mechanical Ventilation.* New York, McGraw-Hill, 1994.
55. Tobin MJ, Perez W, Guenther SM, et al: The pattern of breathing during successful and unsuccessful trials of weaning from mechanical ventilation. *Am Rev Respir Dis* 134:1111–1118, 1986.
56. Tomlinson JR, Miller KS, Lorch DG, et al: A prospective comparison of IMV and T-piece weaning from mechanical ventilation. *Chest* 96:348–352, 1989.
57. Tromans AM, Mecci M, Barrett FH, et al: The use of the BiPAP biphasic positive airway pressure system in acute spinal cord injury. *Spinal Cord* 36:481–484, 1998.
58. Whitehead T, Slutsky AS: The pulmonary physician in critical care. 7: Ventilator induced lung injury. *Thorax* 57:635–642, 2002.
59. Wijdicks EFM, Lawn ND, Fletcher DD: Tracheostomy scars in Guillain-Barré syndrome: a reason for concern? (Letter to the editor.) *J Neurol* 248:527–528, 2001.
60. Wijdicks EFM, Scott JP: Outcome in patients with acute basilar artery occlusion requiring mechanical ventilation. *Stroke* 27:1301–1303, 1996.
61. Wijdicks EFM, Scott JP: Causes and outcome of mechanical ventilation in patients with hemispheric ischemic stroke. *Mayo Clin Proc* 72:210–213, 1997.
62. Yamada S, Nishimiya J, Kurokawa K, et al: Bilevel nasal positive airway pressure and ballooning of the stomach. *Chest* 119:1965–1966, 2001.
63. Yang KL: Inspiratory pressure/maximal inspiratory pressure ratio: a predictive index of weaning outcome. *Intensive Care Med* 19:204–208, 1993.
64. Yang KL, Tobin MJ: A prospective study of indexes predicting the outcome of trials of weaning from mechanical ventilation. *N Engl J Med* 324:1445–1450, 1991.

6

Volume Status and Blood Pressure

Intravascular volume and pressure reflect hemodynamic status and are tightly correlated. Intensive care allows physiologic monitoring of these parameters—most on a continuous basis. Changes in volume and pressure must be interpreted in light of the underlying neurologic disorder.

Hypovolemia is a potential clinical concern in virtually all patients with acute central nervous system injury. The paradigm of current fluid management—that is, aggressive fluid intake with crystalloids or colloids—has taken shape. Once common orders by physicians for fluid restriction in patients with acute catastrophic events have now been modified into skillful limitation of free water or at least maintenance of euvolemic fluid status or modest hypervolemia, often closely guided by pulmonary wedge pressures.[50,52]

Coinciding with this diametrical change in patient fluid management has been a change in the management of acutely increased blood pressure.[19,22,39,51] Careful titration of antihypertensive drugs—but in many instances monitoring of acute hypertension and judicious use of antihypertensive drugs—has become a standard approach in the immediate aftermath of acute neurologic disorders.[19,55]

It is self-evident that a clear understanding of how to govern volume status is necessary. In addition, this chapter makes several arguments for very cautious use of antihypertensive medications in the acute phase.

REGULATION OF BODY WATER

The compartments in which body water settles are defined as the cellular space, or intracellular volume, and the interstitial and intravascular volumes. Although not fixed, the complex mechanisms that control homeostasis locate two-thirds of the body water in the extracellular space. Translocation of body water across these compartments is largely determined by osmotic forces. Solutes that cannot freely cross the cell membrane may produce an osmotic gradient and thus influence the distribution of body water between compartments. This active osmotic state (usually between intracellular and extracellular fluids separated by cell membrane) is called "effective osmolality" or "tonicity." Sodium is a typical example of a solute that cannot move freely across the cellular membrane and increases tonicity. The primary determinant of plasma osmolality is plasma sodium concentration, which is thus a major factor in fluid shifts across the compartments.

Hypovolemia triggers at least three physiologic pathways: antidiuretic hormone, renin, and norepinephrine, all enhancers of sodium reabsorption. At the collecting duct, antidiuretic hormone increases water and sodium absorption by binding to its receptor and activating water channel protein (aquaporin 2). In the proximal tubule cells, sodium absorption is increased by the activation of renin-angiotensin II. Aldosterone also is stimulated, increasing reabsorption of sodium at the distal tubule and collection duct. Finally, norepinephrine and epinephrine decrease the glomerular filtration rate and enhance sodium reabsorption at the proximal tubule.

Hypervolemia, in contrast, stimulates sodium excretion through natriuretic peptides and suppression of the vasopressor hormones mentioned above. The natriuretic peptides have variable natriuretic, diuretic, and vasorelaxant activity[53] (Chapter 31). However, they also suppress sympathetic tone and the renin-angiotensin II-aldosterone axis and block the renal effects of antidiuretic hormone. Atrial natriuretic peptide also inhibits thirst and the appetite for salt and has another central effect due to decreasing sympathetic tone at the brain stem level. Management of hypertonic and hypotonic states is discussed in Chapter 31. Further analysis of this complex regulating system can be found in major texts on renal disorders.

REQUISITES FOR ADEQUATE FLUID BALANCE

Maintenance fluids can be estimated with a precise patient history and clinical examination. A key assumption must be that most patients with an acute intracranial injury of any sort tend to have a certain degree of dehydration. Unmistakably, the initial "stress response" and pain can stimulate the release of antidiuretic hormone, which theoretically may result in volume expansion, but later the circumstances for hypovolemia are much more favorable. Deteriorating critically ill patients admitted to hospital wards and then transferred to the intensive care unit often have a marginal fluid balance. This disproportionately increased risk of dehydration in patients before they enter the NICU has several causes. First, failure to recognize the inability to signal thirst in many patients in stupor may lead to rapid loss in intravascular volume. Second, insensible losses associated with fever are invariably underestimated. Third, profound emesis may contribute. The most compelling reason for

dehydration, however, is that daily data on fluid intake and output are often inaccurate, sometimes mere estimations, and not adjusted to the patient's needs. These factors may all lead to significant accruing fluid losses. Dehydration may come to bear when these patients are placed on mechanical ventilators. The sudden introduction of positive pressure ventilation decreases venous return and thus cardiac output, resulting in hypotension.

The regimen for normal maintenance of fluid intake is based on an estimation of fluid losses and must be carefully monitored by laboratory measurements. These laboratory investigations should include daily serum electrolytes, osmolality, creatinine, blood urea nitrogen, serum glucose, and, when indicated, arterial blood gases.

An initial fluid intake of 150 to 200 mL/hour is appropriate. The crystalloid is 0.9% sodium chloride; glucose-based solutions should have no place in patients with acute neurologic disorders unless severe hypernatremia needs correction (Chapter 31). In an injured or ischemic brain, glucose infusions may worsen stress hyperglycemia and anaerobic cerebral glucose metabolism. This may further produce toxic accumulation of lactate and create intracellular acidosis, which in turn may set off lipid peroxidation and free radical formation. Excitatory amino acids such as glutamate may increase, and edema formation may be exaggerated.[26]

A recent elegant study using perfusion- and diffusion-weighted magnetic resonance imaging documented that nonfasting hyperglycemia (> 8 mmol/L or > 144 mg/dL) may reduce penumbral salvage and increase final infarct size after ischemic stroke.[35] Normoglycemia did result in considerable salvage, and the increase in infarct size quickly became apparent with mild increases in blood glucose. Whether this correlation indicates that intensive insulin therapy could improve outcome is very unclear.

The next step in computation of maintenance fluid is to approximate insensible losses from lungs and skin. Insensible fluid loss is often underestimated. Gastrointestinal losses average 250 mL/day, and evaporative fluid loss through the skin and lungs easily amounts to 750 mL; together they easily account for 1 L of unmeasured fluid loss. In addition, the increased evaporation with fever ranges widely and can mount to 500 mL per degree Celsius. A thermal stimulus drives sweating, but it is dependent on ambient conditions (e.g., humidity) and the state of hydration. Diarrhea associated with gut feeding may result in additional imperceptible continuing losses. Hyperventilation may increase fluid requirements, but when humidified gases are provided in patients on mechanical ventilators, the increase in fluid requirement becomes insignificant. Sweating can be profuse in patients with an acute head injury, typically occurring in association with tachycardia, hyperthermia, and tachypnea (paroxysmal sympathetic storms; see Chapter 23). Dysautonomia in GBS may result in episodic diaphoresis, but the prevalence is low (see Chapter 25).

Guidelines for maintaining volume status in patients with acute neurologic illness are summarized in Table 6–1. Serial body weight and fluid balance remain the most practical clinical indicators. The laboratory test results that indicate adequate volume status are normal values of hematocrit, serum osmolality, and serum sodium. Representative values for adequate fluid status are hematocrit of less than 55%, osmolality of less than 350 mOsm, and serum sodium of less than 150 mEq/L. Any higher value

Table 6–1. Indicators of Volume Status in Patients with Acute Neurologic Illness

Basic principles	Urinary output of 1 mL/kg/hour
	Fluid intake of 30 mL/kg/day
	Fluid balance of 750 to 1000 mL/day excess
	Maintenance of body weight
Monitor	Serum hematocrit
	Serum sodium
	Creatinine, blood urea nitrogen, serum glucose
	Plasma osmolality
	Urine osmolality
	Urine specific gravity
	Pulmonary artery wedge and diastolic pressures, systemic vascular resistance, cardiac output (optional)

indicates dehydration and should result in more fluid intake.

Early signs of volume depletion can be detected by other laboratory measurements that may further guide adjustments. Free water deficit can be calculated by assuming that the total body deficit equals the increase in plasma sodium. The formula for calculation of water deficit is $0.6 \times$ body weight $\times$ (plasma sodium/140) $- 1$ in liters. Urine output remains the pivotal variable by which one should measure the effectiveness of correction of fluid balance. Urine output must total at least 1 mL/kg per hour. Urine output greater than 2 mL/kg may indicate overintake of fluids, but other causes must be considered, particularly diabetes insipidus (see Chapter 31).

Fluid intake should be adjusted accordingly when a patient is receiving enteral feeding (Chapter 7).

FLUID REPLACEMENT PRODUCTS AND STRATEGY

Several types of replacement fluids are available, each with its own characteristics. Pulmonary edema and morbidity do not differ between use of crystalloids and use of colloids for fluid resuscitation in young persons but may differ in elderly patients.[8,12] The use of crystalloids generally is preferred in patients with acute neurologic disorders. Crystalloids are solutions in which sodium is the major osmotically active particle (e.g., isotonic saline, lactated Ringer's solution, hypertonic saline). The prototype is 0.9% sodium chloride (normal saline). This solution is slightly hypertonic to plasma (308 mOsm/kg as opposed to plasma osmolality of 289 mOsm/kg). Lactated Ringer's solution, an electrolyte solution used frequently in patients with polytrauma, is slightly hypotonic (273 mOsm/kg). The major drawback of using isotonic saline and Ringer's solution is redistribution. These fluids remain intravascular for a maximum of 2 hours, barely enough time to have a major effect on volume status, and are clearly insufficient when a sustained effect is warranted. The effect of crystalloids on total body water distribution is marginal.[48] Infusion of isotonic saline or 5% dextrose in water (D5W) results in only a very modest increase in intravascular volume. With D5W and isotonic saline, 250 mL of 3 L and 750 mL of 3 L, respectively, remain in the intravascular space but for only 30 minutes at the most. However, the effect of hypertonic saline is much more significant by means of recruiting fluid from the intracellular space but again is transient[41] (Fig. 6–1). The effect of isotonic saline infusion on more objective variables, such as pulmonary artery wedge pressure and cardiac index, is not measurable, and colloid replacement is more effective in situations requiring rapid correction of intravascular volume. In short, 0.9% sodium chloride accomplishes a satisfactory physiologic state in most critically ill patients in NICUs. Hypertonic saline 3% or 5% has an increasingly important role (Chapter 9), but the response is brief.

The characteristics of colloids are different. The major advantages of fluid replacement with colloids are a smaller infused volume, prolonged plasma expansion, and minimal peripheral edema. Colloids are solutions in which substances of large molecular weight are the major osmotically active particles, which do not easily pass capillary walls. The disadvantages of colloids are not hypothetical and in addition to greater expense (an inconsiderate physician order of "albumin around the clock" may mount to daily costs of $1000) include a reduction in ionized calcium and a small risk of anaphylactoid reactions. Dextran, gelatin, and hydroxyethyl starch may produce clinically relevant coagulopathy by inhibiting platelet aggregation and reducing activation of factor VIII (e.g., dextran 40) after large-volume infusions.[1,16]

Albumin is a very effective solution.[17] Albumin 5% expands intravascular volume by only 15 mL of water per gram, and albumin 25% expands intravascular volume five times more than the infused volume. This difference is explained by a much higher colloid osmotic pressure, the major determinant of fluid distribution. The effect of both types of albumin lasts at least 24 hours.

Hetastarch (HES, hydroxyethyl starch, pentastarch) with sodium chloride (Hespan) is a good alternative colloid and much less costly. Hetastarch is available in the United States and has a median molecular weight of 450 kd. (In Europe and the United Kingdom, different preparations are available.[23]) Hetastarch may affect platelet function through reduced glycoprotein IIb-IIIa expression[45] and prolong activated partial thromboplastin time and prothrombin time.[43] Low-molecular-weight hetastarch (70 kd) appears to have a less significant effect on platelet function.[24] The reported bleeding complications may be due to hemodilution and inhibition of factor VIII (von Willebrand factor). There is no evidence that hetastarch increases postoperative bleeding, and instances of aneurysmal bleeding have been exceptional, with doubtful causality.[12] Contraindications to hetastarch are severe congestive heart failure, renal failure, and hypersensitivity to the agent (e.g., pruritus).[31]

Fluid replacement is best first accomplished by increasing the rate of maintenance infusion. When blood pressure is reduced (systolic pressure less than 100 mm Hg), a bolus of 500 mL of albumin 5% should be administered. The initial effect should become clear within minutes. This fluid challenge is validated by changes in blood pressure (increase), heart rate (decrease), and urine production (increase). In clinical circumstances with hypovolemic shock, hemodynamic measurements are most useful, and a pulmonary artery balloon catheter should be inserted (Chapter 10), particularly if the results of intervention are uncertain. Lack of a persistent effect in hypovolemic patients must without hesitation result in infusion of hypertonic saline 3%, with a suggested rate of 4 mL/kg over 3 minutes. The response can be prolonged when saline is combined with 5% albumin or hetastarch. Blood transfusion must be considered if hemorrhage caused the hypovolemic state. Judicious use of small, incremental quantities may reduce the risk of pulmonary edema in patients who have poor underlying cardiac function. The characteristics of the available plasma expanders are shown in Table 6–2.

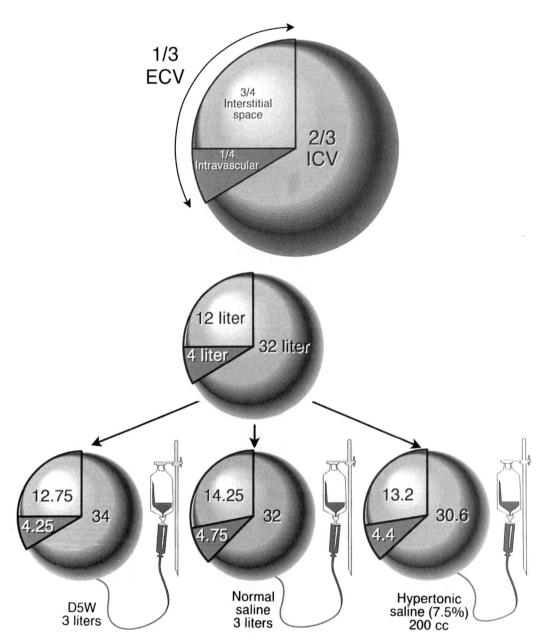

Figure 6–1. Distribution of body water (*top*) and effect of infusion of different solutions on intravascular volume (*bottom*). D5W, 5% dextrose in water; ECV, extracellular volume; ICV, intracellular volume. Note only 200 mL in hypertonic saline as opposed to 3 liters in other infusions. (Modified from Rainey TG, Read CA: Pharmacology of colloids and crystalloids. In Chernow B [ed]: *The Pharmacologic Approach to the Critically Ill Patient*, 3rd ed. Baltimore, Williams & Wilkins, 1994, pp 272–290. By permission of the publisher.

Table 6–2. Volume-Expanding Agents

Agent	Sodium (mEq/L)	Cost°	$T^1/_2$	Side Effects
Isotonic saline	154	D	Minute	None
Albumin 5%	130–160	20D	5–6 hours	Anaphylaxis, pulmonary edema
Albumin 25%	130–160	20D	5–6 hours	Anaphylaxis, pulmonary edema
Lactated Ringer's solution	130	2D	Minute	Hypo-osmolar state
Hypertonic saline	513	D	Minute	Hypernatremia, hyperchloremia, hypokalemia, pulmonary edema
Fresh frozen plasma	170	30D	5–6 hours	Hepatitis, human immunodeficiency virus, anaphylaxis
Dextran 70	154	10D	6 hours	Renal failure, anaphylaxis, pseudohyperglycemia, coagulopathy
Hetastarch	130	10D	12 hours	Coagulopathy, congestive heart failure, vomiting, mild hepatotoxicity

°D is the hospital base price per purchasing contract. The remaining indicators are compared with this price (e.g., 20D = 20 times more expensive).

REGULATION OF BLOOD PRESSURE

The major components of blood pressure are the steady state part of resistance (mean arterial blood pressure) and the pulsatile component of impedance (pulse pressure equals systolic blood pressure minus diastolic blood pressure). Neither threshold of normal has been defined in acute neurologic conditions.

Vasomotor control is centered in the central nervous system. The peripheral afferent and efferent sympathetic nerves and the adrenal medulla, also known as the sympathetic nervous system, are the primary operators in acute hypertension. Acute stimulation of the sympathetic system may cause a sudden increase in systemic vascular resistance and an increase in vasoconstrictor substances, including endothelin.

The central adrenergic efferent impulse follows tracts from the hypothalamus to the medulla and spinal cord and switches to second neurons in the sympathetic ganglia. Norepinephrine is the major neurotransmitter, causing adrenergic receptor stimulation. Stimulation of the α-adrenergic receptor produces vasoconstriction of the arterioles and venules. Stimulation of the β-adrenergic receptor causes vasodilatation, tachycardia, and increased myocardial contractility and metabolism.

Hypertension after acute central nervous system lesions has historically been attributed to ischemia in the pontomedullary region and termed the "Cushing response."[13,14] This response consists of an acute surge in blood pressure associated with bradycardia and change in rhythmic breathing, including apnea. The anatomical location of the hypertensive response is presumptively in the caudal portion of the ventral medulla. The classic explanation is increased intracranial pressure associated with a decrease in cerebral perfusion pressure resulting in brain stem ischemia. This response occurs most commonly in patients with acute lesions in the posterior fossa and in patients with very marginal brain compliance from increased intracranial pressure. Hypertension from the Cushing response is not always associated with bradycardia. Whether a bradycardia response can be mounted depends on whether the vagal nuclei are ischemic as well. In addition, the hypertensive response can be fluctuating and not sustained.[14] Hypertension is common in patients with acute cerebellar hemorrhage or infarct. Distortion of the brain stem is the most probable mechanism.

BLOOD PRESSURE MANAGEMENT

Increase in blood pressure is common in acute central nervous system lesions. For example, a study on the prevalence of hypertensive emergencies and urgencies in the emergency department found that a cerebral infarct was a trigger in one of four patients.[56]

Causes for increased blood pressure may include pain, agitation, and frequent bucking of the ventilator. In every patient with uncontrollable hypertension in the first hours after admission, use of street drugs must be considered (amphetamines, cocaine), certainly in young patients with an acute stroke. However, when confounding factors have been excluded, treatment of hypertension in acute central nervous system lesions is controversial and could be detrimental. The effects of treatment of hypertension on outcome in patients with acute neurologic illness have not been studied prospectively. For example, the effects are unknown in the very early hours after intracerebral hematoma and in patients with large vessel occlusions in a compensatory state requiring recruitment of collaterals and maximal vasodilatation. In addition, the definition of hypertension occurring after acute brain injury is difficult. Moreover, the natural history is favorable, with normalization after 24 hours in the vast majority of patients with acute central nervous system lesions.[5,25]

The weight assigned to the risks and benefits of blood pressure treatment in acute central nervous system catastrophes varies widely.[6,9–11,15,22,49] A tendency to immediately control acute hypertension, unfortunately often seen in emergency departments, is theoretically linked to the possibility of uncontrolled hypertension causing rebleeding (aneurysmal subarachnoid hemorrhage), promoting edema in a lesion with an acutely opened blood–brain barrier (hemispheric stroke), facilitating extension of the volume of intracerebral hematoma (putamen or cerebellum hemorrhage), and possibly causing deterioration from hemorrhagic transformation (hemispheric stroke). These basic premises can be challenged. An additional reason for treatment of hypertension is impending cardiac failure, a reasonable concern in elderly patients with prior coronary artery disease. An aggressive approach in acute hypertension almost certainly has been fostered by all these concerns, which are much more relevant in traditional hypertensive emergencies.[3]

Concerns about sustained hypertension in patients with acute hemorrhagic or ischemic stroke exist. However, a study from Stockholm of patients with untreated very high blood pressures (systolic > 200 mm Hg, diastolic > 115 mm Hg) could not identify an increased risk of progression of symptoms in acute stroke, but mortality was higher.[4] In a post hoc analysis of the International Stroke Trial, outcome was worse when systolic blood pressures fell outside the 120–140 mm Hg range, but the explanation or the practical implications of this association remain uncertain.[28] Untreated hypertension may increase the volume of ganglionic hemorrhages. Although there seems to be no evidence of a periclot ischemic zone in either human or animal experiments,[42,57] concern remains that treatment of increased blood pressure may cause global ischemia or an increased zone of ischemia surrounding the clot.[21,30] This complication is particularly important in patients with ganglionic hemorrhages who have long-standing hypertension that has resulted in narrowing of the lower limit of the autoregulation curve (Chapter 9).

Lowering of the blood pressure could result in a considerable decrease in cerebral perfusion pressure. Some studies suggested that a reduction of mean arterial blood pressure by more than 20% could reduce cerebral blood flow, but a small study in 14 patients with largely ganglionic hematomas showed no appreciable reduction in cerebral blood flow when positron emission tomography studies were done an average of 15 hours after the ictus and blood pressure was reduced to 119 ± 11 mm Hg. The number of patients was limited, and the effect of changes in blood pressure in the most critical physiologic period of the first hours after onset of hemorrhage was not studied.[27,40]

Several studies with retrospective analyses of early rebleeding in putaminal hemorrhages could not demonstrate a relationship with hypertension, but the issue remains unsettled. An interesting study linked extravasation of contrast medium during computed tomographic angiography to increased blood pressure, hematoma size, and coma. Contrast material extravasation (which was loosely interpreted as continuing hemorrhage) was more common in patients with mean arterial blood pressure of more than 120 mm Hg.[2]

Treatment of hypertension in aneurysmal subarachnoid hemorrhage is controversial.[51] The relationship with rebleeding is not established, largely because rebleeding was poorly defined in earlier studies. A recent study claimed that systolic arterial blood pressure of more than 160 mm Hg increased the risk of early rebleeding in aneurysmal subarachnoid hemorrhage. Serious definitional problems with rebleeding criteria were notable.[33]

Management of hypertension after recent use of thrombolytic agents is important, and failure to do so has been linked to hemorrhagic conversion. In a recently published rat model, increased blood pressure correlated with hemorrhagic transformation, which also could be reduced in incidence after treatment with hydralazine.[46] In the National Institute of Neurological Disorders and Stroke (NINDS) trial, the lower rate of intracerebral hemorrhage than that in other thrombolytic trials has been tentatively linked to aggressive management of hypertension.[7]

Postoperative hypertension (for example, in patients with coiling or clipping of an aneurysm or craniotomy for cerebellar hemorrhage) is best managed by relief of pain, hypoxemia, and excessive volume overload, if present.[47] In postoperative patients, blood pressure can be normalized by adjusting the ventilation settings to a more comfortable mode (usually intermittent mandatory ventilation), by sedating the patient with low doses of propofol, and by liberal use of narcotic agents for pain management.

Until results of prospective studies become available, increased blood pressure after acute brain injury probably should be left alone or treated judiciously.[29,37–39] Treatment is reasonable with computed tomography scan evidence of rapidly worsening brain edema and with the use of thrombolytic agents (Chapter 8). The cutoff point in treatment of hypertension (arbitrarily defined as systolic blood pressure > 230 mm Hg or diastolic > 125 mm Hg or mean arterial blood pressure > 130 mm Hg on repeated occasions) is very difficult to define because of lack of hard data on any disorder. It is reasonable to gradually decrease blood pressure with rapid-acting antihypertensive drugs when the mean arterial blood pres-

sure reaches 130 mm Hg or cerebral perfusion pressure is higher than 85 mm Hg. These values closely correspond with the upper limit of autoregulation, and higher pressures may further increase brain edema, if present. These goals should be higher in chronically hypertensive patients (mean arterial pressure ≥ 140 mm Hg).

Treatment of hypertension should also proceed if myocardial ischemia occurs or congestive heart failure develops from significantly increased systemic vascular resistance.[3] If blood pressure cannot be controlled with labetalol or esmolol, fenoldopam has clear advantages over nitroprusside because its onset of action is less abrupt. Fenoldopam should not be used if congestive heart failure or myocardial ischemia has already emerged, and nitroglycerin, 5 to 100 μg/minute intravenously via infusion pump, should be considered because it reduces preload and afterload.[32]

PHARMACOLOGIC CHOICES

The pros and cons of the currently available antihypertensive agents are discussed in this section, and the most pertinent characteristics relevant for clinical practice are summarized in Table 6–3.

β- and α-Blocking Agents

Agents with combined α- and β-adrenergic receptor blocking properties are preferred in the management of acute hypertension. Most experience has been gained with labetalol.[36,54] Although labetalol is a combined α- and β-blocker, the potency of β-blockade is seven times greater with increasing intravenous doses. Its effect results from a decrease in systemic vascular resistance without measurable effect on cardiac output. The absence of an associated tachycardia is caused by β-adrenergic receptor blockade.

Treatment is started with a bolus of 20 mg of labetalol given in 5 minutes, and this may be followed by a double dose of 40 mg or further increase to 80 mg. A bolus of 40 mg may be repeated every 15 minutes, but when a total

Table 6–3. Blood Pressure Management in Acute Central Nervous System Disease

Drug°	Dose†	ACTION		Adverse Effects	Not Recommended
		Onset	Duration		
Esmolol	500 μg/kg bolus, then infusion of 50–300 μg/kg per minute IV	1–2 minutes	10–30 minutes	Hypotension, nausea, bronchospasm	Asthma, chronic obstructive pulmonary disease
Labetalol	20 mg IV bolus, slow 2 minutes, then every 10 minutes 40–80 mg injections	5–10 minutes	3–6 hours	Vomiting, scalp tingling, burning in throat, dizziness, nausea, heart block, liver damage, bronchospasm	Asthma, chronic obstructive pulmonary disease, left ventricular failure
Enalaprilat	0.625 mg IV Slow 5 minutes, then 1.25 mg q6h	15–30 minutes	6 hours	Response variable	
Nitroprusside	0.3–10 μg/kg per minute as IV infusion	Immediate	3–4 minutes	Nausea, vomiting, muscle twitching, sweating, thiocyanate intoxication with prolonged use	Coronary artery disease
Diazoxide	1–3 mg/kg (150 mg max dose), repeat 5–15 min	2–4 minutes	6–12 hours	Nausea, flushing, tachycardia, chest pain	Coronary artery disease
Nicardipine	5 mg IV, max 15 mg/hour	5–10 minutes	1–4 hours	Tachycardia, headache, flushing	Left ventricular failure
Hydralazine	20–40 mg IV	10–20 minutes	3–8 hours	Tachycardia, flushing, headache	
Fenoldopam	0.1 μg/kg per minute; increase 0.05 μg/kg per minute every 15 minutes until effect	5–15 minutes	1–4 hours	Electrocardiographic changes, reflex tachycardia, hypokalemia, headache	Hepatic cirrhosis

°In order of preference.
†Ranges given are lowest possible dose preferred until desired pressure is achieved.

dose of 300 mg is reached, no further benefit should be expected. Continuous intravenous infusion is seldom needed as intervention but if desired can be started in the range of 50–200 mg given at an infusion rate of 2 mg/minute.

Labetalol is relatively easy to use, and an unexpected decrease in blood pressure should not occur in patients whose intravascular system is adequately filled. Side effects, including vomiting, scalp itching, lichenoid skin eruptions, and hepatic failure, are rare but more common with long-term use.

Labetalol is not recommended for patients with asthma, chronic obstructive pulmonary artery disease, or severe left ventricular failure. In these patients, an angiotensin-converting enzyme inhibitor or calcium channel blocker should be the preferred agent.

β-Adrenergic Blockade

The rationale for use of β-blockers is a decrease in central sympathetic nervous activity. (Vasodilatation may be another mechanism by which these agents work.) Use of β-blockade has been considered controversial in acute neurologic injury simply because of the preconceived idea that β-blockers produce sedation. This side effect, however, is extremely rare.

Esmolol is very useful in the NICU because of its short half-life (minutes) and ease of intravenous administration.[9] Its effect is easily titrated and is lost within 15 minutes after administration. Esmolol is cardioselective, producing negative inotropic effects and peripheral vasodilatation. The loading dose is 500 μg/kg in a 1-minute bolus. A maintenance dose of 50 μg/kg per minute may be sufficient, but infusion rates to 300 μg/kg per minute may be needed to control hypertension surges. (One should be aware of the considerable free water load, because esmolol is administered in D5W instead of isotonic saline.) Again, β-blockers are contraindicated in patients with chronic obstructive pulmonary disease.

Angiotensin-Converting Enzyme Inhibitors

With the introduction of enalaprilat (Vasotec I.V.), angiotensin-converting enzyme inhibitors are increasingly used in hypertensive emergencies in the NICU.[18,44] This prodrug has important advantages over many other vasodilators. Angiotensin-converting enzyme inhibitors also do not produce a reflex sympathetic stimulation. Their major drawbacks are a peak plasma concentration of 3 to 4 hours and an early effect after 15 to 30 minutes, considerably longer than those with intravenously administered β-blockers. A unique effect of angiotensin-converting enzyme inhibitors is the ability to reset the autoregulatory curve to lower pressure levels, so that the risk of diffuse cerebral ischemia from lowering blood pressure is reduced.[18] This attribute may make this drug one of the preferred drugs in patients with acute neurologic illness who have marked treatment-refractory hypertension. The starting dose of enalaprilat is 0.625 mg, followed by repeat doses of 1.25 mg every 6 hours.

Miscellaneous Agents

In most instances, hypertension is well controlled with the agents mentioned above. Recently, a dopamine D_1-like receptor agonist, fenoldopam, was introduced for treatment of acute hypertension. Because of rapid onset and short duration of action, absence of coronary artery steal, minimal hypotension overshoot, easy titration, and lack of thiocyanate toxicity, it is a reasonable alternative agent to nitroprusside in hypertensive crises. The initial dose is 0.1 μg/kg per minute, which is increased by 0.05 to 0.1 μg/kg per minute every 15 minutes to a maximum of 1.6 μg/kg per minute.[34]

Other choices are nitroprusside, trimethaphan, and phentolamine.[20] Nitroprusside (starting dose of 0.3 μg/kg per minute), however, may be the last resort when any other type of medication fails and regulation of blood pressure is needed. If the dose reaches 10 μg/kg per minute, thiocyanate toxicity may occur within hours, and other drugs should be tried. Nitroprusside remains a preferred drug in patients with hypertension from use of cocaine, crack, and amphetamines who are admitted with closed head injury, but its use generally is discouraged due to its major side effects. Because of important side effects, reserpine and methyldopa (both produce marked sedation), hydralazine (increases cerebral blood flow), diazoxide (decreases cerebral blood flow), and nicardipine (progressive decrease in blood pressure with marked reflex tachycardia) should all be considered second choices. A study with single-photon emission computed tomography corroborated a marked decrease in mean arterial pressure and cerebral blood flow after use of nicardipine in acute stroke.[29]

With the availability of transdermal patches, clonidine has been used more frequently, but its rebound effect is a major concern. A review of a large series of patients with aneurysmal subarachnoid hemorrhage treated with clonidine in an attempt to control surges of systolic blood pressure found average blood pressures to be higher than in patients not treated with clonidine.[51] Clonidine, however, may have a role when hypertension is related to opiate and alcohol withdrawal.

CONCLUSIONS

- Minimal initial fluid intake in patients with acute central nervous system disorders is 200 mL/hour. The goal is a positive fluid balance of approximately 1000 mL to correct for insensible loss.
- Water deficit in hypovolemic patients can be calculated as follows: 0.6 × body weight × (plasma sodium/140) − 1 in liters.
- Hypertonic saline 3% has some advantages over albumin and is less costly. Adequate fluid replacement is achieved with sodium chloride 3% at a rate of 4 mL/kg over 3 minutes or with an immediate bolus of 500 mL of albumin 5%.
- Treatment of hypertension after acute central nervous system injury is unsettled. A treatment cutoff point of mean arterial pressure of > 130 mm Hg or cerebral perfusion pressure of 85 mm Hg is reasonable in patients without hypertension. Treatment is indicated in patients with persistent extreme surges in blood pressure, rapidly progressing brain edema, or impending congestive heart failure.
- Preferred agents for the treatment of hypertension in patients with acute neurologic illness are esmolol, labetalol, and enalaprilat.

REFERENCES

1. Abramson N: Plasma expanders and bleeding (letter to the editor). Ann Intern Med 108:307, 1988.
2. Becker KJ, Baxter AB, Bybee HM, et al: Extravasation of radiographic contrast is an independent predictor of death in primary intracerebral hemorrhage. Stroke 30:2025–2032, 1999.
3. Blumenfeld JD, Laragh JH: Management of hypertensive crises: the scientific basis for treatment decisions. Am J Hypertens 14:1154–1157, 2001.
4. Britton M, Carlsson A: Very high blood pressure in acute stroke. J Intern Med 228:611–615, 1990.
5. Britton M, Carlsson A, de Faire U: Blood pressure course in patients with acute stroke and matched controls. Stroke 17:861–864, 1986.
6. Broderick J, Brott T, Barsan W, et al: Blood pressure during the first minutes of focal cerebral ischemia. Ann Emerg Med 22:1438–1443, 1993.
7. Brott T, Lu M, Kothari R, et al: Hypertension and its treatment in the NINDS rt-PA Stroke Trial. Stroke 29:1504–1509, 1998.
8. Bunn F, Roberts I, Tasker R, et al: Hypertonic versus isotonic crystalloid for fluid resuscitation in critically ill patients. Cochrane Database Syst Rev 4:CD002045, 2002.
9. Calhoun DA, Oparil S: Treatment of hypertensive crisis. N Engl J Med 323:1177–1183, 1990.
10. Carlberg B, Asplund K, Hägg E: Course of blood pressure in different subsets of patients after acute stroke. Cerebrovasc Dis 1:281–287, 1991.
11. Carlberg B, Asplund K, Hägg E: Factors influencing admission blood pressure levels in patients with acute stroke. Stroke 22:527–530, 1991.
12. Choi PT, Yip G, Quinonez LG, et al: Crystalloids vs. colloids in fluid resuscitation: a systematic review. Crit Care Med 27:200–210, 1999.
13. Cushing H: Concerning a definite regulatory mechanism of the vasomotor centre which controls blood pressure during cerebral compression. Johns Hopkins Hosp Bull 12:290–292, 1901.
14. Cushing H: Some experimental and clinical observations concerning states of increased intracranial tension. Am J Med Sci 124:375–400, 1902.
15. Davalos A, Cendra E, Teruel J, et al: Deteriorating ischemic stroke: risk factors and prognosis. Neurology 40:1865–1869, 1990.
16. de Jonge E, Levi M: Effects of different plasma substitutes on blood coagulation: a comparative review. Crit Care Med 29:1261–1267, 2001.
17. Erstad BL, Gales BJ, Rappaport WD: The use of albumin in clinical practice. Arch Intern Med 151: 901–911, 1991.
18. Fagan SC, Robert S, Ewing JR, et al: Cerebral blood flow changes with enalapril. Pharmacotherapy 12: 319–323, 1992.
19. Fisher M (ed): Stroke Therapy. Boston, Butterworth-Heinemann, 1995.
20. Gifford RW Jr: Management of hypertensive crises. JAMA 266:829–835, 1991.
21. Graham DI: Ischaemic brain following emergency blood pressure lowering in hypertensive patients. Acta Med Scand Suppl 678:61–69, 1983.
22. Hachinski V: Hypertension in acute ischemic strokes. Arch Neurol 42:1002, 1985.
23. Huettemann E: Hetastarch and hydroxyethyl starch are not the same. Anesth Analg 91:1561, 2000.
24. Jamnicki M, Bombeli T, Seifert B, et al: Low- and medium-molecular-weight hydroxyethyl starches: comparison of their effect on blood coagulation. Anesthesiology 93:1231–1237, 2000.
25. Jansen PA, Schulte BP, Poels EF, et al: Course of blood pressure after cerebral infarction and transient ischemic attack. Clin Neurol Neurosurg 89:243–246, 1987.

26. Kagansky N, Levy S, Knobler H: The role of hyperglycemia in acute stroke. *Arch Neurol* 58:1209–1212, 2001.

27. Kuwata N, Kuroda K, Funayama M, et al: Dysautoregulation in patients with hypertensive intracerebral hemorrhage. A SPECT study. *Neurosurg Rev* 18:237–245, 1995.

28. Leonardi-Bee J, Bath PMW, Phillips SJ, et al: Blood pressure and clinical outcomes in the International Stroke Trial. *Stroke* 33:1315–1320, 2002.

29. Lisk DR, Grotta JC, Lamki LM, et al: Should hypertension be treated after acute stroke? A randomized controlled trial using single photon emission computed tomography. *Arch Neurol* 50:855–862, 1993.

30. Loyke HF: Lowering of blood pressure after stroke. *Am J Med Sci* 286:2–11, 1983.

31. Murphy M, Carmichael AJ, Lawler PG, et al: The incidence of hydroxyethyl starch-associated pruritus. *Br J Dermatol* 144:973–976, 2001.

32. Murphy MB, Murray C, Shorten GD: Fenoldopam—a selective peripheral dopamine-receptor agonist for the treatment of severe hypertension. *N Engl J Med* 345:1548–1557, 2001.

33. Ohkuma H, Tsurutani H, Suzuki S: Incidence and significance of early aneurysmal rebleeding before neurosurgical or neurological management. *Stroke* 32:1176–1180, 2001.

34. Oparil S, Aronson S, Deeb GM, et al: Fenoldopam: a new parenteral antihypertensive: consensus roundtable on the management of perioperative hypertension and hypertensive crises. *Am J Hypertens* 12:653–664, 1999.

35. Parsons MW, Barber PA, Desmond PM, et al: Acute hyperglycemia adversely affects stroke outcome: a magnetic resonance imaging and spectroscopy study. *Ann Neurol* 52:20–28, 2002.

36. Patel RV, Kertland HR, Jahns BE, et al: Labetalol: response and safety in critically ill hemorrhagic stroke patients. *Ann Pharmacother* 27:180–181, 1993.

37. Phillips SJ: Pathophysiology and management of hypertension in acute ischemic stroke. *Hypertension* 23:131–136, 1994.

38. Powers WJ: Cerebral hemodynamics in ischemic cerebrovascular disease. *Ann Neurol* 29:231–240, 1991.

39. Powers WJ: Acute hypertension after stroke: the scientific basis for treatment decisions (editorial). *Neurology* 43:461–467, 1993.

40. Powers WJ, Zazulia AR, Videen TO, et al: Autoregulation of cerebral blood flow surrounding acute (6 to 22 hours) intracerebral hemorrhage. *Neurology* 57:18–24, 2001.

41. Prough DS, Johnson JC, Stump DA, et al: Effects of hypertonic saline versus lactated Ringer's solution on cerebral oxygen transport during resuscitation from hemorrhagic shock. *J Neurosurg* 64:627–632, 1986.

42. Qureshi AI, Wilson DA, Hanley DF, et al: No evidence for an ischemic penumbra in massive experimental intracerebral hemorrhage. *Neurology* 52:266–272, 1999.

43. Roberts JS, Bratton SL: Colloid volume expanders. Problems, pitfalls and possibilities. *Drugs* 55:621–630, 1998.

44. Schmidt JF, Andersen AR, Paulson OB, et al: Angiotensin converting enzyme inhibition, CBF autoregulation, and ICP in patients with normal-pressure hydrocephalus. *Acta Neurochir (Wien)* 106:9–12, 1990.

45. Stogermuller B, Stark J, Willschke H, et al: The effect of hydroxyethyl starch 200 kD on platelet function. *Anesth Analg* 91:823–827, 2000.

46. Tejima E, Katayama Y, Suzuki Y, et al: Hemorrhagic transformation after fibrinolysis with tissue plasminogen activator: evaluation of role of hypertension with rat thromboembolic stroke model. *Stroke* 32:1336–1340, 2001.

47. Van Aken H, Cottrell JE, Anger C, et al: Treatment of intraoperative hypertensive emergencies in patients with intracranial disease. *Am J Cardiol* 63:43C–47C, 1989.

48. Virgilio RW, Rice CL, Smith DE, et al: Crystalloid vs. colloid resuscitation: Is one better? A randomized clinical study. *Surgery* 85:129–139, 1979.

49. Wallace JD, Levy LL: Blood pressure after stroke. *JAMA* 246:2177–2180, 1981.

50. Wijdicks EFM, Vermeulen M, Hijdra A, et al: Hyponatremia and cerebral infarction in patients with ruptured intracranial aneurysms: Is fluid restriction harmful? *Ann Neurol* 17:137–140, 1985.

51. Wijdicks EFM, Vermeulen M, Murray GD, et al: The effects of treating hypertension following aneurysmal subarachnoid hemorrhage. *Clin Neurol Neurosurg* 92:111–117, 1990.

52. Wijdicks EFM, Vermeulen M, ten Haaf JA, et al: Volume depletion and natriuresis in patients with a ruptured intracranial aneurysm. *Ann Neurol* 18:211–216, 1985.

53. Wilkins MR, Redondo J, Brown LA: The natriuretic-peptide family. *Lancet* 349:1307–1310, 1997.

54. Wilson DJ, Wallin JD, Vlachakis ND, et al: Intravenous labetalol in the treatment of severe hypertension and hypertensive emergencies. *Am J Med* 75:95–102, 1983.

55. Yatsu FM, Zivin J: Hypertension in acute ischemic strokes. Not to treat. *Arch Neurol* 42:999–1000, 1985.

56. Zampaglione B, Pascale C, Marchisio M, et al: Hypertensive urgencies and emergencies: prevalence and clinical presentation. *Hypertension* 27:144–147, 1996.

57. Zazulia AR, Diringer MN, Videen TO, et al: Hypoperfusion without ischemia surrounding acute intracerebral hemorrhage. *J Cereb Blood Flow Metab* 21:804–810, 2001.

7

Nutrition

Nutritional support in the NICU has distinctive characteristics. Daily care is focused on countering the effects of hypermetabolism and acute gastroparesis and to keep off complications associated with enteral nutrition.[40,44,46] Early feeding of the gut to guarantee adequate nutrition may seem fundamental in patients with any type of acute neurologic illness, but there is a dilemma. To be more precise, feeding prevents gastrointestinal mucosal atrophy, whereas a lag in nutritional support may create a situation in which patients become too weak to effectively cough up secretions, and they may not maximally fend off looming bacterial infections. Outcome studies in patients with severe head injury and stroke suggest that when nutritional support is prompt, mortality is reduced and the number of nosocomial infections is significantly lower.[26,39,41,56-58] In contrast, early nasogastric tube feeding in patients with acute gastroparesis increases the risk of aspiration of retained solutions and gastric acid, both extremely damaging to the lung, increasing mortality in some units.[36] Ventilator-associated pneumonia and *Clostridium difficile* infection were shown to be more common in patients fed immediately.[22] Moreover, nutritional support practices vary. A prospective study in a medical intensive care unit suggested underutilization, with half of the patients receiving suboptimal caloric intake[16] and failing to reach targeted nutritional goals. Gradual increase in infusion rates to reduce gastric distention may be one of the explanations. Randomized studies have been published in head injury, but not in many other conditions, and nutritional support remains based on empirical evidence.[30,56]

The handling of complex nutritional problems may not be the typical neurologist's forte, but critical care neurologists must be comfortable with administering various tube feedings and determining the indications for percutaneous endoscopic gastrostomy. Nutritional care, the details of monitoring the adequacy of nutritional support tailored toward specific acute neurologic disorders, and the handling of devices that deliver nutrition form the major focus of this chapter.

NUTRITIONAL NEEDS AND MAINTENANCE

As a matter of principle, and seemingly obvious, a consensus statement from the American College of Chest Physicians emphasizes that doses of nutrients provided should be compatible with the existing metabolism.[9] The main goals of nutritional support are to preserve muscle mass (lean body mass) and to provide adequate fluids, vitamins, minerals, and fats.[5,32]

Any patient transferred to the NICU needs a full assessment of nutritional status. One of the first objectives is to estimate nutritional needs. The components of clinical nutritional assessment should be partitioned into evaluation of possible underlying malnutrition and estimation of nutritional needs in a patient in a hypermetabolic state. For example, a common misconception is that obese patients should be able to tolerate intervals without feeding.

There is a fundamental difference between starvation and the much more common hypermetabolic state. In starvation, the major physiologic changes are characterized by decreased energy expenditure and utilization of alternative fuel sources. Patients can tolerate extended periods of semistarvation because the body responds to decreased energy intake by reduction of the basal metabolic rate and favors a state in which the fat supplies are used as primary fuel. Patients with a neurologic catastrophe respond differently. The metabolic rate is dramatically increased (hypermetabolism), and rather than depletion of fat, protein stores from lean body mass are rapidly mobilized.[17] The major physiologic changes that are characterized by increased metabolic rate are fever, leukocytosis, hyperglycemia, hypoalbuminemia, and increased blood urea nitrogen.

The physical examination should focus specifically on features of underlying malnutrition. Besides the visible appearance of severe wasting, more subtle clinical features may indicate malnutrition. Typical clinical signs associated with malnutrition are shown in Table 7–1. Many of these signs may suggest deficiency of a specific nutrient. Awareness of the possibility of malnutrition should be very high in emergency admissions of patients with closed head injury and fulminant bacterial meningitis, conditions that are considerably

more common in alcoholics. Vitamin B_1 (thiamine) deficiency should be anticipated not only because intake is poor but also because alcohol reduces thiamine absorption. Reduced erythrocyte transketolase levels can be diagnostic; thiamine deficiency deranges glucose metabolism, and in the pentose phosphate pathway transketolase is the thiamine-dependent step. Large doses of parenteral thiamine (50 mg intravenously initially and 50–100 mg intramuscularly for 5 to 7 days) must be administered to prevent a lapse into a florid Wernicke-Korsakoff syndrome in thiamine-deficient patients, particularly before intravenous carboxyhydrate loads are administered. Magnesium (1 g as undiluted 50% solution intramuscularly) acts as a cofactor for transketolase activity and may have to be administered in addition.[35] Wernicke-Korsakoff syndrome can be recognized by a confusional state, horizontal or vertical nystagmus, gaze palsy, and ataxia of gait or limbs but is seldom manifested by coma. The dose of thiamine in an established Wernicke-Korsakoff syndrome should be 100–200 mg for 3 days, depending on severity and response to therapy. The symptoms, particularly the ophthalmic manifestations, typically disappear within this time period.

Other laboratory values may also help in the interpretation of underlying malnutrition. Hypoalbuminemia is an important marker for malnutrition at the initial presentation. Decrease in plasma albumin in critical illness is a result of decreased hepatic production during the acute phase response. The daily production rate may be substantially decreased, certainly in patients with continuing bacteremia. Cytokines such as interleukin-1 and tumor necrosis factor decrease food intake and have a direct down-regulating effect on the albumin gene. Surveys in surgical intensive care units have emphasized a significantly higher mortality among patients with serum albumin levels below 3.5 g/L from malnutrition. Decreased transferrin and total lymphocyte count—but also albumin-bound calcium, magnesium, and zinc—may indicate protein wasting, but these values are not very reliable in the intensive care unit. Measurement of triceps skin fold thick-

Table 7–1. Physical Signs of Malnutrition

Disorder	Deficiency
Generalized muscle wasting	Any global
Easily plucked, thin, dyspigmented hair	Zinc
Nasolabial seborrhea	Any global
Fissuring of eyelid corners	Vitamin B_2
Angular stomatitis	Vitamin B_{12}
Cheilosis	Vitamin B_{12}
Periodontal disease, mottled enamel, and caries	Any global
Raw and swollen tongue	Niacin and folate
Spoon-shaped nails	Iron
Hyperkeratosis and petechial hemorrhages of the skin	Vitamin C or K

ness remains difficult to perform and less practical.

Malnutrition has a strikingly adverse effect on lung function by impairing respiratory muscles, decreasing ventilatory drive, and diminishing the lung defense mechanism. These effects become important in patients with acute neuromuscular failure and could hamper weaning efforts. However, there may be a fine line, because overfeeding with excess carbohydrate calories (> 3,000/day) may lead to hypercapnia, which also reduces the success of weaning.

Caloric needs can be estimated by weight and approximate 25 to 30 kcal/kg per day. The Harris-Benedict formulas, however, are more accurate in determining caloric needs.[42,48,49] Nutritional needs in patients with neurologic critical illness should be calculated with the Harris-Benedict equation to obtain the basal energy expenditure (BEE) in calories. The Harris-Benedict formulas are based on kilograms of weight (W), centimeters of height (H), and years of age (A). For men, the formula is BEE = $66.5 + 13.8W + 5H - 6.8A$, and for women, BEE = $655 + 9.6W + 1.8H - 4.7A$. This method, although introduced in healthy persons, remains the most practical means of obtaining daily caloric needs. Correcting factors for specific critical disease states, which primarily add a certain percentage to the calculated value, have been proposed, but they increase the inaccuracy of an estimate. More specifically, no correcting factors are known in acute brain injury. It is, however, very reasonable to add a "stress factor" in patients with an acute central nervous system catastrophic event and marked sympathetic manifestations, such as profuse sweating, hyperthermia, hypertension, and tachycardia. Total calories are then calculated by BEE + 20%. In obese patients, 75% of the basal Harris-Benedict calculation based on obese weight seems reasonable.

More accurate measurements can be obtained by indirect calorimetry, which is based on calculation of energy expenditure through measurement of respiratory gas exchange. Metabolism is expressed as oxygen consumption and carbon dioxide production. With the use of portable devices (metabolic carts), the resting energy expenditure can be calculated from $\dot{V}O_2$ (oxygen consumption in liters per minute) and $\dot{V}CO_2$ (carbon dioxide production in liters per minute). The metabolic cart that measures the concentration of O_2 and CO_2 can be connected to the ventilator tubing. (Resting energy expenditure = $3.94\ [\dot{V}O_2] + 1.1[\dot{V}CO_2] \times 1440$ = kcal in 1 day.) Although metabolic carts are expensive to use and calibration is at times questionable, they can be of value in patients who have difficulty in weaning, are morbidly obese, or have been treated with prolonged volume expansion, which makes the estimation of "dry weight" cumbersome. Another method—using the Swan-Ganz catheter in the calculation of the metabolic rate—has seldom been applied in this population.

The estimated energy expenditure subsequently is divided into proteins of 1.5 g/kg per day, and the remaining calories are evenly divided between carbohydrates and lipids. Enteral products in the formulary usually contain 1 kcal/1 mL and 40 g of protein. Glucose should be maintained at a range of 80–110 mg/dL (and certainly when a critical illness such as sepsis emerges[54]), blood urea nitrogen at less than 100 mg/dL, and triglyceride level at less than 500 mg/dL. The simplest way to monitor nutritional support, however, is to weigh patients regularly. A severe catabolic state can be further monitored by nitrogen balance. This can be calculated at intervals of several days, provided that renal function is not changing. Urinary nitrogen is measured in a 24-hour urine collection. The nitrogen balance is calculated as fol-lows: nitrogen balance (grams) = (protein intake/6.25) − (urinary nitrogen + 4). Increased nitrogen secretion results in negative nitrogen balance, and more protein must be delivered.

ASSESSMENT OF ASPIRATION RISK

Patients with head injury may be intoxicated from alcohol or other substances, and swallowing mechanics may be disturbed in patients with a brain stem or hemispheric stroke and in patients with acute neuromuscular disease. Other important risk factors are impaired level of consciousness, vomiting, seizures, obesity, nasogastric feeding, and diabetes-associated gastrointestinal motility disorder (Chapter 29). Aspiration is markedly increased in patients requiring emergency intubation. A similar risk occurs with extubation, and aspiration is increased immediately after a procedure in which anesthetic agents have been used. Premature extubation postoperatively may be dangerous, because many anesthetic agents reduce laryngeal closure.

Aspiration pneumonia can possibly be prevented if patients with abnormal swallowing mechanisms are identified early. The result of any bedside test of swallowing (Table 7–2) that suggests an abnormal mechanism should prompt a more formal evaluation.[13] The gag reflex has a low predictive value and is absent in at least one-third of the normal population. Testing of pharyngeal sensation may be more useful,[14] and studies have confirmed increased risks of aspiration in patients with pharyngeal sensory deficits. Alternative techniques include assessment of laryngeal adductor reflex with air pulse stimulation. Its absence predicts aspiration.[1]

Patients with a high probability of swallowing difficulties should be evaluated with videofluoroscopy.[11] Interpretation requires significant skills. Features, alone or in combination, that can be assessed are bolus formation, residue in oral cavity, oral transit time, triggering of pharyngeal swallowing, laryngeal elevation and epiglottic closure, nasal penetration,

vallecular residue, pharyngeal wall coating, and pharyngeal transit time.[20] Videofluoroscopy may also predict long-term difficulties. A study in 128 patients after stroke found that delayed oral transit and penetration into the laryngeal vestibule predicted poor outcome and failure to resume oral feeding.[34] The incidence of aspiration tends to be higher in patients with nondominant hemispheric ischemic stroke (labeled *quiet aspirators*), explained by ineffective throat clearing, possible neglect, and prolonged pharyngeal response (time between initiation of hyoid excursion and return to rest). However, patients with dominant hemispheric stroke typically have an abnormal oral stage, with uncoordinated labial, lingual, and mandibular movements from apraxia of swallowing and prolonged pharyngeal transit times (arrival of the bolus head at the ramus of the mandible until complete passage through the upper esophageal sphincter opening).[24,45,53] Patients who in addition have aphonia are at particularly high risk.

The immediate consequences of a high risk of aspiration are clear. However, nil per os may not have any measurable influence on gastric volume or pH and therefore should not substantially reduce aspiration. An H_2-antagonist should be administered to patients at high risk of aspiration,[33] but protein pump inhibitors may be more effective. Both agents may reduce gastric volume and increase pH. Positioning at 45° head elevation is an important additional measure. (For more details, see Chapter 29.)

ENTERAL NUTRITION

The integrity of the gut is maintained by enteral feeding and is greatly challenged in parenteral nutrition. The timing of enteral nutrition is not known. However, enteral nutrition is probably required early in patients who are hypermetabolic from the ictus.[9]

An 8 or 16 French gauge tube should be inserted in most patients. The patient is positioned sitting with the head of the bed elevated to 45°. One end of the tube is held with thumb

Table 7–2. Features Suggesting Abnormal Swallowing Mechanism

Abnormal laryngeal rise
Abnormal throat clearing
Abnormal volitional ("coup de glottis") and reflexive cough
Abnormal gag reflex
Abnormal pharyngeal sensation
Abnormal oral motor rapid movement and strength
Abnormal vocal clarity
Abnormal sipping of water and eating of crackers

and index finger behind the ear. The length of the nasogastric tube is estimated by measuring from the ear to the tip of the nose and from the tip of the nose to the xyphoid process. After patency is checked by having the patient breathe through the nose (with one nostril occluded), the feeding tube can be placed. Many techniques may greatly facilitate placement. They include flexion of the neck, generous lubrication of the tube, placement of the tube in an ice water bath to increase rigidity, the Jarmon technique (filling the nostril with lidocaine jelly, which enters the posterior pharynx and relaxes the nasal constrictors), and, as a last resort, direct visualization with a laryngoscope and advancement with a forceps.[6] Alert patients can be asked to swallow water through a straw while the tube is advanced.

The technique of advancing the tube consists of a gentle motion with advancement of at least 3 inches each time the patient swallows. Auscultation of a gurgling sound after pushing air through the tube may not be very reliable, and only aspiration of the gastric contents confirms location within the stomach.[47] Correct placement of a nasogastric tube must be checked by radiography before feeding is started.[37] In combative, agitated patients, the risk of misplacement is obviously higher and the risk of aspiration is significant from self-extubation.

Complications of placement of the nasogastric tube are rare. Occasionally, a feeding tube is placed in the bronchial tree (Fig. 7–1), and if this error is not recognized, a potentially fatal chemical pneumonitis results. One study suggested that connection to a handheld end-tidal carbon dioxide device can identify false placement (presence of a carbon dioxide waveform) and reduce discomfort or formation of an iatrogenic bronchopleural fistula from manipulation.[7] Nonetheless, a chest radiograph is needed to confirm adequate placement. In addition, intracranial placement has been repeatedly reported in patients with very severe facial trauma.[15,31]

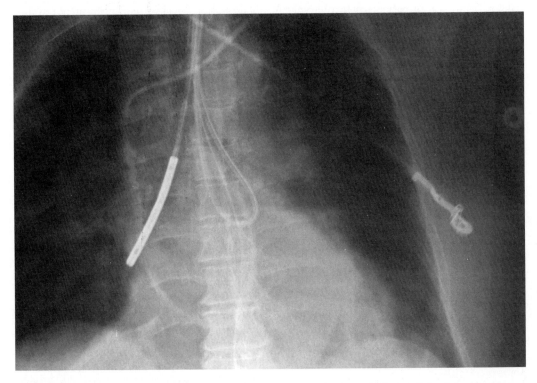

Figure 7–1. Inadvertent placement of nasogastric tube in right lower lobe bronchus.

It is prudent to consider postpyloric feeding in patients with central nervous system catastrophes, because gastric atony increases the risk of aspiration. However, drug absorption in the jejunum may be unreliable. Gastric atony or impaired gastric motility can be anticipated in patients with subarachnoid hemorrhage of poor grade or severe closed head injury.[25] The use of nasoduodenal or nasojejunal tubes may reduce the risk of aspiration. Duodenal placement can be tried by inserting a coiled tube that is at least 10 cm more than the calculated length into the stomach and then waiting 24 hours to allow spontaneous advancement past the pylorus. The right lateral decubitus position may facilitate the motion. Another helpful bedside technique, with a 75% success rate, is air insufflation. A 60 mL syringe is used to pump 500 mL of air into the stomach.

Tubes that fail to pass may be placed fluoroscopically, and this technique is very successful.[19] Additionally, metoclopramide or erythromycin elixir facilitates transpyloric passage.[51] Erythromycin (200 mg) given intravenously in patients with a gastric feeding tube may improve nutritional intake, similar to that in patients fed through a tube placed transpylorically,[4] and could be considered in appropriate patients.

Enteral feeding should preferably be done by continuous infusion with a volumetric pump. Continuous tube feedings have been associated with a positive nitrogen balance and weight gain more often than intermittent tube feedings.[12] A recent successful protocol started feeding at 25 mL/hour and increased the volume by 25 mL/hour every 4 hours until the goal of nutrition was achieved.[43] When a gastric residual volume of more than 250 mL was detected, feeding was held for 4 hours and restarted at the same rate but with a more gradual increase in rate. A prokinetic agent (metoclopramide, cisapride, or domperidone) was mandated. If this approach is not tolerated and residuals are significant, the tube should be relocated into the jejunum. This can be done on a tilting fluoroscopic table with placement beyond the ligament of Treitz. Continuous administration is essential in jejunal feeding because a rapidly formed bolus of a hyperosmolar solution may cause serious cramps and diarrhea.

Feeding can be started with any of the standard commercially available enteral nutrition products. The available formulas provide approximately 1 kcal/mL. However, fluid intake and total volume load could become substantial, and maintenance fluids should be adjusted. We have been using Osmolite and Promote in most patients admitted to the NICU. The enteral formulas should be used as directed and not diluted (see the Appendix for formulary and indications). Bacterial contamination has been reported with nonsterile handling of the formula.

Problems with enteral feeding are frequent.[3,8] The most common is diarrhea, which can be associated with rapid infusion rates and the use of hyperosmolar formulas (see Chapter 32). It is less often due to intolerance to fat, lactulose, and bacterial overgrowth. Nausea, cramps, and abdominal distention are often associated with rapid feeding. Causes in the NICU are shown in Table 7–3. Decreased gastric emptying can be demonstrated if residuals exceed 50% of the amount delivered in the last feeding or are 50% above the flow rate per hour. Intravenously administered metoclopramide (antagonizes dopamine and sensitizes acetylcholine), 10 mg every 6 hours, may be effective in persistent cases that cannot be resolved with changes in the method of delivery.[29] Liver and renal failure should prompt dose adjustment. Erythromycin (acts on motilin receptors), 200 mg intravenously, is the preferred promotility agent.[10,59] Renal failure should prompt dose adjustment. Cisapride has been associated with serious cardiac arrhythmias and death, and use was discontinued in the United States in July 2000.

Table 7–3. Factors Altering Gastric Emptying in the Neurologic Intensive Care Unit

Premorbidity (e.g., diabetes mellitus, prior vagotomy)
Electrolyte abnormalities (e.g., hyperglycemia, hypokalemia)
Drugs (opiates, anticholinergics, cephalosporins)
Sepsis

A consistent problem of enteral feeding is tube obstruction, most commonly in tubes of smaller French size. Clogging of the tube can be resolved by frequent flushing with 50 mL of fluid, but cranberry juice or any carbonated drink (e.g., *Coca-Cola, Mountain Dew,* or *Dr. Pepper*) often loosens the residuals within the tube.

Medication can be administered by this route, and absorption should be sufficient. Mortars and pestles are needed to thoroughly crush tablets. Problems arise with sustained-action release and enteric-coated tablets, which lose their intended function by crushing. Specific absorption problems have been noted with warfarin, phenytoin, and carbamazepine. Absorption of phenytoin with tube feeding is poor, in some patients virtually unmeasurable. One method is to hold feeding 2 hours before administration. This should result in adequate absorption and therapeutic phenytoin plasma levels, but the total dose may still need to be increased. Parenteral administration of phenytoin, however, is then preferable.

In summary, enteral nutrition is not without complications, and the most common are aspiration and diarrhea. The complications are shown in Table 7–4, but most are very uncommon. Diarrhea often is related to enteral formulation, and reducing the flow rate probably is more effective than changing to another formula (Chapter 32). Nosocomial infections (e.g., *Clostridium difficile*) should be considered, particularly when antibiotics are similarly administered (see Chapter 33).

INDICATIONS FOR GASTROSTOMY

The indications for surgical placement of a feeding tube have not been clearly delineated in the patient with critical neurologic illness. The advantages of percutaneous endoscopic gastrostomy (PEG) are great in patients who cannot tolerate nasogastric tubes, who frequently extubate themselves, or who may need long-term enteral feeding largely because of defective swallowing mechanisms.[28] However, nasogastric tubes can be tolerated for months in many patients.

The placement of gastrostomy with the use of endoscopic guidance is often considered in patients with debilitating neurologic disease, particularly when dysphagia persists beyond 2 to 3 weeks. Percutaneous endoscopic gastrostomy placement seems much less attractive in patients with a high probability of death or who are severely disabled. It is very important to note that PEG placement should be postponed if withdrawal of support is anticipated. One should seriously weigh the risks and benefits of gastrostomy, choose wisely, and carefully use this resource.

Patients with anticipated prolonged enteral feeding typically have major hemispheric or, more often, brain stem ischemic stroke or are in prolonged coma from any cause. Its use as an early intervention was studied in patients with severe head injury and Glasgow coma scale scores of less than 8.[27] A gastrostomy device was anchored in the stomach and jejunal tubes placed into the small intestine in 27 patients within 5 days of presentation. In many patients, nitrogen loss was reduced, and complications from having the tube in situ were not noted.[27] Whether this aggressive approach can resolve the caloric loss associated with hypermetabolism is very uncertain. More recently, in 30 patients with acute stroke and persistent dysphagia randomized to PEG or nasogastric tube feeding, gastrostomy tube feeding 2 weeks after acute stroke significantly reduced mortality and aspi-

Table 7–4. Complications of Enteral Feeding

Cause	Events
Mechanical	Malplacement
	Tube clogging
	Nasal mucosal ulceration
	Otitis media
	Pharyngitis
	Pneumothorax
	Reflux esophagitis
Gut	Aspiration of stomach contents
	Bloating, constipation
	Diarrhea, vomiting
Metabolic	Liver function abnormalities
	Dehydration
	Hyperglycemia
	Micronutrient deficiency

ration pneumonia.[39] In our study, however, patients who received PEG after acute stroke remained severely disabled, with at least one-third dying from systemic complications of stroke.[55]

Many techniques of PEG placement have been developed.[18] Antibiotic prophylaxis is standard before placement (1 g of cefazolin in one dose).[23] The percutaneous method begins with an endoscope into a stomach distended with air. An introducer catheter is inserted where the light beam from the endoscope can be seen. The procedural steps of introducing the catheter are shown in Figure 7–2. Several other techniques are known but are outside the scope of the chapter.[2] Complications of PEG are rare (Table 7–5), but bleeding from submucosal vessels of the stomach may occur. Fortunately, iced saline lavage stops the bleeding. Other procedure-related complications are local infection and necrotizing fasciitis, but the morbidity associated with this procedure remains low (less than 10%). Pneumoperitoneum, occurring in 40% of patients, often has no clinical significance. In our study, aspiration

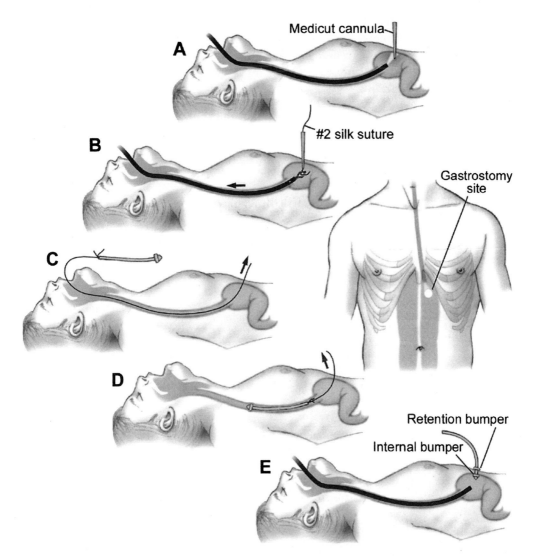

Figure 7–2. Percutaneous endoscopic gastrostomy placement.

Table 7–5. Complications of Percutaneous Endoscopic Gastrostomy and Jejunostomy Placement*

Colocutaneous fistula
Gastric outlet obstruction
Bleeding from submucosal lesions
Ileus
Necrotizing fasciitis
Stoma leakage
Wound and skin infection
Volvulus

*Most complications are minor and occur within the first 3 months of placement.

pneumonia occurred in 1 of 10 patients who had a PEG placement, but occlusion or accidental removal was uncommon. Removal of the PEG tube and oral feeding were possible in one of four patients with acute stroke and equally common in those with hemispheric or brain stem lesions.[55]

PARENTERAL NUTRITION

Parenteral nutrition is not a common procedure in the NICU, although some investigators in clinical nutrition favor early initiation of total parenteral nutrition. The decision depends on the underlying nutritional state and metabolic rate and whether enteral nutrition (the preferred method) is poorly tolerated.[50] Parenteral nutrition is complex, carries many more complications, and requires close monitoring of laboratory variables.

Subclavian vein cannulation on the right side to diminish the risk of damage to the thoracic duct is the preferred access when parenteral nutrition is considered (the approach and procedure are outside the scope of this book). Many institutions use triple-lumen catheters. The care of these catheters must include changing over a guide wire regularly to minimize the risk of catheter-related sepsis. Although recorded data are conflicting on the increased risk of infection in triple-lumen catheters over that in single-lumen catheters, colonization remains low (4% to 5%). (Catheter sepsis is further discussed in Chapter 33.) Maintenance of the catheter includes heparin flushes (10 units/mL), frequent change of transparent adherent dressings, and meticulous skin antisepsis with povidone-iodine.

The composition of a parenteral formula requires consultation from nutritional support services. However, parenteral nutritional solutions are easily available and meet individual patient needs.

Energy requirements are again calculated from the total daily calories estimated by the Harris-Benedict equation or indirect calorimetry. Protein requirements are typically about 1.5 g/kg per day, but in patients with acute dev-

Table 7–6. Formulation of Total Parenteral Nutrition Solution

Base solution	
40%–70% dextrose	500–1500 mL
8.5%–15% crystalline amino acids	500–1500 mL
Intravenous fat emulsion 10%	20–100 g
(200–500 mL 2–7 times/week)	
Add to each 1000 mL	
Sodium chloride	40–50 mEq
Potassium chloride	20–30 mEq
Potassium or sodium acid	15–30 mEq
phosphate (10–20 mm phosphorus)	
Magnesium sulfate	15–18 mEq
Calcium gluconate	4.6–9.2 mEq
Add to daily formulation	
Zinc sulfate, 5–10 mg; copper sulfate, 1–2 mg;	
selenium, 60 μg; chromium chloride, 10–20 μg;	
manganese chloride, 0.5 mg; iron dextran, 5 mg;	
and multivitamin infusion	
Add to any 1 liter 2 times a week	
Vitamin K	10 mg

astating central nervous system disorder, a hypermetabolic state, and insufficient caloric intake by enteral nutrition, protein in doses of 2.0 to 3.5 g/kg per day should be recommended. Fat must be provided in 500 mL aliquots of 10% emulsion, and the total dose of calories must be less than 60% of the total nonprotein calories. The basic components are (1) dextrose 50%, which provides 250 g in a 500 mL solution, (2) amino acid mixture of 8.5% in 500 mL bottles, and (3) 10% fat emulsion in 500 mL bottles. The formula is supplemented with standard electrolyte solutions, daily multivitamins, and trace elements. A basic formula is provided in Table 7–6.

A mechanical or metabolic complication is estimated to occur in approximately 50% of patients with parenteral nutrition.[38] The mechanical complications are often associated with placement of the catheter. The most important are pneumothorax, hemothorax, hydrothorax, chylothorax, and air embolism.

Complex metabolic problems may arise. The most fearful complication is hyperglycemia, often manifested as nonketotic hyperosmolar hyperglycemia. Well-established triggers of hyperglycemia are rapid infusion, decreased insulin output from diabetes, transient glucose resistance, and medication, particularly the use of corticosteroids. Coma from nonketotic hyperglycemia is expected when the serum glucose value reaches 1000 mg/dL and serum osmolarities approach values of 350 mOsm/L. Treatment includes insulin and, more importantly, rehydration and eventually change into a larger proportion of lipids. Hypophosphatemia occasionally occurs and may produce generalized muscle weakness and respiratory failure from diaphragmatic dysfunction. The most common electrolyte abnormality, however, is hyponatremia associated with large infusions of free water. This can be overcome simply by tailoring glucose infusions.[52] Practical guides have been published.[21]

CONCLUSIONS

- Energy requirement in the NICU is calculated by the Harris-Benedict formula and is based on weight, height, and age. Energy expenditure for men = 66.5 + 13.8W + 5H − 6.8A and for women = 655 + 9.6W + 1.8H − 4.7A. A stress factor of 20% can be introduced to counter increased caloric needs.
- Abnormal swallowing during evaluation is characterized by abnormal laryngeal rise, abnormal throat clearing, inefficient coughing, weak tongue protrusion, and abnormal vocal clarity.
- Enteral nutrition with nasogastric or duodenal placement is recommended. Continuous infusion is started at the rate of 25 mL/hour, the rate is gradually increased, and commercially available enteral formulas providing 1 kcal/mL are used.
- Percutaneous endoscopic gastrostomy is indicated in patients with persistent dysphagia for 2 to 3 weeks. The procedure can be considered for patients with repeated nasogastric tube extubations, patients with persistent coma from any cause, and patients with a severe brain stem stroke.
- Parenteral nutrition should be considered in patients who do not tolerate enteral nutrition.

REFERENCES

1. Aviv JE, Spitzer J, Cohen M, et al: Laryngeal adductor reflex and pharyngeal squeeze as predictors of laryngeal penetration and aspiration. *Laryngoscope* 112:338–341, 2002.

2. Baskin WN: Advances in enteral nutrition techniques. *Am J Gastroenterol* 87:1547–1553, 1992.

3. Benya R, Mobarhan S: Enteral alimentation: administration and complications. *J Am Coll Nutr* 10:209–219, 1991.

4. Boivin MA, Levy H: Gastric feeding with erythromy-

cin is equivalent to transpyloric feeding in the critically ill. *Crit Care Med* 29:2029–2030, 2001.

5. Bower RH: Nutritional and metabolic support of critically ill patients. *JPEN J Parenter Enteral Nutr* 14 Suppl:257S–259S, 1990.

6. Boyes RJ, Kruse JA: Nasogastric and nasoenteric intubation. *Crit Care Clin* 8:865–878, 1992.

7. Burns SM, Carpenter R, Truwit JD: Report on the development of a procedure to prevent placement of feeding tubes into the lungs using end-tidal CO_2 measurements. *Crit Care Med* 29:936–939, 2001.

8. Cabre E, Gassull MA: Complications of enteral feeding. *Nutrition* 9:1–9, 1993.

9. Cerra FB, Benitez MR, Blackburn GL, et al: Applied nutrition in ICU patients. A consensus statement of the American College of Chest Physicians. *Chest* 111:769–778, 1997.

10. Chapman MJ, Fraser RJ, Kluger MT, et al: Erythromycin improves gastric emptying in critically ill patients intolerant of nasogastric feeding. *Crit Care Med* 28:2334–2337, 2000.

11. Chen MY, Peele VN, Donati D, et al: Clinical and video-fluoroscopic evaluation of swallowing in 41 patients with neurologic disease. *Gastrointest Radiol* 17:95–98, 1992.

12. Ciocon JO, Galindo-Ciocon DJ, Tiessen C, et al: Continuous compared with intermittent tube feeding in the elderly. *JPEN J Parenter Enteral Nutr* 16:525–528, 1992.

13. Daniels SK, Ballo LA, Mahoney MC, et al: Clinical predictors of dysphagia and aspiration risk: outcome measures in acute stroke patients. *Arch Phys Med Rehabil* 81:1030–1033, 2000.

14. Davies AE, Kidd D, Stone SP, et al: Pharyngeal sensation and gag reflex in healthy subjects. *Lancet* 345:487–488, 1995.

15. Dees G: Difficult nasogastric tube insertions. *Emerg Med Clin North Am* 7:177–182, 1989.

16. De Jonghe B, Appere-DeVechi C, Fournier M, et al: A prospective survey of nutritional support practices in intensive care unit patients: What is prescribed? What is delivered? *Crit Care Med* 29:8–12, 2001.

17. Deutschman CS, Konstantinides FN, Raup S, et al: Physiological and metabolic response to isolated closed-head injury. Part 1: Basal metabolic state: correlations of metabolic and physiological parameters with fasting and stressed controls. *J Neurosurg* 64:89–98, 1986.

18. DiSario JA, Baskin WN, Brown RD, et al: Endoscopic approaches to enteral nutritional support. *Gastrointest Endosc* 55:901–908, 2002.

19. Gutierrez ED, Balfe DM: Fluoroscopically guided nasoenteric feeding tube placement: results of a 1-year study. *Radiology* 178:759–762, 1991.

20. Han TR, Paik NJ, Park JW: Quantifying swallowing function after stroke: a functional dysphagia scale based on videofluoroscopic studies. *Arch Phys Med Rehabil* 82:677–682, 2001.

21. Hamilton H: *Total Parenteral Nutrition: A Practical Guide for Nurses.* Edinburgh: Churchill Livingstone, 2000.

22. Ibrahim EH, Mehringer L, Prentice D, et al: Early versus late enteral feeding of mechanically ventilated patients: results of a clinical trial. *J Parenter Enteral Nutr* 26:174–181, 2002.

23. Jain NK, Larson DE, Schroeder KW, et al: Antibiotic prophylaxis for percutaneous endoscopic gastrostomy. A prospective, randomized, double-blind clinical trial. *Ann Intern Med* 107:824–828, 1987.

24. Johnson ER, McKenzie SW, Rosenquist CJ, et al: Dysphagia following stroke: quantitative evaluation of pharyngeal transit times. *Arch Phys Med Rehabil* 73:419–423, 1992.

25. Kao CH, ChangLai SP, Chieng PU, et al: Gastric emptying in head-injured patients. *Am J Gastroenterol* 93:1108–1112, 1998.

26. Kirby DF: As the gut churns: feeding challenges in the head-injured patient (letter to the editor). *JPEN J Parenter Enteral Nutr* 20:1–2, 1996.

27. Kirby DF, Clifton GL, Turner H, et al: Early enteral nutrition after brain injury by percutaneous endoscopic gastrojejunostomy. *JPEN J Parenter Enteral Nutr* 15:298–302, 1991.

28. Kirby DF, Craig RM, Tsang TK, et al: Percutaneous endoscopic gastrostomies: a prospective evaluation and review of the literature. *JPEN J Parenter Enteral Nutr* 10:155–159, 1986.

29. Kittinger JW, Sandler RS, Heizer WD: Efficacy of metoclopramide as an adjunct to duodenal placement of small-bore feeding tubes: a randomized, placebo-controlled, double-blind study. *JPEN J Parenter Enteral Nutr* 11:33–37, 1987.

30. Klein S, Kinney J, Jeejeebhoy K, et al: Nutrition support in clinical practice: review of published data and recommendations for future research directions. Summary of a conference sponsored by the National Institutes of Health, American Society for Parenteral and Enteral Nutrition, and American Society for Clinical Nutrition. *Am J Clin Nutr* 66:683–706, 1997.

31. Koch KJ, Becker GJ, Edwards MK, et al: Intracranial placement of a nasogastric tube. *AJNR* 10:443–444, 1989.

32. Koretz RL: Nutritional supplementation in the ICU. How critical is nutrition for the critically ill? *Am J Respir Crit Care Med* 151:570–573, 1995.

33. Manchikanti L, Colliver JA, Marrero TC, et al: Ranitidine and metoclopramide for prophylaxis of aspiration pneumonitis in elective surgery. *Anesth Analg* 63:903–910, 1984.

34. Mann G, Hankey GJ, Cameron D: Swallowing function after stroke: prognosis and prognostic factors at 6 months. *Stroke* 30:744–748, 1999.

35. McLean J, Manchip S: Wernicke's encephalopathy induced by magnesium depletion (letter to the editor). *Lancet* 353:1768, 1999.

36. Mentec H, Dupont H, Bocchetti M, et al: Upper digestive intolerance during enteral nutrition in critically ill patients: frequency, risk factors, and complications. *Crit Care Med* 29:2033–2034, 2001.

37. Metheny N: Minimizing respiratory complications of nasoenteric tube feedings: state of the science. *Heart Lung* 22:213–223, 1993.
38. Mughal MM: Complications of intravenous feeding catheters. *Br J Surg* 76:15–21, 1989.
39. Norton B, Homer-Ward M, Donnelly MT, et al: A randomised prospective comparison of percutaneous endoscopic gastrostomy and nasogastric tube feeding after acute dysphagic stroke. *BMJ* 312:13–16, 1996.
40. Norton JA, Ott LG, McClain C, et al: Intolerance to enteral feeding in the brain-injured patient. *J Neurosurg* 68:62–66, 1988.
41. Ott L, McClain C, Young B: Nutrition and severe brain injury. *Nutrition* 5:75–79, 1989.
42. Payne-James J: Enteral nutrition: accessing patients. *Nutrition* 8:223–231, 1992.
43. Pinilla JC, Samphire J, Arnold C, et al: Comparison of gastrointestinal tolerance to two enteral feeding protocols in critically ill patients: a prospective, randomized controlled trial. *JPEN J Parenter Enteral Nutr* 25:81–86, 2001.
44. Ritz MA, Fraser R, Tam W, et al: Impacts and patterns of disturbed gastrointestinal function in critically ill patients. *Am J Gastroenterol* 95:3044–3052, 2000.
45. Robbins J, Levine RL, Maser A, et al: Swallowing after unilateral stroke of the cerebral cortex. *Arch Phys Med Rehabil* 74:1295–1300, 1993.
46. Roubenoff RA, Borel CO, Hanley DF: Hypermetabolism and hypercatabolism in Guillain-Barré syndrome. *JPEN J Parenter Enteral Nutr* 16:464–472, 1992.
47. Salasidis R, Fleiszer T, Johnston R: Air insufflation technique of enteral tube insertion: a randomized, controlled trial. *Crit Care Med* 26:1036–1039, 1998.
48. Sax HC, Souba WW: Enteral and parenteral feedings. Guidelines and recommendations. *Med Clin North Am* 77:863–880, 1993.
49. Schlichtig R, Sargent SC: Nutritional support of the mechanically ventilated patient. *Crit Care Clin* 6:767–784, 1990.
50. Skaer TL: Total parenteral nutrition: clinical considerations. *Clin Ther* 15:272–282, 1993.
51. Stern MA, Wolf DC: Erythromycin as a prokinetic agent: a prospective, randomized, controlled study of efficacy in nasoenteric tube placement. *Am J Gastroenterol* 89:2011–2013, 1994.
52. Sunyecz L, Mirtallo JM: Sodium imbalance in a patient receiving total parenteral nutrition. *Clin Pharm* 12:138–149, 1993.
53. Teasell RW, Bach D, McRae M: Prevalence and recovery of aspiration poststroke: a retrospective analysis. *Dysphagia* 9:35–39, 1994.
54. Van den Berghe G, Wouters P, Weekers F, et al: Intensive insulin therapy in critically ill patients. *N Engl J Med* 345:1359–1367, 2001.
55. Wijdicks EFM, McMahon MM: Percutaneous endoscopic gastrostomy after acute stroke: complications and outcome. *Cerebrovasc Dis* 9:109–111, 1999.
56. Yanagawa T, Bunn F, Roberts I, et al: Nutritional support for head-injured patients. *Cochrane Database Syst Rev* 2:2000.
57. Young B, Ott L, Phillips R, et al: Metabolic management of the patient with head injury. *Neurosurg Clin N Am* 2:301–320, 1991.
58. Young B, Ott L, Yingling B, et al: Nutrition and brain injury. *J Neurotrauma* 9 Suppl 1:S375–S383, 1992.
59. Zaloga GP, Marik P: Promotility agents in the intensive care unit. *Crit Care Med* 28:2657–2659, 2000.

8

Anticoagulation and Thrombolytic Therapy

Two major issues can be emphasized in summarizing the use of anticoagulation and, more recently, thrombolytic agents in the clinical practice of critical care neurology. First, anticoagulants for patients with acute neurologic illness can be divided into prevention of deep venous thrombosis (and its obviously more relevant potential complication of pulmonary embolization) and prevention of further clot formation or propagation in acute embolic occlusion of a major cerebral artery. Appropriate use of anticoagulants is of importance in only a few acute neurologic conditions. The evidence of its effect is not robust, in some conditions relatively weak or nonexistent. Second, intra-arterial thrombolytic agents are becoming a promising intervention at an early stage of acute ischemic stroke, particularly in occlusions involving the posterior cerebral circulation.

This chapter reviews the clinical guidelines for anticoagulation, the daily management of heparin infusion, the use of oral anticoagulants, and the indications for use of thrombolytic agents. Adequate knowledge of the concepts underpinning the use of these agents is needed before they are administered.

INDICATIONS FOR PROPHYLACTIC ANTICOAGULATION

The actual occurrence of venous thrombosis and pulmonary emboli is probably more frequent than the neurologic literature suggests and is, for the most part, preventable. Although the efficacy of heparin in the prevention of deep venous thrombosis is undisputed, in the intensive care unit, the overall risk of deep venous thrombosis with subcutaneous administration of low-dose heparin is 5% to 15% in the first week.[5] The risk of deep venous thrombosis can be substantial in patients with a brief stay in the NICU who did not receive prophylaxis. The risk of deep venous thrombosis may also be determined by the patient mix in the NICU (trauma or nontrauma). Deep venous thrombosis often develops in a paralyzed leg (or legs in Guillain-Barré syndrome or acute spinal cord disorder). Subcutaneous heparin substantially reduces the risk of deep venous thrombosis and pulmonary embolism when given to patients with ischemic stroke.[59] Intracerebral hematomas do not necessarily preclude use of subcutaneous heparin. A study of subcutaneous heparin in patients with intracerebral hematoma found that pulmonary embolism was significantly reduced without increased risk of hemorrhagic complications (deep venous thrombosis was monitored with phleboscintigraphy of erythrocytes labeled in vitro, and pulmonary perfusion scans were done in instances of clinical suspicion).[13]

However, pneumatic compression devices have similarly significantly reduced the incidence of venous thrombosis postoperatively[17,19] but have not been rigorously tested in the NICU population with the exception of elective neurosurgical patients.[101] Pneumatic compression devices compress the calves and markedly increase venous flow velocity.

The reduction in deep venous thrombosis and pulmonary embolus with intermittent pneumatic compression devices is similar to that with low-dose heparin and may be a safer alternative in patients with spontaneous or traumatic hematoma. One study comparing historical controls with stroke patients suggested that these devices should be used in combination with a heparin regimen; with this approach, deep venous thrombosis occurred in 0.2% of 432 patients and there were no pulmonary emboli.[57]

Generally, venous thromboembolism is most effectively prevented with low doses of unfractionated heparin (5000 units subcutaneously every 12 hours) until the patient is ambulatory. Patients with a history of recurrent venous thrombosis should receive the low-molecular-weight heparin enoxaparin, 30 mg subcutaneously every 12 hours. Aspirin, although appealing, or a low dose of warfarin (1 mg) cannot be recommended yet and awaits further evaluation of safety and efficacy.

In most of our patients, however, we have been using pneumatic compression devices to prevent deep venous thrombosis. These devices provide more comfort than twice-daily subcutaneous injections, but they have to remain in place much of the day. (They are disconnected during transport and procedures.) Pneumatic compression devices are generally well tolerated. These devices are probably not sufficient in preventive action in patients with a high risk of venous thromboembolism (previous deep venous thrombosis, underlying malignant disease, or expectation of major surgery, e.g., orthopedic surgery for fractures in patients with multitrauma) or thrombophilia. (Patients with a genetic predisposition to thrombosis usually have the first thrombotic event before age 45.[94]) Subcutaneous heparin is warranted.

INDICATIONS FOR THERAPEUTIC ANTICOAGULATION

The effectiveness of heparin in evolving acute ischemic hemispheric stroke or in acute basilar artery occlusion remains unclear.[69] In approximately 25% of patients, further progression of hemiparesis occurs while activated partial thromboplastin time (APTT) is prolonged.[37] In fact, one critical overview of antithrombotic therapy in acute ischemic stroke did not indicate that heparin is sufficiently effective to prevent further deterioration.[91] The evidence is also less conclusive about the target of APTT.

Not all patients with an acute ischemic stroke need to be treated with intravenous heparin, and treatment depends on the underlying mechanism. Patients with a high likelihood of a cardiogenic embolus are at significant risk for recurrence. Typically, this pertains to patients with atrial fibrillation, acute myocardial infarction, or demonstrated evidence of intracardiac thrombus or a large akinetic ventricular segment.

Heparin must also be considered in patients with a critical stenosis or acute occlusion of the carotid or vertebral artery. Acute carotid occlusion has a risk of embolization from the carotid stump and justifies anticoagulation for at least 4 weeks.[81] For high-grade stenosis of the basilar artery or recent acute basilar artery occlusion in association with recent ischemic stroke in the posterior circulation, heparin administration is considered by many to be standard therapy, but there is virtually no evidence of a beneficial effect. Thrombolytic agents may be much more promising in this clinical situation. Suggested indications for heparinization in acute ischemic stroke are summarized in Table 8–1.

HEPARIN

The main mechanism of action of heparin is binding with antithrombin III. This binding enhances its inhibiting activity of not only throm-

Table 8–1. Indications for Heparin in Patients with Acute Stroke Admitted to the Neurologic Intensive Care Unit

Cardiogenic ischemic stroke
Carotid or vertebral artery dissection
Acute carotid artery occlusion (or high-grade critical stenosis)
Acute basilar artery occlusion (or high-grade critical stenosis)
Crescendo transient ischemic attacks
Cerebral venous thrombosis

bin and factor Xa but also factors IXa, XIa, and XIIa.

Intravenous administration of heparin results in an anticoagulant response that is variable and unpredictable. In the conventional approach, an intravenous bolus of 5000 units is followed by continuous intravenous infusion of heparin (maintenance dose range of 20,000 to 40,000 units per 24 hours). It is universally recommended that heparin be monitored by APTT, with a predefined range of 1.5 to 2.0 times the mean control value. (In most laboratories, this is equivalent to 50 to 75 seconds.)

The most important concerns in use of heparin are the time required to reach this therapeutic range and bleeding complications that result from excessive anticoagulation. Nomograms for adjustment of heparin dose have been suggested. Raschke et al.[88] found that a weight-based nomogram was superior to any other standard care nomogram proposed earlier. In the weight-based nomogram, tested in patients with a wide variety of diagnoses, the mean time to reach the therapeutic range was 8 hours, whereas this time was 20 hours in the standard nomogram. The therapeutic threshold was achieved in 86% of the patients on the first drawn sample for APTT compared with

32% in the standard group. Major bleeding complications did not occur in this comparatively small series of 62 patients treated with this protocol. Confirmatory studies are required in the intensive care unit patient population.

It is well known from hospital audits that dosage of heparin is often inadequate. The bioavailability of heparin is poor through rapid clearance and binding to many plasma proteins when initial therapeutic doses are administered.[28] However, with the use of an intravenous bolus, the biologic half-life increases significantly (Fig. 8–1). Thus, when immediate anticoagulation must be achieved (e.g., pulmonary embolus), it is important to initiate heparin with an intravenous bolus. An example of a dosing regimen is shown in Table 8–2.[25] (An alternative protocol is described by Hirsh et al.[51,52])

The major risk of heparin is hemorrhage, at any site, that can be fatal. It has not been consistently found that excessive prolongation of APTT exclusively increases this risk. Additional predictive factors of heparin-induced bleeding are serious underlying illness, chronic alcohol abuse, renal failure, and administration of heparin by intermittent doses. Bleeding from heparin is possible at any location but often occurs in the gastrointestinal tract. However, acute gastrointestinal bleeding is often associated with ulcers, and endoscopic evaluation may reveal a significant gastrointestinal lesion. A less common, but life-threatening, complication is bilateral adrenal hemorrhage,[47,96] which unfortunately has also been reported with prophylactic use of subcutaneous administration of heparin. It must be considered when shock suddenly develops without overt evidence of blood loss in any anticoagulated patient. Retroperitoneal hemorrhage should be considered in patients with a rapid decrease in hematocrit and no other explanations for labile blood pressure. Retroperitoneal hemorrhage can be spontaneous or, less commonly, associated with cerebral angiography. (An abdominal computed tomography scan usually demonstrates a large-volume hematoma) (Fig. 8–2).

Equally serious hemorrhages are located in the brain and spinal cord. In acute ischemic

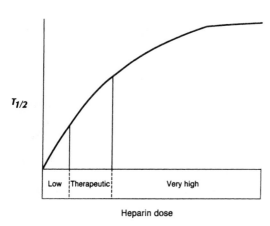

Figure 8–1. Clearance of heparin. Half-time increases with increasing doses. (From Hirsh J, Fuster V: Guide to anticoagulant therapy. Part 1: Heparin. *Circulation* 89:1449–1468, 1994. By permission of the American Heart Association.)

Table 8–2. Weight-Based Heparin Nomogram

Start:	Bolus of heparin, 80 units/kg IV		
	Heparin infusion, 18 units/kg per hour (20,000 units in 500 mL of D5W = 40 units/mL)		
Measure:	APTT 6 hours after bolus		
Adjust:	APTT, second	Bolus, U/kg	New infusion rate, U/kg/hour
	< 35	80	22
	35–45	40	20
	46–70	No	18
	71–90	No	16
	> 90	No	15 (stop after 1 hour)

Administration of warfarin, 10 mg, can be started on the second day of heparin therapy if long-term anticoagulation is warranted. Complete blood cell count with platelet count is done every 3 days.
D5W, 5% dextrose in water; APTT, activated partial thromboplastin time.
Source: Modified from Raschke et al.[88] By permission of the American College of Physicians.

stroke, intracranial hemorrhage has most often been associated with large middle cerebral artery territory involvement, occurring within 24 hours after initiation of heparinization and at times with excessive prolongation of APTT (> 150 seconds) (see Chapter 16). Amyloid an-giopathy, rather than older age alone, may be a predisposing factor.[90] A fatal hemorrhage during anticoagulation has been associated with cerebral amyloid angiopathy.[68] We have also seen heparin-associated intracranial he-matomas in patients with evidence of cav-

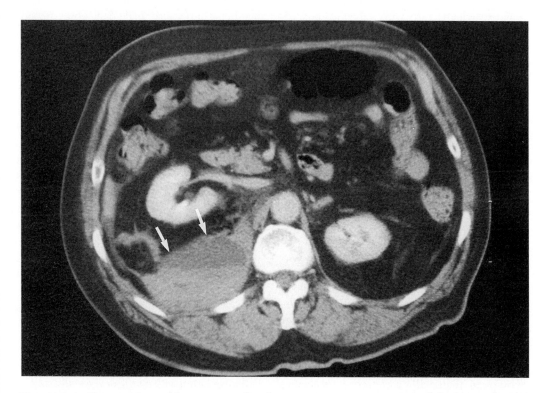

Figure 8–2. Retroperitoneal hematoma after heparin use, causing a marked decline in hematocrit and blood pressure (arrows).

ernous angioma at other locations on magnetic resonance imaging, which may suggest that in some patients an underlying lesion is present under these circumstances.

The safety profile of intravenous heparin in ischemic stroke, particularly the danger of hemorrhagic conversion with clinical progression or development of intracerebral hematoma, has not been well studied. Retrospective studies have suggested that this risk is very low.[6,80,87] The outcome of hemorrhagic conversion of brain infarcts in anticoagulated patients did not differ significantly from that in nonanticoagulated patients.[100] Discontinuation of therapy or adjustment of the heparin dose to a level lower than that aimed at originally is probably appropriate when ischemic infarcts convert to hemorrhagic, often petechial, infarcts.

Thrombocytopenia due to an immunologic drug reaction, another well-established complication of heparin treatment, is usually mild.[11] This complication can occur solely with flushing of an intravenous access with heparin. It is exceedingly rare with subcutaneous administration of heparin.[53] It occurs 5 to 10 days after heparin treatment and more often in patients with previous heparin treatment. The incidence of thrombocytopenia associated with therapeutic use of heparin is approximately 2%. Heparin should be replaced by hirudin (lepirudin) in a loading dose of 0.4 mg/kg by intravenous bolus followed by 0.15 mg/kg per hour intravenously to reach an APTT 1.5 to 2.5 times the normal range.[51]

Although anticoagulation can be greatly simplified with low-molecular-weight heparin (LMWH), the three products (dalteparin, enoxaparin, and ardeparin) available in the United States have been approved only for prophylaxis of deep venous thrombosis.[24,65,77] In 1998, enoxaparin was approved by the Food and Drug Administration for treatment of venous thromboembolism. It is also approved for unstable angina and non-Q-wave myocardial infarction. One study showed that the rate of deep venous thrombosis was 59% less with enoxaparin than with compression stockings alone.[3] The recommended dose of enoxaparin is 30 mg subcutaneously twice daily for pro-

phylaxis of deep venous thrombosis. All three LMWH products have different pharmacologic effects because methods of preparation and molecular structures differ.[12,21,86] The primary mechanism of action of LMWH is binding to antithrombin III. One of the fundamental differences between LMWH and standard heparin is less significant neutralization by platelet factor 4, which is released after platelet activation. (Platelet factor 4 competitively inhibits the binding to antithrombin III, and this effect reduces the anticoagulant effect.)

Low-molecular-weight heparin has greater bioavailability, indicated by longer plasma half-life, less variability in the anticoagulant response, and fewer or equally frequent hemorrhagic complications.[76] Side effects of LMWH are thrombocytopenia (which may be related to the nature of each individual LMWH), transient increase in liver enzymes, and skin necrosis that has been interpreted as toxic epidermal neurolysis.[79] Low-molecular-weight heparin is much easier to use than heparin because single daily doses are sufficient and monitoring is not necessary. Currently, its use in the treatment of deep venous thrombosis and various other cardiovascular diseases, including stroke, is under investigation.[30,84,92] Although a large randomized study of Org-10172 in acute ischemic stroke did not show a benefit, a subgroup of patients with large artery atherosclerosis seemed to benefit.[2] The LMWH certoparin did not improve outcome in ischemic stroke.[29] In a recent study, high-dose tinzaparin was not superior to aspirin and resulted in a higher incidence of intracerebral hematomas.[9] With these credible trials of different LMWHs, these agents have no role in the treatment of stroke. For now, the main objection to LMWH is cost (three times more expensive than standard heparin) unless it can be offset by reduced hospital and intensive care unit stay.

WARFARIN

Anticoagulation with warfarin is usually started 2 or 3 days after initiation of heparin therapy. Coumarins act by inhibiting the synthesis of factors II, VII, IX, and X, but several days are required for these vitamin K-dependent anticoagulants to clear from the plasma. When the international normalized ratio (INR) is therapeutic, an overlap of 2 days with heparin is recommended before administration of heparin is discontinued.

The first- and second-day doses of warfarin are 10 mg and 5 mg, respectively, and subsequent oral doses are adjusted to achieve the desired INR (Table 8–3). (A full report of the Sixth Consensus Conference of the American College of Chest Physicians has been published.[95]) A consensus meeting concluded that in patients with small-to-moderate-sized ischemic strokes, an INR of 2.0 to 3.0 was reasonable, but the recommendation for this range of prothrombin time prolongation is derived from expert opinion only. When ischemic strokes are associated with antiphospholipid antibody syndrome, higher INRs (3.0 to 3.5) are recommended,[61] because the risk of recurrence is high with lower INRs. An INR of 2.5 to 3.5 is recommended in ischemic stroke associated with mechanical valves.[52]

The risk that bleeding will develop in patients receiving warfarin who have an INR of 3.0 or higher is 1 in 14/year (serious hemorrhage, 1 in 50/year). Age is not an important determinant of bleeding until 80 years of age

Table 8–4. Commonly Used Drugs That Potentiate or Interfere with the Action of Warfarin

Potentiator	Inhibitor
Acetaminophen	Barbiturates
Amiodarone	Carbamazepine
Anesthetics	Chlordiazepoxide
Chloramphenicol	Cholestyramine
Cimetidine	Corticosteroids
Diazoxide	Griseofulvin
Erythromycin	Haloperidol
Fluconazole	Meprobamate
Indomethacin	Nafcillin
L-Methyldopa	Rifampin
Metronidazole	Sucralfate
Miconazole	Tetracyclines
Omeprazole	
Phenylbutazone	
Phenytoin	
Piroxicam	
Propranolol	
Tolbutamide	
Trimethoprim- sulfamethoxazole	

or older. Intensity of anticoagulation is a strong predictor of warfarin-associated bleeding, most commonly located in the gastrointestinal tract.[38] A rare complication of warfarin is warfarin-induced skin necrosis, usually 3 days after initiation. This localized patch of tissue necrosis, often in thighs, breasts, and buttocks, may need skin grafting.[20] Another rare complication is "purple toe syndrome" from embolization of microemboli in patients with ulcerated aortic plaques. In occasional patients, an impressive livedo reticularis is seen.[55]

Excessive INRs with warfarin use most commonly indicate vitamin K deficiency or interaction with pharmaceutical agents. Drug interactions with warfarin are numerous, and the most relevant are summarized in Table 8–4.

THROMBOLYTIC THERAPY

Thrombolysis is not a novel therapy, and its applications have included acute myocardial infarction, massive pulmonary embolus, and peripheral arterial thrombi.[41,42,62,66]

Table 8–3. International Normalized Ratio Recommendations for Various Indications

Indication	International Normalized Ratio
Prophylaxis of deep venous thrombosis	2.0–3.0
Treatment of venous thrombosis	2.0–3.0
Treatment of pulmonary embolism	2.0–3.0
Atrial fibrillation	2.0–3.0
Tissue heart valves	2.0–3.0
Acute ischemic stroke or transient ischemic attacks	2.0–3.0
Antiphospholipid antibody syndrome	3.0–3.5
Mechanical prosthetic valves	2.5–3.5

Source: Data from Dalen JE, Hirsh J, Guyatt GH (Guest Editors): Sixth ACCP Consensus Conference on Antithrombotic Therapy. *Chest* 119 Suppl:S1–S430, 2001.

Thrombolytic therapy can induce complete dissolution of emboli. The mechanism of action is activation of the proteolytic enzyme plasminogen followed by fibrin dissolution and increasing fibrinogen degradation products.

The initial results with intravenous thrombolytic agents in acute carotid territory stroke were far from satisfactory because of recanalization in only one-third of the patients and a 10% incidence of clinical deterioration associated with hemorrhagic conversions, including intracerebral hematoma.[27,46,72,102,107] However, intravenous thrombolysis has been studied in several clinical trials, which have yielded important clinically relevant information. Three studies with streptokinase were discontinued prematurely because of a high frequency of bleeding complications and mortality in treated patients.[31,73,74] Recent European studies (European Cooperative Acute Stroke Study and Second European-Australasian Acute Stroke Study) found a threefold increase in parenchymal hemorrhage and only a subtle improvement in functional disability.[43,44]

A study of recombinant tPA in stroke from the National Institute of Neurological Disorders and Stroke further defined the role of tPA in acute stroke.[75] Within 3 hours of onset of stroke, tPA (Activase) was administered intravenously in a dose of 0.9 mg/kg (maximum, 90 mg), 10% of the total dose in a bolus and 90% in a constant infusion for 1 hour. This study consisted of two parts. The first part, which included 291 patients studied in double-blind, randomized fashion without angiographic confirmation, did not show any short-term benefit. In this part of the study, neurologic improvement in 24 hours (defined as complete resolution of a neurologic deficit or an improvement of four points or more in the National Institutes of Health Stroke Scale) did not differ significantly from that in patients treated with placebo. In the second part (333 patients), however, there was a 10% to 13% absolute increase in improvement at 3 months on several disability and handicap scales. Mortality was similar between the groups, but symptomatic intracerebral hematoma within 36 hours occurred significantly more often in the treated

group (6.4%) than in the placebo group (0.6%). These results were confirmed by the European Cooperative Acute Stroke Study I and II trials. Only a small proportion of patients were eligible for intravenously administered tPA. Exclusion was due to uncertain time of onset, interval of more than 3 hours, and clinical improvement.[7] Intravenously administered tPA significantly increased intracerebral hemorrhage when administered more than 3 hours after onset.[16] The thrombolysis meta-analysis by Wardlaw for the Cochrane Stroke Group has recently been published (Fig. 8–3). This analysis concluded that taking into account fatal cerebral hemorrhage, the overall net benefit of intravenous tPA was very significant. It is summarized in a memorable statement: "For every 1000 patients treated with i.v. rt-PA, 57 avoided death or dependence when treated up to 6 hours after stroke, and 140 when treated within 3 hours of stroke."[103]

A more attractive therapy is intra-arterial infusion of a thrombolytic agent aimed directly at the clot.[36] The cerebral angiogram allows for clear visualization of the obstructing clot and thus provides an additional justification for thrombolytic agents. There is much interest in development of laser-mediated thrombus fragmentation, suction thrombectomy, and other mechanical techniques. In our experience, fragmentation of the clot has been feasible in recently formed clots due to an invasive procedure[106] or in those originating from the venous system, such as in a stroke in a patient with patent foramen ovale. Most often, intra-arterial thrombolysis is mastered by interventional neuroradiologists, and they should be available at very short notice. In addition, up to 1 hour may be required to set up an angiographic study and catheterize the clot (Fig. 8–4). After a routine cerebral angiogram, a catheter with multiple side holes to maximize thrombolysis is advanced inside the clot. Recanalization and immediate clinical improvement can be achieved in a much larger proportion of patients. Failure to recanalize can result if the catheter tip is between the clot and the vessel wall, is in a "plaque-dominant" occlusion, or involves a lengthy thrombus[14] (Fig. 8–4).

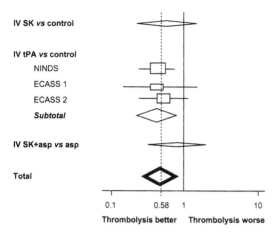

Figure 8–3. Death or dependency (modified Rankin 3-6) by the end of follow-up. Patients were treated within 3 hours of stroke. asp, aspirin; ECASS 1, European Cooperative Acute Stroke Study; ECASS 2, Second European-Australasian Acute Stroke Study; IV, intravenous; NINDS, National Institute of Neurological Disorders and Stroke; SK, streptokinase; tPA, tissue plasminogen activator. (From Wardlaw.[103] By permission of the American Academy of Neurology.)

Theoretically, the risk of hemorrhage should be lower in intra-arterial thrombolysis because uninvolved vessels are not infused, but in 5% to 17% of the patients, an intracerebral hematoma (and not petechial hemorrhagic conversion) complicated the procedure.[22] The mortality is high (83%). Risk factors have not been clearly identified except for hyperglycemia (> 200 mg/dL). (Hyperglycemia may promote vascular rupture after reperfusion or further damages the blood–brain barrier.[58]) Reperfusion may not be the sole mechanism for hemorrhagic conversion, because hemorrhagic conversion has been reported with persistent occlusion.[78] Reperfusion may come from contribution of the collateral circulation (see Chapter 16).

As a general guideline, thrombolysis should be started before 6 hours in the carotid artery territory[104] (Table 8–5) and 12 hours in the vertebrobasilar artery territory[82] (Table 8–6).

However, the interval between presenting symptoms and infusion remains uncertain, and data are based on use of urokinase, no longer commercially available in the United States.

Typically, a baseline activated clotting time is obtained and 2000 U of heparin is administered as a bolus. A heparin bolus is used at 20-minute intervals to maintain the activated clotting time at 180–220 seconds. Usually, an rt-PA infusion of 20 mg is prepared and mixed with normal saline for a total volume of 50 mL. Initially, the infusion rate is 1–5 mg per hour, and more is infused until recanalization. The maximal dose has not been defined, but hemorrhagic complications further increase when the dose of rt-PA reaches 20 mg.

The fibrinogen level can be monitored and should not decrease below 100 mg/dL. Nonetheless, monitoring of thrombolytic therapy

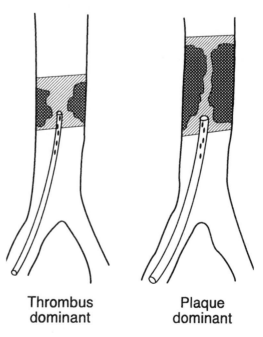

Thrombus dominant **Plaque dominant**

Figure 8–4. Technique of intra-arterial catheterization. A catheter (preferably with multiple side holes) is advanced into the obstructing clot. Two possible occlusions are shown: thrombus dominant and plaque dominant.

Table 8–5. Outcome in Patients Who Have Carotid Territory Stroke Treated with Intra-arterial Thrombolysis

Study	No. of Patients	Agent	Good Outcome (%)*	Dead (%)
Mori et al., 1988[71]	22	UK	70	14
del Zoppo et al., 1988[26]	20	SK/UK	33	11
Theron et al., 1989[98]	12	SK/UK	67	8
Ezura and Kagawa, 1992[35]	11	UK	29	0
Zeumer et al., 1993[108]	33	tPA/UK	32	24
Barnwell et al., 1994[8]	10	UK	71	30
Higashida et al., 1994[48]	27	UK	67	33
Sasaki et al., 1995[93]	35	tPA/UK	46	3
Jahan et al., 1999[56]	26	UK	48	31
Edwards et al., 1999[33]	11	UK	56	27
Suarez et al., 1999[97]	54	UK	48	24
Pillai et al., 2001[83]	27	UK	48	NA
Arnold et al., 2002[4]	100	UK	68	10

NA, not available; SK, streptokinase; tPA, tissue plasminogen activator; UK, urokinase.
*Recanalization only shown; includes patients who improved.
Source: Modified from Wechsler and Jungreis.[104] By permission of WB Saunders Company.

remains difficult, and the predictive value of these blood markers has been poorly studied. (In studies of acute myocardial infarction, levels of plasma fibrinogen, fibrinogen degradation product, and plasminogen did not correlate with hemorrhagic complication. On the other hand, elevation of thrombin-antithrombin III complex [> 6 ng/L] strongly predicted unsuccessful thrombolysis.[50])

The Prolyse in Acute Cerebral Thromboembolism II trial enrolled 180 patients (from 12,323 screened patients and 474 with cerebral angiograms) who had a median National Institutes of Health Stroke Scale score of 17 and M_1 or M_2 middle cerebral artery occlusion.[39] Nine milligrams of recombinant prourokinase and heparin was compared with heparin alone within 6 hours of ictus. At 3 months, 40% of the patients who received thrombolysis had a modified Rankin score of 2 or less (slight or no neurologic disability) compared with 25% in the control group. The frequency of intracranial hematoma was 10% in the treated group and 2% in the control group, and the high frequency may be related to additional use of heparin. Recanalization occurred in 66% of the patients receiving the combination of prourokinase and heparin but in only 19% of the controls.

The treatment of acute occlusion of the intracranial internal carotid artery at the level of its bifurcation (T-type occlusion) has been disappointing. It has led some experts to consider exclusion from thrombolysis.[40] These large emboli are considered of aged thrombotic material that could be less responsive to thrombolytic agents. Nevertheless, we were successful in a young patient with infusion less than 3 hours from stroke onset, and others reported 33% good outcome with this type of occlusion.[85]

An alternative approach is combined intravenous and intra-arterial thrombolysis.[49,60] Intravenously administered tPA in a reduced dose of 0.6 mg/kg over 30 minutes within 3 hours of onset is combined with intra-arterial tPA, 0.3 mg/kg in a 2-hour infusion within 6 hours of onset. The Cincinnati and University of California, Los Angeles, studies both documented feasibility, but safety and outcome remain unknown.[34] The major potential for this intravenous–intra-arterial combination may be provisional treatment of patients transferred to tertiary care centers.

Table 8–6. Summary of Reported Series of Thrombolysis in Vertebrobasilar Occlusion

References	No. of Patients	Agent and Method	RECANALIZATION		GOOD COLLATERAL CIRCULATION		HEMORRHAGIC COMPLICATIONS		GOOD OUTCOME		DEATH	
			No.	*%*	*No.*	*%*	*No.*	*%*	*No.*	*%*	*No.*	*%*
Hacke et al., 1988[45]	43	IA UK and SK	19	44	NA		4	9	10	23	30	70
Matsumoto and Satoh, 1991[67]	10	IA UK	4	40	1	13°	NA		4	40	3	30
Zeumer et al., 1993[108]	28	IA UK and tPA	21	75	NA		2	7	7	25	10	36
Huemer et al., 1995[54]	16	IV tPA	10	63	NA		2	13	3	19	11	69
Becker et al., 1996[10]	12	IA UK	10	83	NA		2	17	3	25	8	67
Brandt et al., 1996[14]	51	IA UK, IA tPA, and IV tPA	26	51	32	63	7	14	10	20	35	69
Wijdicks et al., 1997[105]	9	IA UK	7	78	NA		1	11	5	56	2	22
Cross et al., 1997[23]	20	IA UK	10	50	NA		3	15	4	20	13	65
Gonner et al., 1998[40]	10	IA UK	5	50	5	50	1	10	5	50	4	40
Pillai et al., 2001[83]	10	IA UK	9	90	NA		NA		NA		NA	

IA, intra-arterial; IV, intravenous; NA, not available; SK, streptokinase; tPA, tissue plasminogen activator; UK, urokinase.
°Percentage is based on eight patients because the collateral circulation of two patients was described as unknown by the authors.
Source: Phan and Wijdicks.[82] By permission of WB Saunders Company.

Our experience with intra-arterial thrombolysis is encouraging, and we offer this still very experimental therapy, when appropriate, to patients with occlusion of large intracranial arteries (e.g., middle cerebral artery occlusion and acute basilar artery occlusion). Intravenous tPA therapy should generally be considered in patients with symptoms within 3 hours of onset, but when feasible we commonly proceed with a cerebral angiogram to define the anatomical localization.

The contraindications for thrombolysis are listed in Table 8–7. A hyperdense middle cerebral artery sign in a patient with a major neurologic deficit predicts poor clinical outcome after use of thrombolysis.[99] Hypodensity on CT is associated with much worse outcome, although recent analysis of the PROACT II (Prolyse in Acute Cerebral Thromboembolism) study suggests it is not.[89] How much hypodensity to allow in tPA is unknown, but we are reluctant to proceed in patients with early hemispheric (frontotemporal or cerebellar) edema with early appearance of a hypodensity involving more than a third of the territory. Blood pressure is carefully controlled with intravenous administration of labetalol if readings remain persistently high (e.g., mean arterial pressure >120 mm Hg). The use of thrombolysis is further discussed in Chapters 16 and 17.

Another promising drug is the platelet glycoprotein IIb/IIIa inhibitor abciximab. Abciximab is administered intravenously in a bolus injection of 0.2 mg/kg followed by an infusion at 0.05 μg/kg per minute for 12 hours. A demonstrated beneficial effect in maintaining coronary patency after stenting and thrombolysis in

Table 8–7. Suggested Contraindications for Intra-arterial Thrombolytic Therapy

Interval from onset of stroke: intra-arterial > 6 hours in anterior circulation and > 12 hours in posterior circulation* (intravenous, > 3 hours)
Rapidly resolving neurologic signs
Treatment-refractory hypertension (mean arterial pressure > 120 mm Hg on several occasions)
Diffuse swelling and hypodensity of affected hemisphere‡
Computed tomographic evidence of hemorrhagic conversion
Fibrinogen < 100 mg/dL
Prothrombin time > 15 seconds
Platelets < 100,000
Recent history of gastrointestinal or genitourinary bleeding
Recent lumbar puncture
Pregnancy or lactation‡
Stroke within past 2 months
Surgical procedure within 30 days§

---

*One hour may be required for catheterization.
†The size of the hypodensity is a matter of debate.
‡With early pregnancy, may be given on a compassionate basis, assuming abortion is granted.
§Contraindication recently questioned.[15]

patients with myocardial infarction kindled interest for its potential in ischemic stroke.[70] Two case reports documented dissolution of the thrombus refractory to thrombolysis,[63,64] and a preliminary study in ischemic stroke showed a trend toward improvement.[1] The combination of abciximab and intra-arterial tPA was successful in 2 of 3 patients with occlusion in the posterior circulation.[32] Its role is entirely undetermined, and the drug may increase the risk of hemorrhage after thrombolysis. We and others have used it only in patients with small occlusive emboli during coiling, stenting, or angioplasty procedures.[18]

CONCLUSIONS

- Indications for intravenous heparin in acute ischemic stroke are cardiogenic ischemic stroke, carotid or vertebral artery dissection, acute carotid or basilar artery occlusion or high-grade critical stenosis, crescendo transient ischemic attacks, and cerebral venous thrombosis.
- Deep venous thrombosis can be minimized by 5000 units of heparin given subcutaneously twice a day. Enoxaparin, 30 mg twice a day, must be considered in high-risk patients.
- Heparin therapy is begun with 80 units/kg intravenously and is continued with 18 units/kg per hour. Activated partial thromboplastin time is determined 6 hours after an initial bolus, and the dose is adjusted.

- When indicated, administration of warfarin (10 mg) can be started on the second day of heparin therapy, and the dose is usually adjusted to INR 2.0 to 3.0. An INR of 3.0 to 4.5 is recommended in ischemic stroke associated with mechanical prosthetic valves. An INR of 3.0 to 3.5 is recommended in patients with antiphospholipid antibody syndrome associated with ischemic stroke.
- Intravenous administration of thrombolytic agents in acute carotid territory occlusion should be considered within 3 hours after onset.
- Intra-arterial thrombolysis should be considered in acute ischemic stroke involving large arterial territories if the patient is seen within 3 to 6 hours (anterior cerebral circulation) or 12 hours (posterior cerebral circulation) of onset.

REFERENCES

1. The Abciximab in Ischemic Stroke Investigators: Abciximab in acute ischemic stroke: a randomized, double-blind, placebo-controlled, dose-escalation study. *Stroke* 31:601–609, 2000.
2. Adams HP Jr, Bendixen BH, Leira E, et al: Antithrombotic treatment of ischemic stroke among patients with occlusion or severe stenosis of the internal carotid artery: a report of the Trial of Org 10172 in Acute Stroke Treatment (TOAST). *Neurology* 53:122–125, 1999.
3. Agnelli G, Piovella F, Buoncristiani P, et al: Enoxaparin plus compression stockings compared with compression stockings alone in the prevention of venous thromboembolism after elective neurosurgery. *N Engl J Med* 339:80–85, 1998.
4. Arnold M, Schroth G, Nedeltchev K, et al: Intra-arterial thrombolysis in 100 patients with acute stroke due to middle cerebral artery occlusion. *Stroke* 33:1828–1833, 2002.
5. Attia J, Ray JG, Cook DJ, et al: Deep vein thrombosis and its prevention in critically ill adults. *Arch Intern Med* 161:1268–1279, 2001.
6. Babikian VL, Kase CS, Pessin MS, et al: Intracerebral hemorrhage in stroke patients anticoagulated with heparin. *Stroke* 20:1500–1503, 1989.
7. Barber PA, Zhang J, Demchuk AM, et al: Why are stroke patients excluded from TPA therapy? An analysis of patient eligibility. *Neurology* 56:1015–1020, 2001.
8. Barnwell SL, Clark WM, Nguyen TT, et al: Safety and efficacy of delayed intraarterial urokinase therapy with mechanical clot disruption for thromboembolic stroke. *AJNR Am J Neuroradiol* 15:1817–1822, 1994.
9. Bath PM, Lindenstrom E, Boysen G, et al: Tinzaparin in acute ischaemic stroke (TAIST): a randomised aspirin-controlled trial. *Lancet* 358:702–710, 2001.
10. Becker KJ, Monsein LH, Ulatowski J, et al: Intraarterial thrombolysis in vertebrobasilar occlusion. *AJNR Am J Neuroradiol* 17:255–262, 1996.
11. Becker PS, Miller BT: Heparin-induced thrombocytopenia. *Stroke* 20:1449–1459, 1989.
12. Bick RL, Fareed J: Low molecular weight heparins: differences and similarities in approved preparations in the United States. *Clin Appl Thromb Hemost* 5 Suppl 1:S63–S66, 1999.
13. Boer A, Voth E, Henze T, et al: Early heparin therapy in patients with spontaneous intracerebral haemorrhage. *J Neurol Neurosurg Psychiatry* 54:466–467, 1991.
14. Brandt T, von Kummer R, Müller-Küppers M, et al: Thrombolytic therapy of acute basilar artery occlusion: variables affecting recanalization and outcome. *Stroke* 27:875–881, 1996.
15. Chalela JA, Katzan I, Liebeskind DS, et al: Safety of intra-arterial thrombolysis in the postoperative period. *Stroke* 32:1365–1369, 2001.
16. Clark WM, Alberts GW, Madden KP, et al: The rtPA (Alteplase) 0- to 6-hour acute stroke trial, part A (A0276g). The Thrombolytic Therapy in Acute Ischemic Stroke Study investigators. *Stroke* 31:811–816, 2000.
17. Clarke-Pearson DL, Synan IS, Dodge R, et al: A randomized trial of low-dose heparin and intermittent pneumatic calf compression for the prevention of deep venous thrombosis after gynecologic oncology surgery. *Am J Obstet Gynecol* 168:1146–1153, 1993.
18. Cloft HJ, Samuels OB, Tong FC, et al: Use of abciximab for mediation of thromboembolic complications of endovascular therapy. *AJNR Am J Neuroradiol* 22:1764–1767, 2001.
19. Coe NP, Collins RE, Klein LA, et al: Prevention of deep vein thrombosis in urological patients: a controlled, randomized trial of low-dose heparin and external pneumatic compression boots. *Surgery* 83:230–234, 1978.
20. Cole MS, Minifee PK, Wolma FJ: Coumarin necrosis—a review of the literature. *Surgery* 103:271–277, 1988.
21. Cornelli U, Fareed J: Human pharmacokinetics of low molecular weight heparins. *Semin Thromb Hemost* 25 Suppl 3:57–61, 1999.
22. Cross DT III, Derdeyn CP, Moran CJ: Bleeding complications after basilar artery fibrinolysis with tissue plasminogen activator. *AJNR Am J Neuroradiol* 22:521–525, 2001.
23. Cross DT III, Moran CJ, Akins PT, et al: Relationship between clot location and outcome after basilar artery thrombolysis. *AJNR Am J Neuroradiol* 18:1221–1228, 1997.
24. Cziraky MJ, Spinler SA: Low-molecular-weight heparins for the treatment of deep-vein thrombosis. *Clin Pharm* 12:892–899, 1993.

25. Davydov L, Dietz PA, Lewis P, et al: Outcomes of weight-based heparin dosing based on literature guidelines and institution individualization. *Pharmacotherapy* 20:1179–1183, 2000.

26. del Zoppo GJ, Ferbert A, Otis S, et al: Local intra-arterial fibrinolytic therapy in acute carotid territory stroke. A pilot study. *Stroke* 19:307–313, 1988.

27. del Zoppo GJ, Poeck K, Pessin MS, et al: Recombinant tissue plasminogen activator in acute thrombotic and embolic stroke. *Ann Neurol* 32:78–86, 1992.

28. de Swart CA, Nijmeyer B, Roelofs JM, et al: Kinetics of intravenously administered heparin in normal humans. *Blood* 60:1251–1258, 1982.

29. Diener HC, Ringelstein EB, von Kummer R, et al: Treatment of acute ischemic stroke with the low-molecular-weight heparin certoparin: results of the TOPAS trial. *Stroke* 32:22–29, 2001.

30. Dolovich LR, Ginsberg JS, Douketis JD, et al: A meta-analysis comparing low-molecular-weight heparins with unfractionated heparin in the treatment of venous thromboembolism: examining some unanswered questions regarding location of treatment, product type, and dosing frequency. *Arch Intern Med* 160:181–188, 2000.

31. Donnan GA, Davis SM, Chambers BR, et al: Streptokinase for acute ischemic stroke with relationship to time of administration: Australian Streptokinase (ASK) Trial Study Group. *JAMA* 276:961–966, 1996.

32. Eckert B, Koch C, Thomalla G, et al: Acute basilar artery occlusion treated with combined intravenous abciximab and intra-arterial tissue plasminogen activator: report of 3 cases. *Stroke* 33:1424–1427, 2002.

33. Edwards MT, Murphy MM, Geraghty JJ, et al: Intra-arterial cerebral thrombolysis for acute ischemic stroke in a community hospital. *AJNR Am J Neuroradiol* 20:1682–1687, 1999.

34. Ernst R, Pancioli A, Tomsick T, et al: Combined intravenous and intra-arterial recombinant tissue plasminogen activator in acute ischemic stroke. *Stroke* 31:2552–2557, 2000.

35. Ezura M, Kagawa S: Selective and superselective infusion of urokinase for embolic stroke. *Surg Neurol* 38:353–358, 1992.

36. Ferguson RDG, Ferguson JG, del Zoppo GJ, et al: Cerebral intraarterial fibrinolysis at the crossroads: Is a phase III trial advisable at this time? *AJNR Am J Neuroradiol* 15:1201–1222, 1994.

37. Fieschi C, Argentino C, Lenzi GL, et al: Clinical and instrumental evaluation of patients with ischemic stroke within the first six hours. *J Neurol Sci* 91:311–321, 1989.

38. Fihn SD, Callahan CM, Martin DC, et al: The risk for and severity of bleeding complications in elderly patients treated with warfarin. *Ann Intern Med* 124:970–979, 1996.

39. Furlan A, Higashida R, Wechsler L, et al: Intra-arterial prourokinase for acute ischemic stroke. The PROACT II study: a randomized controlled trial. Prolyse in Acute Cerebral Thromboembolism. *JAMA* 282:2003–2011, 1999.

40. Gonner F, Remonda L, Mattle H, et al: Local intra-arterial thrombolysis in acute ischemic stroke. *Stroke* 29:1894–1900, 1998.

41. Granger CB, Califf RM, Topol EJ: Thrombolytic therapy for acute myocardial infarction. A review. *Drugs* 44:293–325, 1992.

42. Grines CL: Thrombolytic, antiplatelet, and antithrombotic agents. *Am J Cardiol* 70:18I–26I, 1992.

43. Hacke W, Kaste M, Fieschi C, et al: Intravenous thrombolysis with recombinant tissue plasminogen activator for acute hemispheric stroke: The European Cooperative Acute Stroke Study (ECASS). *JAMA* 274:1017–1025, 1995.

44. Hacke W, Kaste M, Fieschi C, et al: Randomised double-blind placebo-controlled trial of thrombolytic therapy with intravenous alteplase in acute ischaemic stroke (ECASS II). Second European-Australasian Acute Stroke Study Investigators. *Lancet* 352:1245–1251, 1998.

45. Hacke W, Zeumer H, Ferbert A, et al: Intra-arterial thrombolytic therapy improves outcome in patients with acute vertebrobasilar occlusive disease. *Stroke* 19:1216–1222, 1988.

46. Haley EC Jr, Levy DE, Brott TG, et al: Urgent therapy for stroke. Part II. Pilot study of tissue plasminogen activator administered 91-180 minutes from onset. *Stroke* 23:641–645, 1992.

47. Hardwicke MB, Kisly A: Prophylactic subcutaneous heparin therapy as a cause of bilateral adrenal hemorrhage. *Arch Intern Med* 152:845–847, 1992.

48. Higashida RT, Halbach VV, Barnwell SL, et al: Thrombolytic therapy in acute stroke. *J Endovasc Surg* 1:4–15, 1994.

49. Hill MD, Barber PA, Demchuk AM, et al: Acute intravenous–intraarterial revascularization therapy for severe ischemic stroke. *Stroke* 33:279–282, 2002.

50. Hirsch DR, Goldhaber SZ: Contemporary use of laboratory tests to monitor safety and efficacy of thrombolytic therapy. *Chest* 101: Suppl 4:98S–105S, 1992.

51. Hirsh J, Anand SS, Halperin JL, et al: Guide to anticoagulant therapy: heparin: a statement for healthcare professionals from the American Heart Association. *Circulation* 103:2994–3018, 2001.

52. Hirsh J, Dalen J, Anderson DR, et al: Oral anticoagulants: mechanism of action, clinical effectiveness, and optimal therapeutic range. *Chest* 119 (Suppl):8S–S21, 2001.

53. Horellou MH, Conard J, Lecrubier C, et al: Persistent heparin induced thrombocytopenia despite therapy with low molecular weight heparin (letter to the editor). *Thromb Haemost* 51:134, 1984.

54. Huemer M, Niederwieser V, Ladurner G: Thrombolytic treatment for acute occlusion of the basilar artery. *J Neurol Neurosurg Psychiatry* 58:227–228, 1995.

55. Hyman BT, Landas SK, Ashman RF, et al: Warfarin-related purple toes syndrome and cholesterol microembolization. *Am J Med* 82:1233–1237, 1987.

56. Jahan R, Duckwiler GR, Kidwell CS, et al: Intraarterial thrombolysis for treatment of acute stroke: expe-

rience in 26 patients with long-term follow-up. *AJNR Am J Neuroradiol* 20:1291–1299, 1999.

57. Kamran SI, Downey D, Ruff RL: Pneumatic sequential compression reduces the risk of deep vein thrombosis in stroke patients. *Neurology* 50:1683–1688, 1998.

58. Kase CS, Furlan AJ, Wechsler LR, et al: Cerebral hemorrhage after intra-arterial thrombolysis for ischemic stroke. The PROACT II trial. *Neurology* 57:1603–1610, 2001.

59. Kelly J, Rudd A, Lewis R, et al: Venous thromboembolism after acute stroke. *Stroke* 32:262–267, 2001.

60. Keris V, Rudnicka S, Vorona V, et al: Combined intraarterial/intravenous thrombolysis for acute ischemic stroke. *AJNR Am J Neuroradiol* 22:352–358, 2001.

61. Khamashta MA, Cuadrado MJ, Mujic F, et al: The management of thrombosis in the antiphospholipid-antibody syndrome. *N Engl J Med* 332:993–997, 1995.

62. Kucinski T, Koch C, Grzyska U, et al: The predictive value of early CT and angiography for fatal hemispheric swelling in acute stroke. *AJNR Am J Neuroradiol* 19:839–846, 1998.

63. Kuker W, Friese S, Vogel W, et al: Incomplete resolution of basilar artery occlusion after intra-arterial thrombolysis: abciximab and heparin prevent early rethrombosis. *Cerebrovasc Dis* 10:484–486, 2000.

64. Lee KY, Heo JH, Lee SI, et al: Rescue treatment with abciximab in acute ischemic stroke. *Neurology* 56:1585–1587, 2001.

65. Lensing AWA, Prins MH, Davidson BL, et al: Treatment of deep venous thrombosis with low-molecular-weight heparins. *Arch Intern Med* 155:601–607, 1995.

66. Levine MN: Thrombolytic therapy in acute pulmonary embolism. *Can J Cardiol* 9:158–159, 1993.

67. Matsumoto K, Satoh K: Topical intra-arterial urokinase infusion for acute stroke. In Hacke W, del Zoppo GJ, Hirschberg M (eds): *Thrombolytic Therapy in Acute Ischemic Stroke*. Berlin, Springer-Verlag, 1991, pp 207–215.

68. Melo TP, Bogousslavsky J, Regli F, et al: Fatal hemorrhage during anticoagulation of cardioembolic infarction: role of cerebral amyloid angiopathy. *Eur Neurol* 33:9–12, 1993.

69. Miller VT, Hart RG: Heparin anticoagulation in acute brain ischemia. *Stroke* 19:403–406, 1988.

70. Montalescot G, Barragan P, Wittenberg O, et al: Platelet glycoprotein IIb/IIIa inhibition with coronary stenting for acute myocardial infarction. *N Engl J Med* 344:1895–1903, 2001.

71. Mori E, Tabuchi M, Yoshida T, et al: Intracarotid urokinase with thromboembolic occlusion of the middle cerebral artery. *Stroke* 19:802–812, 1988.

72. Mori E, Yoneda Y, Tabuchi M, et al: Intravenous recombinant tissue plasminogen activator in acute carotid artery territory stroke. *Neurology* 42:976–982, 1992.

73. The Multicenter Acute Stroke Trial—Europe Study Group: Thrombolytic therapy with streptokinase in acute ischemic stroke. *N Engl J Med* 335:145–150, 1996.

74. Multicentre Acute Stroke Trial—Italy (MAST-I) Group: Randomised controlled trial of streptokinase, aspirin, and combination of both in treatment of acute ischaemic stroke. *Lancet* 346:1509–1514, 1995.

75. The National Institute of Neurological Disorders and Stroke rt-PA Stroke Study Group: Tissue plasminogen activator for acute ischemic stroke. *N Engl J Med* 333:1581–1587, 1995.

76. Nieuwenhuis HK, Albada J, Banga JD, et al: Identification of risk factors for bleeding during treatment of acute venous thromboembolism with heparin or low molecular weight heparin. *Blood* 78:2337–2343, 1991.

77. Noble S, Peters DH, Goa KL: Enoxaparin: a reappraisal of its pharmacology and clinical applications in the prevention and treatment of thromboembolic disease. *Drugs* 49:388–410, 1995.

78. Ogata J, Yutani C, Imakita M, et al: Hemorrhagic infarct of the brain without a reopening of the occluded arteries in cardioembolic stroke. *Stroke* 20:876–883, 1989.

79. Ojeda E, Perez MC, Mataix R, et al: Skin necrosis with a low molecular weight heparin. *Br J Haematol* 82:620, 1992.

80. Pessin MS, Estol CJ, Lafranchise F, et al: Safety of anticoagulation after hemorrhagic infarction. *Neurology* 43:1298–1303, 1993.

81. Pessin MS, Hinton RC, Davis KR, et al: Mechanisms of acute carotid stroke. *Ann Neurol* 6:245–252, 1979.

82. Phan TG, Wijdicks EFM: Intra-arterial thrombolysis for vertebrobasilar circulation ischemia. *Crit Care Clin* 15:719–742, 1999.

83. Pillai JJ, Lanzieri CF, Trinidad SB, et al: Initial angiographic appearance of intracranial vascular occlusions in acute stroke as a predictor of outcome of thrombolysis: initial experience. *Radiology* 218:733–738, 2001.

84. Prins MH, Gelsema R, Sing AK, et al: Prophylaxis of deep venous thrombosis with a low-molecular-weight heparin (Kabi 2165/Fragmin) in stroke patients. *Haemostasis* 19:245–250, 1989.

85. Rabinstein AA, Wijdicks EFM, Nichols DA: Complete recovery after early intra-arterial recombinant tissue plasminogen activator thrombolysis of carotid T occlusion. *AJNR Am J Neuroradiol* 23:1596–1599, 2002.

86. Racine E: Differentiation of the low-molecular-weight heparins. *Pharmacotherapy* 21:62S–70S, 2001.

87. Ramirez-Lassepas M, Quinones MR: Heparin therapy for stroke: hemorrhagic complications and risk factors for intracerebral hemorrhage. *Neurology* 34:114–117, 1984.

88. Raschke RA, Reilly BM, Guidry JR, et al: The weight-based heparin dosing nomogram compared with a "standard care" nomogram. *Ann Intern Med* 119:874–881, 1993.

89. Roberts HC, Dillon WP, Furlan AJ, et al: Computed tomographic findings in patients undergoing intra-

arterial thrombolysis for acute stroke due to middle cerebral artery occlusion: results from the PROACT II trial. *Stroke* 33:1557–1567, 2002.

90. Rosand J, Hylek EM, O'Donnell HC, et al: Warfarin-associated hemorrhage and cerebral amyloid angiopathy: a genetic and pathologic study. *Neurology* 55:947–951, 2000.

91. Sandercock PA, van den Belt AG, Lindley RI, et al: Antithrombotic therapy in acute ischaemic stroke: an overview of the completed randomised trials. *J Neurol Neurosurg Psychiatry* 56:17–25, 1993.

92. Sandset PM, Dahl T, Stiris M, et al: A double-blind and randomized placebo-controlled trial of low molecular weight heparin once daily to prevent deep-vein thrombosis in acute ischemic stroke. *Semin Thromb Hemost* 16 Suppl:25–33, 1990.

93. Sasaki O, Takeuchi S, Koike T, et al: Fibrinolytic therapy for acute embolic stroke: intravenous, intracarotid, and intra-arterial local approaches. *Neurosurgery* 36:246–252, 1995.

94. Seligsohn U, Lubetsky A: Genetic susceptibility to venous thrombosis. *N Engl J Med* 344:1222–1231, 2001.

95. Sixth ACCP Consensus Conference on Antithrombotic Therapy. *Chest* 119 Suppl:1S–370S, 2001.

96. Souied F, Pourriat JL, Le Roux G, et al: Adrenal hemorrhagic necrosis related to heparin-associated thrombocytopenia. *Crit Care Med* 19:297–299, 1991.

97. Suarez JI, Sunshine JL, Tarr R, et al: Predictors of clinical improvement, angiographic recanalization, and intracranial hemorrhage after intra-arterial thrombolysis for acute ischemic stroke. *Stroke* 30:2094–2100, 1999.

98. Theron J, Courtheoux P, Casasco A, et al: Local intraarterial fibrinolysis in the carotid territory. *AJNR Am J Neuroradiology* 10:753–765, 1989.

99. Tomsick T, Brott T, Barsan W, et al: Prognostic value of the hyperdense middle cerebral artery sign and stroke scale score before ultraearly thrombolytic therapy. *AJNR* 17:79–85, 1996.

100. Toni D, Fiorelli M, Bastianello S, et al: Hemorrhagic transformation of brain infarct: predictability in the first 5 hours from stroke onset and influence on clinical outcome. *Neurology* 46:341–345, 1996.

101. Turpie AG, Hirsh J, Gent M, et al: Prevention of deep vein thrombosis in potential neurosurgical patients. A randomized trial comparing graduated compression stockings alone or graduated compression stockings plus intermittent pneumatic compression with control. *Arch Intern Med* 149:679–681, 1989.

102. von Kummer R: Intravenous tissue plasminogen activation in acute stroke. In Hacke W, del Zoppo GJ, Hirschberg M (eds): *Thrombolytic Therapy in Acute Ischemic Stroke.* Berlin, Springer-Verlag, 1991, pp 161–174.

103. Wardlaw JM: Overview of Cochrane thrombolysis meta-analysis. *Neurology* 57 Suppl 2:S69–S76, 2001.

104. Wechsler LR, Jungreis CA: Intra-arterial thrombolysis for carotid circulation ischemia. *Crit Care Clin* 15:701–718, 1999.

105. Wijdicks EFM, Nichols DA, Thielen KR, et al: Intra-arterial thrombolysis in acute basilar artery thromboembolism: the initial Mayo Clinic experience. *Mayo Clin Proc* 72:1005–1013, 1997.

106. Wijdicks EFM, Thielen KR, Reeder GS: Immediate cerebral angiography and mechanical fragmentation of cerebral embolus after percutaneous myocardial revascularization. *Ann Intern Med* 132:846–847, 2000.

107. Yamaguchi T, Hayakawa T, Kikuchi H, et al: Intravenous tissue plasminogen activator ameliorates the outcome of hyperacute embolic stroke. *Cerebrovasc Dis* 3:209, 1993.

108. Zeumer H, Freitag HJ, Zanella F, et al: Local intra-arterial fibrinolytic therapy in patients with stroke: urokinase versus recombinant tissue plasminogen activator (r-TPA). *Neuroradiology* 35:159–162, 1993.

9

Intracranial Pressure

The physiologic principles of increased intracranial pressure (ICP) in patients with acute brain injury are known, but many of the feedbacks and couplings remain unexplored. Studies have begun to clarify the ways in which modulating therapies act on ICP and cerebral perfusion pressure (CPP). With the introduction of fiber-optic probes (Chapter 10), the monitoring of ICP has improved technically. The availability of reliable ICP monitoring devices has facilitated management and often dictates therapies that may become potentially harmful if used indiscriminately and not directed by measurements. For example, uncontrolled use of hyperventilation and osmotic diuretics without laboratory or pressure monitoring may potentially compromise cerebral blood flow and possibly produce cerebral ischemia.

The bony skull does not allow for expansion; therefore, one compartmental increase in volume invariably means a decrease in another. If not, ICP rises quickly, resulting in both brain stem displacement and herniation of brain tissue. A point may be reached beyond which the patient cannot recover from brain stem damage caused by displacement or distortion from encroaching tissue. Eventually, when ICP exceeds mean arterial pressure, cerebral perfusion ceases, and brain necrosis ensues.

The complex interactions among cerebrospinal fluid (CSF) flow and pressure regulation, blood volume, and other hydrodynamic relationships are discussed in this chapter. The main objective is to introduce the physiologic consequences of increased ICP and the essentials of management.

THE INTRACRANIAL COMPARTMENTS: BASIC PRINCIPLES

The relationships of cerebral blood flow, cerebral blood volume, CPP, increased ICP, and mean arterial blood pressure to one another are complex, difficult to grasp, and vexing. A useful starting point is the Monro-Kellie doctrine, which states that although intracranial volume relationships may vary, the total volume is constant. The intracranial volume is determined by the sum of the volumes of brain tissue, CSF, and blood. The volume of the brain parenchyma is 1900 mL in adults, filling approximately 80% of the space. Blood and CSF each contribute 10% of the total volume within the skull. This volume is constant because the skull is rigid and tissues are incompressible, with little elasticity. The ICP at equilibrium is less than 10 mm Hg, and usually no pressure differences exist between regions of the brain.

The introduction of an additional volume in brain parenchyma (e.g., a mass from an intracranial hematoma or swollen, infarcted brain tissue) must, by necessity, be compensated for by changes in the blood or CSF compartment for intracranial volume to remain constant (Fig. 9–1). The same reasoning applies to change in the CSF compartment (e.g., due to an increase in the CSF from hydro-

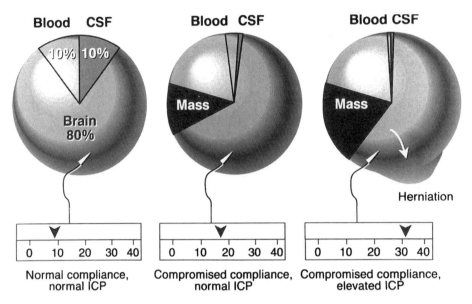

Figure 9–1. Illustration of compartments and compensation of increased intracranial pressure (ICP). CSF, cerebrospinal fluid.

cephalus) or blood compartment, which is largely the venous system (e.g., cerebral venous sinus thrombosis) (Table 9–1). Again, these changes increase the total volume and therefore must be counterbalanced by a reduction in volume of the other compartments.

Several compensatory mechanisms keep ICP within normal limits. An important mechanism is a shift of CSF from the ventricular or subarachnoid space into the spinal compartment. However, the volume distensibility at the spinal compartment is small and may not provide a sufficient escape route for changes in intracranial volume. Cerebral blood volume

Table 9–1. Causes of Intracranial Hypertension

Intracranial mass
Cerebral edema
    Cytotoxic (intracellular)
    Vasogenic (extracellular)
Cerebrospinal fluid hypervolemia
    Decreased absorption
    Obstructed venous outflow
    Overproduction of cerebrospinal fluid
Increased intracranial blood volume
    Cerebral vasodilatation (hypoxia, hypercapnia)
    Obstructed venous outflow

is accommodated mostly in the triangular-shaped dural sinuses and venules. One-third of the total volume is in arterioles. Cerebral blood volume is regulated by changes in the inflow tract (mechanisms that determine cerebral blood flow) and changes in the outflow tract (determined by jugular venous pressure and, eventually, intrathoracic venous pressure). Cerebral blood volume effectively is determined by the caliber of the intracranial vessels, cerebral blood flow, and venous outflow resistance. Thus, the second compensatory mechanism, most likely equally important, is reduction of the intracranial blood volume by collapsing of veins and dural sinuses and by changes in the diameter of cerebral vessels. The diameter in arterioles significantly determines the cerebral blood volume, and changes can be brought on rapidly. These changes in vessel caliber (particularly arterioles) can result in a wide range of total intravascular blood volume (15 to 70 mL), and with introduction of a new volume mass, one may be able to entirely compensate for the increase in volume. The most important regulator of vessel diameter is carbon dioxide tension in arterial blood.

On the whole, the major mechanisms that compensate for an increase in ICP are movement of CSF into the spinal subarachnoid space and removal of blood from the cerebral venous vessels. Cerebrospinal fluid volume may also decrease from increased CSF absorption, largely caused by the low outflow resistance of the arachnoid villi.

If the limits of these compensatory mechanisms are exceeded, the ICP begins to rise, and only a few milliliters in volume may increase the ICP. The pressure-volume curve of the intracranial compartment, shown in Figure 9–2, is biexponential. Displacement of CSF and blood represents the horizontal part. The intracranial compliance, defined as a measure of the distensibility of the intracranial cavity, $\Delta V/\Delta P$, decreases rapidly, however. This results in a substantial increase in pressure with any subtle increase in volume (the exponential curve) (Fig. 9–2). In the steep part of the curve, the compliance is poor, but differences may ex-

ist. The curve may be shifted more to the right in patients with more reserve to compensate for increases in volume (e.g., due to atrophy).

In an intact pressure regulation system, cerebral blood flow is constant, with a CPP between 50 and 150 mm Hg or mean arterial blood pressure between 60 and 160 mm Hg.[17] The main operators of cerebral autoregulation are pressure and resistance; blood flow itself is guided by the changes in pressure. A marked decrease in cerebral perfusion pressure results in a similar decrease in cerebral blood flow, but in an autoregulating system, vasodilatation decreases resistance, maintaining cerebral blood flow despite lower pressures. Conversely, a marked rise in CPP results in increased cerebral blood flow, which is corrected by decreasing arteriolar diameter.

Autoregulation is often impaired in patients with acute brain injury, but impairment is highly variable in different regions of the brain. Diffuse head injury, aneurysmal subarachnoid hemorrhage, and any type of global bihemispheric brain damage may virtually abolish autoregulation. In other clinical situations, focal edema surrounding masses or increased ICP alone may impair the normal regulation between cerebral blood flow and CPP. Marginal blood flow may cause ischemia, but this can be compensated for by increased oxygen extraction of the blood. Further reduction in cerebral blood flow leads to ischemia and infarction.

Basically, autoregulation is mediated through changes in cerebrovascular resistance (cerebral blood flow is CPP divided by cerebrovascular resistance). Disruption of autoregulation results in a linear relation between cerebral blood flow and CPP. Hypercapnia and hypoxemia both cause cerebral vasodilatation and may lower the upper limit of autoregulation. The cerebral vessels, however, are less responsive to changes in P_{O_2} than to those in P_{CO_2}. Little change can be expected in cerebral blood flow until a marked decrease in arterial P_{O_2} occurs, usually to less than 50 mm Hg, a level found almost exclusively in patients with neurogenic pulmonary edema, massive pulmonary emboli,

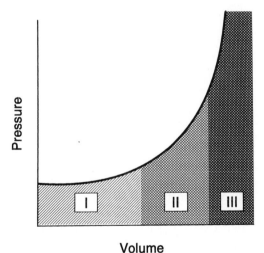

Figure 9–2. Pressure-volume curve. Zone I, compensatory mechanisms are optimal. Zone II, compensatory mechanisms fail. There is a slow rise (period of spatial compensation). Zone III, virtually irreversible increased intracranial pressure and herniations occur. There is a rapid rise (period of spatial decompensation).

or status epilepticus. At that breakpoint, cerebral blood flow increases, almost doubling at a PO_2 of 30 mm Hg. Hyperoxemia does not produce marked changes in cerebral blood flow.

The reactivity with PCO_2 is as follows: In patients with PCO_2 levels above 80 mm Hg, maximal vasodilatation occurs up to 100% of the baseline value, and no significant increase in cerebral blood flow can be expected beyond this point. At the other end of this spectrum, lowering of the PCO_2 below 20 mm Hg does not cause any further decrease in cerebral blood flow, but flow may increase when tissue ischemia causes vasodilatation. Cerebral blood flow generally changes by 2% to 3% for each change in PCO_2 within the range of 20 to 80 mm Hg. An example of the changes associated with PO_2 and PCO_2 is depicted in Figure 9–3.

Many drugs may significantly alter cerebral blood flow and ICP. Barbiturates, for example, are potent vasoconstrictors besides their characteristic of protecting against ischemic insults, but the reduction in ICP may only be partly explained by vasoconstrictive effects. More likely, the reduction in blood flow is due to reduced

Table 9–2. Drug Effects on Intracranial Pressure

Anesthetics and sedatives	
Halothane	++
Enflurane	++
Isoflurane	++
Desflurane	++
Dexmedetomidine	±
Propofol	±
Midazolam	±
Narcotics	
Morphine	0
Alfentanil	±
Vasodilators and calcium channel blockers	
Sodium nitroprusside	+
Hydralazine	+
Nitroglycerin	+
Nifedipine	+
Nicardipine	+
Nimodipine	0

++, significant and clinically relevant; +, significant; ±, not clinically relevant; 0, no change.
Source: Artru AA: Intracranial volume/pressure relationship during desflurane anesthesia in dogs: comparison with isoflurane and thiopental/halothane. *Anesth Analg* 79:751–760, 1994; Hadley MN, Spetzler RF, Fifield MS, et al: The effect of nimodipine on intracranial pressure. Volume-pressure studies in a primate model. *J Neurosurg* 67:387–393, 1987; Michenfelder JD, Milde JH: The interaction of sodium nitroprusside, hypotension, and isoflurane in determining cerebral vasculature effects. *Anesthesiology* 69:870–875, 1988; Papazian L, Albanese J, Thirion X, et al: Effect of bolus doses of midazolam on intracranial pressure and cerebral perfusion pressure in patients with severe head injury. *Br J Anaesth* 71:267–271, 1993; Scheller MS, Todd MM, Drummond JC, et al: The intracranial pressure effects of isoflurane and halothane administered following cryogenic brain injury in rabbits. *Anesthesiology* 67:507–512, 1987; Tateishi A, Sano T, Takeshita H, et al: Effects of nifedipine on intracranial pressure in neurosurgical patients with arterial hypertension. *J Neurosurg* 69:213–215, 1988; Watts AD, Eliasziw M, Gelb AW: Propofol and hyperventilation for the treatment of increased intracranial pressure in rabbits. *Anesth Analg* 87:564–568, 1998; Zornow MH, Scheller MS, Sheehan PB, et al: Intracranial pressure effects of dexmedetomidine in rabbits. *Anesth Analg* 75:232–237, 1992.

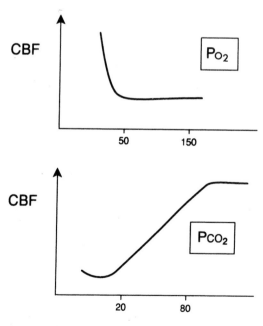

Figure 9–3. Effect of changes in PaO_2 and $PaCO_2$ in cerebral blood flow (CBF).

neuronal metabolism from coupling. Many inhalation anesthetics and antihypertensive drugs cause a change in autoregulation by dilatation of cerebral vessels (Table 9–2). Muscle relaxants do not affect cerebral circulation.

Cerebral blood flow increases in patients who have fever or seizures, and this increase may trigger marked sustained surges in ICP in susceptible patients.

Cerebral blood flow autoregulation in patients with acute intracranial hypertension changes significantly; in particular, the lower limit of autoregulation shifts toward lower CPP levels.[21] This shift is seen only in patients with a marked increase in ICP. The autoregulation curve with moderately increased ICP (approximately 30 mm Hg) remains unchanged. The possible cause of the shift of the lower limit of the autoregulation downward is dilatation of small resistant vessels.

Long-standing hypertension produces a profound change in cerebral autoregulation, resulting in a rightward shift of the entire curve (approximately 20 to 30 mm Hg) (Fig. 9–4). (This compensation is important to counter large increases in blood pressure that would otherwise lead to hypertensive encephalopathy from compromise of the blood–brain barrier.) Again, this shift in the lower limit of autoregulation is important when antihypertensive drug therapy is instituted. Carbon dioxide reactivity in patients with chronic hypertension, however, remains intact.

The ICP waveform is shown in Figure 9–5. Typical features of this waveform, which is of vascular origin, are the first peak (percussion wave), most likely originating from the pulsation of the choroid plexus; the second peak (dicrotic wave), transmitted from pulsations of the major cerebral arteries; and a tidal wave. The first peak is most prominently displayed, but in conditions of decreased brain compliance, the second wave increases in amplitude. This increase may be due to an increase in transmission of pressure

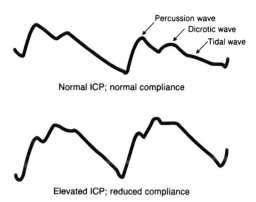

Figure 9–5. Intracranial pressure (ICP) waveform. (From Chesnut RM, Marshall LF: Treatment of abnormal intracranial pressure. *Neurosurg Clin N Am* 2:267–284, 1991. By permission of WB Saunders Company.)

caused by compensatory arterial dilatation. With increasing ICP values, the amplitude of the second and third waves increases without concomitant increases in the first wave, so that the waveform assumes a more rounded configuration. (The three components of the ICP waveform, however, remain distinctively present.)

Next to interpretation of the ICP waveform is interpretation of the trend of the ICP over time. The trend data for ICP values are obtained over hours and may display marked surges in ICP. The most important pressure changes are the so-called plateau waves. A waves, sudden increases in pressure of 50 to 80 mm Hg that may last for 5 to 20 minutes and often decrease rapidly, define the plateau (Fig. 9–6). The origin of the plateau is most likely defined by elevation of the ICP at the beginning of the plateau because of dilatation of the cerebral vessels, and reduction of the ICP because of constriction of the cerebral vessels.[12,50] Marked sluggishness of CSF flow and abnormal CSF absorption may contribute as well to the development of greatly increased ICP during plateau waves.[22,23] Plateau waves must be regarded as strong indicators of failing brain compliance, and they reflect cerebral ischemia.[22,23] Any type of manipulation of the patient may readily trigger these plateau

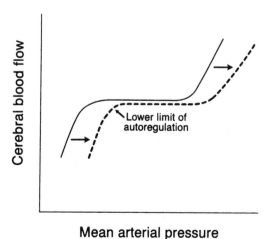

Figure 9–4. Change in autoregulation curve in long-standing hypertension.

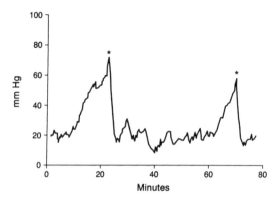

Figure 9–6. Example of plateau (*A*) waves (*asterisks*). (From Chesnut RM, Marshall LF: Treatment of abnormal intracranial pressure. *Neurosurg Clin N Am* 2:267–284, 1991. By permission of WB Saunders Company.)

waves. Prevention of these particularly dangerous surges in ICP is an essential part of management. Tracheal suctioning, repositioning and daily hygiene of the patient, replacement and flushing of indwelling bladder catheters, and changing of central venous catheters over a guidewire in a flat position are well-known triggers. The mechanism of triggering these plateau waves is not always clear from careful scrutiny of the daily chart, but in many patients the manipulations mentioned above cause surges in systolic blood pressure that can be implicated as the main instigators. Preemptive treatment with intravenously administered lidocaine or pentobarbital may considerably mute these responses.[3]

These waves should not be confused with so-called B waves, pressure increases that are seldom higher than 20 mm Hg and that occur one or two times a minute. However, these pressure waves are not innocuous and may be harbingers of plateau waves.

BRAIN TISSUE SHIFT AND HERNIATION

The end result of increased ICP is brain tissue shift with herniation under the falx cerebri, central or diencephalic transtentorial herniation, uncal herniation over the lateral edge of the tentorium, and, in a number of cases, herniation through a craniotomy defect.[44]

The falx and tentorium divide the brain into several compartments but leave openings through which tissue can herniate and wedge. Displacement may occur under the falx, tentorium (uncinate gyrus), and foramen magnum (tentorial pressure cone) (Fig. 9–7). When ICP increases, brain tissue drifts toward a compartment of lower pressure. Unilateral supratentorial lesions carry the thalamus and upper brain stem to the opposite side, opening up the ipsilateral cisterna ambiens, a buffer zone between the midbrain and tentorial free edge. The crowding of the tentorial opening involves herniation of uncal tissue, either passively or forcefully wedged into the opening. It causes compression and elongation of the ipsilateral cerebral peduncle.

No herniation from the opposite side is possible, because of early horizontal displacement of the brain stem. The ipsilateral third nerve is stretched and pulled to the posterior clinoid process, but the opposite third nerve is slackened. Further descent of the herniating mass impinges on the upper surface of the pons and moves the brain stem downward. Uncal herniation is manifested by dilatation (6 to 9 mm) of the ipsilateral pupil, with sluggish constriction to light and sluggish dilatation when the neck skin is pinched (ciliospinal reflex). When the midbrain becomes impaired, the opposite pupil dilates, but both pupils may become fixed in midposition. However, the tentorial notch or aperture varies in width and length and the brain stem may be positioned in different ways, creating different angles and lengths of exiting third cranial nerves. These morphologic variations may impact on the effect of direct pressure by the hippocampal gyrus and explain some of the inconsistencies of pupillary dilation with uncal herniation.[1] When both hemispheres swell or a mass is located medially, the cerebral convolutions become flattened and drive brain tissue through the hiatus of the cerebellar tentorium. The midbrain may move down.

Diencephalic herniation causes bilateral pupillary constriction and can be explained by injury to hypothalamic mydriatic areas. At the midpons–midbrain stage, pupils become wider and

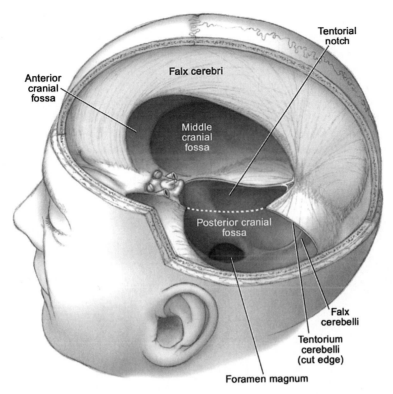

Figure 9–7. Intracranial compartments defined by falx and tentorial blades. Potential outlets for brain tissue shift are shown.

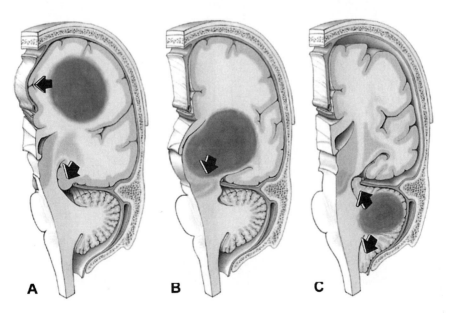

Figure 9–8. The brain herniation syndromes: (*A*) Falcial bowing, subfalcial herniation, and uncal syndrome; (*B*) central or diencephalic syndrome; (*C*) tonsillar syndrome and upward herniation (arrows).

fix at midposition. Rostrocaudal impairment in the brain stem also is evidenced by paratonic resistance ("pseudovoluntary resistance to passive movement") and decorticate (pathologic flexion) and decerebrate (pathologic extension) responses. Breathing becomes ataxic (irregular intervals between breaths and variable tidal volumes), signifying medullary failure (Fig. 9–8). Current neuroimaging techniques can document these pathologic changes, creating the opportunity not only to link clinical features with brain

tissue shift but also prospectively to define "point of no return" abnormalities that portend very poor outcome[68] (Fig. 9–9).

MANAGEMENT OF INCREASED INTRACRANIAL PRESSURE

The indications for placement of the monitoring device are described in Chapter 10. Many consider placement of an ICP monitor stan-

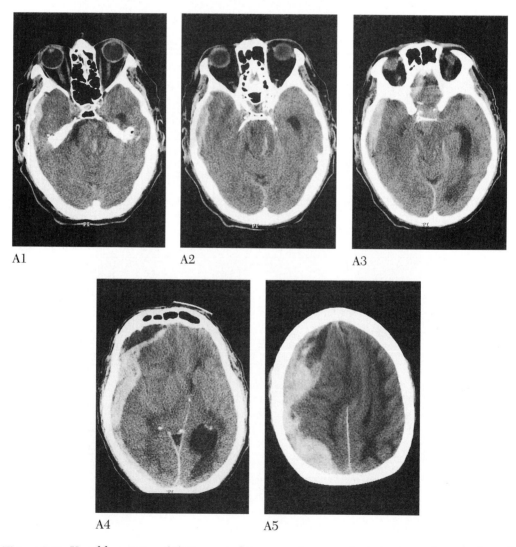

A1   A2   A3

A4   A5

Figure 9–9. Uncal herniation. (*A*) Computed tomography scans depicting typical signs of uncal herniation (note tip of temporal horn, A3), brain stem elongation, contralateral hydrocephalus, and Duret's hemorrhages (A1 and A2) associated with massive subdural hematomas.

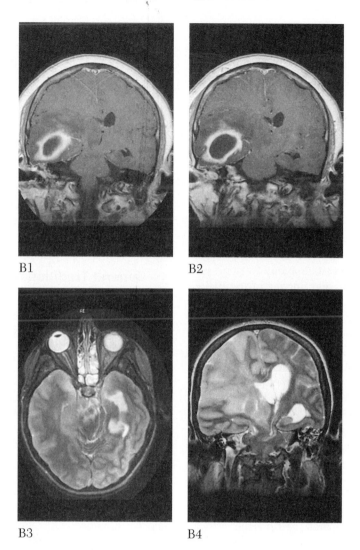

B1

B2

B3

B4

Figure 9–9. (*Continued*) Uncal herniation. (*B*) Magnetic resonance images, coronal and axial views, of different stages of uncal herniation. B1 and B2, earlier stages; B3 and B4, massive herniation and brain stem displacement. (*A* from Wijdicks.[68] By permission of the American Medical Association.)

dard treatment in comatose patients with traumatic head injury, ganglionic hemorrhage of large volume, and massive cerebral edema from infarction, but persistent critics of the clinical utility of ICP monitoring continue to debate the issue. In management of increased ICP, CPP (CPP = mean arterial pressure − ICP) must be considered another important guide for further titration of treatment.

Reduction of increased ICP is governed by attempts to reduce the total intracranial volume. This involves (*1*) CSF withdrawal by ventricular drain, (*2*) reduction of the cerebral tissue volume (e.g., osmotic dehydration), (*3*) reduction of the cerebral blood volume by reduction of cerebral blood flow or by enhancement of cerebral venous drainage, and (*4*) removal or decompression of a mass.

The management of increased ICP involves general measures and more specific treatment modalities. General measures should receive great emphasis before more traditional therapies, such as osmotic diuresis, are started.

Strong arguments have been put forward to place greater emphasis on management of CPP than on management of ICP. This controversial management pertains only to patients with severe traumatic brain injury. Two opposing protocols (Lund and Rosner) exist. The crux of CPP management techniques developed by Rosner et al.[56] is the preservation of cerebral blood flow to prevent cerebral ischemia. Cerebral perfusion is set at a minimum of 70 mm Hg, and to finally arrive at that value, one may need to place a ventriculostomy tube to drain CSF and to use a combination of vasopressor, volume expansion, and nursing of the patient in a flat position. This method posits that decreased cerebral perfusion due to increased ICP or decreased blood pressure will lead to increased vasodilatation, increased cerebral blood volume, and further increase in ICP. Increased ICP reduces CPP, creating a cycle further reducing CPP. Increasing blood pressure breaks the cycle.[56] However, with a high CPP, an abnormal blood–brain barrier may facilitate cerebral edema by driving additional fluids into brain tissue.

The post hoc analysis of the International Selfotel Trial in traumatic brain injury clearly discounted this management protocol. Subsets of patients were compared, and patients with an ICP greater than 20 had a much worse outcome than patients with lower ICP recordings, irrespective of CPP. The same investigators reported prolonged brain swelling in patients with artificially increased CPPs greater than 90 mm Hg.[26]

The crux of ICP management, devised by Lund, is to facilitate interstitial fluid reabsorption by preservation of normal osmotic pressure, to reduce intracapillary hydrostatic pressures, and to reduce cerebral blood volume. This novel but highly unusual approach turns to those forces that move fluids out of the capillaries.

First, colloid osmotic pressure is maintained by transfusion of albumin and by not over-transfusing, maintaining a normovolemic state. Second, hydrostatic pressure is reduced by reduction of mean arterial pressure with metoprolol, 0.2 to 0.3 mg/kg per 24 hours intravenously, and clonidine, 0.4 to 0.8 μg/kg four to six times a day intravenously. Third, cerebral blood volume is further reduced by vasoconstriction of the precapillary resistance vessels (low dose of thiopental sodium) and veins (dihydroergotamine, up to 0.9 μg/kg per hour). Thus, ICP is not managed traditionally with hyperventilation, CSF drainage, or osmotherapy.[15] Neither the Lund nor the Rosner protocol has shown better outcome than traditional ICP–CPP care (aiming at ICP < 20, CPP 60 to 70).

General Traditional Measures

Every patient should be adequately oxygenated, and normal mean arterial blood pressure should be maintained. Mechanical ventilation may be indicated in patients with marginal gas exchange and inability to protect the airway. Fortunately, the mode of mechanical ventilation does not significantly influence ICP. High levels of positive end-expiratory pressure (15 to 20 cm H_2O) may not markedly influence cerebral venous return.[19] Reduction of pulmonary compliance in patients with marked adult respiratory distress syndrome (the typical situation in which positive end-expiratory pressure is indicated) does not appear to influence ICP. Nonetheless, positive end-expiratory pressure may interfere with systemic arterial pressure by induction of arteriolar vasodilatation.

Fever, after being investigated thoroughly (Chapter 29), should be treated aggressively with cooling blankets. In patients with autonomic storms (sudden episodes of tachycardia, tachypnea, increase in temperature up to 41°C, and marked shivering), a combination of morphine and bromocriptine is indicated.

Head position should be neutral to reduce any possible compression of the jugular veins that could lead to a decrease in intracranial venous outflow.[51,55] Whether the head should be elevated remains somewhat controversial, but many intensive care neurologists consider head elevation of 30° standard. This position is further supported by a careful study in 22 patients with head injury, most of whom had marked reduction in ICP.[16] Elevation of the head, however, may cause a reduction in arterial pressure, particularly if the patient has orthostatic hypotension from diabetes mellitus or has marked hypovolemia or orthostasis from psychotropic drugs used to counter agitation (e.g., phenothiazines). Trendelenburg's position should be avoided except in overt life-threatening shock. Intracranial pressure should be monitored closely in patients in the supine position at the time of procedures such as placement of a catheter in the jugular or subclavian vein or fiber-optic bronchoscopy.[29]

Any patient with increased ICP should be made comfortable and become rested. Pain, bladder distention, and agitation should be minimized by codeine, placement of a Foley catheter and maintenance of unobstructed flow, and small doses of propofol (Chapter 4). Episodes of agitation may be caused by fighting the ventilator, and the mode of ventilation may need to be adjusted. Bronchial suctioning should be performed regularly to reduce hypoxemia, but the number of passages through the endotracheal tube should be limited to one. When a marked increase in ICP is observed during bronchial suctioning, a bolus of lidocaine (1 mg/kg) could be administered intravenously to mute this response. Deepening the level of sedation is another technique and easier to apply.

One should identify possible, seemingly trivial, triggers in the intensive care unit that may increase ICP. Pain and frequent stimulation by such maneuvers as washing and change of position are factors that may contribute to agitation and increased ICP.

In patients with increased ICP, a euvolemic state is preferred. Fluid restriction is not a recognized treatment of increased ICP. Moreover, dehydration associated with fluid restriction causes hypotension and hemoconcentration with increased viscosity and may for that reason have a deleterious effect.

Seizures are associated with hypoxemia and hypercapnia and may greatly increase ICP through cerebral vasodilatation. Seizures may result in respiratory acidosis, aspiration, and pro-longed hypoxemia. Prophylaxis with antiepileptic drugs in patients treated for increased ICP is debatable, but intravenous loading with phenytoin should be strongly considered in patients assumed to have a marginally compliant brain parenchyma and in patients at comparably high risk for seizures.

In general, vasodilators such as hydralazine and nitroprusside which may increase ICP to unacceptable levels should be avoided (Table 9–2).[20]

Cerebrospinal Fluid Drainage

Ventricular drainage remains a very rational solution to increased ICP and is perhaps the best option. Its use is predominantly focused on patients with acute obstructive hydrocephalus after aneurysmal subarachnoid hemorrhage or acute expanding cerebellar masses. In traumatic brain injury, however, its use is very controversial, but some trauma centers almost routinely insert ventricular catheters.[53] In patients with head injury, drainage can be significantly compromised by a large volume of intraventricular blood and compression of the frontal horns to slitlike proportions from surrounding edema. The use of ventricular catheters is discussed in more detail in Chapter 10.

Cerebrospinal fluid drainage may also potentially facilitate bulk flow from edematous brain tissue, moving fluid from an area of high pressure to one of low pressure. Whether drainage of CSF improves cerebral perfusion pressure or has any effect on ICP reduction remains very uncertain, because most of the increase in ICP is from cerebrovascular compartments. In a study of patients with traumatic brain injury, CSF drainage produced a transient decrease in ICP but no change in cerebral blood flow velocities on regional cerebral oximetry.[28]

Hyperventilation

Use of hyperventilation after any insult to the central nervous system and particularly after severe closed head injury has been criticized for its potential long-term adverse effects.[43]

Nonetheless, acute hyperventilation remains a very effective way of reducing ICP.

Acute hyperventilation causes a reduction in ICP by cerebral vasoconstriction, which in turn reduces cerebral blood flow. Vasoconstriction is mediated by a change in the pH of CSF, and a narrow response to hyperventilation exists. Cerebral blood flow decreases 40% approximately 30 minutes after reduction of the $PaCO_2$ by 15 to 20 mm Hg. After several hours, an increase in cerebral blood flow to approximately 90% of the baseline value is seen, with a potential overshoot of cerebral blood flow. The effects of hyperventilation on cerebral blood flow and ICP are therefore not significant after several hours. Predominantly bicarbonate is responsible for rapid buffering of alkalotic CSF.[52]

A major question is whether hyperventilation is potentially harmful. In a prospective study, patients with severe traumatic brain injury were randomized to treatment with prophylactic hyperventilation for 5 days after the injury with an average $PaCO_2$ of 25 mm Hg or to management without hyperventilation with $PaCO_2$ goals of 35 mm Hg.[35] At 3 and 6 months, patients in the hyperventilation group with initial Glasgow coma motor scores of 4 or 5 had significantly worse outcomes. A recent study that monitored brain tissue oxygen found that even a small reduction in $PaCO_2$ caused a decrease in cerebral oxygenation in comatose patients with traumatic brain injury and also minimal cerebral vessel reactivity to $PaCO_2$ from day 2 to 5 after the insult.[9] It appears that aggressive hyperventilation can cause cerebral blood flow to closely approach an ischemic threshold, and this may explain a potentially more harmful outcome.

The true effect of acute hyperventilation in the setting of severe head injuries had not been studied carefully until recently.[63] Two groups[13,25] found contradictory results. Both studies were limited by the small number of patients, but the resulting data were novel. Diringer et al[13] found that when a brief period of hyperventilation was introduced, cerebral blood flow, as expected, was reduced substantially. However, in most patients, cerebral

metabolism was not impaired because of increased oxygen extraction. With the use of PET technology for the first time in this particular setting, a $PaCO_2$ of 30 mm Hg did not change global or regional cerebral metabolism. Similar results were obtained in a small subset of patients with more aggressive hyperventilation ($PaCO_2$ less than 25 mm Hg). These investigators found that even when cerebral blood flow decreased to only 10 mL per 100 g per minute, cerebral metabolism was still preserved. In contrast, Imberti et al[25] studied in a more indirect way the consequences of hyperventilation using a measurement of cerebral tissue PO_2 and jugular venous oxygen saturation. Both brain tissue PO_2 and the jugular vein oxygenation were reduced with hyperventilation. Whether brain tissue PO_2 and metabolic rate are directly correlated remains uncertain. Other studies have found that moderate hyperventilation may significantly increase accumulation of lactate and extracellular fluid.[7]

All these studies indicate that the consequence of hyperventilation may be deleterious to the already injured brain, but it is difficult to define a clear, safe threshold. Thiagarajan et al[62] found that hyperoxia during acute hyperventilation may further improve oxygen delivery to the brain, and this may be the best compromise. If necessary, hyperventilation to a $PaCO_2$ of 30 mm Hg, with preoxygenation or increasing the oxygen delivery, may protect the brain in certain areas but at the risk of ischemia.

Hyperventilation can also be potentially harmful in patients with emphysema and marked obesity associated with carbon dioxide retention. Sudden reduction in $PaCO_2$ may cause very significant hypotension. Other adverse effects of hypocapnea are decreased myocardial oxygen supply and increased myocardial oxygen demand. Hypocapnia may promote development of cardiac arrhythmia.[30]

Most of the available recommendations are based on work in severe head injury, and fine-grain plans of action in other conditions are not exactly known. There is a growing consensus that osmotic agents should be used first and that hyperventilation should become a second method of treatment only if brief, rapid reduction of ICP is necessary.

When hyperventilation is instituted, the change in ventilation should be derived largely from a change in respiratory rate. The respiratory rate can be increased to approximately 20 breaths per minute while a normal tidal volume of 12 mL/kg is maintained. Increasing minute ventilation by changing both components may potentially lead to high airway pressures, barotrauma, and, at the extreme, pneumothorax. End-tidal carbon dioxide can be used to approximate $PaCO_2$, but arterial blood gas is more reliable, and $PaCO_2$ may remain relatively stable after a certain mode of ventilation is set.

Weaning the patient from hyperventilation should be gradual; minute ventilation is reduced by two breaths per minute during careful monitoring of ICP. An increase in or, less likely, a rebound of ICP occurs in some patients with normalization of $PaCO_2$ but in many instances is simply not distinguishable from an increase due to progressive clinical neurologic deterioration. Cerebral vessels adapt in patients with prolonged hyperventilation.[36] Experimental animal studies have found that eventually normalization of the vessel diameter occurs. Restoration of $PaCO_2$ to normocapnia, therefore, can be "read" as relative hypercapnia and may induce vasodilatation with a subsequent increase in both cerebral blood volume and ICP. This increase in ICP can be associated with marked deterioration in the motor response, and some patients may have brief extensor posturing during this manipulation.

Jugular venous oxygen saturation can be monitored (see also Chapter 10) to titrate depth of hyperventilation (cerebral ischemia from vigorous hyperventilation is reflected in increased oxygen extraction and increased arteriovenous oxygen saturation difference).

Osmotic Diuresis

The basic principle of osmotherapy is decrease of brain water. For osmotic agents to work, an osmotic gradient and intact blood–brain barrier are needed. Consequently, osmotic agents shrink mostly brain tissue that has not been damaged. Brain water filters from a compartment with low osmolality to a compartment with high osmolality. The available diuretic agents for treatment of increased ICP are mannitol, hypertonic saline, albumin, glycerol and urea, and furosemide.[48,65,67,71] In most institutions, either mannitol or hypertonic saline is used to decrease ICP. The mechanism of mannitol has traditionally been attributed to movement of brain water into the vascular space. This osmotic gradient remains the overriding principle, but other mechanisms of action are increased cerebral blood flow from transient hypervolemia and hemodilution resulting in a decrease in blood viscosity.[8,34,37] Cerebral blood volume, however, remains much the same from a compensatory reflex vasoconstriction of the cerebral arterioles. Mannitol also probably increases CSF absorption.[48] Cerebrospinal fluid production is reduced by a high dose (2 g/kg) and continuous infusion.[14] Trials are lacking comparing different doses of mannitol or modes of administration, and bolus versus continuous infusion.[57] Nonetheless, the effect of mannitol in pathologic areas with a breached blood–brain barrier is not known and is not necessarily absent. Mannitol may enter damaged brain tissue and decrease the osmotic gradient, in fact reverse the osmotic gradient, causing worsening of swelling. An animal study found that a single dose of mannitol was very effective, but administration of multiple doses reversed the blood–brain barrier gradient and increased cerebral edema by 3%.[27]

The potential for an increasing shift from reducing counterpressure from the unaffected compartment has not been substantiated.[18,64] A recent study with serial magnetic resonance imaging in patients with hemispheric stroke did not document increased brain shift.[33] A follow-up study, however, found that noninfarcted brain tissue shrank more, but the difference was sufficient to determine a measurable shift on MRI.[64]

Mannitol may exert its effect through free radical scavenging capabilities rather than through reduction of edema. An experimental study in rats found that mannitol administered at 6-hour intervals of ischemia reduced the number of histologically apparent ischemic neurons.[31]

Mannitol is typically used in its 20% solution. Elimination follows first-order kinetics (estimated half-life between 30 and 60 minutes), no metabolism occurs, and the agent is excreted entirely through the kidneys. Proportionally more water is lost than sodium, and profound diuresis may result in hypovolemia and hypernatremia. Mannitol should be administered in an initial dose of 1 g/kg, which can be tapered to various amounts for maintenance (0.25 to 0.50 g/kg). Rarely, higher doses (up to 2 g/kg) are needed to reduce ICP. The reduction in ICP with mannitol administration should be apparent after 15 minutes, and failure of ICP to respond to mannitol should be considered a poor prognostic sign. The maximum effect approximates 60 minutes. The goal for serum osmolarity should be 310 to 320 mOsm/L.[52,54] An increase in serum osmolarity of more than 325 mOsm/L ultimately leads to significant renal failure from dehydration and renal vasoconstriction. Osmolality can be calculated, and a difference of less than 10 mOsm/kg between measured and calculated osmolality (osmolality = 2 Na + glucose/18 + blood urea nitrogen/2.8) can be used to guide the need for an additional bolus of mannitol. The adverse reactions of mannitol, including congestive heart failure and profound pulmonary edema, are a result of rapid intravascular expansion. Hypotension is due to the rate of infusion and can be avoided. Movement of intracellular water to the extracellular space may cause hyponatremia, but typically this occurs only if mannitol is administered to patients with renal failure. Hyperkalemia may become significant only after infusion of high doses; the underlying physiologic mechanism is unknown.[32]

Rebound after mannitol use has been considered a possible concern. Rebound after mannitol is tentatively explained by influx of mannitol into brain tissue, reversing osmosis. A "rebound" to higher ICP values after discontinuation of mannitol was found in 12% of 65 patients but could not be explained by higher doses or rapid infusion rates. In addition, factors such as changed fluid management and worsening brain contusion have confounded the results.[41] No rebound effect was found in a recent study of ischemic infarction in a rat model.[42] The ICP-reducing activity of mannitol diminishes over time and becomes ineffective, and cumulatively higher doses are needed to keep the ICP within acceptable limits. The rebound effect of mannitol thus remains an imprecisely defined condition.

If there is no response to mannitol treatment with 2 g/kg and enlargement of a potentially removable mass on computed tomography scan is excluded, another treatment should be tried. Furosemide with albumin or hypertonic saline 3%, 50 mL in 10 minutes, can be given.[71] Studies of combined mannitol and furosemide have been done, but the risk of significant reduction of blood pressure from dehydration is great.[45,67] However, 40 mg of furosemide can be administered to patients with severe congestive heart failure who may not tolerate this volume load from mannitol.

There has been renewed fascination with the use of hypertonic saline as a hyperosmolar solution. The osmolarity of 3% saline (1026 mOsm/L) is approximately similar to that of 20% mannitol (1375 mOsm/L), but it is considerably higher in 7.5% saline (2565 mOsm/L) and 23.4% saline (8008 mOsm/L).[46,47] This characteristic may be responsible for a much stronger fluid shift directed toward the capillaries and reversal of brain swelling. Despite promising animal experiments, it remains uncertain whether hypertonic saline has more benefits than a hardly significant prolonged duration of action. A recent small study suggested that repeated bolus infusions of 7.5% saline at a dose of 2 mL/kg of body weight and an infusion rate of 20 mL/minute had a lowering effect on ICP in patients with brain injury from trauma.[24] In none of these patients could ICP be lowered with mannitol or other common measures. In another study, 75 mL of hypertonic saline (this time 10%) reduced ICP in patients with stroke failing to respond to mannitol.[59] Thus, hypertonic saline could be reserved for use in these circumstances. The potentially adverse effects of hypertonic saline should be carefully monitored; they include, as expected, hypokalemia and hyperchloremic acidemia, hypernatremia (and associated risk of seizures), and congestive heart failure due to volume expansion. These side effects, insufficiently studied in a systematic fashion, may eventually reduce the enthusiasm for the use of hypertonic saline.

Tromethamine

Tromethamine (THAM) has been introduced as an agent to control increased ICP. (Tromethamine is a buffer that is commonly used to correct metabolic acidosis associated with cardiac bypass surgery or cardiac arrest.) The advantage of tromethamine is that it alkalizes without increasing $PaCO_2$ and plasma sodium. The dose of tromethamine is 1 mL/kg per hour. Besides local tissue irritation and necrosis, respiratory depression and hypoglycemia have been described. Tromethamine has been compared with mannitol for ICP control, and one small, nonrandomized trial found it to be at least as effective. Larger studies in patients with head injury found that fluctuations in ICP could be better controlled, but outcome was similar.[69] Tromethamine should be used for patients in whom mannitol is contraindicated (e.g., renal failure). Tromethamine may also have a place in countering rebound from hyperventilation.

Barbiturates

The use of barbiturates has been proposed, particularly in severe head injury, as a last resort for patients with refractory intracranial hypertension.[40,49,70] Unfortunately, barbiturates often have been used in patients close to fulfilling clinical criteria of brain death, making later organ retrieval very problematic, if not impossible. Barbiturate therapy could be useful in reduction of ICP and may certainly decrease mortality in patients with uncontrollable ICP refractory to all other standard medical

and surgical treatments. The position of the American Association of Neurosurgeons joint session on neurotrauma and critical care has been published and underscores extreme caution with its use.[6] The number of patients eventually considered for barbiturate treatment is very small, because usually standard therapies or removal of a mass reduces ICP. Moreover, treatment with barbiturates is a challenge. Myocardial depression and hypothermia are major concerns. There is an increased risk of nosocomial infections,[39] particularly pneumonia, from depression of mucociliary clearance in patients receiving barbiturate treatment.[52] Approximately 50% of the patients treated with barbiturates need inotropic agents to control hypotension.[49,70] In many patients, combinations of dobutamine and epinephrine are needed as well as additional fluids. These patients require a Swan-Ganz catheter with regular hemodynamic monitoring and frequent determination of serum barbiturate levels.

Barbiturate treatment is started with pentobarbital, 10 mg/kg intravenously over 30 minutes.[2] The maintenance dose is generally 1 to 3 mg/kg per hour by constant intravenous infusion. A higher dose (5 mg/kg per hour) can be used initially for several hours to obtain adequate loading. Adequate volume can be achieved by monitoring pulmonary capillary wedge pressure, which should be within the normal range of 12 to 14 mm Hg. Blood pressure can be maintained with dopamine infusion (5 to 10 μg/kg per minute). Suppression of the electroencephalogram is usually seen when serum barbiturate levels are approximately 30 to 40 mg/dL. Serum levels should be checked regularly and one should aim at the lowest possible dose for control of ICP. It is not necessary to proceed to a burst-suppression pattern. The dose of barbiturates that produces a burst-suppression pattern is typically associated with hypotension; therefore, a lower dose may reduce the need for vasopressors and still control ICP. Common practice is to maintain barbiturate treatment for 2 to 3 days. When computed tomography scanning does not show any new findings or progression of findings and ICP is well controlled, barbiturate therapy can be withdrawn slowly by reduction of the infusion rate by 50% each day.

Hypothermia

A possible adjunctive measure to reduce ICP is induction of moderate hypothermia (core temperature, 33°C) for 24 hours by use of cooling blankets above and below the patient and other measures such as ice water gastric lavage (see Chapter 16, Fig. 9A). In an elegant study, ICP was reduced (mean, 10 mm Hg) and CPP increased (mean, 14 mm Hg) in 16 patients. No increase in bacterial infection was found, but premature ventricular contractions occurred in 40% of the hypothermic patients. Moreover, one patient had hypovolemic shock and another had a rapid increase in ICP during rewarming.[61]

Moderate hypothermia has been studied in traumatic brain injury but has not been effective in improving outcome.[10] Analysis of its effect on ICP and CPP did not show a significant difference from that of normothermia. Absence of a major effect on outcome was corroborated by a Japanese study of mild hypothermia, which also found significant systemic complications, including pneumonia, meningitis, leukocytopenia, thrombocytopenia, hyponatremia, hypokalemia, and increased amylase.[60]

Its effect in stroke is not known, although early experience suggests cerebral swelling can be abated. A carefully studied cohort showed a possible effect on ICP in patients with infarction of the middle cerebral artery

distribution, but pressure increased after rewarming.[58]

Miscellaneous Options

The use of corticosteroids has been tested in large prospective trials. In patients with severe head injury, high-dose dexamethasone (100 mg/day) and methylprednisolone (30 mg/kg) do not improve outcome.[5] The adverse effects of corticosteroids are significant and include hyperglycemia, sepsis, and an increased risk of gastrointestinal bleeding. High doses of corticosteroids may only be helpful in patients with a malignant brain tumor or metastases and could reduce swelling and intracranial pressure (dexamethasone, 4–6 mg p.o. or IV q.i.d.)

Many alternative anesthetic agents, including lidocaine and, more recently, propofol, have been tried to control the increase in ICP.[11,52,53] As noted earlier, lidocaine can be used in a dose of 1 mg/kg given slowly over 1 minute to blunt ICP response in patients with marked surges of ICP during nursing care, nasotracheal suctioning, or procedures such as fiber-optic broncho-scopy. An alternative option, treatment with a 4% lidocaine nebulizer, is not successful in reducing ICP.[29]

Propofol is an effective hypnotic drug. Long-term infusion of propofol may produce significant adrenal depression, with an increased risk of nosocomial infection. The use of propofol as a sedative has been accepted as effective (see Chapter 4), but the reduction in blood pressure and associated decrease in CPP when higher doses are needed may seriously limit its

Table 9–3. Initial Treatment of Increased Intracranial Pressure

Method	Procedure	Monitoring
Ventricular catheter	Ventricular right frontal placement with subcutaneous tunneling	CSF pressures, changes in waveform Daily calibration Drip chamber at 15–20 cm H_2O Consider prophylactic antibiotics
Hyperventilation	Increase respiratory rate to 20 breaths/minute alone	Pco_2, 25–30 mm Hg Daily chest radiograph for possible pneumothorax
Osmotic diuresis	Mannitol 20%, 1 g/kg Hypertonic saline 3%, 50 mL/10 minutes	Plasma osmolarity, 310–320 mOsm/L BUN, creatinine, sodium, potassium Urine output

BUN, blood urea nitrogen; CSF, cerebrospinal fluid.

use for ICP control. Propofol administration can begin with an infusion of 1 to 3 mg/kg per hour. A bolus of 1 mg/kg may transiently lower the ICP without the marked change in blood pressure typically observed with propofol infusion. Rates higher than 5 mg/kg per hour may induce cardiac failure.

A preliminary study suggested considerable success with a bolus of indomethacin (a cyclooxygenase inhibitor; 50 mg in 20 minutes) in patients with increased ICP refractory to therapy. Sudden discontinuation, however, led to a marked rebound effect.[4]

Surgical management of increased ICP has come into vogue, especially in patients with swelling from large middle cerebral artery in-farcts. Interest in decompressive craniotomy in traumatic brain injury has been recently rekindled.[38,66] The procedure may reduce ICP and reopen compressed basal cisterns, and some early data suggest improved outcome and increased compensatory reserve. Suboccipital decompressive craniotomy and ventriculostomy for hydrocephalus—both highly effective therapies for mass lesions in the posterior fossa—are discussed in Chapters 14 and 18. Salvage has also been claimed with extensive craniotomy in subarachnoid hemorrhage associated with massive edema, but the operation is hard to defend in these cases.

Management of increased ICP is summarized in Table 9–3.

CONCLUSIONS

- ICP must be monitored for recognition of plateau waves (A waves)—sudden increases in ICP of 50 to 80 mm Hg lasting several minutes—which indicate failing brain compliance. Plateau waves can be muted by a change in nursing techniques and by increasing depth of sedation or intravenous administration of lidocaine or pentobarbital.
- Hypercapnia, hypoxemia, inhalation anesthetics, fever, and seizures all may increase ICP.
- The first measures to decrease ICP are head elevation to 30°, treatment of agitation, and maintenance of patient comfort during mechanical ventilation.
- Traditional measures for treatment of increased ICP are CSF drainage in patients with obstructive hydrocephalus, administration of mannitol, and hyperventilation. Osmotic diuresis is the preferred first treatment. Administration of mannitol 20% is started with 1 g/kg, aiming at a serum osmolarity of 310 mOsm/L. Hyperventilation should be added for only brief moments.
- Tromethamine infusion, 1 mL/kg per hour, should be considered a second line of treatment and, if not effective, may be followed by propofol (up to 3 mg/kg per hour) or barbiturates (pentobarbital, 10 mg/kg over 30 minutes).

REFERENCES

1. Adler DE, Milhorat TH: The tentorial notch: anatomical variation, morphometric analysis, and classification in 100 human autopsy cases. *J Neurosurg* 96:1103–1112, 2002.
2. Bayliff CD, Schwartz ML, Hardy BG: Pharmacokinetics of high-dose pentobarbital in severe head trauma. *Clin Pharmacol Ther* 38:457–461, 1985.
3. Bedford RF, Persing JA, Pobereskin L, et al: Lidocaine or thiopental for rapid control of intracranial hypertension? *Anesth Analg* 59:435–437, 1980.
4. Biestro AA, Alberti RA, Soca AE, et al: Use of indomethacin in brain-injured patients with cerebral perfusion pressure impairment: preliminary report. *J Neurosurg* 83:627–630, 1995.
5. Braakman R, Schouten HJ, Blaauw-van Dishoeck M, et al: Megadose steroids in severe head injury. Results of a prospective double-blind clinical trial. *J Neurosurg* 58:326–330, 1983.
6. The Brain Trauma Foundation: The American Association of Neurological Surgeons. The Joint Section of Neurotrauma and Critical Care. Use of Barbiturates in the control of intracranial hypertension. *J Neurotrauma* 17:527–530, 2000.
7. Bullock R: Hyperventilation. J Neurosurg 96:157–158, 2002.
8. Burke AM, Quest DO, Chien S, et al: The effects of

mannitol on blood viscosity. *J Neurosurg* 55:550–553, 1981.

9. Carmona Suazo JA, Maas AI, van den Brink WA, et al: CO_2 reactivity and brain oxygen pressure monitoring in severe head injury. *Crit Care Med* 28:3268–3274, 2000.

10. Clifton GL, Miller ER, Choi SC, et al: Lack of effect of induction of hypothermia after acute brain injury. *N Engl J Med* 344:556–563, 2001.

11. Cremer OL, Moons KG, Bouman EA, et al: Long-term propofol infusion and cardiac failure in adult head-injured patients. *Lancet* 357:117–118, 2001.

12. Czosnyka M, Smielewski P, Piechnik S, et al: Hemo-dynamic characterization of intracranial pressure plateau waves in head-injury patients. *J Neurosurg* 91:11–19, 1999.

13. Diringer MN, Videen TO, Yundt K, et al: Regional cerebrovascular and metabolic effects of hyperventila-tion after severe traumatic brain injury. *J Neurosurg* 96:103–108, 2002

14. Donato T, Shapira Y, Artru A, et al: Effect of manni-tol on cerebrospinal fluid dynamics and brain tissue edema. *Anesth Analg* 78:58–66, 1994.

15. Eker C, Asgeirsson B, Grande PO, et al: Improved out-come after severe head injury with a new therapy based on principles for brain volume regulation and pre-served microcirculation. *Crit Care Med* 26:1881–1886, 1998.

16. Feldman Z, Kanter MJ, Robertson CS, et al: Effect of head elevation on intracranial pressure, cerebral per-fusion pressure, and cerebral blood flow in head-injured patients. *J Neurosurg* 76:207–211, 1992.

17. Florence G, Seylaz J: Rapid autoregulation of cerebral blood flow: a laser-Doppler flowmetry study. *J Cereb Blood Flow Metab* 12:674–680, 1992.

18. Frank JI: Large hemispheric infarction, deterioration, and intracranial pressure. *Neurology* 45:1286–1290, 1995.

19. Georgiadis D, Schwarz S, Baumgartner RW, et al: In-fluence of positive end-expiratory pressure on in-tracranial pressure and cerebral perfusion pressure in patients with acute stroke. *Stroke* 32:2088–2092, 2001.

20. Gopinath SP, Robertson CS: Management of severe head injury. In Cottrell JE, Smith DS (eds): *Anesthe-sia and Neurosurgery*. 3rd ed. St Louis, Mosby-Year Book, 1994, pp 661–684.

21. Hauerberg J, Juhler M: Cerebral blood flow autoreg-ulation in acute intracranial hypertension. *J Cereb Blood Flow Metab* 14:519–525, 1994.

22. Hayashi M, Handa Y, Kobayashi H, et al: Plateau-wave phenomenon (I). Correlation between the appearance of plateau waves and CSF circulation in patients with intracranial hypertension. *Brain* 114:2681–2691, 1991.

23. Hayashi M, Kobayashi H, Handa Y, et al: Plateau-wave phenomenon (II). Occurrence of brain herniation in patients with and without plateau waves. *Brain* 114:2693–2699, 1991.

24. Horn P, Münch E, Vajkoczy P, et al: Hypertonic saline solution for control of elevated intracranial pressure in

patients with exhausted response to mannitol and bar-biturates. *Neurol Res* 21:758–764, 1999.

25. Imberti R, Bellinzona G, Langer M: Cerebral tissue PO_2 and $SjvO_2$ changes during moderate hyperventi-lation in patients with severe traumatic brain injury. *J Neurosurg* 96:155–157, 2002.

26. Juul N, Morris GF, Marshall SB, et al: Intracranial hy-pertension and cerebral perfusion pressure: influence on neurological deterioration and outcome in severe head injury. The Executive Committee of the Inter-national Selfotel Trial. *J Neurosurg* 92:1–6, 2000.

27. Kaufmann AM, Cardoso ER: Aggravation of vasogenic cerebral edema by multiple-dose mannitol. *J Neuro-surg* 77:584–589, 1992.

28. Kerr EM, Marion D, Sereika MS, et al: The effect of cerebrospinal fluid drainage on cerebral perfusion in traumatic brain injured adults. *J Neurosurg Anesthe-siol* 12:324–333, 2000.

29. Kerwin AJ, Croce MA, Timmons SD, et al: Effects of fiberoptic bronchoscopy on intracranial pressure in pa-tients with brain injury: a prospective clinical study. *J Trauma* 48:878–882, 2000.

30. Laffey JG, Kavanagh BP: Hypocapnia. *N Engl J Med* 347:43–53, 2002.

31. Luvisotto TL, Auer RN, Sutherland GR: The effect of mannitol on experimental cerebral ischemia, revisited. *Neurosurgery* 38:131–139, 1996.

32. Manninen PH, Lam AM, Gelb AW, et al: The effect of high-dose mannitol on serum and urine electrolytes and osmolality in neurosurgical patients. *Can J Anaesth* 34:442–446, 1987.

33. Manno EM, Adams RE, Derdeyn CP, et al: The ef-fects of mannitol on cerebral edema after large hemi-spheric cerebral infarct. *Neurology* 52:583–587, 1999.

34. Muizelaar JP, Lutz HA III, Becker DP: Effect of man-nitol on ICP and CBF and correlation with pressure autoregulation in severely head-injured patients. *J Neu-rosurg* 61:700–706, 1984.

35. Muizelaar JP, Marmarou A, Ward JD, et al: Adverse effects of prolonged hyperventilation in patients with severe head injury: a randomized clinical trial. *J Neu-rosurg* 75:731–739, 1991.

36. Muizelaar JP, van der Poel HG, Li ZC, et al: Pial ar-teriolar vessel diameter and CO_2 reactivity during pro-longed hyperventilation in the rabbit. *J Neurosurg* 69:923–927, 1988.

37. Muizelaar JP, Wei EP, Kontos HA, et al: Cerebral blood flow is regulated by changes in blood pressure and in blood viscosity alike. *Stroke* 17:44–48, 1986.

38. Münch E, Horn P, Schürer L, et al: Management of severe traumatic brain injury by decompressive craniectomy. *Neurosurgery* 47:315–322, 2000.

39. Neuwelt EA, Kikuchi K, Hill SA, et al: Barbiturate in-hibition of lymphocyte function. Differing effects of various barbiturates used to induce coma. *J Neurosurg* 56:254–259, 1982.

40. Nordby HK, Nesbakken R: The effect of high dose bar-biturate decompression after severe head injury. A con-

trolled clinical trial. *Acta Neurochir (Wien)* 72:157–166, 1984.

41. Paczynski RP: Osmotherapy. Basic concepts and controversies. *Crit Care Clin* 13:105–129, 1997.

42. Paczynski RP, He YY, Diringer MN, et al: Multiple-dose mannitol reduces brain water content in a rat model of cortical infarction. *Stroke* 28:1437–1443, 1997.

43. Patel PM: Hyperventilation as a therapeutic intervention: Do the potential benefits outweigh the known risks? *J Neurosurg Anesthesiol* 5:62–65, 1993.

44. Plum F, Posner JB: *The Diagnosis of Stupor and Coma*. 3rd ed. Philadelphia, FA Davis Company, 1982.

45. Pollay M, Fullenwider C, Roberts PA, et al: Effect of mannitol and furosemide on blood-brain osmotic gradient and intracranial pressure. *J Neurosurg* 59:945–950, 1983.

46. Qureshi AI, Suarez JI: Use of hypertonic saline solutions in treatment of cerebral edema and intracranial hypertension. *Crit Care Med* 28:3301–3313, 2000.

47. Qureshi AI, Wilson DA, Traystman RJ: Treatment of elevated intracranial pressure in experimental intracerebral hemorrhage: comparison between mannitol and hypertonic saline. *Neurosurgery* 44:1055–1063, 1999.

48. Ravussin P, Abou-Madi M, Archer D, et al: Changes in CSF pressure after mannitol in patients with and without elevated CSF pressure. *J Neurosurg* 69:869–876, 1988.

49. Rea GL, Rockswold GL: Barbiturate therapy in uncontrolled intracranial hypertension. *Neurosurgery* 12:401–404, 1983.

50. Risberg J, Lundberg N, Ingvar DH: Regional cerebral blood volume during acute transient rises of the intracranial pressure (plateau waves). *J Neurosurg* 31:303–310, 1969.

51. Ropper AH, O'Rourke D, Kennedy SK: Head position, intracranial pressure, and compliance. *Neurology* 32:1288–1291, 1982.

52. Ropper AH, Rockoff MA: Physiology and clinical aspects of raised intracranial pressure. In Ropper AH (ed): *Neurological and Neurosurgical Intensive Care*. 3rd ed. New York, Raven Press, 1993, pp 11–27.

53. Rosner MJ: Pathophysiology and management of increased intracranial pressure. In Andrews BT (ed): *Neurosurgical Intensive Care*. New York, McGraw-Hill Book Company, 1993, pp 57–112.

54. Rosner MJ, Coley I: Cerebral perfusion pressure: a hemodynamic mechanism of mannitol and the postmannitol hemogram. *Neurosurgery* 21:147–156, 1987.

55. Rosner MJ, Coley IB: Cerebral perfusion pressure, intracranial pressure, and head elevation. *J Neurosurg* 65:636–641, 1986.

56. Rosner MJ, Rosner SD, Johnson AH: Cerebral perfusion pressure: management protocol and clinical results. *J Neurosurg* 83:949–962, 1995.

57. Schierhout G, Roberts I: Mannitol for acute traumatic brain injury. *Cochrane Database Syst Rev* 2:2000.

58. Schwab S, Schwartz S, Spranger M, et al: Moderate hypothermia in the treatment of patients with severe middle cerebral artery infarction. *Stroke* 29:2461–2466, 1998.

59. Schwarz S, Georgiadis D, Aschoff A, et al: Effects of hypertonic (10%) saline in patients with raised intracranial pressure after stroke. *Stroke* 33:1166–1167, 2002.

60. Shiozaki T, Hayakata T, Taneda M, et al: A multicenter prospective randomized controlled trial of the efficacy of mild hypothermia for severely head injured patients with low intracranial pressure. Mild Hypothermia Study Group in Japan. *J Neurosurg* 94:50–54, 2001.

61. Shiozaki T, Sugimoto H, Taneda M, et al: Effect of mild hypothermia on uncontrollable intracranial hypertension after severe head injury. *J Neurosurg* 79:363–368, 1993.

62. Thiagarajan A, Goverdhan PD, Chari P, et al: The effect of hyperventilation and hyperoxia on cerebral oxygen saturation in patients with traumatic brain injury. *Anesth Analg* 87:850–853, 1998.

63. Thomas SH, Orf J, Wedel SK, et al: Hyperventilation in traumatic brain injury patients: inconsistency between consensus guidelines and clinical practice. *J Trauma* 52:47–52, 2002.

64. Videen TO, Zazulia AR, Manno EM, et al: Mannitol bolus preferentially shrinks non-infarcted brain in patients with ischemic stroke. *Neurology* 57:2120–2122, 2001.

65. Wald SL, McLaurin RL: Oral glycerol for the treatment of traumatic intracranial hypertension. *J Neurosurg* 56:323–331, 1982.

66. Whitfield PC, Patel H, Hutchinson PJ, et al: Bifrontal decompressive craniectomy in the management of posttraumatic intracranial hypertension. *Br J Neurosurg* 15:500–507, 2001.

67. Wilkinson HA, Rosenfeld SR: Furosemide and mannitol in the treatment of acute experimental intracranial hypertension. *Neurosurgery* 12:405–410, 1983.

68. Wijdicks EFM: Uncal herniation in acute subdural hematoma: point of no return. *Arch Neurol* 59:305, 2002.

69. Wolf AL, Levi L, Marmarou A, et al: Effect of THAM upon outcome in severe head injury: a randomized prospective clinical trial. *J Neurosurg* 78:54–59, 1993.

70. Woodcock J, Ropper AH, Kennedy SK: High dose barbiturates in non-traumatic brain swelling: ICP reduction and effect on outcome. *Stroke* 13:785–787, 1982.

71. Worthley LI, Cooper DJ, Jones N: Treatment of resistant intracranial hypertension with hypertonic saline. Report of two cases. *J Neurosurg* 68:478–481, 1988.

PART II

EQUIPMENT AND TECHNOLOGIES

10

Monitoring Devices

Patients in NICUs are monitored differently from those in other medical or surgical intensive care units. The emphasis should remain on the clinical neurologic examination and knowledge of the causes of clinical deterioration in any acute central nervous system injury. Monitoring of critically ill neurologic patients requires correct interpretation of changes in brain stem reflexes and motor responses to pain and awareness of the early signs of brain herniation. Any of these changes may have immediate clinical relevance.

Devices are important to monitor neurologic deterioration, to assist in intracranial pressure (ICP) management, to control fluid management, and to assess gas exchange. Before it carves out a niche in the NICU, the performance of any new device should demonstrate that the expected benefits are balanced against the costs and the possible risks of monitoring, and it should be validated for its predictive value. "High-tech" neurologic intensive care may be questionable if the thresholds of interventions have not been defined. Moreover, a high level of monitoring creates a great number of alarms. There are too many loud, false, and irrelevant alarms, many of which in daily practice are not always identified as "critical sounds."[15]

In this chapter, the most frequently used monitoring devices in the NICU are discussed. Monitoring ICP changes is the main theme of the chapter.

MONITORING NEUROLOGIC DETERIORATION (COMA SCALES)

Previously published studies of neurologic deterioration more or less arbitrarily used changes in the Glasgow coma sum score (e.g., a two-point change in sum score defined deterioration in supratentorial intracerebral hemorrhage[34]) or changes in the motor score of the Glasgow coma scale (e.g., a one-point change in deteriorating patients with aneurysmal subarachnoid hemorrhage[63]). The Glasgow coma scale, introduced in 1974 by Teasdale and Jennett,[62] was originally devised to facilitate communication between nurses working in the unit, junior inexperienced physicians, and, particularly, nonneurologic staff working in other medical or surgical units. The scale proved to be more useful in communication (e.g., during transfer from another hospital or from the field) than any other previously used descriptive term for decreased level of consciousness (such as "somnolent," "nonarousable," "unresponsive," or "half asleep"). Subsequent studies, however, emphasized that clinical experience in using the Glasgow coma scale is very important, and substantial errors may occur with inexperienced observers.[54]

The Glasgow coma scale remains one of the most commonly used monitoring tools in the NICU, and any new scale must be tested against this scale. The Glasgow coma scale is shown in Table 10–1. The best response is recorded, and

Table 10–1. Glasgow Coma Scale

Eye opening	4	Spontaneous
	3	To speech
	2	To pain
	1	None
Best verbal response	5	Oriented
	4	Confused conversation
	3	Inappropriate words
	2	Incomprehensible sounds
	1	None
Best motor response°	6	Obeying
	5	Localizing pain
	4	Withdrawal
	3	Abnormal flexing
	2	Extensor response
	1	None

The Glasgow coma sum score is 3 to 15. Coma is often defined as a sum score ≤ 8.
°Upper limbs.
Source: Jennett B, Teasdale G: *Management of Head Injuries.* Philadelphia: FA Davis Company, 1981. By permission of Oxford University Press.

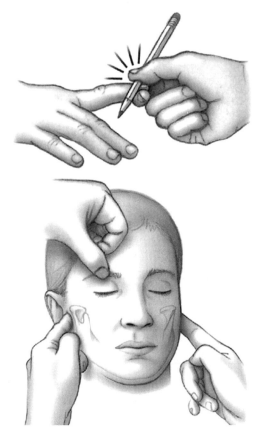

Figure 10–1. Methods of proper pain stimuli used to obtain the Glasgow coma score consist of compression of the nail bed, supraorbital nerve, and temporomandibular joint.

pain stimuli should be standardized. Following commands can be tested by having the patient squeeze hard or wiggle the toes, but higher degrees of wakefulness are present if the patient when asked can show a thumbs up, fist, or victory sign, particularly in a set order.[68] An ideal pain stimulus in the assessment of comatose patients must respect the patient and not be associated with significant bruising. Proper stimuli are sternal rubbing, rubbing the knuckles against the ribs in the axilla, and pressure on the supraorbital nerve. Deep pressure with a blunt object against the nail bed has become standard but may cause nail bed hematoma in anticoagulated patients or those with an underlying coagulopathy. Alternatively, deep pressure on both condyles at the level of the temporomandibular joint can be considered[67] (Fig. 10–1). Eye opening to pain and the type of motor response (upper limbs) are the most important components for monitoring changes over time.

Neurologic deterioration is frequently subtle. Changes often involve vigilance first, and these changes are not always clearly reflected in changes of individual components of the Glasgow coma scale. We have found that within maximal Glasgow coma scores, variations in wakefulness exist that can be detected by asking the patient to raise a hand every time a certain letter is heard in a standardized sentence (e.g., the letter "a" in "Schools *a*nd highw*a*ys cost money; we *a*ll p*a*y for them through t*a*xes," for which the correct answer is five hand raises).[68] It is also useful in patients who are intubated and patients with facial trauma, clinical situations that usually make the Glasgow coma scale less useful. Its limitation is that patients need to be literate and have reasonable spelling skills.

MONITORING OF INCREASED INTRACRANIAL PRESSURE

Monitoring of changes in ICP and, equally important, calculated cerebral perfusion pressure has been criticized because no currently available study clearly shows improved outcome in

Table 10–2. Guidelines for Monitoring Intracranial Pressure

Disorder	Specific Indications
Traumatic brain injury	Any patient with motor response ≤ 4 on Glasgow coma scale
	Bifrontal lobe contusion and edema
	Temporal lobe contusion and edema
	Polytrauma and need for neuromuscular blockade
Intracranial hemorrhage	Lobar or ganglionic hemorrhage with motor response ≤ 4 on Glasgow coma scale or shift on computed tomography
Middle cerebral artery territory stroke	Brain swelling with shift on computed tomography
Herpes simplex encephalitis	Motor response ≤ 4 on Glasgow coma scale; necrotic mass, temporal lobe
Aneurysmal subarachnoid hemorrhage	Acute hydrocephalus
Cerebellar stroke	Acute hydrocephalus

monitored patients. (Similar discussions apply to pulmonary artery balloon catheters, pulse oximeters, routine use of arterial blood gases, daily chest radiographs, frequent monitoring of mechanical ventilators by respiratory therapists, and repeat electrocardiography in patients with uncertain myocardial ischemia.) Important in this debate is whether the observed change is accurate, whether the observed variable leads to a therapeutic intervention, whether this therapeutic intervention favorably changes the clinical course, and whether this monitoring device is not potentially associated with major complications.

Guidelines for monitoring ICP in neurologic critical care practice are summarized in Table 10–2. Intracranial pressure monitoring is considered in comatose patients with a high probability of increased ICP, and often is anticipated on the basis of initial readings of CT images (edema, mass with shift of midline structures). Intracranial pressure monitoring is also used in patients who have had large cerebral tumors removed or frontal lobectomy for seizure control, because of the risk of postoperative swelling. The rationale for ICP monitoring is further detailed in chapters on specific clinical entities.

In most patients, a fiber-optic parenchymal monitor of ICP is placed, but ventriculostomy is preferred if obstructive hydrocephalus is present.

INTRAPARENCHYMAL MONITORS

Fiber-optic, transducer-tipped monitors (Camino Laboratories) are used in most NICUs.[10,11,55] Experience with this device is broad. Its easy

maintenance, reliable waveforms, lack of significant drift, and simple insertion techniques at the bedside have added to the popularity and convinced many skeptics to use ICP monitoring.[16,41,55] The disadvantages with this system are sizable costs from investment in equipment, fragility of the fiber-optic device, and, most importantly, inability to withdraw cerebrospinal fluid. Newer generations of fiber-optic monitors may have electrochemical pH and temperature sensors that may have relevance for treatment.[25] The monitor is calibrated before insertion, and resetting is not possible after placement. The monitor is advanced toward the white matter, 2 to 3 cm into the brain parenchyma, after a very small bur hole is placed in the right frontal area. The correct distance is indicated on the probe itself, and the bolt can be tightly screwed when this indicator line touches the outside of the bolt.

The monitor with its metal transducer is shown in Figure 10–2. Light is transmitted by one of the fiber optic bundles and reflected by a metal pleated-like probe. The change in this metal configuration from pressure outside the system is transduced in a pressure reading and displayed as a typical waveform (see Chapter 9 for interpretations of waveform). The waveform can be displayed through hardware provided by the manufacturer, but most modern bedside monitors should have the capability to enter the ICP recordings and also calculate the cerebral perfusion pressure. The accuracy of the system was tested by comparison with ventricular catheters, and most studies found acceptable variations over a range of 2 to 5 mm

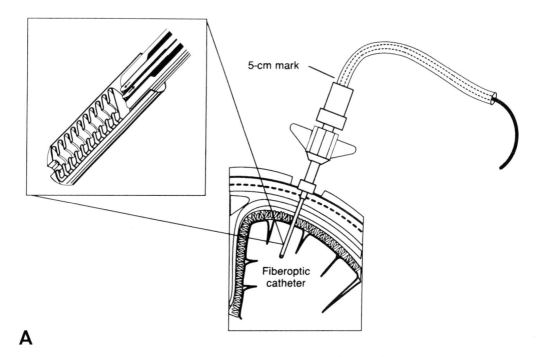

5-cm mark

Fiberoptic
catheter

A

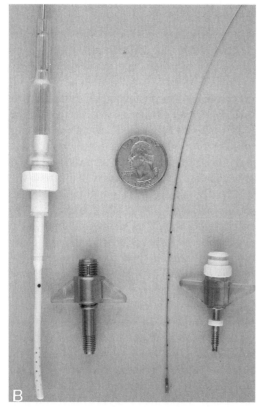

B

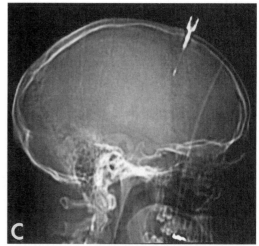

C

Figure 10–2. (*A*) Intraparenchymal placement of Camino intracranial pressure monitor. *Inset*, Metal pleated-like transducer tip. (*B*) True dimensions of the ventricular catheter (*left*) and intraparenchymal monitor (*right*) (both Camino Laboratories) with matching bolts compared with a quarter. (*C*) Skull radiograph showing fiber-optic monitor in situ.

Hg in both directions. The monitor could drift after approximately 5 days (actual daily drift of 2 to 3 mm Hg) and needs to be replaced if large variations occur and monitoring is still indicated, but recent experience found minimal underreading and overreading.[44] The metallic fixation bolt causes a substantial magnetic resonance artifact, and the monitor may move in magnetic resonance fields of 2 tesla.[69] Technical complications were reported in up to 32% of patients, including dislocation of the probe screw and breakage of the optic fiber, mostly after prolonged monitoring. Bacterial colonization occurred in 13%, and as expected, *Staphylococcus epidermidis* was frequent.[5,40]

INTRAVENTRICULAR MONITORING

Intraventricular pressure monitoring devices have been used less frequently since the introduction of intraparenchymal fiber-optic devices. Currently, the indications for placement of intraventricular catheters are more often conditions in which decompression of the ventricular system is urgently indicated. Examples are acute hydrocephalus in aneurysmal subarachnoid hemorrhage and obstructive hydrocephalus in ischemic or hemorrhagic stroke in the cerebellum obliterating the 4th ventricle. However, some trauma centers routinely place ventricular catheters in patients with severe closed head injury (Chapter 9).[53]

The ventricular catheters are connected to an external transducer that allows continuous ICP readings. We and others[4] use the Becker intraventricular external drainage and monitoring system (PS Medical, Goleta, CA). One sideport is used for continuous drainage and sampling. The external pressure transducer can be connected to the main system stopcock, which is level with the patient's ear, a zero reference level that approximates the catheter tip location at the foramen of Monro. The drip chamber can be moved up and down and placed at a desired level against the zero reference level stopcock. The drip chamber at the end of the drain line is typically fixed by a 15 cm length of pressure tubing to secure

drainage in the drip chamber when the ICP rises above 15 mm Hg (Fig. 10–3).

As a practical rule, abnormal resorption of cerebrospinal fluid can be assumed when the daily yield of cerebrospinal fluid approximates 200 mL with a drip chamber at a level of 20 cm H_2O.

An intraventricular catheter based on a fluid-filled system has the major disadvantage of dampening of the system, which makes readings less reliable. This may become a problem when progressive cerebral edema collapses the ventricles, positioning the catheter against the ventricular wall. More commonly, the system becomes blocked when filled with blood. An occluded catheter can be irrigated with small amounts of sterile isotonic saline. Frequently, however, dampening of the waveform suggests an air bubble. Air bubbles in the system can be eliminated by withdrawing air from the monitoring line but only after the system to the patient is closed.

Intravenous administration of antibiotics (cefotaxime, 8 g/day) is preferred while the ventricular catheter is in situ and up to 3 days after removal. Antibiotic prophylaxis should certainly be considered in patients with intraventricular blood, which is a well-recognized risk factor for ventriculitis. The benefit of this prophylactic measure is not exactly known, but it should be emphasized that ventriculitis is associated with considerable morbidity and mortality. The risk of sterilizing cultures and the risk of infection with a therapy-resistant infectious agent seem acceptably low. However, in a recent randomized study in 228 patients, the infection rate was reduced from 11% to 3%, but emergence of methicillin-resistant *Staphylococcus aureus* and *Candida* pathogens increased.[46] Subcutaneous tunneling may also considerably reduce the risk of ventriculitis. (For further guidance and details, see Chapter 33.)

If CSF yield is low in the collecting bag, clamping of the catheter for 24 hours can be tried. The catheter is pulled when no clinical change is observed and when repeat CT scanning does not show a significant increase in ventricular size. If continuous ventricular drainage

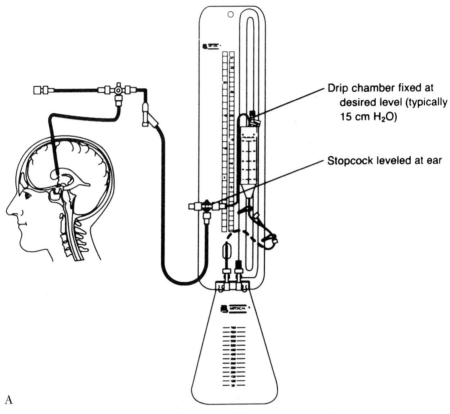

Drip chamber fixed at
desired level (typically
15 cm H$_2$O)

Stopcock leveled at ear

A

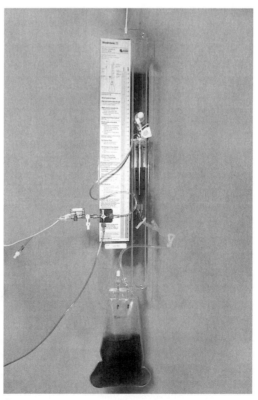

B

134

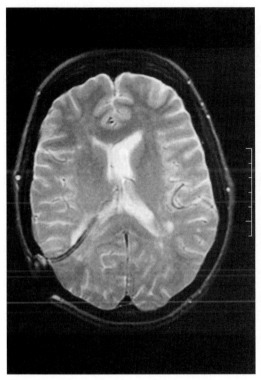
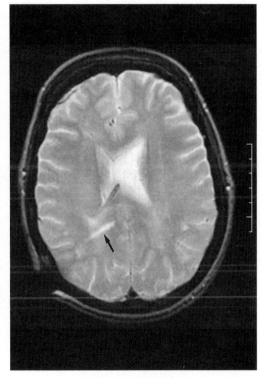

C

Figure 10–3. (*A*) Becker intraventricular external drainage and landmarks for calibrating. (*B*) Device in use in patient with subarachnoid hemorrhage. (*C right* and *left*) Magnetic resonance images showing ventriculostomy drain in situ. Note additional track from prior placement attempt (*arrow*).

is indicated, because either clamping fails or the cause of obstruction in the ventricular system is not expected to reverse within 10 days, a permanent ventricular–peritoneal catheter is placed, but only if no blood sediments are observed. The risk of ventriculitis is too high (despite subcutaneous tunneling of the catheter and prophylactic antibiotics) to permit long-term external drainage.[60] Intraventricular Camino probes caused ventriculitis in 3% of patients when still in place after 10 days.[33]

EPIDURAL AND SUBDURAL MONITORING

Epidural monitors are less reliable than intraparenchymal monitors[66] (Fig. 10–4). They are preferred over parenchymal or ventricular catheters in patients with a need for ICP monitoring but underlying coagulopathy that cannot be easily reversed with platelets or fresh frozen plasma (e.g., cerebral hematomas associated with hematologic malignant lesions or head injury in patients with liver failure). The adverse consequences of invasive monitoring of ICP in patients with severe coagulopathy are not well known but can be extrapolated from experience in fulminant hepatic failure. The incidence of fatal intracerebral hematomas decreased significantly when epidural devices were used in patients with brain edema and fulminant hepatic failure. In these patients with significant coagulopathy, 3% with epidurally placed ICP catheters had intracranial hemorrhages, half of which were fatal; in contrast, the incidences of intracranial hematoma associated with subdural and intraparenchymal catheters were 17% and 13%, respectively.[7]

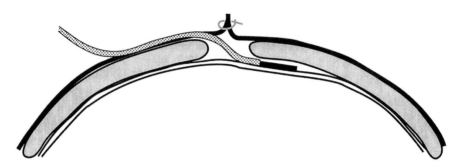

Figure 10–4. Epidural monitor of intracranial pressure.

Many NICUs use the Ladd fiber-optic monitors. Subdural monitors placed directly above the subarachnoid space, often used postoperatively in neurosurgical patients, and since the introduction of intraparenchymal catheters, are less in favor because of spurious readings.

MONITORING OF HEMODYNAMIC PARAMETERS AND BRAIN OXYGEN SUPPLY

Invasive monitoring devices can access the arterial or venous circulatory system and provide the potential for optimization of treatment. None of this equipment is without risk or procedural complications. Use of pulmonary artery catheters is expected to increase in the NICU. The usefulness of fiber-optic oxygen saturation catheters positioned in the jugular bulb has been demonstrated, but the technology is in routine use in only a few centers, usually those with a high volume of patients with head injury.[24,58] Use of the pulmonary artery catheter requires considerable skill and knowledge of the engineering principles—from basic zeroing and leveling of the transducer to understanding of the dynamic responses. (The reader is referred to critical care textbooks and a handbook.[43]) Its efficacy and safety in surgical and medical intensive care units have been seriously questioned.[21,33,45] How pulmonary artery catheter measurements alter decisions in the NICU and whether these decisions affect outcome are not known. Even analysis of the hemodynamic data is difficult, and disagreement among physicians

is common. A recent survey even found that 1 in 3 physicians suggested potentially harmful interventions due to misinterpretation of the data sets.[59] At this juncture, the benefits of certain devices in the NICU should be studied in prospective cohorts. This section is divided into subsections on arterial and venous invasive monitoring devices and closes with information on noninvasive instruments.

Radial Artery Catheter

Radial artery catheterization is considered in patients with unstable blood pressure and thus is much more common in general medical and surgical intensive care units.[22] In the NICU, common indications are use of vasoactive drugs, antihypertensive agents that potentially lower blood pressure (such as midazolam or propofol in status epilepticus), and the need for multiple blood sampling in, for example, mechanically ventilated patients. Oscillometric blood pressure measurements are quite unreliable, and typically the displayed blood pressure is 15 to 30 minutes old (frequency of measurement is arbitrarily set from 1 minute to 1 hour).[9,70] A recent study with different cuff sizes found a discrepancy of more than 20 mm Hg in one-third of almost 1500 measurement pairs, a result favoring radial artery cannulation.[9]

The technique of arterial cannulation is simple and in the United States is often performed by respiratory therapists. Generally, an 85% success rate is achieved with attempted cannulation. Catheter colonization is low, but radial artery thrombosis (asymptomatic) is high (up to 31% obstruction).[32] Frequent changing of arterial cannulas does not prevent these complications, and the cannulas may remain in place for a week or longer. Patency is maintained by flushing with small volumes of saline for 5 seconds.

Pulmonary Artery Catheter

The pulmonary artery balloon flotation catheter (PA catheter) is useful in several circumstances in the NICU (Table 10–3). Fortunately, the interpretation of PA-catheter-derived values and its pitfalls is less problematic in patients with acute neurologic injury, who seldom have acute pulmonary edema, pulmonary hypertension, complicated cardiogenic or septic shock, or acute cardiac disorders, all of which are more common problems in other medical or surgical intensive care units.

Placement of a PA catheter requires expertise, and some complications are directly related to faulty placement.[23] From several studies that have calculated the risks of serious complications, it has become apparent that the benefits outweigh the risks. Prospective studies on complications in PA catheter placement in neurologic patients are not available, but there is no reason to assume that the complication rate is different. Overall, with the most experienced personnel, the complication rate remains 3% to 5% for major complications (such as ventricular tachycardia, bacteremia, and pulmonary infarction) and 15% to 25% for minor complications (Table 10–4).

The indications for placement of a PA catheter should constantly be reviewed. The catheter

Table 10-3. Monitoring Indications for Pulmonary Artery Catheterization in the Neurologic Intensive Care Unit

Adequacy of volume status	Aneurysmal subarachnoid hemorrhage
	Traumatic brain injury or polytrauma
	Dysautonomia in Guillain-Barré syndrome
Effect of medication	Vasodilator medications
	Vasopressor medications
	Inotropic medications

Table 10-4. Complications of Pulmonary Artery Balloon Catheter Placement

Major
  Pneumothorax, pneumomediastinum
  Air embolism
  Thoracic duct injury
  Hemothorax
  Cardiac dysrhythmias
  Pulmonary artery rupture
  Sepsis
Minor
  Ventricular or atrial premature contractions
  Hematomas at puncture site

should be removed when not justifiably indicated and certainly when therapeutic measures are not based strictly on obtained values.[12]

The placement of the catheter is shown in Figure 10–5A. The most common problem with PA catheter insertion is cardiac arrhythmia. Pharmaceutical agents should be ready at the time of placement (for ventricular tachycardia, lidocaine intravenously in a bolus of 1 mg/kg is considered, and for paroxysmal atrial tachycardia or any supraventricular arrhythmia, verapamil intravenously in a bolus of 2.5 mg). The PA catheter is inserted into the internal jugular vein through large introducer sheath catheters. After the catheter is passed through the introduction catheter, the balloon is inflated with air to its maximal capacity of 1.5 mL. During passage of the catheter, the pressure waveforms are closely monitored, and they help in navigation through the right side of the heart. During catheter insertion, the pulmonary valve is at risk for damage, but the more important risk is that supraventricular or ventricular arrhythmias may be triggered at any time during advancement.

The first part of the journey is in the low-pressure venous system and the right atrium. The configuration of the pressure wave has a typically venous pattern, but when the catheter floats in the right ventricle, there is a clearly visible, abrupt change to a much higher systolic pressure, with pressure waves of approximately 20 to 30 mm Hg (Fig. 10–5A). After passage through the pulmonary valve, the pressure configuration changes again because of an increase in the diastolic component. The typical systolic

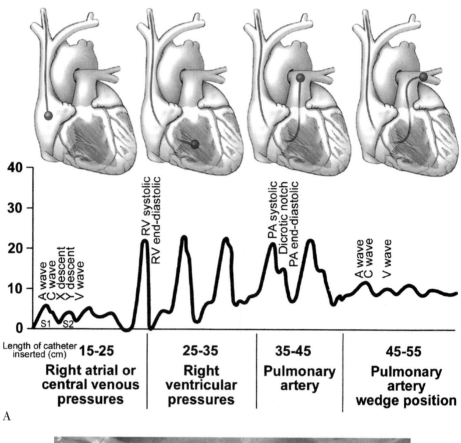

A

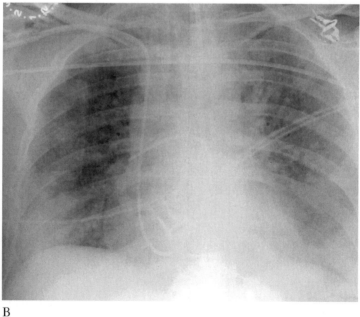

B

Figure 10–5. (*A*) Advancement of pulmonary artery balloon flotation catheter, and characteristic tracings during placement. PA, pulmonary artery; RV, right ventricular; S1, first heart sound; S2, second heart sound. (*B*) Chest radiograph showing accurate placement.

pressure peaks of the right ventricle have decreased, and the diastolic pressures have increased, with pressures of 10 to 20 mm Hg, creating the characteristic dicrotic notch. Further advancement into the pulmonary artery wedges the catheter into a pulmonary artery branch (usually at an insertion of 50 to 55 cm). At this moment, the systolic component disappears, and a virtually flat line appears with a pressure of 6 to 12 mm Hg. When this change is observed on the monitor, the balloon is immediately deflated and inflated again only when measurements are needed. The pulmonary artery wedge pressure is recorded on paper, and the actual pressure is read, by convention, at the end of expiration, usually the lowest point on the paper tracing if the patient is mechanically ventilated. Normal pulmonary artery wedge pressures vary from 6 to 12 mm Hg. If wedge pressures are not reliable, pulmonary artery diastolic pressures can be used as approximations of pulmonary artery wedge pressures.

It is important that the catheter float in the third zone. The pulmonary zones are defined by alveolar pressure, pulmonary artery pressure, and pulmonary capillary pressure. In the third zone, pulmonary artery pressure is greater than pulmonary capillary pressure, which is greater than alveolar pressure, and because the capillary pressure exceeds the alveolar pressure, the pressure at the balloon reflects the atrial pressure. In other pulmonary zones, the pressures do not accurately reflect atrial pressures, and the measurements are thus not reliable. Usually, the catheter floats

toward the third, most dependent, zone, simply because blood flow is greater. The position of the catheter tip is verified by a chest radiograph, and a lateral chest radiograph must show that the catheter is below the right atrium (Fig. 10–5B). Another method of verification is aspiration of blood to determine that oxygen saturation is 95%. The data derived from the PA catheter are usually correct, but the system may not work. Suggestions for troubleshooting are shown in Table 10–5.

The pulmonary artery wedge pressure is a measurement of the pressure in the left atrium. The assumption is that occlusion of a small-caliber pulmonary catheter produces a static column of blood. Thus, with no pulmonary blood flow and no pressure gradient across the pulmonary capillaries, the assumption is made that pulmonary artery wedge pressure equals left atrial pressure and equals left ventricular end-diastolic pressure; therefore, monitoring of the pulmonary capillary wedge pressure accurately reflects left ventricular end-diastolic pressure.

Cardiac output is usually measured with a thermodilution method. In brief, a cold saline solution injected through the proximal port of the PA catheter mixes with the blood in the right heart chambers and lowers the temperature of the blood, which is recorded by a thermistor at the distal end of the pulmonary artery.

Many variables can be calculated with the PA balloon catheter; the formulas are found in the Appendix. The PA catheter can be very useful to discriminate among several hemodynamic profiles. The most commonly encoun-

Table 10–5. Common Causes of Abnormal Waveform with the Pulmonary Artery Catheter

Problem	What To Do
No waveform identifiable	Flush catheter, check pressure bag device (pressure > 300 mm Hg), reassemble connections
Dampened waveforms	Flush catheter for air bubbles or clotting, check possible kinking of tube, recalibrate, reposition catheter to reduce tip placement against vessel wall
Pressure readings too low	True hypovolemia
	Calibrate, check zero reference point, check connections
Persistent PAOP	Withdraw catheter (catheter is advanced too far)
No PAOP	Advance catheter with inflated balloon, consider balloon rupture
Extreme variations in pressure tracings	Reposition catheter or replace

PAOP, pulmonary artery occlusion pressure.

Table 10–6. Pulmonary Artery Catheter Profiles

Condition	PCWP	CO	SVR	Therapy
Cardiac stunning (left ventricular failure)	High	Low	High	Dobutamine
Pulmonary edema				
Diastolic heart failure	High	Normal	Normal	Nitroglycerin
Neurogenic	Normal	Normal or low	Normal	PEEP
Sepsis				
Early	Low	High	Low	Volume expansion
Late	Normal	Normal	High	Dobutamine
Hypovolemia	Low	Low	High	Albumin
Massive pulmonary embolism	Normal	Low	High	Thrombolysis

CO, cardiac output; PCWP, pulmonary capillary wedge pressure; PEEP, positive end-expiratory pressure; SVR, systemic vascular resistance.
For normal values, see the Appendix.

tered conditions in the NICU are summarized in Table 10–6. Most often, the PA catheter is placed to monitor the potential existence of hypovolemia or to titrate to a hypervolemic state. Measurement of pulmonary artery wedge pressure is also useful in determination of neurogenic pulmonary edema (normal) or cardiac pulmonary edema (increased). Pulmonary artery catheter placement can also be useful in patients with congestive heart failure. In most neurologic patients, control over fluid replacement is the major indication for measurement of pulmonary wedge pressures.[47] Pulmonary occlusion pressure is increased to 12 to 15 mm Hg, but beyond this level, further increases in fluid volume minimally increase the ventricular preload defined by the Frank-Starling curve. Cardiac output can increase only if a vasodilator or inotropic agent is added.

Hypervolemia soon results in pulmonary edema, which is displayed by progressive radiologic abnormalities on sequential chest radiographs. At this juncture, a hypervolemic intravascular filling state can be achieved only by adding dobutamine.

Monitoring of Jugular Venous Oxygen Saturation

A technique made possible by the introduction of fiber-optic catheters may be useful in monitoring cerebral metabolism.[2] (In many ways, it is similar to the oximetric Swan-Ganz catheters.) It has been claimed that monitoring of jugular venous deterioration may identify secondary insults to the brain. Most of the studies have been performed in a few centers, specifically in patients with severe head injury and patients with subarachnoid hemorrhage and intracerebral hematomas.[64] The physiologic assumptions are as follows.

Cerebral blood flow is closely linked to the cerebral metabolic rate of oxygen, and its relationship is determined by the Fick equation. The Fick equation defines the oxygen uptake as the product of cardiac output (substituted by cerebral blood flow) and the arteriovenous difference in oxygen content. Studies by Robertson et al.[50–52] showed a close relationship between cerebral blood flow and jugular venous saturation ($SjvO_2$). When cerebral blood flow falters, it is compensated by increasing cerebral oxygen extraction, which results in a decrease in $SjvO_2$. Cerebral blood flow is significantly reduced when one or more episodes of jugular desaturation of oxygen are recorded. The normal $SjvO_2$ is 50% to 65%, and values below 50% for 15 minutes indicate ischemia. Cerebral blood flow can be reduced by many causes, including vasospasm, intracranial hypertension, induced hypocapnia, and hypotension, all of which reduce oxygen delivery to the brain. In addition, reduced hemoglobin may further reduce oxygen delivery.

The monitoring device is placed inside the jugular bulb. The catheter is preferably

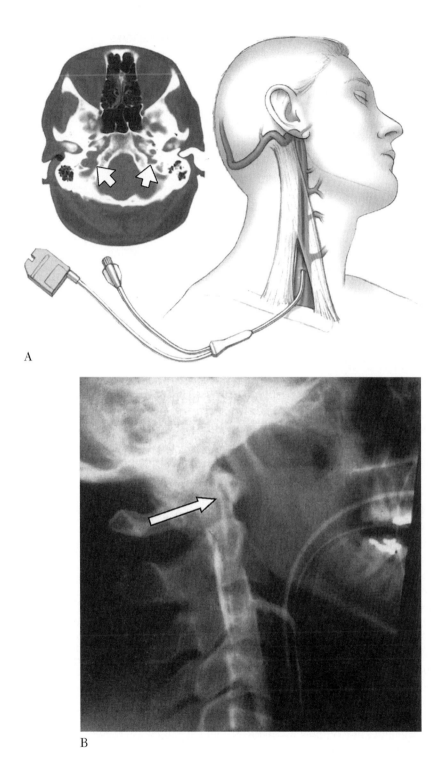

A

B

Figure 10–6. Jugular oxygen saturation catheter. (*A*) Placement of catheter, and jugular foramen on computed tomography scan. Right is typically larger than left (*arrows*). (*B*) Correct catheter tip position is above C1–2 (*arrow*). (*B* from Macmillan and Andrews.[30] By permission of Springer-Verlag.)

placed at the site of the largest jugular foramen (Fig. 10–6A) (dominance of venous flow)
on CT scan. Its position should ideally be cranial to a line connecting the mastoid processes[3] on a plain anteroposterior skull radiograph (Fig. 10–6B).

In previous studies, many abnormal readings were false alarms, with the potential to
encourage nursing staff and attending physicians to ignore abnormal values. In one study,
the sensitivity for detection of jugular bulb
saturation was 45% to 50%, with a specificity
of 98% to 100%, but only after repositioning
or flushing.[14] The monitoring technique,
however, should not be easily discarded as
unreliable and may still have considerable
promising value. A significant limitation is
that a low-intensity reading ($SjvO_2 < 50\%$)
may have its origin in poor positioning of the
probe against the wall as a result of collapse
of the internal jugular vein by decreased central nervous system pressure. One study confirmed false-positive findings in more than
half of these measurements.[58] The observed
oxygen desaturation must therefore be confirmed by measurement of blood withdrawn
from the catheter, and unfortunately this may
be necessary with every other saturation measurement. In addition, arterial hypoxemia or
anemia from whatever source should be excluded as a possible cause of oxygen desaturation. It is also important to calculate the arteriovenous difference in oxygen, which
should move in the opposite direction[58] (see
Appendix). Trends may be more important
(Fig. 10–7).

Complications such as infections, accidental
misplacement, and carotid puncture were very
uncommon, whereas jugular bulb venous
thrombosis was found in 40% of 44 monitored
patients.[13]

The therapeutic interventions in patients
with markedly decreased $SjvO_2$ are (1) adjustment of the depth of hypocapnia, (2) more frequent administration of mannitol boluses, (3)
correction of anemia, and (4) adjustment of
mean arterial blood pressure.[17-20] A guideline
proposed by Macmillan and Andrews[30] is

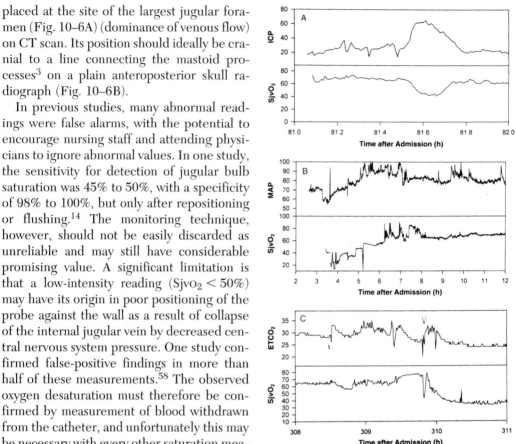

Figure 10–7. Example of trend recordings of
jugular venous oxygen saturation ($SjvO_2$). (*Top*)
Increased intracranial pressure (ICP). (*Middle*)
Hypotension. (*Bottom*) Hypocapnia. $ETCO_2$,
end-tidal carbon dioxide concentration; MAP,
mean arterial pressure. (From Feldman Z,
Robertson CS: Monitoring of cerebral hemo-
dynamics with jugular bulb catheters. *Crit
Care Clin* 13:51–77, 1997. By permission of
WB Saunders Company.)

shown in Figure 10–8. No study has determined the effect of these corrections on outcome in the patients considered for monitoring, but $SjvO_2$ desaturation has been correlated
with poor outcome in head injury.

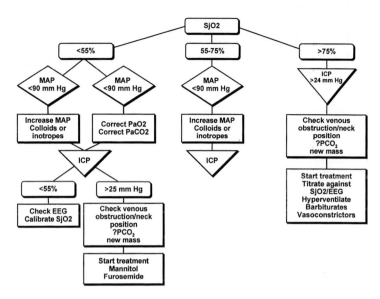

Figure 10–8. Clinical guidelines for jugular bulb saturation (SjO₂). EEG, electroencephalogram; ICP, intracranial pressure; MAP, mean arterial pressure. (Modified from Macmillan and Andrews.[30] By permission of Springer-Verlag.)

Pulse Oximetry

Pulse oximetry is based on spectrophotometric principles. Emitted light is subsequently reflected by hemoglobin; different hemoglobin configurations reflect different wavelengths. With pulse oximetry, two wavelengths are used to determine the relative concentration of oxyhemoglobin and reduced hemoglobin. Several factors, such as anemia, nail polish, hypothermia, and dark-pigmented skin, can produce inaccurate results.[57] Pulse oximetry is accurate in patients with dysrhythmias and a pulse deficit.

Noninvasive oximetry is widely considered to be one of the most important technical advances in monitoring respiratory status and has reduced the number of arterial blood gas determinations. Prospective studies have clearly demonstrated a 19-fold increase in the detection of hypoxemia (pulse oximeter saturation of oxygen < 90%) in postoperative patients.[36,37] However, when audited, pulse oximetry appeared less useful in certain studies. One study found that the number of arterial blood gas measurements decreased by only 3% in me-

chanically ventilated patients monitored by pulse oximetry.[1] In another study, no mention of hypoxemic episodes was made in clinical notes in many patients with desaturation values below 85%.[8] In the NICU we routinely use pulse oximetry and find it particularly useful in monitoring of patients with trauma, patients with any type of acute ischemic or hemorrhagic stroke (particularly when Cheyne-Stokes breathing intervenes), patients with Guillain-Barré syndrome who have diaphragmatic failure, and patients undergoing the apnea test. Pulse oximetry has repeatedly guided us to increase oxygen intake or to proceed with intubation.

Near-Infrared Spectroscopy

Near-infrared spectroscopy can monitor changes in cerebral oxygenation and blood volume by measuring concentrations of oxyhemoglobin and deoxyhemoglobin.[42,48,61] Although superficially similar to pulse oximetry, near-infrared spectroscopy is fundamentally different because of different wavelengths and greater tissue penetration. The principle is shown in Figure 10–9.

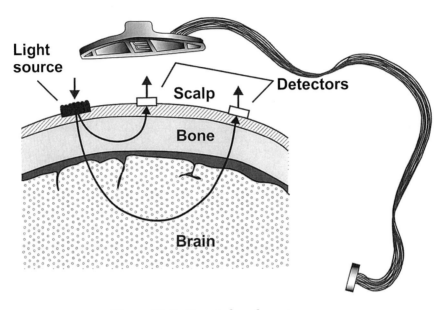

Figure 10–9. Near-infrared spectroscopy.

The absorbance measured by detectors is predominantly that of venous blood, and the findings would thus be equivalent to, for example, those of jugular bulb saturation.

The main assumption is that concentrations of oxyhemoglobin and hemoglobin and oxidized cytochrome oxidase (considered negligible) change with change in cerebral perfusion and oxygenation. Near-infrared light (650 to 1000 nm) penetrates the scalp to a depth of 2.5 cm. The path of the photons is parabolic, and the depth of the tissue penetrated is related to the distance between limited light and detector. The proximal receiver thus detects light passed through tissue outside the cortex. Both signals (proximal and distal detectors) are subtracted, and the ratio gives a value for cerebral oxygen saturation.

Major problems are unreliability due to extracerebral blood and extradural hematoma, difficulty in establishing criteria of ischemia by comparative methods such as electroencephalography and somatosensory evoked potentials, and general problems with replication of results.[6,27–29,39,65] With further generations, the device may become clinically useful.

FUTURE DIRECTIONS

The availability of reliable ICP monitors and the frequent use of Swan-Ganz catheters have changed monitoring of patients in the NICU. Noninvasive monitoring of cerebral well-being remains a holy grail. New noninvasive approaches have included cerebrovenous oxygen monitoring,[30] venous transcranial Doppler ultrasonography (venous blood is pooled to larger venous vessels, and venous maximal blood flow velocity increases),[56] measurement of tympanic membrane pressure (changes in ICP change the hydrostatic pressure of the cochlea and displace the tympanic membrane),[49] ophthalmodynamometry (pressure in the central retinal vein correlates linearly with ICP),[38] pupillometry ("sluggish pupil" reduction in constriction velocity may herald an increase in ICP),[31] and tissue resonance analysis (ultrasonography obtains echopulsograms from the third ventricle equivalent to intracranial pressure waves.[35] Each device should be evaluated for its role in patient care. Neurologic intensive care specialists will continue to face difficult choices in whether to use new technology, and progress is slow. Whether multimodal monitoring (combining the benefits of different devices) is useful is not exactly known, but the concept is certainly exciting.[26] Although it may combine benefits, it may also multiply false readings and create greater confusion. Nonetheless, noninvasive monitoring of brain function should be a focus of meticulous research rather than naive enthusiasm over a new device.

CONCLUSIONS

- Coma scales are useful in monitoring neurologic deterioration. The Glasgow coma scale should be considered the standard scale.
- Fiber-optic monitors are the most contemporary and reliable devices for intraparenchymal monitoring of ICP. Ventriculostomy should be reserved for patients with acute hydrocephalus. Epidural catheters are used only in patients with coagulopathy, to reduce the risk of complications.
- Jugular venous oxygen saturation may identify further insults to the brain, monitor depth of hypocapnia, and could lead to adjustment of mean arterial blood pressure.
- PA catheters are indicated for patients with subarachnoid hemorrhage of poor grade, for patients who have congestive heart failure and ischemic or hemorrhagic stroke, for patients with Guillain-Barré syndrome who have dysautonomia, and for monitoring the effect of vasopressor medication.

REFERENCES

1. Alford PT, Hawkins P, Sherrill TR, et al: Impact of pulse oximetry on demand for arterial blood gases in an ICU (abstract). *Chest* 96 Suppl:288S, 1989.
2. Andrews PJD, Dearden NM, Miller JD: Jugular bulb cannulation: description of a cannulation technique and validation of a new continuous monitor. *Br J Anaesth* 67:553–558, 1991.
3. Bankier AA, Fleischmann D, Windisch A, et al: Position of jugular oxygen saturation catheter in patients with head trauma: assessment by use of plain films. *AJR Am J Roentgenol* 164:437–441, 1995.
4. Barnett GH: Intracranial pressure monitoring devices: principles, insertion, and care. In Ropper AH (ed): *Neurological and Neurosurgical Intensive Care.* 3rd ed. New York, Raven Press, 1993, pp 53–68.
5. Bavetta S, Norris JS, Wyatt M, et al: Prospective study of zero drift in fiberoptic pressure monitors used in clinical practice. *J Neurosurg* 86:927–930, 1997.
6. Beese U, Langer H, Lang W, et al: Comparison of near-infrared spectroscopy and somatosensory evoked potentials for the detection of cerebral ischemia during carotid endarterectomy. *Stroke* 29:2032–2037, 1998.
7. Blei AT, Olafsson S, Webster S, et al: Complications of intracranial pressure monitoring in fulminant hepatic failure. *Lancet* 341:157–158, 1993.
8. Bowton DL, Scuderi PE, Harris L, et al: Pulse oximetry monitoring outside the intensive care unit: Progress or problem? *Ann Intern Med* 115:450–454, 1991.
9. Bur A, Hirschl MM, Herkner H, et al: Accuracy of oscillometric blood pressure measurement according to the relation between cuff size and upper-arm circumference in critically ill patients. *Crit Care Med* 28:371–376, 2000.
10. Chambers KR, Kane PJ, Choksey MS, et al: An evaluation of the Camino ventricular bolt system in clinical practice. *Neurosurgery* 33:866–868, 1993.
11. Chesnut RM, Marshall LF: Management of head injury. Treatment of abnormal intracranial pressure. *Neurosurg Clin N Am* 2:267–284, 1991.
12. Coles NA, Hibberd M, Russell M, et al: Potential impact of pulmonary artery catheter placement on short-term management decisions in the medical intensive care unit. *Am Heart J* 126:815–819, 1993.
13. Coplin WM, O'Keefe GE, Grady MS, et al: Thrombotic, infectious, and procedural complications of the jugular bulb catheter in the intensive care unit. *Neurosurgery* 41:101–107, 1997.
14. Coplin WM, O'Keefe GE, Grady MS, et al: Accuracy of continuous jugular bulb oximetry in the intensive care unit. *Neurosurgery* 42:533–539, 1998.
15. Cropp AJ, Woods LA, Raney D, et al: Name that tone. The proliferation of alarms in the intensive care unit. *Chest* 105:1217–1220, 1994.
16. Crutchfield JS, Narayan RK, Robertson CS, et al: Evaluation of a fiberoptic intracranial pressure monitor. *J Neurosurg* 72:482–487, 1990.
17. Cruz J: Combined continuous monitoring of systemic and cerebral oxygenation in acute brain injury: preliminary observations. *Crit Care Med* 21:1225–1232, 1993.

18. Cruz J: On-line monitoring of global cerebral hypoxia in acute brain injury. Relationship to intracranial hypertension. *J Neurosurg* 79:228–233, 1993.

19. Cruz J, Miner ME, Allen SJ, et al: Continuous monitoring of cerebral oxygenation in acute brain injury: injection of mannitol during hyperventilation. *J Neurosurg* 73:725–730, 1990.

20. Cruz J, Raps EC, Hoffstad OJ, et al: Cerebral oxygenation monitoring. *Crit Care Med* 21:1242–1246, 1993.

21. Dalen JE: The pulmonary artery catheter—friend, foe, or accomplice? *JAMA* 286:348–350, 2001.

22. Frezza EE, Mezghebe H: Indications and complications of arterial catheter use in surgical or medical intensive care units: analysis of 4932 patients. *Am Surg* 64:127–131, 1998.

23. Gnaegi A, Feihl F, Perret C: Intensive care physicians' insufficient knowledge of right-heart catheterization at the bedside: Time to act? *Crit Care Med* 25:213–220, 1997.

24. Gopinath SP, Robertson CS, Contant CF, et al: Jugular venous desaturation and outcome after head injury. *J Neurol Neurosurg Psychiatry* 57:717–723, 1994.

25. Grant SA, Bettencourt K, Krulevitch P, et al: Development of fiber optic and electrochemical pH sensors to monitor brain tissue. *Crit Rev Biomed Eng* 28:159–163, 2000.

26. Kirkpatrick PJ, Czosnyka M, Pickard JD: Multimodal monitoring in neurointensive care. *J Neurol Neurosurg Psychiatry* 60:131–139, 1996.

27. Kirkpatrick PJ, Lam J, Al-Rawi P, et al: Defining thresholds for critical ischemia by using near-infrared spectroscopy in the adult brain. *J Neurosurg* 89:389–394, 1998.

28. Kirkpatrick PJ, Snielewski P, Czosnyka M, et al: Near-infrared spectroscopy use in patients with head injury. *J Neurosurg* 83:963–970, 1995.

29. Lewis SB, Myburgh JA, Thornton EL, et al: Cerebral oxygenation monitoring by near-infrared spectroscopy is not clinically useful in patients with severe closed-head injury: a comparison with jugular venous bulb oximetry. *Crit Care Med* 24:1334–1338, 1996.

30. Macmillan CS, Andrews PJ: Cerebrovenous oxygen saturation monitoring: practical considerations and clinical relevance. *Intensive Care Med* 26:1028–1036, 2000.

31. Marshall LF: Head injury: recent past, present, and future. *Neurosurgery* 47:546–561, 2000.

32. Martin C, Saux P, Papazian L, et al: Long-term arterial cannulation in ICU patients using the radial artery or dorsalis pedis artery. *Chest* 119:901–906, 2001.

33. Martinez-Manas RM, Santamarta D, de Campos JM, et al: Camino intracranial pressure monitor: prospective study of accuracy and complications. *J Neurol Neurosurg Psychiatry* 69:82–86, 2000.

34. Mayer SA, Sacco RL, Shi T, et al: Neurologic deterioration in noncomatose patients with supratentorial intracerebral hemorrhage. *Neurology* 44:1379–1384, 1994.

35. Michaeli D, Rappaport ZH: Tissue resonance analysis; a novel method for noninvasive monitoring of intracranial pressure. *J Neurosurg* 96:1132–1137, 2002.

36. Moller JT, Johannessen NW, Espersen K, et al: Randomized evaluation of pulse oximetry in 20,802 patients: II. Perioperative events and postoperative complications. *Anesthesiology* 78:445–453, 1993.

37. Moller JT, Pedersen T, Rasmussen LS, et al: Randomized evaluation of pulse oximetry in 20,802 patients: I. Design, demography, pulse oximetry failure rate, and overall complication rate. *Anesthesiology* 78:436–444, 1993.

38. Motschmann M, Muller C, Kuchenbecker J, et al: Ophthalmodynamometry: a reliable method for measuring intracranial pressure. *Strabismus* 9:13–16, 2001.

39. Muellner T, Schramm W, Kwasny O, et al: Patients with increased intracranial pressure cannot be monitored using near infrared spectroscopy. *Br J Neurosurg* 12:136–139, 1998.

40. Münch E, Weigel R, Schmiedek P, et al: The Camino intracranial pressure device in clinical practice: reliability, handling characteristics and complications. *Acta Neurochir* 140:1113–1119, 1998.

41. O'Sullivan MG, Statham PF, Jones PA, et al: Role of intracranial pressure monitoring in severely head-injured patients without signs of intracranial hypertension on initial computerized tomography. *J Neurosurg* 80:46–50, 1994.

42. Owen-Reece H, Smith M, Elwell CE, et al: Near infrared spectroscopy. *Br J Anaesth* 82:418–426, 1999.

43. Perret C, Tagan D, Feihl F, et al (eds): *The Pulmonary Artery Catheter in Critical Care: a Concise Handbook*. Oxford, Blackwell Science, 1996.

44. Poca MA, Sahuquillo J, Arribas M, et al: Fiberoptic intraparenchymal brain pressure monitoring with the Camino V420 monitor: reflections on our experience in 163 severely head-injured patients. *J Neurotrauma* 19:439–448, 2002.

45. Polanczyk CA, Rohde LE, Goldman L, et al: Right heart catheterization and cardiac complications in patients undergoing noncardiac surgery: an observational study. *JAMA* 286:309–314, 2001.

46. Poon WS, Ng S, Wai S: CSF antibiotic prophylaxis for neurosurgical patients with ventriculostomy: a randomised study. *Acta Neurochir Suppl (Wien)* 71:146–148, 1998.

47. Pritz MB, Goldenberg TM: Usefulness of a fiber optic Swan-Ganz catheter to monitor oxygen transport during volume expansion in a patient with ischemic neurologic deficits from aneurysmal subarachnoid hemorrhage. *Surg Neurol* 41:125–130, 1994.

48. Prough DS, Pollard V: Cerebral near-infrared spectroscopy: Ready for prime time? *Crit Care Med* 23:1624–1626, 1995.

49. Reid A, Marchbanks RJ, Burge DM, et al: The relationship between intracranial pressure and tympanic membrane displacement. *Br J Audiol* 24:123–129, 1990.

50. Robertson CS, Contant CF, Gokaslan ZL, et al: Cerebral blood flow, arteriovenous oxygen difference, and outcome in head injured patients. *J Neurol Neurosurg Psychiatry* 55:594–603, 1992.

51. Robertson CS, Grossman RG, Goodman JC, et al: The predictive value of cerebral anaerobic metabolism with cerebral infarction after head injury. *J Neurosurg* 67:361–368, 1987.

52. Robertson CS, Narayan RK, Gokaslan ZL, et al: Cerebral arteriovenous oxygen difference as an estimate of cerebral blood flow in comatose patients. *J Neurosurg* 70:222–230, 1989.

53. Rosner MJ, Daughton S: Cerebral perfusion pressure management in head injury. *J Trauma* 30:933–940, 1990.

54. Rowley G, Fielding K: Reliability and accuracy of the Glasgow Coma Scale with experienced and inexperienced users. *Lancet* 337:535–538, 1991.

55. Schickner DJ, Young RF: Intracranial pressure monitoring: fiberoptic monitor compared with the ventricular catheter. *Surg Neurol* 37:251–254, 1992.

56. Schoser BG, Riemenschneider N, Hansen HC: The impact of raised intracranial pressure on cerebral venous hemodynamics: a prospective venous transcranial Doppler ultrasonography study. *J Neurosurg* 91:744–749, 1999.

57. Severinghaus JW, Kelleher JF: Recent developments in pulse oximetry. *Anesthesiology* 76:1018–1038, 1992.

58. Sheinberg M, Kanter MJ, Robertson CS, et al: Continuous monitoring of jugular venous oxygen saturation in head-injured patients. *J Neurosurg* 76:212–217, 1992.

59. Squara P, Bennett D, Perret C: Pulmonary artery catheter: does the problem lie in the users? *Chest* 121:2009–2015, 2002.

60. Sundbarg G, Nordstrom CH, Soderstrom S: Complications due to prolonged ventricular fluid pressure recording. *Br J Neurosurg* 2:485–495, 1988.

61. Tateishi A, Maekawa T, Soejima Y, et al: Qualitative comparison of carbon dioxide-induced change in cerebral near-infrared spectroscopy versus jugular venous oxygen saturation in adults with acute brain disease. *Crit Care Med* 23:1734–1738, 1995.

62. Teasdale G, Jennett B: Assessment of coma and impaired consciousness. A practical scale. *Lancet* 2:81–84, 1974.

63. Vermeulen M, van Gijn J, Hijdra A, et al: Causes of acute deterioration in patients with a ruptured intracranial aneurysm. A prospective study with serial CT scanning. *J Neurosurg* 60:935–939, 1984.

64. von Helden A, Schneider GH, Unterberg A, et al: Monitoring of jugular venous oxygen saturation in comatose patients with subarachnoid haemorrhage and intracerebral haematomas. *Acta Neurochir Suppl (Wien)* 59:102–106, 1993.

65. Wahr JA, Tremper KK, Samra S, et al: Near-infrared spectroscopy: theory and applications. *J Cardiothorac Vasc Anesth* 10:406–418, 1996.

66. Weinstabl C, Richling B, Plainer B, et al: Comparative analysis between epidural (Gaeltec) and subdural (Camino) intracranial pressure probes. *J Clin Monit* 8:116–120, 1992.

67. Wijdicks EFM: Temporomandibular joint compression in coma. *Neurology* 46:1774, 1996.

68. Wijdicks EFM, Kokmen E, O'Brien PC: Measurement of impaired consciousness in the neurological intensive care unit: a new test. *J Neurol Neurosurg Psychiatry* 64:117–119, 1998.

69. Williams EJ, Bunch CS, Carpenter TA, et al: Magnetic resonance imaging compatibility testing of intracranial pressure probes. Technical note. *J Neurosurg* 91:706–709, 1999.

70. Young CC, Mark JB, White W, et al: Clinical evaluation of continuous noninvasive blood pressure monitoring: accuracy and tracking capabilities. *J Clin Monit* 11:245–252, 1995.

11

Diagnostic Procedures

Common diagnostic tests in the NICU are transcranial Doppler ultrasonography (TCD), electrodiagnostic tests (such as electroencephalography, continuous electroencephalographic and video monitoring, and evoked potentials), and CSF examination. Neurologists who care for patients with a critical neurologic illness commonly perform or interpret neuroimaging studies (particularly CT, magnetic resonance imaging [MRI], magnetic resonance angiography, and cerebral angiography), and expert interpretation is necessary to minimize erroneous clinical decisions. The most pertinent neuroradiologic features in acute neurologic conditions are discussed and illustrated in the chapters of Part III of this book. Many clinical decisions (emergency surgery, ventriculostomy) are a result of prompt resolve, and these extrapolating skills have been acquired gradually over the years.

Neurointensivists should have a thorough knowledge of these diagnostic studies and must know what can be expected in deteriorating patients. Close review with the interventional neuroradiologist and neurosurgeon is often necessary to plan care.

This chapter reviews diagnostic procedures performed by neurointensivists at the bedside and assesses their relative advantages but also their imperfections.

GRADING OF COMPUTED TOMOGRAPHY SCAN OF THE BRAIN

In an effort to quantify abnormalities on CT scans, grading scales have been proposed. It matters much if these scales, once developed, are imprecise, and they may fail to become mainstream scoring systems when they lack ease of use. Others argue that the inaccuracies of visual inspection can only be overcome by software-based quantification. None of the scales presented here has clearly dominated over others, and all are commonly used. Any new scale must be validated in other data sets, different scanners, and different institutions.

Scales in Subarachnoid Hemorrhage

Fisher developed one of the first grading systems for subarachnoid hemorrhage (SAH). The *Fisher scale,* although deeply ingrained in NICU jargon, remains a gross estimate of the amount of subarachnoid blood with significant interobserver variability. This scale (Table 11–1), which emphasizes the presence or absence of thick clot in specific locations, predicts the development of delayed cerebral ischemia. In a prospective study, subarachnoid clots (grades 2 and 3) predicted severe vasospasm in 20 of 22 patients.[49]

Another method was developed by Hijdra et

Table 11–1. Computed Tomography Findings in the Fisher Scale

Grade	Finding
1	No detectable subarachnoid blood on CT
2	Diffuse blood, no clots > 3 mm thick or vertical layers > 1 mm thick
3	Localized clot > 5 × 3 mm in subarachnoid space, or > 1 mm in vertical cisterns (interhemispheric, ambient, lateral sylvian cisterns)
4	Intracerebral or intraventricular hemorrhage with diffuse or no subarachnoid blood

CT, computed tomography.

Source: Data from Kistler JP, Crowell RM, Davis KR, et al: The relation of cerebral vasospasm to the extent and location of subarachnoid blood visualized by CT scan: a prospective study. *Neurology* 33:424–436, 1983.

al.[39] (Fig. 11–1). A sum score of greater than 20 is considered predictive of vasospasm. Initial studies of agreement among three observers documented very satisfactory results, but these results could not be confirmed in a separate set of CT scans scored by "expert raters."[91] An expanded scale (Table 11–2), proposed by Claassen et al.,[14] incorporating the Hijdra scale into a 4-point scale, was found superior to the Fisher scale.

We have developed a possibly widely applicable method to quantify subarachnoid hemorrhage on CT scan. Using the Analyze image analysis program (Biomedical Imaging Resource, Mayo Clinic, Rochester, MN), we traced the border of the partitioned hemorrhage on all pertinent images (Fig. 11–2). A threshold of cisternal hemorrhagic volume existed, above which delayed cerebral ischemia developed (> 20 cm³) (Fig. 11–3). The software is inexpensive and can be used on a standard personal computer running a Windows-based operating system. Quantification takes 20 minutes. Prospective evaluation of this method is under way.[29]

Grading in Cerebral Hemorrhage

Assessment of the volume of lobar or ganglionic hemorrhage provides a baseline from which to assess possible enlargement. When compared with computerized methods, the so-called ABC/2 method provides a very useful quantification. This method assumes the hematoma is an ellipsoidal mass in which A is the greatest diameter on the largest hemorrhagic slice, B is the diameter perpendicular to A, and C is the number of axial slices with hemorrhage multiplied by the slice thickness. The product ABC is divided by 2. The volume is expressed in cubic centimeters. Small hematomas (Fig. 11–4) have been arbitrarily considered less than 30 cm³ and large hemorrhages greater than 60 cm³. Intraventricular extension is roughly estimated as sedimentation only or

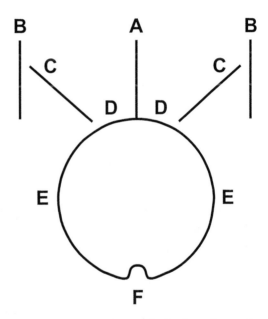

Figure 11–1. Hijdra method of grading subarachnoid hemorrhage. The diagram identifies 10 basal cisterns and fissures: (A) frontal interhemispheric fissure; (B) sylvian fissure, lateral parts; (C) sylvian fissure, basal parts; (D) suprasellar cistern; (E) ambient cisterns; and (F) quadrigeminal cistern. The amount of blood in each cistern and fissure is graded 0, no blood; 1, small amount of blood; 2, moderately filled with blood; and 3, completely filled with blood. The sum score is 0 to 30 points. (From Hijdra A, Brouwers PJAM, Vermeulen M, et al: Grading the amount of blood on computed tomograms after subarachnoid hemorrhage. *Stroke* 21:1156–1161, 1990. By permission of the American Heart Association.)

Table 11–2. Subarachnoid Hemorrhage Computed Tomography Rating Scale

			FREQUENCY (%)	
Grade	Criteria	Patients (%)	Vasospasm	Cerebral Infarction
0	No SAH or IVH	5	0	0
1	Minimal/thin SAH, no IVH in both lateral ventricles	30	12	6
2	Minimal/thin SAH, *with* IVH in both lateral ventricles	5	21	14
3	Thick SAH,° no IVH in both lateral ventricles	43	19	12
4	Thick SAH,° *with* IVH in both lateral ventricles	17	40	28

IVH, intraventricular hemorrhage; SAH, subarachnoid hemorrhage.
°Completely filling ≥ 1 cistern or fissure on the basis of Hijdra criteria.
Source: Claassen J, Bernardini GL, Kreiter K, et al: Effect of cisternal and ventricular blood on risk of delayed cerebral ischemia after subarachnoid hemorrhage: the Fisher scale revisited. *Stroke* 32:2012–2020, 2001. By permission of the American Heart Association.

frank ("packed") hemorrhage in each of the ventricles. More subtle grading of intraventricular blood has not been tested. The value of measuring volume in cerebellar hematoma has not been established, and diameters of more than 3 cm have been considered cutoff values for surgery (Chapter 14).

Diringer et al.[20] suggested a hydrocephalus score. This method grades each of the eight parts of the ventricular system independently into four categories: normal (0), mild (1), moderate (2), and marked (3) enlargement. Enlargement of the parts is defined as follows: frontal horn—increased radius, decreased ventricular angle, and sulcal effacement of the frontal lobe; posterior horn—rounding of the horn with sulcal effacement of the parieto-occipital lobe; temporal horn—increased width; third ventricle—increased width and ballooning of the anterior recess; and fourth ventricle—

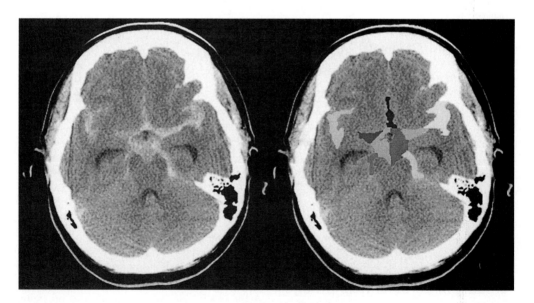

Figure 11–2. Representative images of unsegmented (*left*) and segmented (*right*) computed tomography series. Each region is represented by a different shade. *Source:* Friedman JA, Goerss SJ, Meyer FB, et al: Volumetric quantification of Fisher Grade 3 aneurysmal subarachnoid hemorrhage: a novel method to predict symptomatic vasospasm on admission computerized tomography scans. *J Neurosurg* 97:401–407, 2002. By permission of the American Association of Neurological Surgeons.

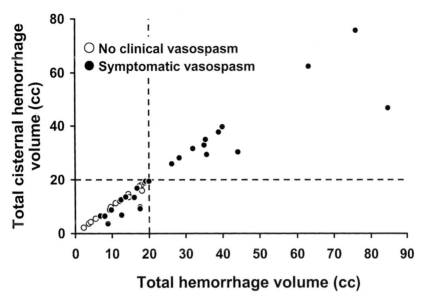

Figure 11–3. Absolute values of total cisternal hemorrhage volume by total hemorrhage volume. Note that at greater than 20 cc of cisternal hemorrhage volume, symptomatic vasospasm developed in all patients. *Source:* Friedman JA, Goerss SJ, Meyer FB, et al: Volumetric quantification of Fisher Grade 3 aneurysmal subarachnoid hemorrhage: a novel method to predict symptomatic vasospasm on admission computerized tomography scans. *J Neurosurg* 97:401–407, 2002. By permission of the American Association of Neurological Surgeons.

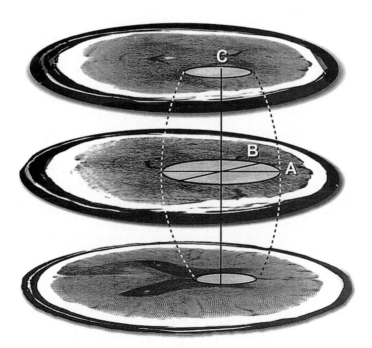

Figure 11–4. Ellipsoid method (ABC/2) for assessing the volume of cerebral hematomas. *A* is the greatest diameter on the largest hemorrhagic slice, *B* is the diameter perpendicular to A, and *C* is the number of axial slices with hemorrhage multiplied by the slice thickness. The product ABC is divided by 2, with the volume expressed in cubic centimeters.

bulging. The score for each ventricle is summed. A maximum score of 24 is considered marked hydrocephalus of all ventricles.

Scales in Head Injury

Computed tomography scan classification systems have been rather scarce, perhaps a reflection of the impossibility of categorizing the multiplicity of findings after a major traumatic impact. Certainly, the difficulty in reliably attaching a certain prognostic measure to one or more CT scan findings has discouraged development of a system. Marshall et al.[61] developed a reasonable working system (Table 11–3), but it has been criticized because the perimesencephalic cisterns were only partly addressed. In another system, grades were defined by widening of the perimesencephalic cisterns, obliteration of these cisterns, deformity of the brain stem in the anteroposterior axis, and density changes, particularly hemorrhagic findings.[58] Deformation of the brain stem and density changes in one study predicted very poor outcome.[58]

TRANSCRANIAL DOPPLER ULTRASONOGRAPHY

The use of TCD in the NICU has generated both enthusiasm and criticism. The precise clinical implications of results obtained by TCD are not always clear. Currently, data are obtained with a single examination. Future studies using continuous TCD monitoring (the probe is cradled in a tight headset) may increase its practical use.

General Principles of Transcranial Doppler Ultrasonography Examination

The technique of TCD is easy to master, and the learning curve is steep. The three-dimensional planes of the circle of Willis must be known to the examiner. Insonation from a temporal window is started first. Several strategies can be tried to obtain adequate TCD signals. The probe is positioned directly above the zygomatic arch, with the transducer often resting on the zygomatic arch midway from the helix of the ear to the orbital rim (Fig. 11–5). A reliable signal can be obtained by pressing the transducer with acoustic gel to the temporal bone. A slow circular movement of the end of the transducer without a change in contact may help in finding a signal. A signal identifying the middle cerebral artery (MCA) can be obtained at a starting depth of 55 mm. If a signal is not found, the probe is shifted more anteriorly toward the orbital rim. If a signal is still not found, the probe is moved upward at the crossing of the zygomatic bone and the lateral orbital margin. Approximately 10% of patients do not have a temporal window, and failure to find a signal cannot be attributed to technique. (Reviews by Newell and Aaslid[67] and Arnolds and von Reutern[2] can

Table 11–3. Diagnostic Categories of Types of Abnormalities Visualized on Computed Tomography Scanning (Marshall Grading System)

Category	Definition
Diffuse injury I (no visible pathology)	No visible intracranial pathology seen on CT scan
Diffuse injury II	Cisterns are present with midline shift 0–5 mm and/or lesion densities present, no high- or mixed-density lesion > 25 cm³; may include bone fragments and foreign bodies
Diffuse injury III (swelling)	Cisterns compressed or absent with midline shift 0–5 mm, no high- or mixed-density lesion > 25 cm³
Diffuse injury IV (shift)	Midline shift > 5 mm, no high- or mixed-density lesion > 25 cm³
Evacuated mass lesion	Any lesion surgically evacuated
Nonevacuated mass lesion	High- or mixed-density lesion > 25 cm³, not surgically evacuated

CT, computed tomography.
Source: From Marshall LF, Marshall SB, Klauber MR, et al: A new classification of head injury based on computerized tomography. *J Neurosurg* 75:514, 1991. By permission of the American Association of Neurological Surgeons.

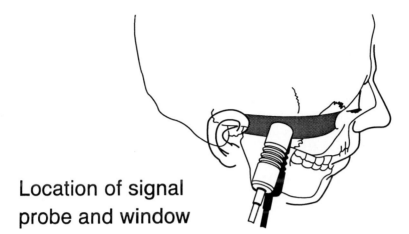

Location of signal probe and window

Figure 11–5. Transcranial Doppler ultrasonography: localization of the temporal window.

be consulted for further refinements in the examination technique.) Doppler examination can proceed only when a reliable signal is identified. No particular prerequisites are necessary. The patient must be immobilized and not continuously moving or speaking. Hyperventilation decreases the mean MCA velocities by 5 cm/second, an amount often too small to measure.

The typical Doppler waveform (Fig. 11–6) portrays the peak systolic velocity (PSV) and end-diastolic velocity (EDV) needed to measure the mean velocity (PSV − EDV/3 +

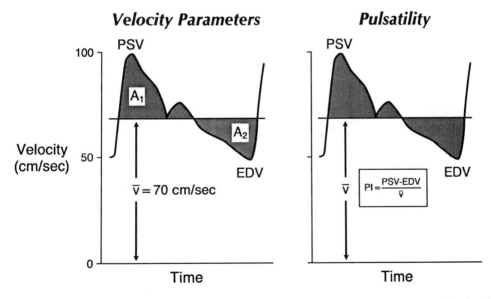

Figure 11–6. Typical Doppler waveform and measurement of mean velocity ($\bar{v}$) and pulsatility index (PI). (*Left panel*) A cursor is placed so that the area above the cursor (A_1, defined by the peak velocity display) is equal to the area below the cursor (A_2, defined by the diastole display). (*Right panel*) The pulsatility index, usually automatically calculated on most modern transcranial Doppler machines, is the difference between the maximal and the minimal velocities divided by the mean velocity. PSV, peak systolic velocity; EDV, end-diastolic velocity.

EDV). The pulsatility index indicates the resistance in the system.

An obstructive lesion proximal to the point of insonation has a lengthened rise time and dampening of the peak systolic and end-diastolic components from loss of pressure across the proximal obstruction. Increased pulsatility index typically occurs proximal to the lesion, because maximal vasodilatation from intact autoregulation produces less resistance and therefore increased pulsation. Abnormalities in absolute values, relative difference of more than 50% from each side, and turbulence, if present, producing a cracked or harsh sound and localized focal reversal of the signal should be noted.

A common technique is to start identifying the MCA signal at 55 mm (Fig. 11–7A). Flow is directed toward the probe, and typical mean velocities are in the range of 50 to 60 cm/second. Next, the probe is held constant while the depth is advanced incrementally to 60 to 65 mm. A bidirectional signal becomes apparent, identifying the bifurcation of the MCA and

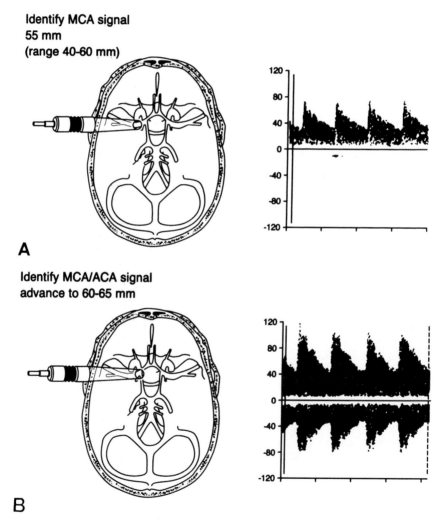

Figure 11–7. Transcranial Doppler ultrasonography: temporal window technique. (*A*) Middle cerebral artery (MCA) signal. (*B*) Bifurcation of the MCA and anterior cerebral artery (ACA) signal.

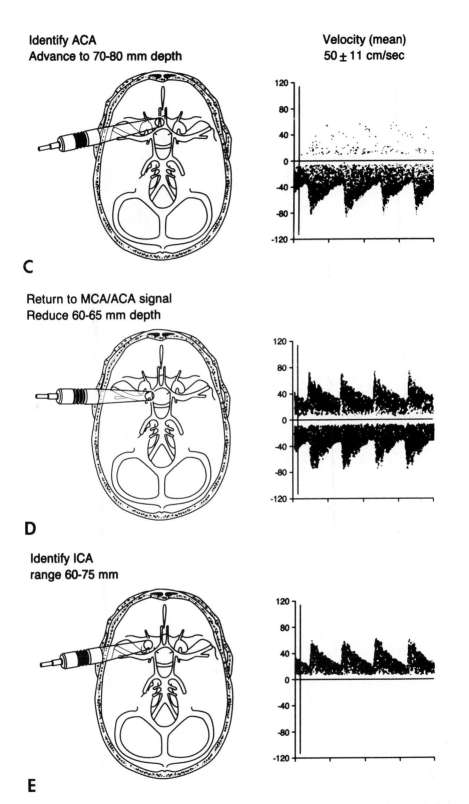

Figure 11–7. (*Continued*) (*C*) ACA signal. (*D*) Relocation of the MCA–ACA signal. (*E*) Internal carotid artery (ICA) signal.

Relocate MCA/ACA signal

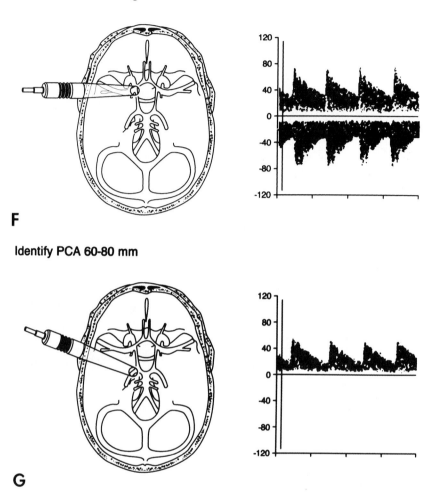

F

Identify PCA 60-80 mm

G

Figure 11–7. (*Continued*) (*F*) Relocation of the MCA–ACA signal. (*G*) Posterior cerebral artery (PCA) signal.

the anterior cerebral artery (ACA) (Fig. 11–7B). The ACA signal is further investigated by minor repositioning of the probe upward and anteriorly and by an increase in depth to between 70 and 80 mm. The ACA velocities (50 cm/second) are slightly lower than the MCA velocities (Fig. 11–7C).

Subsequently, the internal carotid artery (ICA) is identified by reducing the depth of the probe to 60 to 65 mm and adjusting the angle of the probe to relocate the MCA–ACA signal (Fig. 11–7D). From this important landmark, the probe is angulated downward but this time

without any change in depth. The ICA is characterized by flow directed toward the probe. The velocities of the terminal part of the ICA are lower (40 cm/second) (Fig. 11–7E).

The last vessel to be insonated, the posterior cerebral artery (PCA), is found by again relocating the bifurcation signal, MCA–ACA (Fig. 11–7F), and angling the probe downward and toward the occiput, with only minimal increments (5 mm) in depth but to a total depth of up to 80 mm. The PCA signal can be confused with the MCA because of its similar characteristics, but the sound of the PCA signal is lower pitched (Fig. 11–7G). When the result is in doubt during bedside examination, compression of the carotid artery often dampens the MCA signal, or use of a very bright light can reveal increased flow in the PCA signal.

Although less in vogue and considered obsolete by some, examination of the carotid siphon is done through the orbit. The signal of the siphon can provide additional information when no signal can be found through tempo-ral windows. For example, this may be of benefit in patients with acute carotid artery occlusion (to estimate the extent of the thrombus) and in patients who become brain dead (when no second window is available). The probe is placed over the closed eyelid and against the glabella. Information can be obtained from the ophthalmic artery at a depth of 35 mm (Fig. 11–8A) and of the siphon at 50 to 70 mm (Fig. 11–8B).

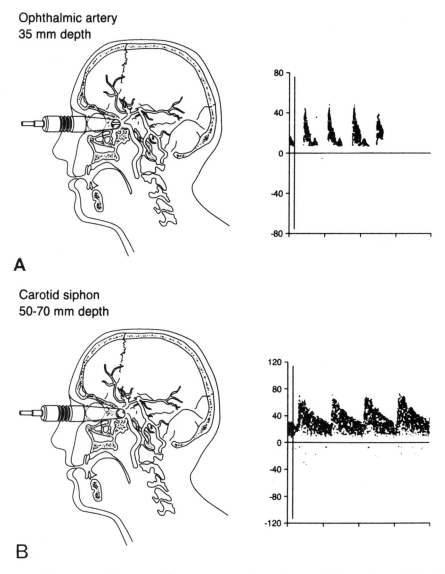

Figure 11–8. Transcranial Doppler ultrasonography through the orbital window. (*A*) Ophthalmic artery. (*B*) Carotid siphon.

Examination of the posterior circulation by TCD is useful in patients with acute basilar artery occlusion and in those with ruptured basilar aneurysm with vasospasm. The probe is placed just under the occipital crest in the midline with the patient in the side-lying position. The posterior window through the foramen magnum can be opened only with considerable head flexion, which may be limited in patients with neck stiffness from subarachnoid hemor-rhage. The probe is advanced to a depth of 60 mm, where the vertebral artery is identified (Fig. 11–9A). As expected, flow is away from the probe on both sides. Advancing the depth to 120 mm insonates the major part of the basi-lar artery (Fig. 11–9B).

Carotid artery dissection can be investigated by TCD as well. The technique with a sub-mandibular approach is demonstrated in Figure 11–10.

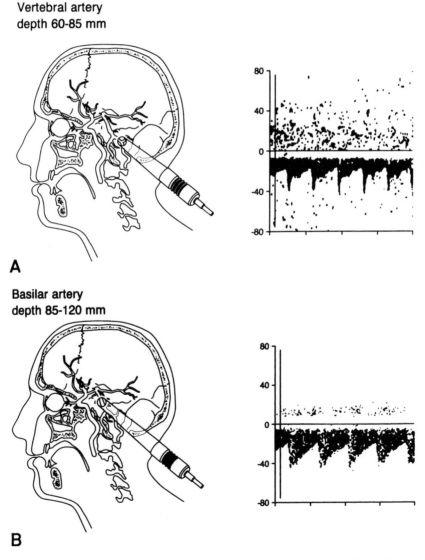

Figure 11–9. Transcranial Doppler ultrasonography through the occipital window. (A) Verte-bral artery. (B) Basilar artery.

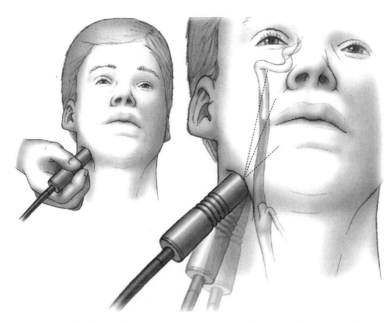

Figure 11–10. Submandibular technique. Insonation at the mandibular angle may identify increased flow velocities in patients with carotid artery stenosis and in patients with carotid artery dissection.

Transcranial Doppler Ultrasonography in Specific Acute Neurologic Conditions

There is sufficient evidence that TCD findings complement clinical assessment in acute neurologic conditions.[72,88] This section describes the usefulness and limitations of TCD in specific clinical neurologic disorders.

Aneurysmal Subarachnoid Hemorrhage

Cerebral vasospasm is very common after SAH, and angiographic studies have reported incidences of up to 50%.[47] By TCD criteria, vasospasm has been reported in 30% of patients with SAH.[32,33] This marked difference in frequency has been explained by the inability of TCD to assess the distal vasculature but in some studies may also reflect a selection of patients with SAH at low risk of delayed cerebral ischemia. The sensitivity of TCD for vasospasm in the middle cerebral artery is 60% to 80%, with virtually 95% specificity in several studies.[55,68,81,84] The sensitivity for vasospasm in the ACA in SAH is only approximately

20%.[56] Sensitivities of TCD for the basilar and vertebral arteries are 77% and 44%, respectively, and specificities, 79% and 88%.[59] A recent unconfirmed study suggested that age may affect mean flow velocity, and thus older patients may have comparatively lower thresholds for TCD-associated vasospasm.[87]

Unfortunately, strict criteria for cerebral vasospasm have not been clearly established, and consensus statements are not yet available. Most laboratories accept the following criteria: MCA mean velocity of ≥ 120 cm/second, Lindegaard MCA–ICA velocity ratio of > 3, marked turbulence (brief low frequent components in the mirror image of the TCD spectrum located close to the zero line and musical sounds in the insonated arteries with increased velocities). With a higher cutoff of at least 130 cm/second, others have found that the specificity is 100% in ICA and 87% in MCA.[9] At the extreme, one group believes that only flow velocities of more than 200 cm/second reliably predict angiographically significant vasospasm (positive predictive value of 87%).[95] A typical example of developing cerebral vasospasm in SAH on TCD is shown in Figure 11–11. Increased flow velocities on TCD strongly indicate cerebral vasospasm on angiography, but their presence often does not precede clinical deterioration from cerebral vasospasm. It has been suggested, however, that a relative increase in MCA velocities in the first days has some predictive value for the development of symptomatic vasospasm. A study from Southern General Hospital in Glasgow found that delayed cerebral ischemia developed in more than 60% of patients with a relative velocity increase of 50 cm/second in the MCA segment within 24 hours.[34]

Important practical questions remain on how to use TCD in the daily assessment of patients with SAH. Routine TCD may lead to a change in management in almost half of the cases,[96] but its effect on outcome (see similar discussion on pulmonary artery catheterization in Chapter 10) is not clear. It is not known exactly whether TCD reduces the need for an-

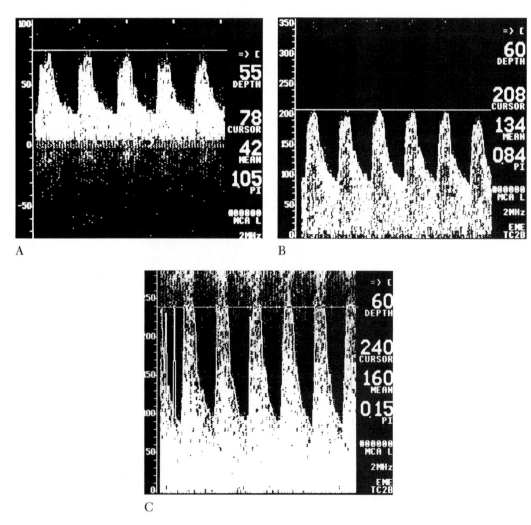

A   B

C

Figure 11–11. Sequential transcranial Doppler ultrasonography in subarachnoid hemorrhage. (*A*) Normal velocities in middle cerebral artery (MCA). (*B*) Two days later, mean velocities are increased. (*C*) Further increases in velocities. (The patient remained asymptomatic during all three recordings.)

giography. This has become an important issue because the use of cerebral angiography has increased in the management of SAH since the introduction of interventional neuroradiologic procedures. Angioplasty has been advocated for patients with focal vasospasm and intra-arterial papaverine for those with diffuse vasospasm (see Chapter 12). The predictive value of TCD in focal symptomatic vasospasm is not known, although one small series suggested a possible connection.[42] Unfortunately, angiographic studies in several of our patients with a suggestion of unilateral ACA or MCA spasm on TCD found diffuse cerebral vasospasm without any clear focal segments that could be eligible for angioplasty.

Another important clinical question is whether initial TCD findings of cerebral vasospasm should call for more aggressive fluid management. Although this approach is unproven and potentially leads to more complications associated with hypervolemia, we often feel the need to deliberately increase fluid intake to the maximal pulmonary artery wedge pressure in patients with large amounts of cisternal blood on CT and a recent increase in MCA velocities (more than 50 msec between studies) (see Chapter 12 for SAH management). Manipulation of blood pressure may increase TCD velocities in the insonated MCA segment, and this effect should not be misinterpreted as worsening vasospasm. In one study, 53% of patients had an increase in TCD velocities of more than 15%.[60] A recent study, however, found no difference in cerebral vasospasm assessed by TCD or single-photon emission computed tomography when prophylactic hypervolemic hypertensive hemodilution therapy was instituted.[25]

Transcranial Doppler ultrasonographic findings of cerebral vasospasm theoretically may influence timing of surgery. Some neurosurgeons are reluctant to clip an aneurysm if TCD supports cerebral vasospasm, and others ignore the findings. However, timing of surgery remains dependent on the World Federation of Neurological Surgeons' clinical grade at admission. The findings on TCD alone probably should not influence planning of aneurysmal clipping or coil placement.

Rebleeding in SAH has been diagnosed by TCD. In extreme circumstances a patient rebleeds during a routine examination. Rebleeding results in a massive surge in intracranial pressure and produces a reversible TCD pattern with small systolic peaks and diastolic reversal, findings that strongly mimic patterns seen in brain death. (In many patients with rebleeding, these brain death patterns on TCD may be real and remain.)

Transcranial Doppler ultrasonographic findings in postoperative patients with successful clipping of an aneurysm are notoriously difficult to interpret. Postoperative TCD may demonstrate increased velocities from hyperemia or aggressive hypervolemic treatment. On the other hand, the effect of surgery alone has been studied, and only minor increases in velocity may be seen, rarely above 120 cm/second. Therefore, in postoperative patients with secondary deterioration in the first 24 hours, swelling from prolonged retraction is difficult to differentiate from cerebral vasospasm by TCD. Normal TCD values or improved velocities if results of previous studies are available for comparison preclude vasospasm and may defer cerebral angiography; but in any other patient with decreased level of consciousness or new focal signs and increased TCD velocities, cerebral angiography is indicated (management of delayed cerebral ischemia is discussed in Chapter 12).

Head Injury

Studies of TCD in head injury have shown potential usefulness.[31] However, the experience with TCD in head injury is very limited, and in most instances the diagnosis of vasospasm by TCD criteria has been made in patients with large amounts of traumatic subarachnoid blood.[78,83] One study in 66 patients with head injury showed an increase in MCA velocities at a maximum of 5 to 7 days after the impact. In this study, cerebral angiographic confirmation of possible cerebral vasospasm was not available and, more importantly, clinical deterioration from cerebral infarction did not follow.[83]

Noninvasive measurement of intracranial pressure by TCD in traumatic brain injury has been a disappointing experience. Only in patients with a considerable increase in intracranial pressure (more than 60 mm Hg) are changes expected in the TCD waveform configuration. These changes include a decrease in cerebral perfusion pressure resulting in an increase in PSV and a decrease in diastolic pressure. The pulsatility index increases, but the relationship between pulsatility index and intracranial pressure is weak.[83] Transcranial Doppler ultrasonography is of value only in a patient with a steep systolic fall-off and marked reduction in diastolic flow, but again this situation usually occurs at a point when intracranial pressure equals diastolic blood pressure (Fig. 11–12). Transcranial Doppler ultrasonography, therefore, may have limited value in the assessment of comatose patients with head injury to determine in which patient an intracranial monitoring device is placed. Transcranial Doppler ultrasonography has been used in experimental settings, however, to study defective autoregulation.[16] Transcranial Doppler ultrasonography in head injury could even be diagnostic for development of swollen contusional masses. Reduced velocities and high pulsatility index were found in a small series of patients with head injury, and these findings require further study using continuous TCD monitoring.[65]

In clinical practice, TCD therefore has very limited value in patients with severe head injury. Its use is justified in those at risk for cerebral vasospasm; but when increased values are found, it is virtually impossible to distinguish between cerebral vasospasm and hyperemia from vasomotor paralysis.[31] TCD may have some value in estimating intracranial pressure.

Acute Ischemic Stroke

Transcranial Doppler ultrasonography can be used to demonstrate intracranial ICA stenosis (70% to 90% sensitivity), MCA main stem obstructions (70% to 100% sensitivity), and vertebral artery stenosis (70% sensitivity).[10,12,48,52,57] In these patients, TCD demonstrates significantly increased velocities on the side of the stenosis, with a decreased pulsatility index at the level of the stenosis. The normal physiologic direction should be maintained. In general, a marked increase in velocity indicates a focal intracranial stenosis. Lesions producing greater than 60% stenosis should be detectable by TCD. Middle cerebral artery stenosis in general produces velocities greater than 100 cm/second; a basilar artery stenosis is within the range of 50 to 150 cm/second.

The diagnostic capability of TCD in vertebral and carotid dissection is promising. (In one study, 8 of 10 patients with vertebral dissection had abnormalities, largely a high-resistance signal.[40]) However, in many of these patients, cerebral angiography is indicated. Transcranial

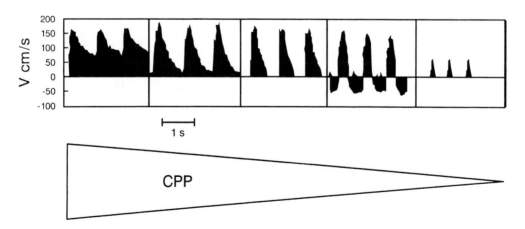

Figure 11–12. Progressive transcranial Doppler changes in patients with increased intracranial pressure. CPP, cerebral perfusion pressure.

Doppler ultrasonography may also have a role in monitoring thrombolysis.[46] Transcranial Doppler ultrasonography in a small group of patients with acute middle cerebral artery occlusion could document recanalization during intravenous tPA and suggested infusion could be halted when recanalization and clinical improvement occurred.[27]

Brain Death

Patients who fulfill the clinical criteria of brain death have waveforms similar to those in patients with markedly increased intracranial pressure. Insonation of both MCA segments is required. Typical brain death patterns are reversal of flow in diastole with a sharp systolic upstroke, systolic spike waveforms (Fig. 11–13), and occasionally complete absence of flow in a patient with previously demonstrated TCD signal through the same temporal window.[3,21,35,71,76]

The criteria for brain death have been substantially expanded and are not yet endorsed by other societies. The TCD criteria for brain death were summarized in a consensus statement of the World Federation of Neurology.[22]

1. Cerebral circulatory arrest bilaterally; two examinations, 30 minutes apart.

2. Systolic spikes or oscillating flow in any cerebral artery in the anterior or posterior circulation.

3. Above findings confirmed by extracranial bilateral recording of the common carotid, internal carotid, and vertebral arteries.

4. Disappearance of intracranial flow can be accepted as proof of circulatory arrest.

5. Exclusion of patients with a ventricular drain or large craniotomy.

ELECTRODIAGNOSTIC STUDIES

There are divergent opinions on the best way to monitor patients with an acute neurologic disorder. On the presumption that clinical features of deterioration are less reliable, some investigators examined continuous electroencephalographic (EEG) monitoring in the NICU.[44,45,70] Electrodiagnostic monitoring undoubtedly has potential value in critically ill neurologic patients. It is possible that EEG is underutilized, particularly in patients worsening from aneurysmal subarachnoid hemorrhage or massive hemispheric stroke and in patients with fluctuating level of consciousness after a single seizure.

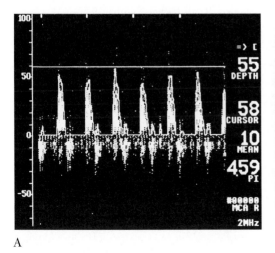
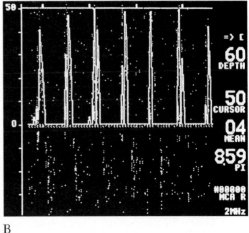

A   B

Figure 11–13. (A) Reverberating flow and (B) typical small systolic peaks on transcranial Doppler ultrasonography diagnostic of brain death. Note significant reduction in mean velocity (mean) and increase in pulsatility index (PI).

The possibility that a relatively simple technique of continuous EEG monitoring may increase early recognition of nonconvulsive status epilepticus and confirm worsening of cerebral blood flow and ischemia is understandably exciting. In addition, EEG may have some prognostic value.[93] Unfortunately, consistent data of a major role of EEG in monitoring patients in the NICU are lacking. Moreover, in monitored patients with a wide spectrum of acute neurologic disorders, EEG may not contribute to an already clinically evident changing situation. In addition, enthusiasm must be tempered because some of the EEG abnormalities may not have clinical relevance. Nonetheless, the use of continuous EEG monitoring has increased our awareness of the possibility of nonconvulsive status epilepticus in patients with acute neurologic catastrophes, although in our experience, the number of well-documented cases is very low.

On the basis of our preliminary experience, continuous EEG monitoring is helpful only in patients who had earlier seizures recognized clinically or during management of status epilepticus (Fig. 11–14). In our unit, we have the capability of video monitoring of patients at risk for seizures, and we found that continuous EEG monitoring is useful in selected patients.

Intraoperative EEG monitoring is common practice during carotid endarterectomy (Chapter 28), but the predictive value of intraoperative changes for perioperative stroke is quite poor, with a sensitivity of 50% and specificity of 70%.[43,63] Serial EEGs or evoked potentials may continue to have significant value in a variety of acute neurologic disorders. In this section, EEGs and evoked potentials are discussed as useful diagnostic tests rather than as means for monitoring.

Electroencephalography

In patients with critical neurologic illness, the EEG continues to be a useful adjunct to clinical observation and in the proper situation supports the clinical diagnosis.

Stroke

A preliminary study found deterioration in EEG patterns before clinical deterioration in patients with ischemic stroke. These EEG abnormalities consisted of increasing focal slow activity, onset of epileptiform activity, or appearance of generalized slowing. The nature of these abnormalities was not clear, although they were tentatively attributed to worsening ischemia. Indeed, earlier studies suggested that an increase in mean arterial pressure to the extreme value of 150 mm Hg resulted in clinical and EEG improvement. This observation needs further refinement and confirmation before EEG abnormalities should prompt the additional use of inotropes.[98]

Electroencephalography, however, has some use in prognostication. A study found that prominent continuous and polymorphic delta activity together with slowing or depression of the alpha or beta activity in the ischemic hemisphere predicted poor functional outcome.[13] Recovery was more likely with absence of slow activity and no decrease in alpha frequency or mu rhythm.

Figure 11–14. (A) Mobile electroencephalographic (EEG) monitoring cart with simultaneous video replay capabilities (video camera is mounted on the ceiling). (B) through (D) Example of focal seizure detected with continuous EEG/video monitoring in a patient with craniotomy for an extracranial mass. (B) Right arm is resting on abdomen. No epileptic discharge is recorded on EEG. (C) Fifteen minutes later, head turns to middle and hand moves to left and clenches (polyspike waves in the left frontocentral region become visible on EEG). (D) Eight seconds later, arm is lifted, head is turned more to the right, and tonic-clonic movements begin in right arm (movement is muted by restraint). Up to six seizures were recorded per hour, only half detectable clinically. Treatment with midazolam infusion alone was successful.

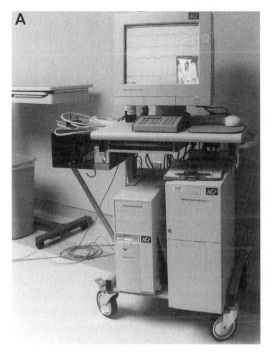

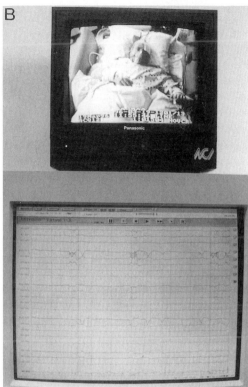

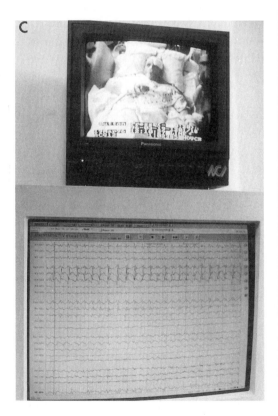

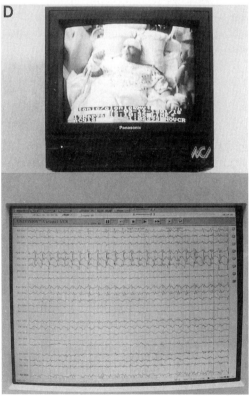

Encephalitis

The EEG has an important role in the early diagnosis of encephalitis, particularly herpes simplex encephalitis. Most patients with a presumed diagnosis of viral encephalitis are admitted to the NICU with impaired level of consciousness or coma, often unable to protect their airway and in need of intubation and mechanical ventilation. Magnetic resonance imaging cannot be performed easily in these patients, and in some patients CSF findings are nondiagnostic or equivocal. Fairly early in herpes simplex encephalitis, the EEG shows polymorphic delta activity over the temporal lobes, which suggests preferential involvement of these regions. Although nonspecific for herpes simplex encephalitis, focal or lateralized sharp- or slow-wave complexes emerge early and eventually become periodic, usually after 1 or 2 days of illness (Fig. 11–15). Sharp waves may occur almost continuously or several seconds apart and may evolve into more distinctive seizure discharges, recognized by repetitive sharp and slow waves or bursts of spike waves. Periodic complexes in the acute phase may indicate a poor prognosis.[79]

Many other encephalitides have diffuse slow-wave abnormalities, and the degree of slowing is often directly related to the severity of the infection.

Seizures and Status Epilepticus

Acute structural lesions of the central nervous system may be accompanied by or present with seizures. Focal seizures are somewhat more common and may be therapy-resistant. The EEG may show transient epileptic discharges, but often these occur in large hemispheric strokes with a significant CT scan hypodensity (Fig. 11–16).

At the time of recording of status epilepticus, most EEG tracings show continuous epileptic discharges (Fig. 11–17) or periodic lateralized epileptiform discharges (PLEDs). These periodic discharges may be associated with focal twitches in the eyelids, face, arm, or leg, but more often PLEDs are interictal phenomena. Patients with generalized tonic-clonic seizures that evolve into status epilepticus and that are not controlled with intravenous phenytoin loading alone are often further managed with midazolam, propofol, or barbiturates. During this episode, EEG recording is very helpful in titration of the antiepileptic agent. These drugs generally are titrated to seizure-free EEG recordings rather than to a burst-

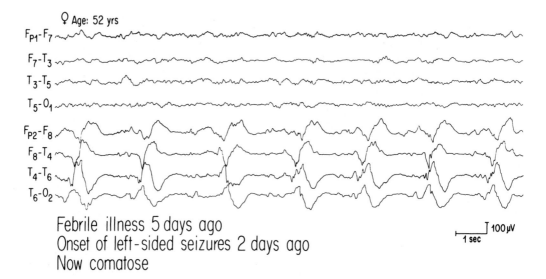

Figure 11–15. Typical periodic lateralized sharp waves in herpes simplex encephalitis. (Courtesy of Dr. B. F. Westmoreland.)

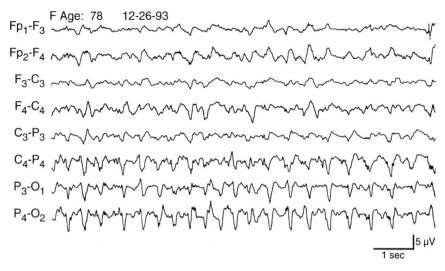

Figure 11–16. Seizure discharge associated with middle cerebral artery infarct.

suppression pattern. Further titrating to a burst-suppression or isoelectric EEG (Fig. 11–17B) is indicated only when clinical seizures persist, but it may seriously complicate hemodynamic stability.

Breakthrough seizures during treatment of status epilepticus may be very subtle and not recognized clinically. Patients may display brief forced gaze that is not appreciated with the eyelids closed or barely noticeable eyelid twitching. Breakthrough seizures were successfully managed with titration of midazolam to burst-suppression patterns in a small series of patients.[15]

Recurrence of electrographic status epilepticus after at least two trials of midazolam, propofol, or barbiturates is associated with a poor outcome. In many of these patients, electrographic seizures are not associated with clinical manifestations, and they remain comatose, only to later awaken severely disabled.

Head Injury

A single EEG has limited value in patients with severe closed head injury.[6,7,18] Earlier classic studies of EEG in head injury commonly showed a generalized widespread slowing (theta and delta range of frequencies) that was associated with poor outcome if it persisted in the first 2 days after injury. The EEG has some

prognostic value in comatose survivors of severe head injury but no pattern, except for isoelectric EEG, has been convincing enough to withdraw support. Spindle coma—characterized by paroxysmal activity in the vertex and rolandic regions, but also more widespread, on a background of theta and delta waves—may potentially indicate a favorable prognosis. However, alpha coma, burst-suppression, triphasic waves, and reduced alpha variability within 5 days of injury are electrographic patterns that indicate significant damage and possibly secondary brain stem distortion.[93]

In 22% of 94 patients, continuous EEG monitoring (from admission to 2 weeks) detected convulsive and nonconvulsive status epilepticus that was not recognized clinically in more than half the patients. All patients with status epilepticus after traumatic brain injury died; therefore, the value of monitoring for therapeutic intervention is very uncertain. The EEG features in these patients may reflect severe brain injury rather than a treatable disorder.[94]

Brain Death

The diagnosis of brain death is a clinical diagnosis, and confirmatory tests in adults are necessary only when certain components of clinical testing are less reliable (Chapter 34). Many countries in the world mandate EEG or serial

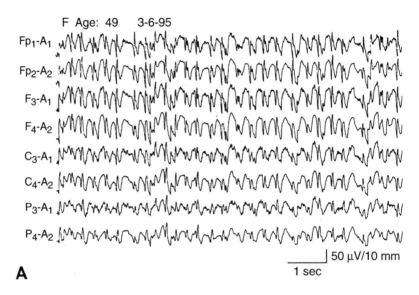

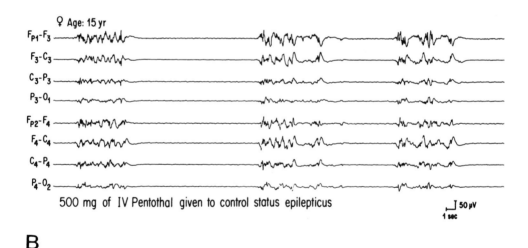

Figure 11–17. Typical status epilepticus. (Courtesy of Dr. B. F. Westmoreland.)

EEG recordings. Electroencephalography remains a useful test, and the long-term experience with interpretation in brain death is a major advantage over other tests.

Electrocerebral silence is defined as no electrical activity when high instrument activity is used (Fig. 11–18). The recording should be done by an experienced technician.

The current recommendations published by the American Electroencephalographic Society are

1. A minimum of eight scalp electrodes
2. Interelectrode impedances between 100 and 10,000 Ω
3. Interelectrode distance of at least 10 cm

4. Sensitivity increase up to 2 μV and time constant of 0.3 to 0.4 seconds
5. Recording of 30 minutes
6. Testing of EEG reactivity to pain stimuli and flashlight

Noise signals on EEG in the NICU are significant because recordings are made with the sensitivity set high. These artifacts are associated with many electrical devices, such as mechanical ventilator, heating blanket to correct hypothermia, and intravenous infusion equipment.

Persistent EEG activity is still compatible with the clinical diagnosis of brain death, and residual activity may be observed in 20% of pa-

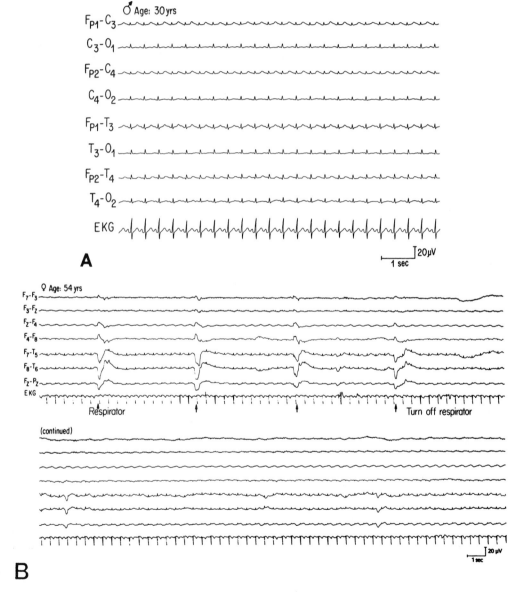

Figure 11–18. Electroencephalograms in brain death. Note (A) electrocardiographic artifact and (B) respirator artifact. (B courtesy of Dr. B. F. Westmoreland.)

tients (see Chapter 34). In patients with brain death from a destructive pontine hemorrhage or acute basilar artery occlusion, a typical alpha coma (8 to 10 Hz; 15 to 50 μV) occurs, with widely distributed activity but little spontaneous variability and no response to pain or visual stimuli.[97] In other patients with destructive brain stem lesions, spindle and diffuse delta activity alternating with alpha coma is observed.[69,97]

Evoked Potentials

Evoked potentials are used sparingly in critically ill patients with neurologic disorders. Future developments may make continuous monitoring possible, a potentially promising application for somatosensory potentials. Of the available techniques, somatosensory evoked potential (SSEP) is most often used, and the additional value of brain stem auditory evoked potential (BAEP) and visual evoked potential in the clinical assessment of patients with acute neurologic illness has been disappointing. Currently, SSEPs are most often used for prognosis in head injury and anoxic-ischemic encephalopathy. The recent development of motor evoked potentials may have promise, although currently no studies in critically ill patients are available.

Auditory stimulation to the acoustic nerve (usually clicks through headphones) generates BAEPs with a typical waveform. The wave I latency (distal portion of the acoustic nerve), wave I–III interpeak latency (tract of the proximal eighth nerve to the inferior pons), and wave III–IV interpeak latency (tract between caudal pons and midbrain) are used for interpretation (Fig. 11–19).

The applications of BAEPs in patients with acute neurologic illness are limited to head injury and confirmation of the clinical diagnosis of brain death. Brain stem auditory evoked potentials have recently been explored in patients with brain stem compression from a large supratentorial mass. Several studies, however, have suggested that BAEPs can be useful in testing brain stem integrity. In a study by Nagao et al.[66] in patients with uncal herniation, a correlation was found between wave V abnormalities and brain stem compression, abnor-

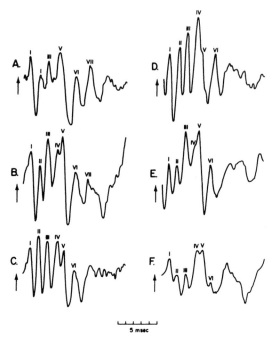

Figure 11–19. Typical brain stem auditory evoked potential response. (From Chiappa KH, Gladstone KJ, Young RR: Brain stem auditory evoked responses: studies of waveform variations in 50 normal human subjects. *Arch Neurol* 36:81–87, 1979. By permission of the American Medical Association.)

malities that reversed after intracranial pressure was controlled. Whether BAEPs provide important information not already known from the clinical examination or intracranial monitoring remains to be investigated. Indeed, one study in patients with deteriorating hemispheric mass lesions suggested marginal additional predictive value.[51]

Another potential use is assessment of brain stem function in patients with head injuries who are comatose and who need barbiturate treatment for control of intracranial pressure. Brain stem auditory evoked potentials can also be helpful in patients who have lost most of their clinical brain stem function from presumed intoxication, in which case the results of BAEP studies are normal.

The prognostic value of BAEPs has been studied in large series of patients with head injury.

Abnormalities are usually signaled by complete absence of the late responses. Wave I must remain identifiable, because deafness from damage to the cochlea or peripheral nerve at the temporal bone may eliminate the potential. The most important study, from Tsubokawa et al.,[90] claimed that patients who lost waves III and IV died or remained in a vegetative state. Two other studies found less accurate results but claimed that patients with bilaterally absent BAEP responses had a much higher likelihood of poor outcome and death.[51,66] (It should be noted that most patients in a persistent vegetative state have normal BAEP responses.)

Brain stem auditory evoked potential testing has also been examined in patients who fulfill the clinical criteria for brain death. Abnormal BAEP findings, however, may also be seen in patients with a central nervous system catastrophe who do not yet fulfill the clinical criteria for brain death. A combined examination with SSEP may have more confirmatory value, particularly in patients with preserved EEG activity.[30]

Somatosensory evoked potentials may have more practical value in the NICU. Electrical stimulation of the median or tibial nerve results in an afferent volley that can be recorded at the cortex. Median nerve stimulation is easier to perform and generally provides the information needed. The electrodes record from Erb's point, over the cervical spine process at C6, and on the scalp. The typical waveform is shown in Figure 11–20. It is assumed that the N13 waveform identifies the dorsal columns and nuclei and that the scalp potentials are correlated with the thalamocortical radiations. A major advantage of SSEP recordings is that the waveforms can be recorded unchanged in patients in whom barbiturate treatment is producing isoelectric EEGs. The bilateral absence of scalp potentials is a measure of poor prognosis.[11] In coma after cardiac resuscitation and head injury (both conditions often appear together in resuscitated trauma patients), this finding has been associated with a permanent vegetative state. Surprisingly, in a systematic review of SSEP in traumatic brain injury, 12 of 777 patients with bilaterally absent scalp potentials had a favorable outcome.[11]

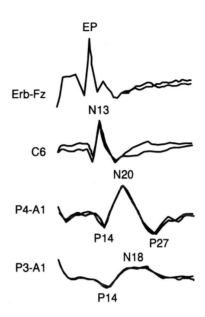

Figure 11–20. Typical somatosensory evoked potential (EP) with normal responses. Erb's point, cervical spine, and bilateral scalp recordings represent the thalamocortical components from upper to lower tracings. Electrode positions: Erb, Erb's point (shoulder); Fz, midfrontal; C6, middle back of neck over C6 cervical vertebra; P4-A1 and P3-A1, scalp overlying the sensoriparietal cortex (odd numbers are left); A, earlobe.

As alluded to previously, SSEP can be useful in brain death. In a study from the Massachusetts General Hospital, 27 patients who fulfilled the clinical criteria for brain death were tested with both SSEP and BAEP. In 16 patients, BAEP and central conduction responses were absent on SSEP; 2 patients had only BAEP wave I and no SSEP; 1 patient had BAEP waves I and II and no SSEP; and the remaining patients had no identifiable waves at all.[30]

SINGLE-PHOTON EMISSION COMPUTED TOMOGRAPHY

Single-photon emission computed tomography (SPECT) requires a rotating gamma camera and usually technetium ^{99m}Tc hexametazime.

Acquisition can be performed 5 minutes after injection and be repeated the next day. Mechanical ventilation and vital signs of the patient can be easily monitored. Single-photon emission computed tomography demonstrates hypoperfusion and not ischemia. Whether hypoperfusion is compensated by increased metabolism and increased oxygen extraction therefore remains unknown. Positron emission tomography scanning can overcome this limitation, but experience is limited to experimental studies.

Acute Stroke

Regional cerebral blood flow measurement with SPECT has been applied in acute ischemic and hemorrhagic stroke as well as in SAH. The SPECT study is helpful in the time zone in which CT scan and magnetic resonance imaging do not reveal abnormalities.[38,74] Its potential uses in ischemic stroke pertain to demonstration of a more significant hypoperfusion than that suggested by CT scan, definition of the penumbra, and possible prediction of prognosis.[36,53] In addition, after intravenous administration of acetazolamide, hypoperfusion may become more apparent in patients with hemodynamically significant carotid artery stenosis.[50] In patients with intracerebral hematoma, studies have demonstrated diminished perfusion surrounding the clot, but the nature of the abnormality is not clear and can be explained by edema, ischemia, or diaschisis.[77] We noted persistent SPECT abnormalities in surrounding areas of the hematoma but with resolving clinical findings (Fig. 11–21).

One disorder in which SPECT is particularly helpful is aneurysmal SAH. After the initial observation that angiography correlated well with ^{99m}Tc-hexametazime SPECT in the evaluation of vasospasm, larger studies were performed in SAH. Studies have found that SPECT is more sensitive than CT in evaluating ischemic com-

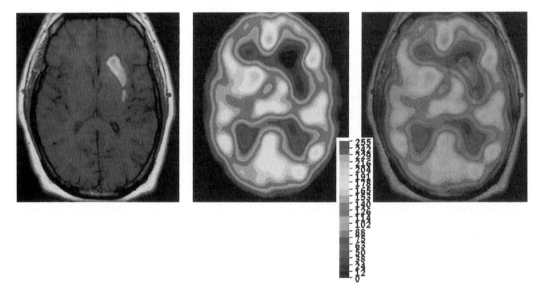

Figure 11–21. Technetium Tc 99m ethyl cysteinate dimer single-photon emission computed tomography (SPECT) scan of the brain performed on the day of admission, when the patient had profound Wernicke's aphasia, coregistered for anatomical localization to the patient's T1-weighted magnetic resonance brain scan by use of a surface-matching technique.[41] This demonstrated marked hypoperfusion in the region of the putaminal hemorrhage but also showed a significant decrease in perfusion to the left lateral frontal and temporal cortex. Hypoperfusion persisted on subsequent SPECT scans, but aphasia completely resolved.

plications. The most common pattern in SAH and cerebral vasospasm is mixed hypoperfusion.[17,82,89] A recent study showed that SPECT abnormalities were common in patients with TCD abnormalities suggestive of vasospasm. Hypoperfusion of SPECT correlated reasonably well with TCD (concordance of 64%).[73]

In our use of SPECT in patients with SAH and normal TCD findings, we occasionally could demonstrate cerebral hypoperfusion, which resulted in a change in management (Fig. 11–22). Serial SPECT may also be useful in patients with abnormal TCD velocities since presentation and new onset of impaired consciousness.

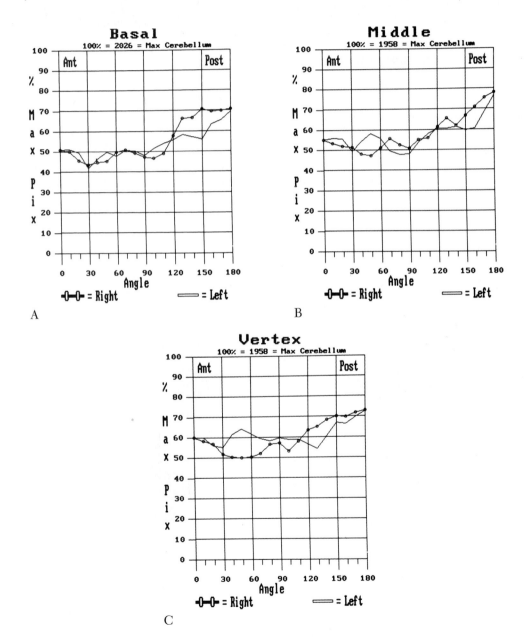

Figure 11–22. Single-photon emission computed tomography in subarachnoid hemorrhage showing global hypoperfusion.

Single-photon emission computed tomography has been used to discriminate cerebral vasospasm from acute hydrocephalus, but experience has been limited. In patients with acute hydrocephalus, decreased uptake of ^{99m}Tc-hexametazime was found, particularly in the basal parts of the brain and in areas surrounding the ventricles; uptake improved after CSF drainage.[37]

Miscellaneous Disorders

Diminished tracer activity is seen after a seizure, particularly in the median temporal lobe (hippocampus). Currently, SPECT is used in comparison with MRI for lesion localization.[8]

Single-photon emission computed tomography has been investigated in closed head injury, but studies are limited.[1,75] It has been suggested that SPECT may be useful in the detection of contrecoup lesions (producing local areas of hypoperfusion) and the prognostication of coma (producing disorganized patterns of tracer uptake).

Single-photon emission computed tomography has been very useful in confirming brain death. Typically, a "hollow skull" or "empty lightbulb" sign consistent with absent tracer uptake is seen (Fig. 11–23), and its predictive value for brain death is similar to that of cerebral angiography but with less cost and dye load.

CEREBROSPINAL FLUID ANALYSIS

In infections of the central nervous system, CSF examination is a pivotal diagnostic procedure. In patients with a highly suspicious history of thunderclap headache, lumbar puncture is typically performed after a CT scan is unrevealing. The alleged risks of lumbar puncture include cerebral herniation in pyogenic

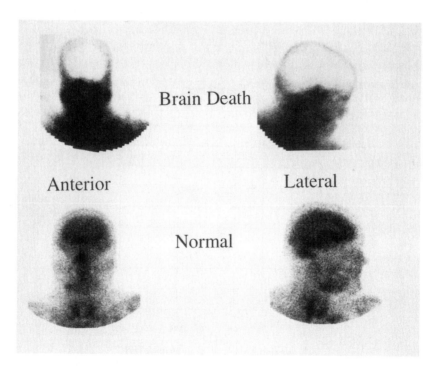

Figure 11–23. Single-photon emission computed tomography (planar technetium Tc 99m hexametazime images) in brain death ("hollow skull") compared with normal uptake.

meningitis, subdural empyema, cerebellar hematoma, and rebleeding in SAH, but concerns about causality remain. The risk of epidural hematoma is substantial in patients with anticoagulation or blood dyscrasias, and platelet count, prothrombin time, or partial thromboplastin time is required. Dural puncture headache is reduced by 26% with use of atraumatic (blunt) needles.[85] The frequency of traumatic lumbar puncture could be reduced from 10% to 3.5% with fluoroscopy-guided lumbar puncture, which should be strongly considered in patients with thunderclap headache and normal CT scan findings.[26]

This section provides a review of the pathologic findings in patients with acute neurologic disorders. The reader is also referred to a review paper[86] or a monograph.[28]

Acute Ischemic Stroke and Subarachnoid Hemorrhage

Cerebrospinal fluid analysis in ischemic stroke is seldom performed but could be done to exclude the possibility of an inflammatory or infectious cause. Acute ischemic stroke may increase CSF protein mildly. The magnitude of the increase is possibly directly associated with the extent of cerebral infarction and subsequent opening of the blood–brain barrier. Some degree of pleiocytosis, seldom more than 50 cells/mm^3 but generally less than 100 mg/dL, is seen.

In patients with vasculitis of the central nervous system, cell count may increase to 100 to 200 lymphocytic cells/mm^3, and the changes often persist after repeat CSF examination. In some patients with a biopsy-proven diagnosis of cerebral vasculitis, the cell count value is within normal limits, but normal CSF findings have a high negative predictive value.[80]

Cerebrospinal fluid examination may also show an increase in cell count if a generalized seizure or, more commonly, a flurry of seizures has occurred at the time of presentation. In most patients, CSF findings remain normal. A small proportion (less than 5%) have an increased cell count, with rapid resolution within 1 to 2 days. Cell counts may increase up to 28 cells/mm^3.[4]

Rarely, lumbar puncture is performed in patients with a strong suspicion of SAH but normal findings on CT scan. Yellow discoloration due to conversion of oxyhemoglobin to bilirubin (xanthochromia) does occur after hemorrhage into the CSF. A classic in vitro study in which intact human erythrocytes were placed in CSF found visible xanthochromia after 4 hours and a marked increase after 12 to 24 hours of incubation.[62] Thus, lumbar puncture ideally should be deferred to at least 4 hours after the ictus to allow the red cells to lyse in CSF and the characteristic xanthochromia to develop in the supernatant. In patients with a normal CT scan and atypical onset of headache, patients in whom the headache profile is uncertain, and possibly immunosuppressed patients with sudden development of headache, lumbar puncture should be performed without much hesitation. Xanthochromia can be demonstrated in most patients up to 2 weeks after the ictus and in a large percentage of patients 3 weeks after the ictus.[92]

The distinction between a traumatic puncture and bloody CSF from SAH is also possible with spectrophotometry,[5] which directly demonstrates oxyhemoglobin or bilirubin (Fig. 11–24). We rarely use spectroscopy, and only in cases with no blood on CT scan, a characteristic thunderclap headache, and the dubious presence of xanthochromia. Visual inspection for xanthochromia remains common practice at most U.S. laboratories.[24]

It has been suggested that D-dimer determination may distinguish between SAH and a traumatic lumbar puncture.[54] We found that D-dimer was not specific and was present in many other neurologic disorders (unpublished observation). D-dimer determination should therefore not be recommended.

Other methods, such as sequential tube tests ("the three-tube test") with decreasing red blood cell counts, hematocrit, and white cell counts and erythrophagocytosis, are possibly differentiating. Hemorrhages in the subarachnoid space may result in 1000 to 10,000 erythrocytes/mm^3, and thus the quantity is not

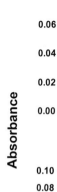
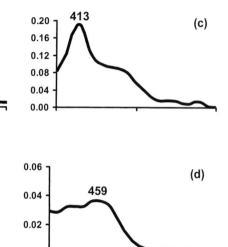

Figure 11–24. Spectrophotometric scans of (*a*) normal cerebrospinal fluid (CSF), (*b*) oxyhemoglobin in CSF, (*c*) oxyhemoglobin and bilirubin in CSF, and (*d*) bilirubin in CSF. All plots were obtained by use of a Cecil CE 6600 Double Beam Spectrophotometer, bandwidth of 2.0 nm and scan speed of 5 nm/second, and were reproduced from original tracings. Wavelengths (nm) of peak maxima are indicated where appropriate. (Modified from Beetham et al.[5] By permission of the Association of Clinical Biochemists.)

a solidly reliable indication of a traumatic puncture.[64]

Bacterial Meningitis

Cerebrospinal fluid examination has the highest priority in the diagnosis of acute bacterial meningitis. Mortality from delayed antibiotic treatment in acute bacterial meningitis is 10 to 20 times greater than the risk of complications associated with lumbar puncture. Computed tomography scan may be performed at a later stage or when the suspicion for a bacterial abscess is very high. Typical findings in the spinal fluid are thousands of leukocytes with predominating polymorphonuclear cells, an increased protein value, and decreased glucose to less than 50% of the serum glucose concentration. In a traumatic puncture, the leukocyte count can be estimated by subtracting 1 leukocyte for every 700 erythrocytes. Alternatively, a more reliable ratio can be calculated: true

leukocytes (CSF) = actual leukocytes (CSF) − leukocytes (serum) × erythrocytes (CSF)/erythrocytes (serum).

Cerebrospinal fluid cultures remain positive in many patients, even after hours of intravenous antibiotic treatment. One study found positive CSF cultures in 43% of those treated with ceftriaxone and in 58% of those treated with ampicillin or chloramphenicol when CSF samples were obtained 4 to 12 hours after treatment.[19] Blood cultures should be obtained as well, because 50% of patients with bacterial meningitis have positive blood cultures. Bacterial antigens, however, may be detected by CSF counterimmunoelectrophoresis and CSF latex agglutination, with high sensitivity. Cerebrospinal fluid abnormalities abate after successful antibiotic therapy, and a significant decrease in the total cell count is expected after the third day of treatment. The protein level stays elevated in many patients for 2 weeks. However, there is no compelling need to repeat CSF examination after successful treatment, because in some clinically improved patients, the CSF has not entirely normalized. One study showed a median of 38 cells/mm³ (range, 0 to 480) in a series of 157 treated and clinically cured patients.[23]

Table 11–4. Infectious and Inflammatory Causes of Acute Bacterial Meningitis Stratified by Cerebrospinal Fluid Findings

Predominantly Polymorphonuclear Leukocytes and Decreased Glucose°

Partially treated bacterial meningitis (most common)
Listeria
Herpes simplex encephalitis
Sarcoidosis
Early syphilis
Early tuberculosis
Amebic meningoencephalitis
Drug-induced meningitis
Acute hemorrhagic leukoencephalitis
Chemical meningitis
Mollaret's meningitis
Behçet's syndrome
Septic emboli

Predominantly Lymphocytes and Normal Glucose

Partially treated bacterial meningitis
Sarcoidosis
Lyme disease
Human immunodeficiency virus
Leptospirosis
Rocky Mountain spotted fever
Viral meningitis
Tuberculous meningitis
Fungal meningitis
Parasitic meningitis (*Toxoplasma*, trichinosis, cysticercosis)
Carcinomatous meningitis
Vogt-Koyanagi-Harada syndrome
Systemic lupus erythematosus
Isolated central nervous system vasculitis

Predominantly Lymphocytes and Decreased Glucose

Partially treated bacterial meningitis
Tuberculous meningitis
Fungal meningitis
Sarcoidosis
Mumps
Enteroviral meningitis
Listeria monocytogenes
Leptospirosis
Syphilis
Carcinomatous meningitis

°Normal glucose may be observed in patients with epidural abscess, subdural empyema, brain abscess, and bacterial endocarditis. The Gram stain is negative in these conditions.

Encephalitis

Spinal fluid is almost invariably diagnostic in encephalitis. Most often, CSF shows a pleocytosis of 50 to 1000 cells/mm³ with lymphocyte dominance. Polymorphonuclear cells may initially overshadow the typical CSF formula but only in the first days and in the phase of prodromal symptoms. The protein value tends to be normal or marginally increased. Erythrocytes are found in the CSF of patients with herpes simplex encephalitis, and when they are present, MRI often has already revealed necrotic (and hemorrhagic) lesions in predilection sites (Chapter 21). Normal spinal fluid findings have been reported in biopsy-proven herpes simplex encephalitis. The development of a very sensitive and very specific polymerase chain reaction has practically eliminated the need for brain biopsy in herpes simplex encephalitis (see Chapter 21). Arbovirus encephalitis is very common in the United States, especially in the early fall, when mosquito populations peak. The CSF often demonstrates a pleocytosis of about 50 cells/mm³, and the glucose and protein concentrations are normal. The specific diagnosis rests on a serologic increase in complement fixation anti-

Table 11–5. Cerebrospinal Fluid Tests in Patients with a Central Nervous System Infection of Undetermined Origin

India ink stain for *Cryptococcus* antigen
PCR for HSV, VZV, EBV, HHV-6, CMV enteroviruses, West Nile, ehrlichiosis
Acid-fast test for *Nocardia* and atypical mycobacteria
Wet mount for *Amoeba*
Latex agglutination test for *Cryptococcus neoformans*
Serology for *Toxoplasma* (immunofluorescence, Sabin-Feldman dye test, enzyme-linked immunosorbent assay titer)
Serology for mosquito-borne viruses
Fluorescent treponemal antibody absorption test
Cultures (multiple) for fungi, including *Coccidioides immitis, Cryptococcus neoformans, Histoplasma capsulatum, Blastomyces, Sporothrix schenckii*
Cultures for mycobacterial organisms
Culture for *Brucella*
Cultures for anaerobic organisms (corynebacteria, *Listeria monocytogenes*)
Cultures for *Leptospira*
Cultures for *Rickettsia*

CMV, cytomegalovirus; EBV, Epstein-Barr virus; HHV, human herpesvirus; HSV, herpes simplex virus; PCR, polymerase chain reaction; VZV, varicella-zoster virus.

bodies, hemagglutinating antibodies, and neutralizing antibodies in the second or third week after the beginning of the febrile response. The isolation rates of several viruses differ significantly. Most viruses (herpes simplex encephalitis, eastern equine encephalomyelitis, western equine encephalomyelitis, St. Louis encephalitis) are rarely isolated. The isolation of enteroviruses, mumps, and varicella is comparatively high.

The differential diagnosis of CSF findings is summarized in Table 11–4. Additional tests in patients with presumed central nervous system infection are listed in Table 11–5, but these should be tailored toward each patient rather than ordered all together.

CONCLUSIONS

- TCD is most useful in the detection of cerebral vasospasm in SAH and in the diagnosis of brain death. Typical features of cerebral vasospasm are increased mean velocities ($\geq$ 120 cm/second) and turbulence.
- EEG is most useful in the NICU for the diagnosis of herpes simplex encephalitis, monitoring in status epilepticus, and guidance in therapy.
- Evoked potentials currently can be used only for prognostication. Poor outcome can be expected in patients with characteristic BAEP (III and IV waves absent) and SSEP (scalp potentials absent) abnormalities.
- SPECT has value in SAH to confirm hypoperfusion. SPECT is as useful as angiography in confirmation of brain death.

REFERENCES

1. Abdel-Dayem HM, Sadek SA, Kouris K, et al: Changes in cerebral perfusion after acute head injury: comparison of CT with Tc-99m HM-PAO SPECT. *Radiology* 165:221–226, 1987.
2. Arnolds BJ, von Reutern GM: Transcranial Doppler sonography. Examination technique and normal reference values. *Ultrasound Med Biol* 12:115–123, 1986.
3. Azevedo E, Teixeira J, Neves JC, et al: Transcranial Doppler and brain death. *Transplant Proc* 32:2579–2581, 2000.
4. Barry E, Hauser WA: Pleocytosis after status epilepticus. *Arch Neurol* 51:190–193, 1994.
5. Beetham R, Fahie-Wilson MN, Park D: What is the role of CSF spectrophotometry in the diagnosis of subarachnoid haemorrhage? *Ann Clin Biochem* 35:1–4, 1998.
6. Bickford RG, Klass DW: Acute and chronic EEG findings after head injury. In Caveness WF, Walker AE (eds): *Head Injury: Conference Proceedings*. Philadelphia, JB Lippincott Company, 1966, pp 63–88.
7. Bricolo AP, Turella GS: Electrophysiology of head injury. In Vinken PJ, Bruyn GW, Klawans HL (eds): *Handbook of Clinical Neurology*. Vol 57; Revised Series 13. Amsterdam, Elsevier Science Publishers, 1990, pp 181–206.
8. Brinkmann BH, O'Brien TJ, Mullan BP, et al: Subtraction ictal SPECT coregistered to MRI for seizure focus localization in partial epilepsy. *Mayo Clin Proc* 75:615–624, 2000.

9. Burch CM, Wozniak MA, Sloan MA, et al: Detection of intracranial internal carotid artery and middle cerebral artery vasospasm following subarachnoid hemorrhage. *J Neuroimag* 6:8–15, 1996.
10. Camerlingo M, Casto L, Censori B, et al: Transcranial Doppler in acute ischemic stroke of the middle cerebral artery territories. *Acta Neurol Scand* 88:108–111, 1993.
11. Carter BG, Butt W: Review of the use of somatosensory evoked potentials in the prediction of outcome after severe brain injury. *Crit Care Med* 29:178–186, 2001.
12. Cher LM, Chambers BR, Smidt V: Comparison of transcranial Doppler with DSA in vertebrobasilar ischaemia. *Clin Exp Neurol* 29:143–148, 1992.
13. Cillessen JP, van Huffelen AC, Kappelle LJ, et al: Electroencephalography improves the prediction of functional outcome in the acute stage of cerebral ischemia. *Stroke* 25:1968–1972, 1994.
14. Claassen J, Bernardini GL, Kreiter K, et al: Effect of cisternal and ventricular blood on risk of delayed cerebral ischemia after subarachnoid hemorrhage: the Fisher scale revisited. *Stroke* 32:2012–2020, 2001.
15. Claassen J, Hirsch LJ, Emerson RG, et al: Continuous EEG monitoring and midazolam infusion for refractory nonconvulsive status epilepticus. *Neurology* 57:1036–1042, 2001.
16. Czosnyka M, Smielewski P, Piechnik S, et al: Cerebral autoregulation following head injury. *J Neurosurg* 95:756–763, 2001.

17. Davis S, Andrews J, Lichtenstein M, et al: A single-photon emission computed tomography study of hypoperfusion after subarachnoid hemorrhage. *Stroke* 21:252–259, 1990.

18. Dawson RE, Webster JE, Gurdjian ES: Serial electroencephalography in acute head injury. *J Neurosurg* 8:613–630, 1951.

19. del Rio MA, Chrane D, Shelton S, et al: Ceftriaxone versus ampicillin and chloramphenicol for treatment of bacterial meningitis in children. *Lancet* 1:1241–1244, 1983.

20. Diringer MN, Edwards DF, Zazulia AR: Hydrocephalus: a previously unrecognized predictor of poor outcome from supratentorial intracerebral hemorrhage. *Stroke* 29:1352–1357, 1998.

21. Ducrocq X, Braun M, Debouverie M, et al: Brain death and transcranial Doppler: experience in 130 cases of brain dead patients. *J Neurol Sci* 160:41–46, 1998.

22. Ducrocq X, Hassler W, Moritake K, et al: Consensus opinion on diagnosis of cerebral circulatory arrest using Doppler-sonography: Task Force Group on Cerebral Death of the Neurosonology Research Group of the World Federation of Neurology. *J Neurol Sci* 159:145–150, 1998.

23. Durack DT, Spanos A: End-of-treatment spinal tap in bacterial meningitis. Is it worthwhile? *JAMA* 248:75–78, 1982.

24. Edlow JA, Bruner KS, Horowitz GL: Xanthochromia. *Arch Pathol Lab Med* 126:413–415, 2002.

25. Egge A, Waterloo K, Sjoholm H, et al: Prophylactic hyperdynamic postoperative fluid therapy after aneurysmal subarachnoid hemorrhage: a clinical, prospective, randomized, controlled study. *Neurosurgery* 49:593–605, 2001.

26. Eskey CJ, Ogilvy CS: Fluoroscopy-guided lumbar puncture: decreased frequency of traumatic tap and implications for the assessment of CT-negative acute subarachnoid hemorrhage. *AJNR Am J Neuroradiol* 22:571–576, 2001.

27. Felberg RA, Okon NJ, El-Mitwalli A, et al: Early dramatic recovery during intravenous tissue plasminogen activator infusion: clinical pattern and outcome in acute middle cerebral artery stroke. *Stroke* 33:1301–1307, 2002.

28. Fishman RA: *Cerebrospinal Fluid in Diseases of the Nervous System.* 2 ed. Philadelphia, WB Saunders Company, 1992.

29. Friedman JA, Goerss SJ, Meyer FB, et al: Volumetric quantification of Fisher grade 3 aneurysmal subarachnoid hemorrhage: a novel method to predict symptomatic vasospasm on admission computerized tomography scan. *J Neurosurg* 97:401–407, 2002.

30. Goldie WD, Chiappa KH, Young RR, et al: Brainstem auditory and short-latency somatosensory evoked responses in brain death. *Neurology* 31:248–256, 1981.

31. Gomez CR, Backer RJ, Bucholz RD: Transcranial Doppler ultrasound following closed head injury: Vasospasm or vasoparalysis? *Surg Neurol* 35:30–35, 1991.

32. Grosset DG, Straiton J, du Trevou M, et al: Prediction of symptomatic vasospasm after subarachnoid hemorrhage by rapidly increasing transcranial Doppler velocity and cerebral blood flow changes. *Stroke* 23:674–679, 1992.

33. Grosset DG, Straiton J, McDonald I, et al: Angiographic and Doppler diagnosis of cerebral artery vasospasm following subarachnoid haemorrhage. *Br J Neurosurg* 7:291–298, 1993.

34. Grosset DG, Straiton J, McDonald I, et al: Use of transcranial Doppler sonography to predict development of a delayed ischemic deficit after subarachnoid hemorrhage. *J Neurosurg* 78:183–187, 1993.

35. Hadani M, Brok B, Ram Z, et al: Application of transcranial Doppler ultrasonography for the diagnosis of brain death. *Intensive Care Med* 25:822–828, 1999.

36. Hanson SK, Grotta JC, Rhoades H, et al: Value of single-photon emission-computed tomography in acute stroke therapeutic trials. *Stroke* 24:1322–1329, 1993.

37. Hasan D, van Peski J, Loeve I, et al: Single photon emission computed tomography in patients with acute hydrocephalus or with cerebral ischaemia after subarachnoid haemorrhage. *J Neurol Neurosurg Psychiatry* 54:490–493, 1991.

38. Hellman RS, Tikofsky RS: An overview of the contribution of regional cerebral blood flow studies in cerebrovascular disease: Is there a role for single photon emission computed tomography? *Semin Nucl Med* 20:303–324, 1990.

39. Hijdra A, Brouwers PJAM, Vermeulen M, et al: Grading the amount of blood on computed tomograms after subarachnoid hemorrhage. *Stroke* 21:1156–1161, 1990.

40. Hoffmann M, Sacco RL, Chan S, et al: Noninvasive detection of vertebral artery dissection. *Stroke* 24:815–819, 1993.

41. Hogan RE, Cook MJ, Kilpatrick CJ, et al: Accuracy of coregistration of single-photon emission CT with MR via a brain surface matching technique. *AJNR Am J Neuroradiol* 17:793–797, 1996.

42. Hurst RW, Schnee C, Raps EC, et al: Role of transcranial Doppler in neuroradiological treatment of intracranial vasospasm. *Stroke* 24:299–303, 1993.

43. Illig KA, Burchfiel JL, Ouriel K, et al: Value of preoperative EEG for carotid endarterectomy. *Cardiovasc Surg* 6:490–495, 1998.

44. Jordan KG: Continuous EEG and evoked potential monitoring in the neuroscience intensive care unit. *J Clin Neurophysiol* 10:445–475, 1993.

45. Jordan KG: Neurophysiologic monitoring in the neuroscience intensive care unit. *Neurol Clin* 13:579–626, 1995.

46. Karnik R, Stelzer P, Slany J: Transcranial Doppler sonography monitoring of local intra-arterial thrombolysis in acute occlusion of the middle cerebral artery. *Stroke* 23:284–287, 1992.

47. Kassell NF, Sasaki T, Colohan AR, et al: Cerebral vasospasm following aneurysmal subarachnoid hemorrhage. *Stroke* 16:562–572, 1985.

48. Kelley RE, Namon RA, Mantelle LL, et al: Sensitivity and specificity of transcranial Doppler ultrasonography

in the detection of high-grade carotid stenosis. *Neurology* 43:1187–1191, 1993.

49. Kistler JP, Crowell RM, Davis KR, et al: The relation of cerebral vasospasm to the extent and location of subarachnoid blood visualized by CT scan: a prospective study. *Neurology* 33:424–436, 1983.

50. Knop J, Thie A, Fuchs C, et al: ^{99m}Tc-HMPAO-SPECT with acetazolamide challenge to detect hemodynamic compromise in occlusive cerebrovascular disease. *Stroke* 23:1733–1742, 1992.

51. Krieger D, Jauss M, Schwarz S, et al: Serial somatosensory and brainstem auditory evoked potentials in monitoring of acute supratentorial mass lesions. *Crit Care Med* 23:1123–1131, 1995.

52. Kushner MJ, Zanette EM, Bastianello S, et al: Transcranial Doppler in acute hemispheric brain infarction. *Neurology* 41:109–113, 1991.

53. Laloux P, Richelle F, Jamart J, et al: Comparative correlations of HMPAO SPECT indices, neurological score, and stroke subtypes with clinical outcome in acute carotid infarcts. *Stroke* 26:816–821, 1995.

54. Lang DT, Berberian LB, Lee S, et al: Rapid differentiation of subarachnoid hemorrhage from traumatic lumbar puncture using the D-dimer assay. *Am J Clin Pathol* 93:403–405, 1990.

55. Laumer R, Steinmeier R, Gonner F, et al: Cerebral hemodynamics in subarachnoid hemorrhage evaluated by transcranial Doppler sonography. Part 1. Reliability of flow velocities in clinical management. *Neurosurgery* 33:1–8, 1993.

56. Lennihan L, Petty GW, Fink ME, et al: Transcranial Doppler detection of anterior cerebral artery vasospasm. *J Neurol Neurosurg Psychiatry* 56:906–909, 1993.

57. Ley-Pozo J, Ringelstein EB: Noninvasive detection of occlusive disease of the carotid siphon and middle cerebral artery. *Ann Neurol* 28:640–647, 1990.

58. Liu H-M, Tu Y-K, Su C-T: Changes of brainstem and perimesencephalic cistern: dynamic predictor of outcome in severe head injury. *J Trauma* 38:330–333, 1995.

59. Lysakowski C, Walder B, Costanza MC, et al: Transcranial Doppler versus angiography in patients with vasospasm due to a ruptured cerebral aneurysm: a systematic review. *Stroke* 32:2292–2298, 2001.

60. Manno EM, Gress DR, Schwamm LH, et al: Effects of induced hypertension on transcranial Doppler ultrasound velocities in patients after subarachnoid hemorrhage. *Stroke* 29:422–428, 1998.

61. Marshall LF, Marshall SB, Klauber MR, et al: A new classification of head injury based on computerized tomography. *J Neurosurg* 75:S14, 1991.

62. Matthews WF, Frommeyer WB. The in vitro behaviour of erthrocytes in human cerebrospinal fluid. *J Lab Clin Med* 45:508–515, 1955.

63. McCarthy WJ, Park AE, Koushanpour E, et al: Carotid endarterectomy. Lessons from intraoperative monitoring—a decade of experience. *Ann Surg* 224:297–305, 1996.

64. McMenemey WH: The significance of subarachnoid bleeding. *Proc R Soc Med* 47:701–704, 1954.

65. McQuire JC, Sutcliffe JC, Coats TJ: Early changes in middle cerebral artery blood flow velocity after head injury. *J Neurosurg* 89:526–532, 1998.

66. Nagao S, Kuyama H, Honma Y, et al: Prediction and evaluation of brainstem function by auditory brainstem responses in patients with uncal herniation. *Surg Neurol* 27:81–86, 1987.

67. Newell DW, Aaslid R (eds): *Transcranial Doppler.* New York, Raven Press, 1992.

68. Newell DW, Winn HR: Transcranial Doppler in cerebral vasospasm. *Neurosurg Clin N Am* 1:319–328, 1990.

69. Niedermeyer E, Lopes da Silva FH (eds): *Electroencephalography: Basic Principles, Clinical Applications, and Related Fields.* 3rd ed. Baltimore, Williams & Wilkins, 1993.

70. Nuwer MR: Continuous EEG monitoring in the intensive care unit. *Electroencephalogr Clin Neurophysiol* 50:Suppl 150–155, 1999.

71. Petty GW, Mohr JP, Pedley TA, et al: The role of transcranial Doppler in confirming brain death: sensitivity, specificity, and suggestions for performance and interpretation. *Neurology* 40:300–303, 1990.

72. Petty GW, Wiebers DO, Meissner I: Transcranial Doppler ultrasonography: clinical applications in cerebrovascular disease. *Mayo Clin Proc* 65:1350–1364, 1990.

73. Rajendran JG, Lewis DH, Newell DW, et al: Brain SPECT used to evaluate vasospasm after subarachnoid hemorrhage: correlation with angiography and transcranial Doppler. *Clin Nucl Med* 26:125–130, 2001.

74. Raynaud C, Rancurel G, Tzourio N, et al: SPECT analysis of recent cerebral infarction. *Stroke* 20:192–204, 1989.

75. Reid RH, Gulenchyn KY, Ballinger JR, et al: Cerebral perfusion imaging with technetium-99m HMPAO following cerebral trauma. Initial experience. *Clin Nucl Med* 15:383–388, 1990.

76. Ropper AH, Kehne SM, Wechsler L: Transcranial Doppler in brain death. *Neurology* 37:1733–1735, 1987.

77. Rubens AB, Coslett HB: Cerebrovascular disease. In Van Heertum RL, Tikofsky RS (eds): *Cerebral SPECT Imaging.* 2nd ed. New York, Raven Press, 1995, pp 53–56.

78. Sander D, Klingelhofer J: Cerebral vasospasm following post-traumatic subarachnoid hemorrhage evaluated by transcranial Doppler ultrasonography. *J Neurol Sci* 119:1–7, 1993.

79. Siren J, Seppalainen AM, Launes J: Is EEG useful in assessing patients with acute encephalitis treated with acyclovir? *Electroencephalogr Clin Neurophysiol* 107:296–301, 1998.

80. Siva A: Vasculitis of the nervous system. *J Neurol* 248:451–468, 2001.

81. Sloan MA, Rigamonti D, Rothman M, et al: Sensitivity and specificity of transcranial Doppler for detection of basilar artery vasospasm (abstract). *Stroke* 23:469, 1992.

82. Soucy JP, McNamara D, Mohr G, et al: Evaluation of vasospasm secondary to subarachnoid hemorrhage with technetium-99m-hexamethyl-propyleneamine oxime (HM-PAO) tomoscintigraphy. *J Nucl Med* 31:972–977, 1990.

83. Steiger HJ, Aaslid R, Stooss R, et al: Transcranial Doppler monitoring in head injury: relations between type of injury, flow velocities, vasoreactivity, and outcome. *Neurosurgery* 34:79–85, 1994.

84. Suarez JI, Qureshi AI, Yahia AB, et al: Symptomatic vasospasm diagnosis after subarachnoid hemorrhage: evaluation of transcranial Doppler ultrasound and cerebral angiography as related to compromised vascular distribution. *Crit Care Med* 30:1348–1355, 2002.

85. Thomas SR, Jamieson DRS, Muir KW: Randomised controlled trial of atraumatic versus standard needles for diagnostic lumbar puncture. *BMJ* 321:986–990, 2000.

86. Thompson EJ: Cerebrospinal fluid. *J Neurol Neurosurg Psychiatry* 59:349–357, 1995.

87. Torbey MT, Hauser TK, Bhardwaj A, et al: Effect of age on cerebral blood flow velocity and incidence of vasospasm after aneurysmal subarachnoid hemorrhage. *Stroke* 32:2005–2011, 2001.

88. Totaro R, Marini C, Cannarsa C, et al: Reproducibility of transcranial Doppler sonography: a validation study. *Ultrasound Med Biol* 18:173–177, 1992.

89. Tranquart F, Ades PE, Groussin P, et al: Postoperative assessment of cerebral blood flow in subarachnoid haemorrhage by means of ^{99m}Tc-HMPAO tomography. *Eur J Nucl Med* 20:53–58, 1993.

90. Tsubokawa T, Nishimoto H, Yamamoto T, et al: Assessment of brainstem damage by the auditory brainstem response in acute severe head injury. *J Neurol Neurosurg Psychiatry* 43:1005–1011, 1980.

91. van der Jagt M, Hasan D, Bijvoet HW, et al: Interobserver variability of cisternal blood on CT after aneurysmal subarachnoid hemorrhage. *Neurology* 54: 2156–2158, 2000.

92. Vermeulen M, Hasan D, Blijenberg BG, et al: Xanthochromia after subarachnoid haemorrhage needs no revisitation. *J Neurol Neurosurg Psychiatry* 52:826–828, 1989.

93. Vespa PM, Boscardin WJ, Hovda DA, et al: Early and persistent impaired percent alpha variability on continuous electroencephalography monitoring as predictive of poor outcome after traumatic brain injury. *J Neurosurg* 97:84–92, 2002.

94. Vespa PM, Nuwer MR, Nenov V, et al: Increased incidence and impact of nonconvulsive and convulsive seizures after traumatic brain injury as detected by continuous electroencephalographic monitoring. *J Neurosurg* 91:750–760, 1999.

95. Vora YY, Suarez-Almazor M, Steinke DE, et al: Role of transcranial Doppler monitoring in the diagnosis of cerebral vasospasm after subarachnoid hemorrhage. *Neurosurgery* 44:1237–1247, 1999.

96. Wardlaw JM, Offin R, Teasdale GM, et al: Is routine transcranial Doppler ultrasound monitoring useful in the management of subarachnoid hemorrhage? *J Neurosurg* 88:272–276, 1998.

97. Westmoreland BF, Klass DW, Sharbrough FW, et al: Alpha-coma. Electroencephalographic, clinical, pathologic, and etiologic correlations. *Arch Neurol* 32:713–718, 1975.

98. Wood JH, Polyzoidis KS, Epstein CM, et al: Quantitative EEG alterations after isovolemic-hemodilutional augmentation of cerebral perfusion in stroke patients. *Neurology* 34:764–768, 1984.

PART III

MANAGEMENT of SPECIFIC DISORDERS in CRITICAL CARE NEUROLOGY

12

Aneurysmal Subarachnoid Hemorrhage

The incidence of aneurysmal SAH varies but overall is 10.5 cases per 100,000 persons per year (doubled in Finland and Japan). The risk is nearly two times higher in women than in men and in blacks than in whites. Subarachnoid hemorrhage is more common in patients with a family history of SAH, polycystic kidney disease, systemic lupus erythematosus, or Ehlers-Danlos disease.[38,39,76,110,133] After aneurysmal rupture, 10% of patients die suddenly before ever receiving medical attention. A pathologic study in Rochester, Minnesota, found that many of these patients had marked intraventricular extension of the hemorrhage and acute pulmonary edema, both reasons for sudden death.[115] Of the patients who reach the emergency department or NICU, from 20% to 30% arrive comatose, of whom half die within 3 months.[54]

The critical steps in management of SAH are to surgically clip the aneurysm or occlude the sac by inserting platinum coils, to treat clinical neurologic deterioration early, and to manage major systemic complications. The patient with SAH most likely to benefit from early aggressive surgery or coiling is a formerly healthy person with a normal level of consciousness.

Admission to the NICU is indicated for any patient with aneurysmal SAH. Admission to the ward (e.g., for patients in very good clinical condition) should be strongly discouraged, even when beds in the NICU are in short supply. The opportunities for rapid, successful resuscitation may not be optimal. Patients with SAH who are in excellent clinical condition face the risk of catastrophic rebleeding, rapidly developing hydrocephalus, and potentially life-threatening cardiac arrhythmias that can be better monitored in an NICU.

CLINICAL RECOGNITION

Aneurysmal SAH may be manifested in many ways. Typically, an unexpected instantaneous headache warns the patient of a very serious disorder and is often described as excruciating and overwhelming. (While taking the history, one may use a handclap to illustrate to the patient the acute onset of the headache.) The headache persists in its severity but may be reduced or even briefly disappear with pain medication. The abruptness of the headache is not specific for SAH, because it may occur in conditions such as arterial dissection, pituitary apoplexy, hypertensive encephalopathy, spontaneous intracranial hypotension, and cerebral venous thrombosis.[21,27,111,114,123] Some patients briefly lose consciousness, and commonly they vomit at least once. Inappropriate behavior and agitation or a soporific state may occur. Localizing neurologic findings, although transient, may indicate the site of the ruptured aneurysm. For example, patients with a ruptured middle cerebral artery aneurysm may have transient or persistent aphasia. In patients with a ruptured middle cerebral artery aneurysm and intraparenchymal extension, hemiparesis often is found. Abulia most often occurs as a complication of a rupture of an aneurysm of the anterior communicating artery. Generalized tonic-clonic seizures are not quite so often seen at the time of rupture, and it is possible that extensor posturing or brief shivering may be mistaken for a seizure. These clinical features in SAH are identical whether or not an aneurysm is detected. Different presentation is expected, however, in an established benign variant of nonaneurysmal SAH, so-called pretruncal SAH. The patients are almost exclusively alert. Loss of consciousness is seldom observed and seizures are absent, but the onset of headache is less acute—in minutes rather than a second.[104]

Neurologic examination reveals neck stiffness in most patients except those seen early after the initial event and those who are comatose. Retinal subhyaloid hemorrhages, present in approximately 25% of the patients, may be associated with reduced visual acuity if they extend into the vitreous cavity (Terson's syndrome) (Fig. 12–1), but more often this is observed in comatose patients and after rebleeding.[36,95] A potentially ominous sign is a developing third nerve palsy due to a compressing posterior communicating artery (Fig. 12–2). The pupil is typically dilated, but the light reflex may be spared. Ptosis may be complete. Cranial nerve abnormalities occur infrequently in SAH unless a giant basilar artery aneurysm (third nerve palsy, sixth nerve palsy,

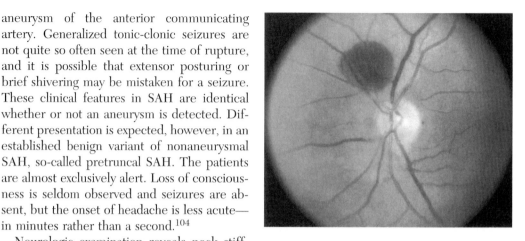

Figure 12–1. Terson's syndrome.

ataxia) or a large carotid artery aneurysm (chiasmal syndromes) directly compresses surrounding structures. Oculomotor palsy is expected to occur in 30% of patients after clipping of a basilar aneurysm.[60]

A simple clinical grading system proposed by the World Federation of Neurological Surgeons (WFNS) introduced the Glasgow coma scale in SAH grading[29] (Table 12–1). Grading of aneurysmal SAH remains useful and for practical reasons the severity is graded as good (WFNS I–III) or poor (WFNS IV, V). A strong correlation between outcome and initial grading level exists. The WFNS grade may

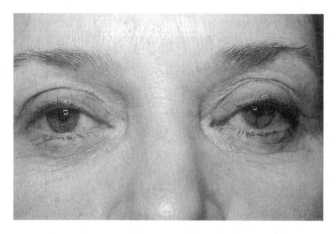

Figure 12–2. Subtle ptosis of the left eye from a ruptured posterior communicating aneurysm.

Table 12–1. Grading System Proposed by the World Federation of Neurological Surgeons for the Classification of Subarachnoid Hemorrhage

WFNS Grade	Glasgow Coma Scale Score	Motor Deficit
I	15	Absent
II	14–13	Absent
III	14–13	Present
IV	12–7	Present or absent
V	6–3	Present or absent

WFNS, World Federation of Neurological Surgeons.

also guide timing of surgery. Craniotomy for clipping could be deferred in patients with WFNS V.

When patients are comatose (Glasgow coma scale score < 8) at presentation, it is largely due to the initial rise in intracranial pressure with reduction of cerebral blood flow and, as a consequence, diffuse bihemispheric ischemia and global cerebral edema.[15] However, one should try to make a distinction between the direct effects of the initial impact and early neurologic deterioration due to other causes. Acute hydrocephalus may have developed in the interim, and placement of a ventricular drain could markedly improve the level of consciousness. Patients admitted days after the ictus may have symptomatic cerebral vasospasm, and focal signs and symptoms may not be present. Coma may be caused by brain tissue shift from a large expanding hematoma in the sylvian fissure. Removal of the hematoma and repair of the aneurysm may result in marked improvement. Systemic metabolic factors may contribute, and each of them should be excluded. Measurements of arterial blood gas, electrolytes, and serum glucose must be obtained rapidly in every patient who enters the NICU with SAH.

NEUROIMAGING AND LABORATORY TESTS

Subarachnoid hemorrhage shows on CT scan (Fig. 12–3). When CT scan is done within hours after the event, the sensitivity in aneurys-

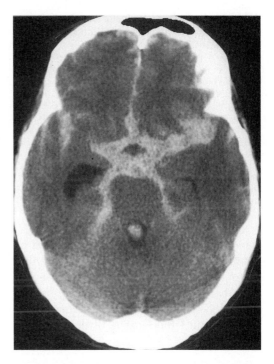

Figure 12–3. Subarachnoid hemorrhage with complete filling of the basal cisterns, creating a "crablike" cast.

mal SAH is very high and may approach 95%.[10,58] In 2% to 5% of the patients, subarachnoid blood has completely "washed out" on CT scans within 24 hours. The proportion of patients with true SAH but normalized CT scan increases in the following week to approximately 10% on day 3 and 50% on day 7.[10] In many patients, subarachnoid blood has disappeared on CT scans after 10 days, but intraventricular and intraparenchymal hematomas take more time to resolve.[10] Reportedly negative CT scans in patients in whom SAH is strongly suspected must be carefully scrutinized for subtle signs of subarachnoid blood. There are several reasons why an SAH may not be recognized on CT scans (Table 12–2).

Infrequently, the aneurysm itself is noted on an unenhanced CT scan, and if it appears, it is of considerable size. Occasionally a thrombosed aneurysm may not fill with contrast during angiography, and its presence is only suggested on CT or MRI. Important information

Table 12–2. Reasons for Failure to Recognize Subarachnoid Hemorrhage on Computed Tomography Scans

Blood in prepontine cistern is not visualized but is present on repeat CT scan
Blood in a part of the pentagon is not visualized from tilting of the gantry but is present on repeat CT scan
Absent unilateral sylvian fissure from isodense SAH
Sedimentation of blood in dependent part of the posterior ventricular horns
Blood in basal cisterns misinterpreted as contrast enhancement
Blood on tentorium misinterpreted as calcification

CT, computed tomography; SAH, subarachnoid hemorrhage.

pointing to a certain site can be gathered by careful inspection of CT scans. The distribution of the subarachnoid blood on CT scan may suggest the location of the aneurysm, but despite subtle differences, CT scanning cannot reliably predict the location of the aneurysm

with a diffuse scattering of cisternal blood.[130] Generally, patients with diffuse distribution of blood in cisterns and fissures often have a basilar artery or anterior communicating artery aneurysm. However, patients with a concentration of blood in the interhemispheric fissure may have an aneurysm of the anterior cerebral artery, and patients with cisternal blood surrounding the perimesencephalic cisterns most likely harbor a basilar artery aneurysm. Likewise, sylvian fissure hemorrhages are mostly from an aneurysm of the middle cerebral artery.

The additional presence of an intracerebral hematoma, however, has more localizing value. Hematomas may be found in the frontal lobe (anterior communicating artery aneurysm), in the medial part of the temporal lobe (internal carotid artery aneurysm), and within the sylvian fissure extending into the temporal lobe (middle cerebral artery aneurysm) (Fig. 12–4).

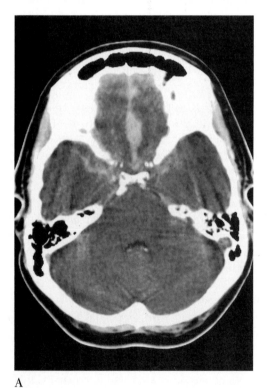 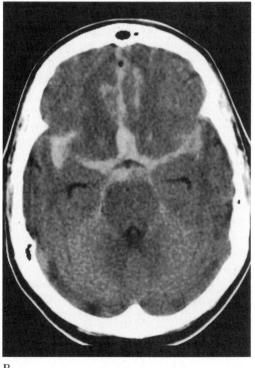

A   B

Figure 12–4. Computed tomography scan patterns in subarachnoid hemorrhage suggesting specific aneurysm locations (*A* and *B*). Hematoma in frontal lobe from anterior cerebral artery aneurysm.

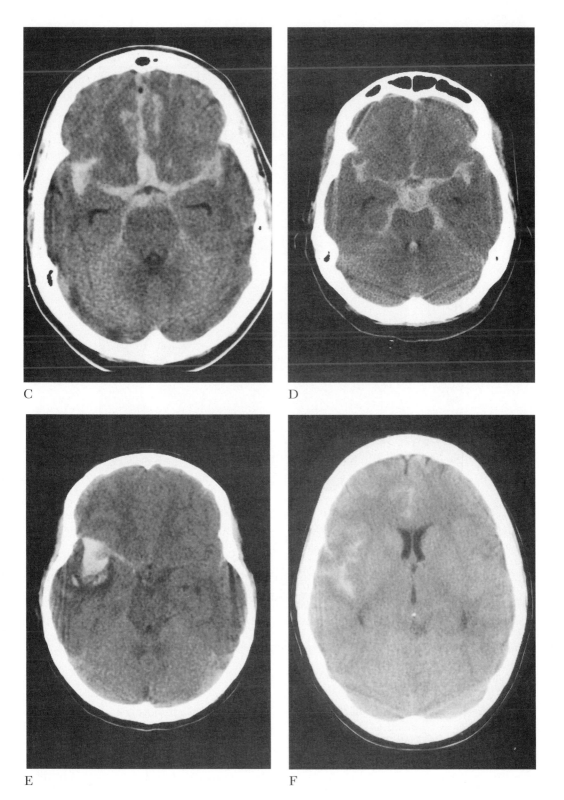

C

D

E

F

Figure 12–4. (*Continued*) (*C*) Mixed density hematoma in temporal lobe indicative of a carotid artery aneurysm. (*D*) Prepontine hematoma from a basilar aneurysm. (*E* and *F*) Blood and hematoma in sylvian fissure from middle cerebral artery aneurysm.

189

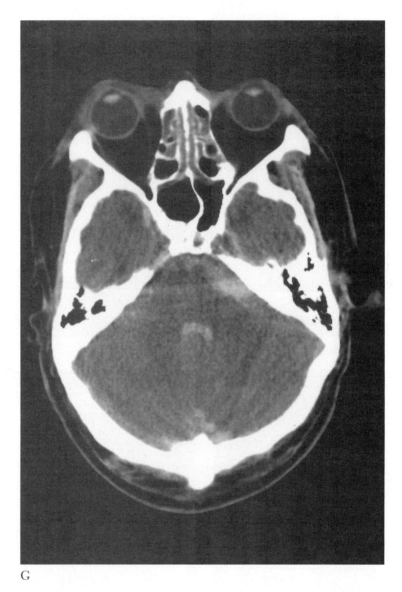

G

Figure 12–4. (*Continued*) (*G*) Premedullary hematoma indicative of a posterior inferior cerebellar artery aneurysm.

A benign form of SAH has been reported in which bleeding is confined to the cisterns in front of the brain stem without evidence of an aneurysm in the posterior cerebral circulation—so-called pretruncal SAH (previously called *perimesencephalic hemorrhage*).[112,134,144,146] True perimesencephalic hemorrhages are either purely traumatic or due to a P2 aneurysm or spinal dural arteriovenous fistula.[48] Typically, in this variant blood clots do not extend to the lateral sylvian fissures or to the anterior interhemispheric fissure. Some extension to the basal part of the sylvian fissure is possible when CT scanning is performed very early. Intraventricular hemorrhage is absent except for some sedimentation in the posterior horns.[144]

Magnetic resonance imaging is helpful in localization of the blood clot in front of the brain stem, but MRI of both the brain and the cervical spine has not revealed a source[145] (Fig. 12–5).

The cause of this perplexing benign form of SAH remains entirely speculative. Rupture of a dilated vein in the prepontine cistern is a possible explanation, but a clinicopathologic correlation has not yet been described. Exploratory surgery in patients with nonaneurysmal pretruncal hemorrhage has yielded negative results. We recently suggested that intramural hematoma from an arterial dissection may be the main cause[113] and could explain the "focal vasospasm" in the basilar artery seen in some patients. Pretruncal hemorrhage may closely mimic a ruptured basilar artery aneurysm, and therefore a full 4-vessel cerebral angiogram is warranted. This pattern of distribution of SAH may appear in approximately 10% of ruptured aneurysms of the posterior circulation.[65] We have also found unusual aneurysms, such as a P2 aneurysm.[116] If the first study is unrevealing, a second cerebral angiogram may be needed if studies of the posterior circulation are technically inadequate or a strong family history of SAH exists. Cerebral angiography in pretruncal nonaneurysmal SAH performed after the first week of rupture may document diffuse vasospasm in both the anterior and the posterior circulation,[118] but the clinical significance is not known. We repeat the cerebral angiogram if it is present because it may not

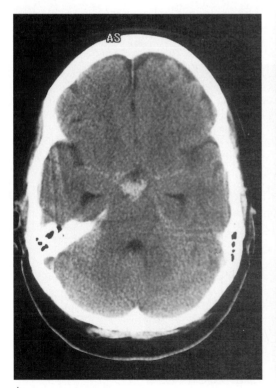

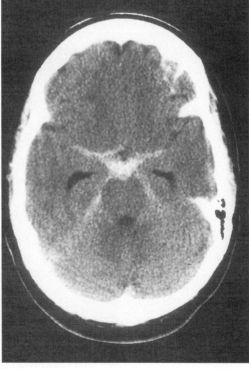

A   B

Figure 12–5. (*A–D*) Computed tomography scan patterns and (*E*) magnetic resonance imaging characteristics of pretruncal nonaneurysmal hemorrhage. (From Wijdicks et al.[146] By permission of Mayo Foundation for Medical Education and Research.)

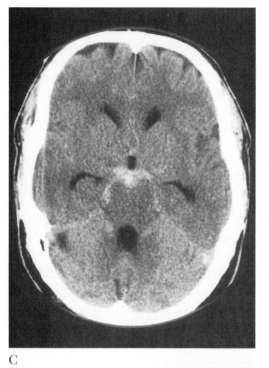

C

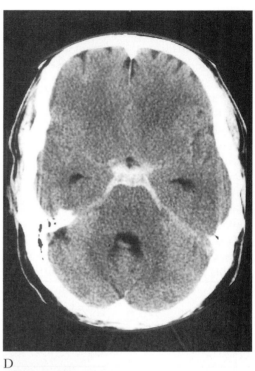

D

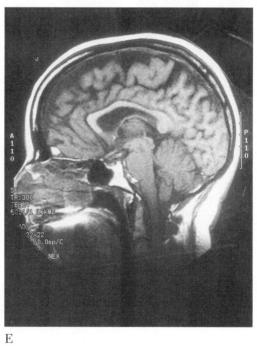

E

Figure 12–5. (*Continued*)

fully exclude a ruptured aneurysm if the feeding arteries are in vasospasm.

Localized blood in the sulci alone is unusual in aneurysmal SAH and often indicates trauma or coagulopathy. We have seen two patients presenting with this localization of SAH due to central nervous system vasculitis.[72] Subarachnoid blood caused by trauma also is most often confined to the vertex and superficial cortical sulci[23] or accumulates in the ambient cisterns at the level of the tentorium.[102] Computed tomography scans should be scrutinized for fractures on bone windows when physical examination shows other signs of trauma, for example, skin bruising or a soft tissue swelling. When blood is in the sylvian fissure, a reliable distinction from a ruptured middle cerebral aneurysm cannot be made on clinical grounds or by CT scan, and four-vessel cerebral angiography is needed.

Intraventricular blood on CT scans signals a severe SAH. Aneurysms of the anterior communicating artery have a proclivity to rupture into the ventricular system. Massive intraventricular hemorrhage in patients with SAH may also suggest rerupture. Subdural hematomas are seen in 1% of patients with SAH, often with cisternal blood and very rarely in isolation. Most often, a carotid artery aneurysm can be demonstrated on the angiogram, a suggestion that previous bleeding resulted in adhesion of the aneurysm to the arachnoid and dura.[88]

An important feature on CT scanning is acute hydrocephalus. Enlargement of the lateral ventricles is often asymptomatic in acute SAH,[132] but acute hydrocephalus as an explanation for drowsiness is more convincing if progression on sequential CT scans can be demonstrated or if the ventricles are very plump. The CT scan characteristics in SAH with the most important predictive features are shown in Table 12–3.

When results of CT scanning are negative, a lumbar puncture should be performed. It is not known whether lumbar puncture carries the risk of rebleeding.[30] Moreover, the risk in patients with a normal CT scan (and highly likely no SAH) is probably negligible. It is doubtful practice to proceed immediately with cerebral angiography without demonstrating actual SAH. At a later stage, MRI can be performed to detect hemosiderin, but the study is not very useful in the acute stage.[2]

Blood-stained CSF may have a traumatic origin. As alluded to, the number of patients with a negative CT scan but blood pigments in the CSF from SAH is small (2–5%),[35,131] and the probability that "bloody" CSF represents a traumatic puncture is higher. Traumatic lumbar puncture and true SAH can be differentiated by centrifuging CSF and inspecting the supernatant for xanthochromia (see Chapter 11).

Patients with a normal examination and who have negative results both on CT scan and on

Table 12–3. Interpretation of Computed Tomography Scans in Subarachnoid Hemorrhage

Feature	Suggests or Predicts
Completely filled suprasellar cistern *and* anterior interhemispheric fissure *and* ambient cistern	High probability of cerebral ischemia from vasospasm[55]
Massive intraventricular bleeding	Early rebleeding[57]
Intracerebral hematoma	
Frontal lobe	Anterior cerebral artery aneurysm
Temporal lobe (medial)	Internal carotid or posterior communicating artery aneurysm
Temporal lobe (lateral)	Middle cerebral artery aneurysm
Enlarged third ventricle	Development of hyponatremia[147]
Subdural hematoma	Carotid aneurysm (suggests rebleeding)[88]
Focal prepontine hemorrhage	Nonaneurysmal SAH[23,72,102]
SAH in sulci only	Trauma, coagulopathy, vasculitis

SAH, subarachnoid hemorrhage.

lumbar puncture most likely had a "thunderclap headache syndrome," and cerebral angiography is not warranted.[26,77,143] The results of large retrospective and prospective studies strongly suggest that these patients do not have a "missed SAH,"[77,143] and it is very uncertain whether these patients need cerebral angiography. It is prudent to perform MRI and magnetic resonance angiography, but the yield of finding an explanation for this explosive headache is not known. Cerebral angiography seems reasonable only if CSF examination or CT scan is performed more than 2 weeks after the ictus.

Cerebral angiography remains the unchallenged gold standard for the diagnosis of cerebral aneurysm. Before cerebral angiography is undertaken, plasma creatinine concentration should be determined. The most important risk factor for contrast-induced nephrotoxicity is preexisting renal failure. The risk is also increased in patients with reduced intravascular volume and in patients using drugs that impair renal responses, such as angiotensin-converting enzyme inhibitors and nonsteroidal anti-inflammatory drugs. In patients with preexisting renal impairment, defined as a creatinine value of more than 1.8 mg/dL, 0.45% saline should be given intravenously at a rate of 1 mL/kg of body weight per hour beginning 12 hours before the scheduled angiography. Further addition of mannitol or furosemide is not needed. Contrast neurotoxicity may occur, most often in patients with aneurysms that seem difficult to demonstrate and in patients who have platinum coils placed (in both situations, large doses of contrast agent are used). The typical features of central nervous system contrast neurotoxicity are agitated behavior (see Chapter 4), language difficulties characterized by anomia alone, transient global amnesia,[63] and, most striking, cortical blindness. Treatment with corticosteroids and mannitol is sufficient, and most signs resolve within 24 hours (Chapter 4). The risk of a permanent stroke after cerebral angiography is very low (0.07%).[16,50]

The timing of four-vessel cerebral angiography is less clear, but one can argue for early angiography in every patient, including those with poor-grade SAH. These patients may have aneurysms that can be occluded through endovascular techniques.

Cerebral angiography by the transfemoral approach may demonstrate aneurysms at typical locations (Fig. 12–6). Standard examination should include anteroposterior and lateral views, but because overlapping is significant, oblique views are often necessary.[121] The neuroradiologist may be guided by the findings on CT scan and should frequently use additional oblique views in evaluating the circle of Willis. Important additional views are submentovertex views (particularly useful for demonstrating the neck of an anterior communicating aneurysm) and transorbital projection (neck of the middle cerebral artery). Towne's projection is important to visualize the tip of the basilar artery. Failure to demonstrate an aneurysm may be related to inadequate projection or incomplete study (three-vessel study), and a second angiogram at a slightly different angle may uncover an aneurysm. Three-dimensional image volume generated by digital fluorography with rotational image acquisition could improve detection.

Multiple aneurysms may be found, and it is virtually impossible to predict which aneurysm has bled. However, additional clues (next to CT scan patterns) may be present, such as irregularity of the wall of the aneurysm produced by the sealing clot, vasospasm in the vicinity of the aneurysm, and size between 5 and 15 mm.

When an angiogram is negative, a second cerebral angiogram may demonstrate an aneurysm in approximately 10% of cases. The second cerebral angiogram should be particularly carefully scrutinized for a posterior circulation aneurysm, which could have been "missed" on the first angiogram. Whether craniotomy is needed in patients with a high suspicion of an aneurysm (presence of subarachnoid blood and intracranial hematoma) is very unclear even though some explorations have been successful in detecting the ruptured aneurysm.[25,62]

Spiral (helical) CT scanning has been used in patients with large aneurysms to better doc-

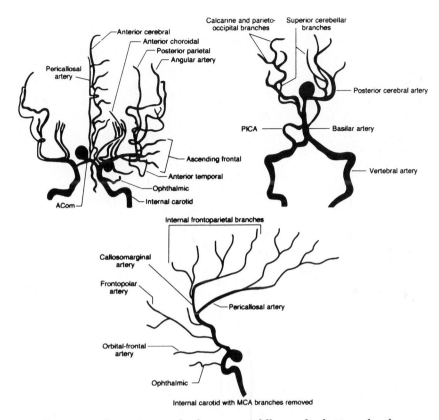

Figure 12–6. Drawings of anterior cerebral artery, middle cerebral artery, basilar artery tip, and posterior communicating artery aneurysms on cerebral angiogram in their optimal projections. ACom, anterior communicating artery; MCA, middle cerebral artery; PICA, posterior inferior cerebellar artery.

ument anatomical configuration (Fig. 12–7), in patients with an initial negative cerebral angiogram (as a means of follow-up), and as the only additional diagnostic test in patients with pretruncal SAH in some European centers.[136] Computed tomography angiography may detect aneurysms not seen on conventional cerebral angiography.[154] It may be useful to further assess vascular anatomy before surgery.[137] Its place in diagnostic evaluation of patients with an SAH is unclear. Moreover, the less than perfect sensitivity of 97% (87% in aneurysms < 3 mm) and specificity of 86% may have medicolegal implications.[47,153] Anatomical bulges of the basilar tip and pituitary stalk mistaken for aneurysms and incorrect three-dimensional reconstruction

of overlapping middle cerebral arteries are some of the reasons for false-positive results. The large amount of iodinated contrast medium required is another potential concern.[152]

FIRST STEPS IN MANAGEMENT

Initial management in patients with aneurysmal SAH can be adapted to the initial grade. Subarachnoid hemorrhage of WFNS grade I to III should be differentiated from poor-grade SAH (WFNS grade IV or V), assuming that the poor clinical grade is caused by the initial impact alone.

The initial management in aneurysmal SAH is summarized in Table 12–4. Continuous as-

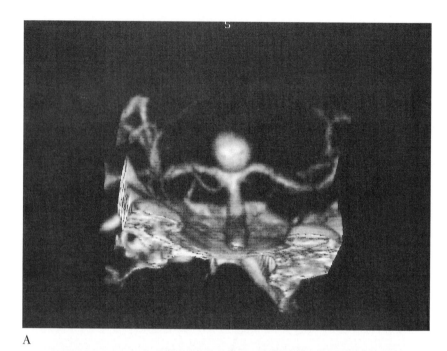

A

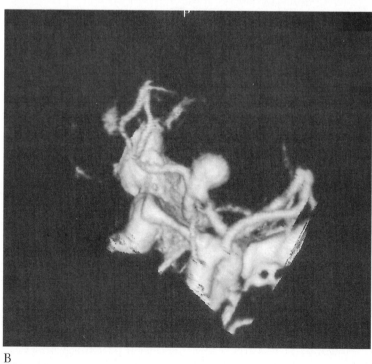

B

Figure 12–7. (*A* and *B*) Spiral computed tomography scans of basilar tip aneurysm.

Table 12–4. Initial Management in Subarachnoid Hemorrhage

Airway management	Intubation and MV if patient has severe hypoxemia, GCS motor score of withdrawal, or worse
	IMV mode (8–10 breaths/minute), PEEP 5 cm H_2O
	Assist-control mode if patient is moribund or there is progression to brain death
	Consider pressure-controlled ventilation if patient has significant aspiration pneumonitis or early ARDS
Fluid management	2–3 L of 0.9% NaCl per 24 hours
	Fludrocortisone acetate, 0.2 mg in 200 mL of glucose 5% b.i.d., if patient has hyponatremia
Blood pressure management	Accept MAP of $\leq$ 130 mm Hg; if MAP > 130, labetalol 20–40 mg IV or esmolol IV, 500 μg/kg in 1 minute, or enalapril, 1–5 mg IV
Nutrition	Enteric nutrition with continuous infusion on day 2
Additional measures	Nimodipine, 60 mg six times a day for 21 days
	Stool softener
	Pneumatic compression devices
	Codeine 30–60 mg every 4 hours as needed
	Tramadol, 50–100 mg p.o. q4h, for pain management
	Phenytoin loading, 20 mg/kg, if seizures have occurred

ARDS, adult respiratory distress syndrome; GCS, Glasgow coma scale; IMV, intermittent mechanical ventilation; IV, intravenously; MAP, mean arterial pressure; MV, mechanical ventilation; NaCl, sodium chloride; PEEP, positive end-expiratory pressure.

sessment of alertness and performance remains important. Experienced nurses in neurologic intensive care usually are familiar with the peak time of cerebral ischemia and the first clinical signs of acute hydrocephalus.

An important component of management in SAH is the relief of pain. Severe headache is best treated by acetaminophen with codeine. Many patients benefit from the calming effect of these agents, but others do not tolerate opioids and may vomit excessively. Tramadol may be helpful in this situation.

Respiratory care is largely supportive, and serial chest radiographs should be reviewed for signs of gastric aspiration or pulmonary edema. Intubation and mechanical ventilation are often indicated in poor-grade SAH. The ventilatory mode chosen should provide adequate minute ventilation at the lowest possible airway pressure—in most instances, an intermittent mandatory ventilation mode.[141]

Cardiac stunning tends to develop in patients with poor-grade SAH, and it can be observed clinically and on repeat echocardiograms. It may be a cause for the development of pulmonary edema[80] (see Chapter 30 for further details).

Adequate fluid intake is an essential part of the management of SAH. Approximately one-third of the patients have a decrease in plasma volume of more than 10% during the perioperative period, often detected by negative fluid balance.[149] Initially, most patients are probably best managed with 3 L of isotonic saline (infusion of 125 mL/hour). Fever (> 38.5°C) is more common in poor-grade intubated patients and those who have had ventriculostomy and is associated, in the absence of any infection, with development of cerebral vasospasm. The effect of aggressive reduction of fever on outcome is not known, but fluid intake must be adjusted.[92]

The management of hypertension after SAH is difficult (Chapter 7), and a fine line for antihypertensive treatment separates necessity from harm. A retrospective study suggested that the incidence of cerebral infarction is increased in patients treated with antihypertensive drugs (largely clonidine).[148] On the other hand, earlier studies suggested that rebleeding and death from rebleeding are increased in patients with persistently increased systolic blood pressure of 160 mm Hg or greater,[151] but, as discussed earlier, rebleeding was loosely defined (Chapter 7).

Hypertension after SAH is difficult to define, but when a mean arterial blood pressure of approximately 130 mm Hg persists and hypertension is not typically associated with increased pain, anxiety, or fighting off the ventilator, the tendency is to decrease blood pressure with labetalol or esmolol.[12]

Nutrition can usually be deferred until the second day. Enteral feedings in patients with critical neurologic illness are not always tolerated, and poor gastric emptying may lead to aspiration. However, placement of a nasoenteric feeding tube into the duodenum or jejunum may overcome these problems. Usually, concentrated commercial solutions infused at a low rate are administered (see Appendix).

Patients with SAH may be combative and require sedation. Agitation may be directly related to placement of the endotracheal tube and to inappropriate mechanical ventilator settings (e.g., high-frequency assist-control in an alert patient). Not infrequently, these patients can be extubated without any difficulty, which resolves the distress and agitation.

Combative and agitated patients (usually patients with large frontal hematomas from a ruptured anterior communicating artery aneurysm) can be best treated with propofol infusion. Stool softeners are prescribed, particularly for patients who regularly require opiates. Prophylaxis of deep venous thrombosis is provided by stockings and pneumatic compression devices. Pantoprazole is provided only for patients who have a history of gastric ulcers or have been using nonsteroidal anti-inflammatory agents or aspirin and in patients on the mechanical ventilator. Patients who have a decreased level of consciousness need an indwelling bladder catheter. The use of intermittent catheterization may decrease the incidence of urinary tract infection, but the procedure is too stressful for patients with acute SAH.

Nimodipine is administered in all patients with SAH to prevent delayed cerebral ischemia; it can be crushed and applied through the nasogastric tube.[1,91,94,96,97] A regimen of nimodipine (60 mg six times a day orally) is instituted for 21 days on the basis of significant reduction in the incidence of delayed cerebral ischemia and mortality.[3] A review of 90 patients treated with nimodipine for 15 days or less did not suggest an increase in delayed cere-

bral ischemia, but there is no reason to shorten the period of administration.[126] Nimodipine can be discontinued when cerebral angiographic findings are negative. In recent trials, no other agents have been found to reduce cerebral ischemia, including the 21-aminosteroid tirilazad mesylate[43,127] and the antioxidant ebselen.[108]

Anecdotal studies have suggested that placement of recombinant tissue plasminogen activator in the cisterns after aneurysm clipping may enhance resolution of clot and reduce delayed cerebral ischemia. However, a randomized study in 100 patients found no justification for the use of intracisternal recombinant tissue plasminogen activator.[33]

The use of prophylactic antiepileptic medication is very questionable, and such therapy should only be initiated if seizures occurred at the time of the rupture. The incidence of seizures after acute SAH is very low,[45,90] and most seizures recur during rerupture. The risk of late seizures may theoretically be increased in patients who have a temporal lobe or frontal lobe hematoma and large amounts of blood on CT,[11] but again no hard data are available to specifically justify prophylactic antiepileptic agents.

Currently, antifibrinolytic therapy is not used routinely. Antifibrinolytic therapy is very effective in preventing rebleeding and significantly reduces the risk of rebleeding. However, a reciprocal increase in delayed cerebral ischemia results in no overall benefit.[138] A pilot study in which tranexamic acid was given for only 4 days produced the reverse of the desired result, with no effect on the incidence of rebleeding and an increase in the incidence of cerebral ischemia.[142] A recent randomized study combined antifibrinolytic treatment with nimodipine but did not document improvement in outcome despite reduction in rebleeding.[105] A possible increase in pulmonary emboli in patients treated with antifibrinolytic agents was of concern. However, a better outcome, including reduction of rebleeding risk, was evident in a subgroup of patients with normal Glasgow coma scores after SAH.[105] This finding leaves open the possibility that antifibrinolytic agents can be used in alert patients who have small amounts of subarachnoid hemorrhage but a giant aneurysm while they await careful planning of surgical repair.

Emergency or early surgery is indicated in patients with evidence of rebleeding or intracerebral hematoma in the temporal lobe and tissue shift and, at the opposite end of the spectrum, any patient in good prior health with WFNS grade I–III. Elective surgery with provision for cardiopulmonary bypass to perform clipping of the aneurysm under hypothermic conditions should be considered in patients with giant aneurysms. Surgery can be temporarily withheld in patients in WFNS grade IV or V with packed intraventricular hemorrhage and hydrocephalus. Ventriculostomy could produce improvement in such patients. Surgery may also be postponed in patients with symptomatic vasospasm. Endovascular therapy may be an alternative option.

For eligible patients, cerebral angiography should be performed as soon as feasible and should be followed by surgical clipping of the aneurysm (operative techniques and neuroanesthesia are outside the scope of this book). A cooperative study group found in a large survey that no major differences existed between early and late surgery but that outcome was worse when surgery was performed between days 7 and 10.[67]

The development of detachable coils (Guglielmi detachable platinum coils) has modified current practices (currently already 20%–30% of ruptured aneurysms treated).[13,86,140] A direct electrical current disconnects the coil, and the positive electrical charge increases thrombus formation. The procedure of multiple coil placement is very time-consuming, taking several hours, and needs anesthesia monitoring.[87] Coil placement has become a reasonable consideration in patients with a ruptured basilar artery aneurysm, irrespective of the WFNS grade.[5,41,135] Other locations of saccular aneurysms are much more difficult to approach for placement of coils, but one study of 173 patients with anterior circulation aneurysms demonstrated successful coil insertion and aneurysm occlusion.[140] In the ISAT study,[61] preliminary results found benefit from use of coils in good-

grade patients with small anterior circulation aneurysms, but no sufficient proof in other patients with SAH. Large series of patients from France reported good outcomes in many patients with poor-grade SAH.[6,13] Long-term outcome is not yet available, and concern about imperfect repair remains. A review of 509 patients with treated ruptured aneurysms found ischemic complications in 7% and aneurysm perforation in 3%, with procedure-related mortality of 1%.[9] The estimated morbidity related to the technique is 9%, with an overall mortality of 6%.[140] A considerable drawback to the technique is rebleeding from a remnant aneurysm (reported rebleeding rates from 6% to 25%).

Experience with endovascular coil placement in acute ruptured aneurysm is mounting but the decision to "clip or coil" remains arbitrary and could be determined by whoever has the upper hand in multidisciplinary communication. In a recent trial,[61] the involved physicians did not square with each other in more than two-thirds of cases. Certain criteria have emerged that are based on the width of the neck and size and location of the aneurysm. Selection for coiling is often determined by location of the aneurysm in the posterior circulation, width of neck less than 5 mm, and a dome-to-neck ratio greater than 2[22,28] (Fig. 12–8). Platinum coil placement is illustrated in Figure 12–9.

DETERIORATION: CAUSES AND MANAGEMENT

Most often, patients with SAH are prone to deterioration from delayed cerebral ischemia,[55] rebleeding,[57] acute hydrocephalus,[46] and enlargement of a temporal lobe hematoma.[7]

The risk of rebleeding after the first rupture is approximately 30% in the first month. Many patients rebleed within 24 hours after the first bleeding.[37,57] The clinical presentation of rerupture is dramatic. The typical clinical features of rebleeding are loss of consciousness associated with loss of several brain stem reflexes, including pupillary light response and oculocephalic responses. In most patients, respiratory arrest or gasping breathing occurs, neces-

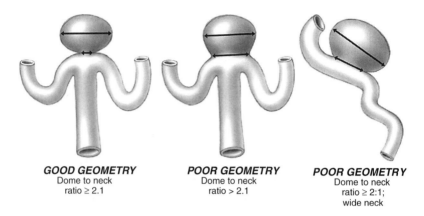

GOOD GEOMETRY
Dome to neck
ratio ≥ 2.1

POOR GEOMETRY
Dome to neck
ratio > 2.1

POOR GEOMETRY
Dome to neck
ratio ≥ 2:1;
wide neck

Figure 12–8. Using the neck:dome ratio to assess the feasibility of coil placement.

sitating immediate endotracheal intubation and mechanical ventilation. Computed tomography scanning very often demonstrates fresh blood, more common in the ventricular system (Fig. 12–10), or less often a new intracerebral hematoma that causes marked brain stem distortion. Recovery from rebleeding is difficult to predict, but many patients begin to fight the ventilator within hours,[56] and very often recovery is also signaled by a return of most brain stem reflexes. These patients may improve rapidly up to the point of self-extubation.

Rebleeding can be much less dramatic in patients presenting with acute headache alone. In some fortunate patients, rebleeding begins with sudden emergence of fresh blood in the collection bag of the ventricular drain, and rapid evacuation of intraventricular blood is often lifesaving. Management of rebleeding is essentially supportive, with intravenous (fos)phenytoin loading (20 mg/kg) if seizures have occurred. Emergency clipping of the aneurysm must be strongly considered, since most patients will have a second rebleeding, which is associated with very high mortality. The initial mortality of rebleeding is 50%. Rerupture often occurs in the same week, and the total mortality from initial rebleeding and from complications associated with persistent coma is 80% in 3 months.[57] Patients with a devastating rebleeding may progress to brain death. This clinical course is most likely in patients with massive hydrocephalus and ventricles packed with blood clots.

Delayed cerebral ischemia or symptomatic vasospasm is manifested by a gradual decrease in level of consciousness in most patients[53,55,84] and in some is associated with hemiparesis, mutism, and, less frequently, apraxia. Very unusual presentations, such as paraparesis and right hemiparesis without aphasia, have been described as well.[34,40] Delayed cerebral ischemia may cause sudden deterioration and coma and then often massive brain swelling, and bihemispheric infarction is detectable on a repeat CT scan. Patients with delayed cerebral ischemia may become apathetic and cut short answers to questions and have initial weakness of one leg or both legs, indicating infarction in both territories of the anterior cerebral arteries.[34,40] Early recognition of the decrease in level of consciousness remains crucial. Some patients have a fluctuating level of consciousness: days with daytime sleep (barely arousable) intermingled with days of appropriate behavior and better responsiveness. Risk factors for delayed cerebral ischemia include a large number of cisternal and ventricular clots, poor WFNS clinical grade, hyperglycemia, and early surgery.[8] The incidence of cerebral vasospasm in patients who have endovascular treatment is not known exactly, but our review suggests significantly less symptomatic vasospasm than

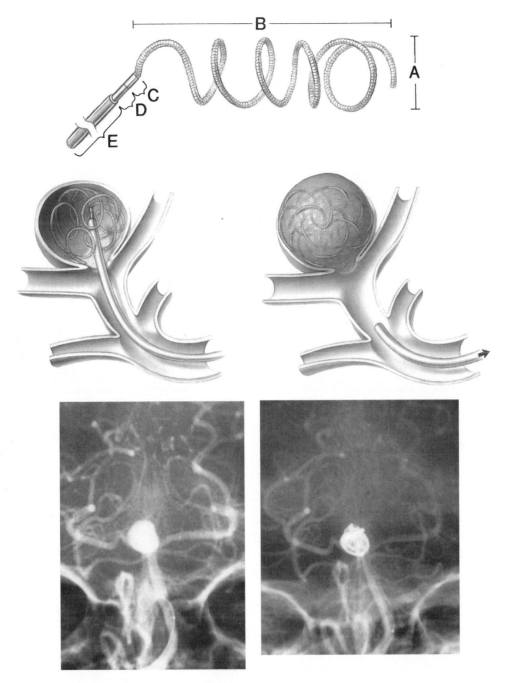

Figure 12–9. Occlusion of aneurysm with Guglielmi detachable platinum coil. (*Top*) Diagram of coil showing (*A*) helical diameter of coil, (*B*) length of coil (4 to 40 cm if straightened), (*C*) microsolder connecting distal stainless steel wire to platinum coil, (*D*) uninsulated segment of stainless steel wire, and (*E*) proximal polytef-insulated stainless steel wire. (*Left middle*) Placement of coil through guide wire positioned inside aneurysmal sac. (*Right middle*) Completion of treatment. Aneurysm is filled and excluded from intracranial circulation by combination of thrombus and multiple coils. Microcatheter is being withdrawn from basilar artery (*arrow*). (*Bottom left*) Large aneurysm at tip of basilar artery before coiling. (*Bottom right*) Coiled aneurysm. (*Top, left middle, right middle* from Nichols et al.[87] Reproduced by permission of Mayo Foundation for Medical Education and Research.)

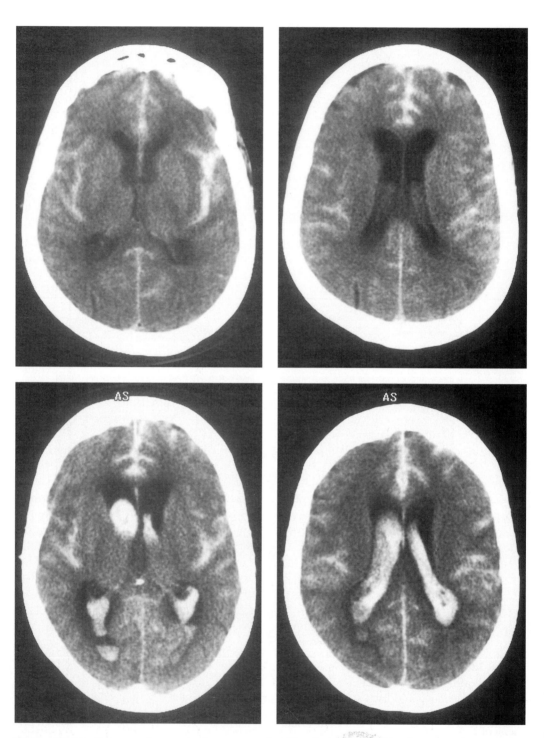

Figure 12–10. Computed tomography scans with rebleeding. (*Top row*) Admission images. (*Bottom row*) Clinical deterioration with significant intraventricular clot.

that with clipping of the aneurysm.[101] Additional laboratory testing (e.g., transcranial Doppler ultrasonography, single-photon emission computed tomography, or cerebral angiography) often confirms cerebral vasospasm (Chapter 11).

Diffusion-weighted MRI can detect abnormalities and a reduction in diffusion coefficients. It is unknown whether these abnormalities are potentially reversible with therapeutic intervention. Currently, limited experience suggests a role in the diagnosis of delayed cerebral ischemia. Reported studies have shown scattered multiple hyperintense signals highly consistent with the diffuse nature of cerebral vasospasm.[19,106]

We recognize the difficulties in timely acquisition of these tests. A recent study reported use of diffusion-weighted MRI in patients with vasospasm. All 10 patients with Doppler-confirmed vasospasm had diffusion-weighted imaging abnormalities, whereas 4 control patients without vasospasm had no such abnormalities.[19] Interestingly, 7 of the 10 patients with vasospasm were asymptomatic, and some of the diffusion-weighted abnormalities were reversible. Another study, in six patients with angiographic vasospasm, reported that diffusion- and perfusion-weighted imaging and hemodynamically weighted imaging tracked a rapid gadolinium bolus during its first pass through the brain. On diffusion-weighted imaging, this technique showed multiple ischemic lesions that were associated with a large surrounding area of decreased cerebral blood flow.[106] We noted diffusion-weighted abnormalities on MRI in a patient with patho-logically proven infarction and normal findings on transcranial Doppler ultrasonography (Fig. 12–11). Diffusion-weighted imaging is a promising new technique to diagnose vasospasm and should be thoroughly explored.

Management of cerebral vasospasm has been guided by a medical attempt first and then endovascular intervention. Current published data on the best approach are unconvincing because systematic measurements of variables are lacking, with different methods used in each of the cohorts.[73,75,81,93] Claims of hypervolemic therapy in some of the studies may not amount to much. We are gathering data from a new management strategy, as outlined below, but acknowledge that no data exist to suggest an "optimal" management strategy. The areas of uncertainty are the timing of hemodynamic augmentation, the variable to be augmented (perfusion pressure or cardiac output), the countering of a concomitant cerebral salt-wasting syndrome, and the timing of endovascular procedures. The protocol is outlined in Table 12–5. Our protocol starts with preload augmentation. Cardiac index augmentation is associated with a greater increase in myocardial oxygen demand and a risk of cardiac arrhythmia. The optimized intravascular state is defined when the flat part of the Starling curve is reached. (The Starling curve is the relationship between stroke volume and left end-diastolic ventricular pressure or pulmonary wedge pressure. With increasing preload—related to the patient's volume status and ventricular compliance—stroke volume increases steeply but reaches a maximum.) Intravascular volume expansion can be enhanced by fludrocortisone acetate, 0.2 mg twice a day.[44,85,150] The fluid balance is carefully calculated every hour and scrutinized for changes in urinary output. Weight change is essentially equivalent to change in body water, and therefore the daily availability of body weight is useful in adjusting fluid intake. Commonly used hemodynamic agents are shown in Table 12–6.

Particular care is warranted in patients with significant electrocardiographic changes, and induced hypertension may possibly trigger cardiac arrhythmias. It remains uncertain whether hypertensive-hypervolemic therapy is safe. A review from Barnes Hospital NICU found no major systemic complications when this therapy was administered by experienced personnel.[83]

When patients do not improve with these measures, we proceed with a cerebral angiogram. Angioplasty can be considered if adequate volume expansion has not resulted in marked clinical improvement.[24,71] Cerebral va-

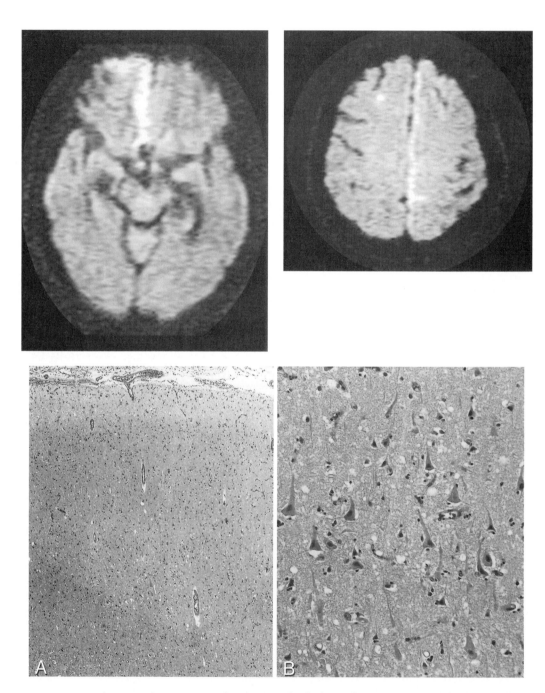

Figure 12–11. (*Top row*) Deteriorated patient with abulia and paraparesis. Diffusion-weighted magnetic resonance images showing hyperintensity in the territory of the anterior cerebral artery. (*A* and *B*) Corresponding necrosis is shown on microscopy from a sample of the frontal lobe. An area of pallor and mild vacuolation in the cerebral cortex is consistent with acute infarction. Most of the neurons, shrunken and with pyknotic nuclei, have the appearance of acutely ischemic "red" neurons.

Table 12–5. Mayo Clinic Protocol for Hemodynamic Augmentation in the Treatment of Cerebral Vasospasm in Aneurysmal Subarachnoid Hemorrhage

---

SAH, clinically asymptomatic but TCD or CT evidence of diffuse cerebral vasospasm
   Place central venous catheter
   Obtain hourly readings of fluid balance and body weight
   Accomplish volume repletion with crystalloids
   Note end points of volume resuscitation: CVP ≥ 8 mm Hg, urine output > 250 mL/hour
   Avoid antihypertensive and diuretic agents
SAH, secured aneurysm, clinical evidence of cerebral vasospasm°
   Notify interventional neuroradiologist for possible cerebral angiography
   Place pulmonary artery catheter
   Give crystalloid bolus or albumin 5% until increase in stroke volume index is < 10% for every 2 mm Hg increase
      in pulmonary capillary wedge pressure
   Match fluid input with urine output
   When urine output is > 250 mL/hour, start administration of fludrocortisone acetate, 0.2 mg b.i.d.
   Wait 1 hour for clinical improvement
   If no improvement, start administration of phenylephrine, 10–30 μg/min, with increase in MAP 25% above
      baseline or > 120 mm Hg
   Start administration of dobutamine, 5–15 μg/kg/min, to increase cardiac index > 3.5 L/minute/m²
   Consider replacing phenylephrine with norepinephrine if desired effect is not attained
   If no effect, perform cerebral angiography for angioplasty or papaverine infusion

---

CT, computed tomography; CVP, central venous pressure; MAP, mean arterial pressure; SAH, subarachnoid hemorrhage; TCD, transcranial Doppler ultrasonography.
°See text p. 203. Typically, fluctuation in level of consciousness or a localizing sign such as aphasia, hemiparesis, paraparesis, or apraxia.

sospasm can be arbitrarily categorized as mild, moderate, or severe with 50% luminal narrowing. Focal cerebral vasospasm indicates vasospasm in one cerebral artery; in diffuse cerebral vasospasm, multiple vessels are involved. Angioplasty of focal spastic segments is a potentially effective treatment for cerebral vasospasm.[20] Neurologic improvement was described in 60% to 70% of patients who did not have a response to hypervolemic hypertensive treatment, but most of the patients had clipped aneurysms, and these results seem too optimistic.[20,24,71] A more recent study of 30 patients showed improvement in only 4 patients despite good angiographic results.[99]

An additional advantage of cerebral angiography is that intra-arterial papaverine can be considered when cerebral vasospasm is diffuse or involves distal segments beyond A1, M1, or P1.[64] Papaverine is an opium alkaloid that relaxes vascular smooth muscle from phosphodiesterase inhibition. Intra-arterial papaverine

Table 12–6. Commonly Used Hemodynamic Agents in Subarachnoid Hemorrhage*

Agent	Action	Dose	Side Effect
Dobutamine	β_1 agonist (↑ CO) β_2 stimulation (↓ SVR)	5–15 μg/kg/min (up to 40)	Tachycardia (often when hypovolemic)
Dopamine	Low dose (1–2 μg/kg/min) → renal vasodilatation → small decrease in BP High dose (2–5 μg/kg/min) (↑ β_1 receptors) → increase in CO → increase in BP	1–5 μg/kg/min (up to 15)	Tachyarrhythmia (common)
Phenylephrine	α_1 agonist (↑ SVR) No effect on CO	10–30 μg/min	Reflex bradycardia

BP, blood pressure; CO, cardiac output; SVR, systemic vascular resistance.
*See the Appendix for dosage schedule.

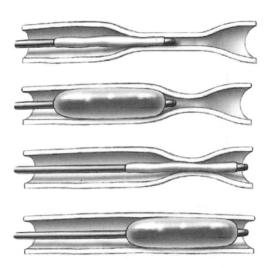

Figure 12–12. Technique of angioplasty.

cur with overdistention or distal placement in the artery.[78] Except for this caveat, most interventional neuroradiologists treat all accessible vasospastic arteries at once.[31]

Histopathologic studies showed that compression and expansion of the intima caused considerable stretching of the vessel to diameters larger than original.[59] Intimal damage appeared minimal. Angioplasty can be performed without major complications, although at least one case of vessel perforation is on record.[124] Virtually no patients have subsequent infarcts in the territory of the perforators of the middle cerebral artery, most likely because there is no intimal damage.

Angioplasty can be combined with intra-arterial papaverine (Fig. 12–13B). Papaverine administration is at a rate of 5 mg/minute for 45 minutes,[17] considerably lengthening the angiographic procedure. Failure of angioplasty or papaverine has been linked to delay in treatment. A large study suggested that angioplasty within 2 hours after failure of medical management resulted in an increase in patients with clinical improvement.[107] The effect may be short-lived. The side effects are not exactly known, but ipsilateral pupillary dilatation for 15 minutes after the infusion, which at first may suggest third nerve palsy, has been described. Progressive loss of brain stem reflexes (fixed pupils, no doll's eyes, and no corneal reflexes) has been described, with resolution 3 hours after discontinuation of the infusion.[4,52] In addition, significant progression of cerebral vasospasm immediately after infusion of papaverine, interpreted as possible paradoxical aggravation by papaverine, has been noted.[18]

During and after angioplasty or papaverine infusion, maintenance of an adequate fluid balance remains the mainstay of treatment of delayed cerebral ischemia. One should anticipate that the procedure may last hours, and fluid management should continue during cerebral

was shown to be effective in a small series,[66] but the infusion is time-consuming, and there is considerable concern that cerebral vasospasm will return after the infusion is discontinued. Intra-arterial verapamil is currently being investigated.[32]

Angioplasty of the major cerebral arteries is performed with a silicone balloon catheter.[24,71] After proper placement, the balloon is gently inflated to a 1.0 atmosphere and almost immediately deflated and advanced 1 cm to the next segment. The technique most commonly used is shown in Figure 12–12. The middle cerebral, anterior cerebral, posterior cerebral, and vertebral arteries are eligible for angioplasty (Fig. 12–13). More distal arteries are technically accessible, but the risk of rupture from overextension is real. Angioplasty of a feeding artery of a recently ruptured aneurysm is contraindicated unless the aneurysm is secured first with coils or clips. Risk of rupture of the artery itself is low, but rupture may oc-

Figure 12–13. (A) Successful angioplasty in middle cerebral artery segment vasospasm. (B) Papaverine infusion with improvement in degree of vasospasm.

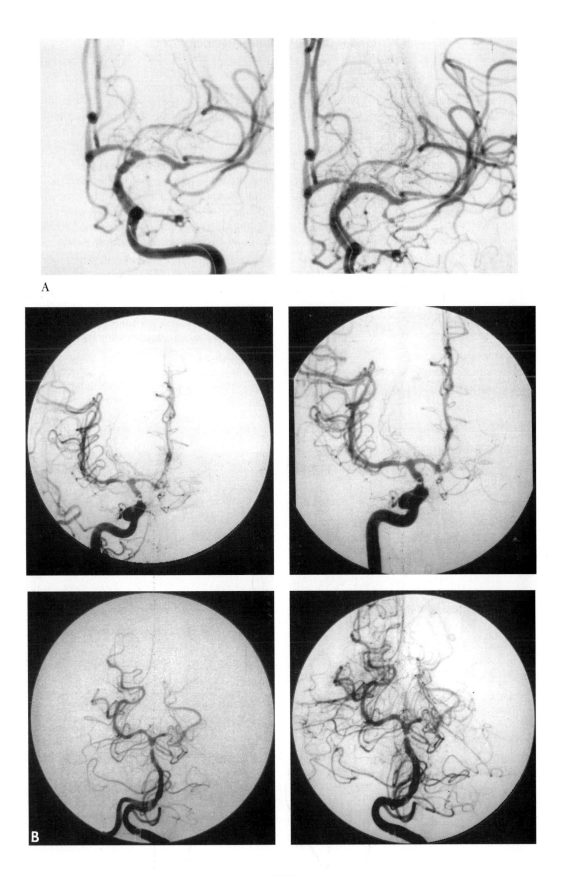

angiography. (It is not unusual for patients to have received insufficient fluids while outside the intensive care unit.) If a negative fluid balance continues to develop or hyponatremia develops, fludrocortisone acetate (Florinef), 0.2 mg twice daily, can be added. The side effects of fludrocortisone acetate (marked hypertension and pulmonary edema) rarely occur. Serum potassium concentration should be regularly checked, and hypokalemia should be corrected. (Hypokalemia together with a positive fluid balance indicates that fludrocortisone is effective.)

Failure to reverse clinical deficits most commonly indicates cerebral infarction. Computed tomography scanning may be helpful but if done early may give only a limited view of the area that is infarcted. Not infrequently, only a single arterial territory appears affected, but multifocal infarction may become apparent on subsequent CT scans or at autopsy. (One should be aware that multiple small hypodensities on CT scan, particularly in the cere-bellum, thalamus, and cortical areas, may be related to complications from cerebral angiography.) Mass effect from large hemispheric infarction may occur and often is fatal (Fig. 12–14). Temporal lobectomy may salvage the patient but at the price of severe disability. It may be an option only in young patients.

Finally, a particularly difficult problem arises when a patient's condition deteriorates in the days after clipping of the aneurysm. Drowsiness is common in patients who have had early surgery, and whether lifting and retraction causing swelling of the brain or vasospasm is the cause of neurologic deterioration is notoriously difficult to determine. Transcranial Doppler ultrasonography

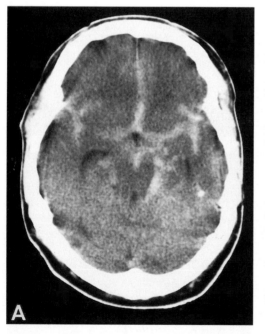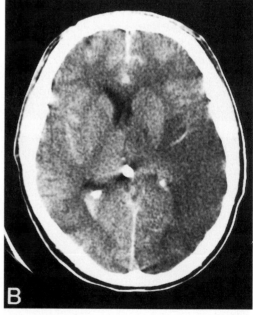

Figure 12–14. Subarachnoid hemorrhage with cerebral infarct from vasospasm. (*A*) Blood in the basal cistern with asymmetrical distribution in the suprasellar region and ambient cistern. (*B*) Five days later, progressive coma with hypodensity of a major part of the middle cerebral territory, with mass effect and brain shift.

or SPECT may distinguish between the two possibilities. In patients with postoperative swelling, transcranial Doppler ultrasonography findings are within normal limits, and most of these patients improve over days (Chapter 11).

The clinical presentation of acute hydrocephalus is characterized by progressive impairment of consciousness. In many patients, this has already occurred before admission to the NICU. Patients become much more drowsy, are tachypneic, and may not be able to protect the airway or cough up secretions. Most patients cannot follow complex commands, and only vigorous pain stimuli open the eyes and cause localization of a pain stimulus. Pinpoint pupils and downward deviation of the eyes may develop, most often in patients with dramatic enlargement of the ventricular system. The diagnosis of acute hydrocephalus becomes clear when serial CT scans show further enlargement of the ventricular system (Fig. 12–15).

Placement of a ventricular drain is indicated in patients with intraventricular blood and clinical deterioration. Earlier study has suggested that the risk of rebleeding is increased in patients with ventricular drainage, often days after ventriculostomy.[46] Our study in SAH failed to show an increased incidence of rebleeding when preoperative ventriculostomy was done within 24 hours after SAH.[82]

Ventriculostomy is often performed when enlarged hemoventricles are present in comatose patients, but we have not seen dramatic improvement in poor-grade SAH. The ventricles may become smaller after drainage, but this effect may also be seen in association with swelling from infarction (Fig. 12–16). Late hydrocephalus may be more common in patients with large hemoventricles, and 20% to 50% may need a permanent shunt.[119]

Subarachnoid hemorrhage in a patient admitted with a temporal lobe hematoma, almost invariably associated with a middle cerebral artery aneurysm, is relatively unusual but potentially life-threatening.[74] The hematoma usually is large, and virtually no blood is present in the cisterns other than the suprasellar cistern. Acute deterioration with massive enlargement of the hematoma may occur with rebleeding, most often diagnosed when additional intraventricular hemorrhage is found (Fig. 12–17). Early neurosurgical intervention is indicated and besides evacuation of the clot includes repair of the aneurysm.[51] It is difficult to decide whether patients with drowsiness alone should have emergency neurosurgical evacuation, but one may opt for emergency angiography in this situation and proceed with clipping of the aneurysm soon after presentation. A study of intracerebral hematoma in aneurysmal SAH showed that intracranial hemorrhage on CT scan alone was more often associated with a poor outcome.[49] In another study, rebleeding occurred statistically more often in patients with SAH-associated intracranial hematomas.[125] Therefore, patients with intracerebral hemorrhage should be scheduled for early angiographic study and emergency surgery, irrespective of the Glasgow coma score on admission. However, cerebral angiography should be deferred if deterioration ensues, and craniotomy should proceed immediately.

Subarachnoid hemorrhage may be the first manifestation of a ruptured giant aneurysm. Rebleeding rates are not different from those in patients with smaller sized aneurysms, and rebleeding may occur at any time from the first rupture.[68,98] Sudden deterioration in a patient with a giant aneurysm may indicate thrombus formation, and extension to the parent vessel may cause infarction.[69] Timing of surgery and planning of techniques, including hypothermic cardiopulmonary bypass, may take additional days after admission.[98] The management mortality has been estimated to be about 21%, with perioperative mortality reaching 9%. Temporary occlusion of a patent vessel is needed in two-thirds of the cases.

Of all possible systemic complications, hyponatremia is the most common but is seldom a cause of deterioration. It is more common in patients with hydrocephalus, par-

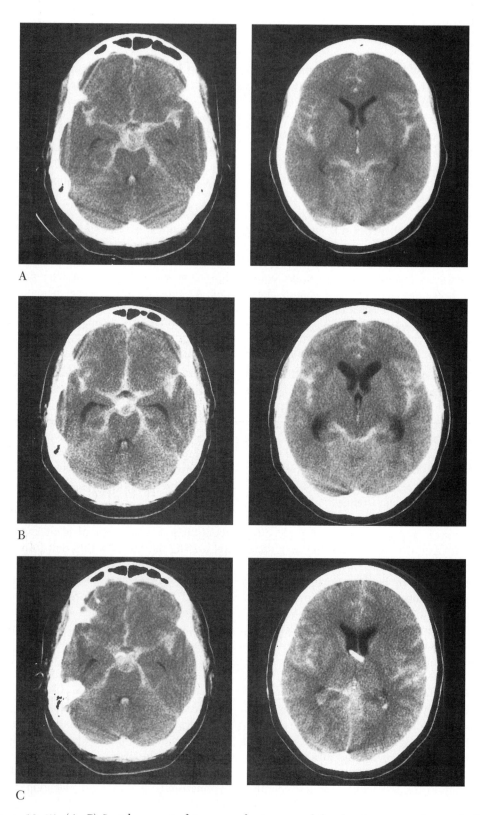

Figure 12–15. (*A–C*) Serial computed tomography images of the development of acute hydrocephalus and resolution with ventricular drainage.

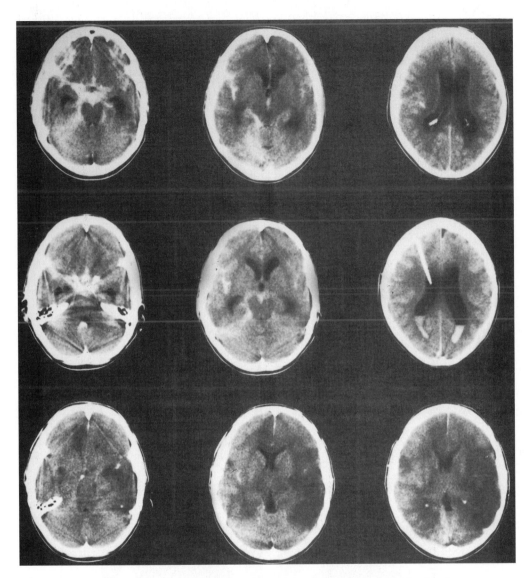

Figure 12–16. Acute hydrocephalus with developing massive cerebral infarction.

ticularly enlargement of the third ventricle.[147] A mild degree of hyponatremia (125 to 134 mmol/L) is usually well tolerated and self-limiting. Acute symptomatic hyponatremia requires urgent treatment with 3% saline but is very rare after SAH. If hyponatremia is persistent, fludro-cortisone can be added (400 μg/day in two doses)[44,150] (see Chapter 31).

An unusual but well-documented cause of sudden deterioration is acute cardiac arrhythmia with a significant decrease in blood pressure. Well-known life-threatening cardiac arrhythmias are brief ventricular tachycardia, asystole, and torsades de pointes (see Chapter 30).

Seizures may cause sudden deterioration, but most are observed at the initial rupture or

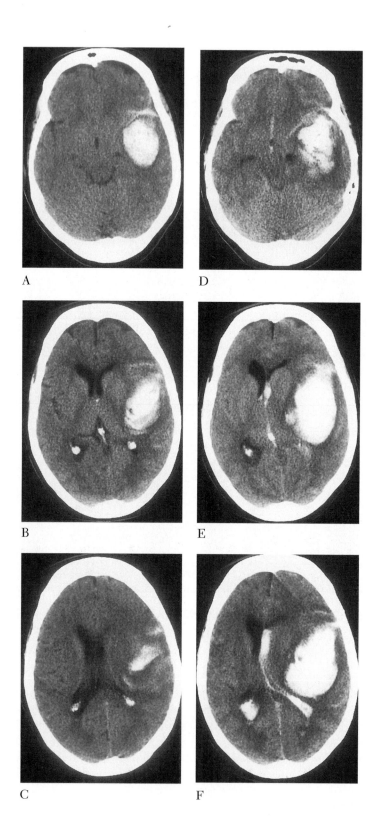

A

D

B

E

C

F

Figure 12–17. (*A–F*) Temporal lobe hematoma due to a middle cerebral artery aneurysm and early rebleeding.

during rebleeding. Failure to fully awaken after a generalized tonic-clonic seizure may point to nonconvulsive status epilepticus, but this cause of deterioration is very unusual.

An uncommon cause of sudden deterioration is fatal pulmonary embolism. The risk is increased after craniotomy and in patients who have leg paralysis predisposing to deep venous thrombosis (often after clipping of the anterior cerebral artery). Sudden death from pulmonary embolism may occur in the first 2 weeks after successful clipping of the aneurysm.

In summary, acute, often transient, deterioration in SAH remains unexplained in 20% to 30% of patients.[139] It is certainly possible that unwitnessed seizures, drug effects (e.g., from large doses of opioids for pain management), or swelling surrounding a parenchymal hema-

toma can be implicated in some instances, but the cause often remains elusive.

OUTCOME

Several outcome studies have shown that in patients with SAH who reach the hospital, the initial grade and presentation and the Glasgow coma score determine outcome (Fig. 12–18). Failure to improve in neurologic grade within 24 to 48 hours in poor-grade SAH (IV or V) despite mannitol and ventriculostomy is associated with a very high likelihood of poor outcome, particularly in patients with intraventricular hemorrhage and ventriculomegaly.[120,122] Many of these patients die from systemic complications if they do not awaken

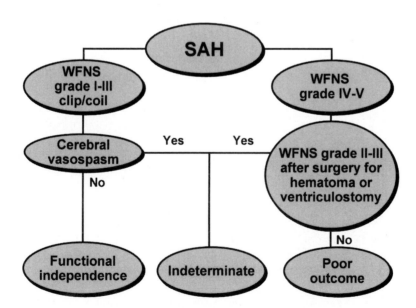

Figure 12–18. Outcome algorithm. SAH, subarachnoid hemorrhage; WFNS, World Federation of Neurological Surgeons. Functional independence: no assistance needed, minor handicap may remain. Indeterminate: any statement would be a premature conclusion. Poor outcome: severe disability or death, vegetative state.

from coma 2 weeks after admission. Some studies suggest that changes in management and timing of surgery lead to improved outcome, but only in patients with a good grade.[14] Many other factors also contribute, such as amount of blood on CT scan, aneurysm site (particularly the posterior circulation[117]), and size, age, and further neurologic deterioration, all of which determine a less satisfactory outcome. In a study from Australia, seizures at onset emerged as an independent risk factor for late seizures and poor outcome.[11]

Patients who have a supposedly good outcome after SAH could have neuropsychologic deficits characterized by disturbed concentration, disturbed mood, short-term memory lapses, and difficulty with information processing.[89,100,109] This condition may be more prevalent in patients with surgery for anterior circulation aneurysms.[79] In many of these patients, extensive neuropsychologic battery tests are needed to demonstrate these findings. Mood changes may remain at 1 year after SAH.[42]

A recently published randomized study from Finland of 109 patients found comparable clinical and cognitive outcome when surgical clipping within 3 days was compared with endovascular occlusion.[70]

Patients with normal angiograms have a much better outcome, but only if they have a pretruncal pattern on CT scan.[103] One study found that patients with normal angiograms and so-called aneurysmal patterns on CT scan (diffuse localized blood in all cisterns rather than more focal perimesencephalic hemorrhage) did as poorly as patients with aneurysmal hemorrhage, whereas patients with pretruncal nonaneurysmal hemorrhage did not have any major cognitive deficits, rebleeding, or delayed cerebral ischemia.[103]

Recurrence of SAH after satisfactory obliteration of the aneurysm by surgical clipping is low. In a large study from Japan with a median follow-up of 11 years (range, 3 to 21 years), recurrence approximated 3%.[129] The risk of regrowth of a previously clipped aneurysm was 0.26% annually. De novo formation of aneurysms after clipping of an aneurysm was 0.89% annually and, as expected, more common in patients with prior multiple aneurysms.[128]

CONCLUSIONS

- Preferably, SAH is graded by the WFNS classification: I, Glasgow coma scale 15; II, 14-13; III, 14-13 with motor deficit; IV, 12-7 with or without motor deficit; V, 6-3 with or without motor deficit.
- CT scans are normal in 2% to 5% of patients when imaging is done on the first day of acute headache. The probability of a nondiagnostic CT scan due to washout of cisternal blood is 10% after day 3, 50% after day 7, and almost 100% on day 10.
- Basic management in SAH consists of (1) endotracheal intubation if patients cannot protect their airway, have aspirated, or have acquired neurogenic pulmonary edema; (2) adequate fluid management with 2 or 3 L of 0.9% sodium chloride; (3) no antihypertensive agents unless mean arterial pressure is more than 130 mm Hg or 160 mm Hg systolic; (4) nimodipine, 60 mg six times a day; and (5) pneumatic compression devices and pain management with codeine.
- The management of rebleeding consists of mechanical ventilation, antiepileptic agents if seizures occurred and emergency angiography on recovery, and early clipping.
- Delayed cerebral ischemia is managed by hemodynamic augmentation and, if this is unsuccessful, angioplasty or intra-arterial administration of papaverine.
- Ventriculostomy is indicated in acute hydrocephalus and hemoventricles.

REFERENCES

1. Allen GS, Ahn HS, Preziosi TJ, et al: Cerebral arterial spasm—a controlled trial of nimodipine in patients with subarachnoid hemorrhage. *N Engl J Med* 308:619–624, 1983.

2. Atlas SW: MR imaging is highly sensitive for acute subarachnoid hemorrhage . . . not! *Radiology* 186:319–322, 1993.

3. Barker FG II, Ogilvy CS: Efficacy of prophylactic nimodipine for delayed ischemic deficit after subarachnoid hemorrhage: a metaanalysis. *J Neurosurg* 84:405–414, 1996.

4. Barr JD, Mathis JM, Horton JA: Transient severe brain stem depression during intraarterial papaverine infusion for cerebral vasospasm. *AJNR Am J Neuroradiol* 15:719–723, 1994.

5. Bavinzski G, Killer M, Gruber A, et al: Treatment of basilar artery bifurcation aneurysms by using Guglielmi detachable coils: a 6-year experience. *J Neurosurg* 90:843–852, 1999.

6. Bracard S, Lebedinsky A, Anxionnat R, et al: Endovascular treatment of Hunt and Hess grade IV and V aneurysms. *AJNR Am J Neuroradiol* 23:953–957, 2002.

7. Brandt L, Sonesson B, Ljunggren B, et al: Ruptured middle cerebral artery aneurysm with intracerebral hemorrhage in younger patients appearing moribund: Emergency operation? *Neurosurgery* 20:925–929, 1987.

8. Brilstra EH, Rinkel GJ, Algra A, et al: Rebleeding, secondary ischemia, and timing of operation in patients with subarachnoid hemorrhage. *Neurology* 55:1656–1660, 2000.

9. Brilstra EH, Rinkel GJ, van der Graaf Y, et al: Treatment of intracranial aneurysms by embolization with coils: a systematic review. *Stroke* 30:470–476, 1999.

10. Brouwers PJ, Wijdicks EFM, Van Gijn J: Infarction after aneurysm rupture does not depend on distribution or clearance rate of blood. *Stroke* 23:374–379, 1992.

11. Butzkueven H, Evans AH, Pitman A, et al: Onset seizures independently predict poor outcome after subarachnoid hemorrhage. *Neurology* 55:1315–1320, 2000.

12. Calhoun DA, Oparil S: Treatment of hypertensive crisis. *N Engl J Med* 323:1177–1183, 1990.

13. Casasco AE, Aymard A, Gobin YP, et al: Selective endovascular treatment of 71 intracranial aneurysms with platinum coils. *J Neurosurg* 79:3–10, 1993.

14. Cesarini KG, Hardemark HG, Persson L: Improved survival after aneurysmal subarachnoid hemorrhage: review of case management during a 12-year period. *J Neurosurg* 90:664–672, 1999.

15. Claassen J, Carhuapoma JR, Kreiter KT, et al: Global cerebral edema after subarachnoid hemorrhage: frequency, predictors, and impact on outcome. *Stroke* 33:1225–1232, 2002.

16. Cloft HJ, Joseph GJ, Dion JE: Risk of cerebral angiography in patients with subarachnoid hemorrhage, cerebral aneurysm, and arteriovenous malformation: a meta-analysis. *Stroke* 30:317–320, 1999.

17. Clouston JE, Numaguchi Y, Zoarski GH, et al: Intraarterial papaverine infusion for cerebral vasospasm after subarachnoid hemorrhage. *AJNR Am J Neuroradiol* 16:27–38, 1995.

18. Clyde BL, Firlik AD, Kaufmann AM, et al: Paradoxical aggravation of vasospasm with papaverine infusion following aneurysmal subarachnoid hemorrhage: case report. *J Neurosurg* 84:690–695, 1996.

19. Condette-Auliac S, Bracard S, Anxionnat R, et al: Vasospasm after subarachnoid hemorrhage: interest in diffusion-weighted MR imaging. *Stroke* 32:1818–1824, 2001.

20. Coyne TJ, Montanera WJ, Macdonald RL, et al: Percutaneous transluminal angioplasty for cerebral vasospasm after subarachnoid hemorrhage. *Can J Surg* 37:391–396, 1994.

21. de Bruijn SF, Stam J, Kappelle LJ: Thunderclap headache as first symptom of cerebral venous sinus thrombosis. CVST Study Group. *Lancet* 348:1623–1625, 1996.

22. Debrun GM, Aletich VA, Kehrli P, et al: Selection of cerebral aneurysms for treatment using Guglielmi detachable coils: the preliminary University of Illinois at Chicago experience. *Neurosurgery* 43:1281–1295, 1998.

23. Demirçivi F, Özkan N, Büyükkeçeci S, et al: Traumatic subarachnoid haemorrhage: analysis of 89 cases. *Acta Neurochir (Wien)* 122:45–48, 1993.

24. De Roux PD, Newell DW, Eskridge J, et al: Severe symptomatic vasospasm: the role of immediate postoperative angioplasty. *J Neurosurg* 80:224–229, 1994.

25. Di Lorenzo N, Guidetti G: Anterior communicating aneurysm missed at angiography: report of two cases treated surgically. *Neurosurgery* 23:494–499, 1988.

26. Dodick DW: Thunderclap headache. *J Neurol Neurosurg Psychiatry* 72:6–11, 2002.

27. Dodick DW, Wijdicks EFM: Pituitary apoplexy presenting as a thunderclap headache. *Neurology* 50:1510–1511, 1998.

28. Dovey Z, Misra M, Thornton J, et al: Guglielmi detachable coiling for intracranial aneurysms: the story so far. *Arch Neurol* 58:559–564, 2001.

29. Drake CG: Report of World Federation of Neurological Surgeons Committee on a Universal Subarachnoid Hemorrhage Grading Scale (letter to the editor). *J Neurosurg* 68:985–986, 1988.

30. Duffy GP: Lumbar puncture in spontaneous subarachnoid haemorrhage. *Br Med J [Clin Res]* 285:1163–1164, 1982.

31. Elliott JP, Newell DW, Lam DJ, et al: Comparison of balloon angioplasty and papaverine infusion for the treatment of vasospasm following aneurysmal subarachnoid hemorrhage. *J Neurosurg* 88:277–284, 1998.

32. Feng L, Fitzsimmons B-F, Young WL, et al: Intraarterially administered verapamil as adjunct therapy for cerebral vasospasm: safety and 2-year experience. *AJNR Am J Neuroradiol* 23:1284–1290, 2002.

33. Findlay JM, Kassell NF, Weir BKA, et al: A randomized trial of intraoperative, intracisternal tissue plasminogen activator for the prevention of vasospasm. *Neurosurgery* 37:168–176, 1995.

34. Fisher CM, Roberson GH, Ojemann RG: Cerebral vasospasm with ruptured saccular aneurysm—the clinical manifestations. *Neurosurgery* 1:245–248, 1977.

35. Foot C, Staib A: How valuable is a lumbar puncture in the management of patients with suspected subarachnoid haemorrhage? *Emerg Med* 13:326–332, 2001.

36. Frizzell RT, Kuhn F, Morris R, et al: Screening for ocular hemorrhages in patients with ruptured cerebral aneurysms: a prospective study of 99 patients. *Neurosurgery* 41:529–533, 1997.

37. Fujii Y, Takeuchi S, Sasaki O, et al: Ultra-early rebleeding in spontaneous subarachnoid hemorrhage. *J Neurosurg* 84:35–42, 1996.

38. Goodman BP, Wijdicks EFM, Schievink WI: Systemic lupus erythematosus and intracranial aneurysms (abstract). *Ann Neurol* 50 Suppl:S15, 2001.

39. Graf S, Schischma A, Eberhardt KE, et al: Intracranial aneurysms and dolichoectasia in autosomal dominant polycystic kidney disease. *Nephrol Dial Transplant* 17(5):819–823, 2002.

40. Greene KA, Marciano FF, Dickman CA, et al: Anterior communicating artery aneurysm paraparesis syndrome: clinical manifestations and pathologic correlates. *Neurology* 45:45–50, 1995.

41. Gruber DP, Zimmerman GA, Tomsick TA, et al: A comparison between endovascular and surgical management of basilar artery apex aneurysms. *J Neurosurg* 90:868–874, 1999.

42. Hackett ML, Anderson CS: Health outcomes 1 year after subarachnoid hemorrhage: an international population-based study. The Australian Cooperative Research on Subarachnoid Hemorrhage Study Group. *Neurology* 55:658–662, 2000.

43. Haley EC Jr, Kassell NF, Apperson-Hansen C, et al: A randomized, double-blind, vehicle-controlled trial of tirilazad mesylate in patients with aneurysmal subarachnoid hemorrhage: a cooperative study in North America. *J Neurosurg* 86:467–474, 1997.

44. Hasan D, Lindsay KW, Wijdicks EFM, et al: Effect of fludrocortisone acetate in patients with subarachnoid hemorrhage. *Stroke* 20:1156–1161, 1989.

45. Hasan D, Schonck RS, Avezaat CJ, et al: Epileptic seizures after subarachnoid hemorrhage. *Ann Neurol* 33:286–291, 1993.

46. Hasan D, Vermeulen M, Wijdicks EFM, et al: Management problems in acute hydrocephalus after subarachnoid hemorrhage. *Stroke* 20:747–753, 1989.

47. Hashimoto H, Iida J, Hironaka Y, et al: Use of spiral computerized tomography angiography in patients with subarachnoid hemorrhage in whom subtraction angiography did not reveal cerebral aneurysms. *J Neurosurg* 92:278–283, 2000.

48. Hashimoto H, Iida J, Shin Y, et al: Spinal dural arteriovenous fistula with perimesencephalic subarachnoid haemorrhage. *J Clin Neurosci* 7:64–66, 2000.

49. Hauerberg J, Eskesen V, Rosenørn J: The prognostic significance of intracerebral haematoma as shown on CT scanning after aneurysmal subarachnoid haemorrhage. *Br J Neurosurg* 8:333–339, 1994.

50. Heiserman JE, Dean BL, Hodak JA, et al: Neurologic complications of cerebral angiography. *AJNR Am J Neuroradiol* 15:1401–1407, 1994.

51. Heiskanen O, Poranen A, Kuurne T, et al: Acute surgery for intracerebral haematomas caused by rupture of an intracranial arterial aneurysm. A prospective randomized study. *Acta Neurochir (Wien)* 90:81–83, 1988.

52. Hendrix LE, Dion JE, Jensen ME, et al: Papaverine-induced mydriasis. *AJNR Am J Neuroradiol* 15:716–718, 1994.

53. Heros RC, Zervas NT, Varsos V: Cerebral vasospasm after subarachnoid hemorrhage: an update. *Ann Neurol* 14:599–608, 1983.

54. Hijdra A, van Gijn J: Early death from rupture of an intracranial aneurysm. *J Neurosurg* 57:765–768, 1982.

55. Hijdra A, Van Gijn J, Stefanko S, et al: Delayed cerebral ischemia after aneurysmal subarachnoid hemorrhage: clinicoanatomic correlations. *Neurology* 36:329–333, 1986.

56. Hijdra A, Vermeulen M, van Gijn J, et al: Respiratory arrest in subarachnoid hemorrhage. *Neurology* 34:1501–1503, 1984.

57. Hijdra A, Vermeulen M, van Gijn J, et al: Rerupture of intracranial aneurysms: a clinicoanatomic study. *J Neurosurg* 67:29–33, 1987.

58. Hillman J: Should computed tomography scanning replace lumbar puncture in the diagnostic process in suspected subarachnoid hemorrhage? *Surg Neurol* 26:547–550, 1986.

59. Honma Y, Fujiwara T, Irie K, et al: Morphological changes in human cerebral arteries after percutaneous transluminal angioplasty for vasospasm caused by subarachnoid hemorrhage. *Neurosurgery* 36:1073–1081, 1995.

60. Horikoshi T, Nukui H, Yagishita T, et al: Oculomotor nerve palsy after surgery for upper basilar artery aneurysms. *Neurosurgery* 44:705–710, 1999.

61. International Subarachnoid Aneurysm Trial (ISAT) of neurosurgical clipping versus endovascular coiling in 2143 patients with ruptured intracranial aneurysms: a randomised trial. *Lancet* 360:1267–1274, 2002.

62. Iwanaga H, Wakai S, Ochiai C, et al: Ruptured cerebral aneurysms missed by initial angiographic study. *Neurosurgery* 27:45–51, 1990.

63. Jackson A, Stewart G, Wood A, et al: Transient global amnesia and cortical blindness after vertebral angiography: further evidence for the role of arterial spasm. AJNR Am J Neuroradiol 16 Suppl 4:955–959, 1995.

64. Kaku Y, Yonekawa Y, Tsukahara T, et al: Superselective intra-arterial infusion of papaverine for the treatment of cerebral vasospasm after subarachnoid hemorrhage. J Neurosurg 77:842–847, 1992.

65. Kallmes DF, Clark HP, Dix JE, et al: Ruptured vertebrobasilar aneurysms: frequency of the nonaneurysmal perimesencephalic pattern of hemorrhage on CT scans. Radiology 201:657–660, 1996.

66. Kassell NF, Helm G, Simmons N, et al: Treatment of cerebral vasospasm with intra-arterial papaverine. J Neurosurg 77:848–852, 1992.

67. Kassell NF, Torner JC, Jane JA, et al: The International Cooperative Study on the Timing of Aneurysm Surgery. Part 2: Surgical results. J Neurosurg 73:37–47, 1990.

68. Khurana VG, Piepgras DG, Whisnant JP: Ruptured giant intracranial aneurysms. Part I. A study of rebleeding. J Neurosurg 88:425–429, 1998.

69. Khurana VG, Wijdicks EFM, Parisi JE, et al: Acute deterioration from thrombosis and rerupture of a giant intracranial aneurysm. Neurology 52:1697, 1999.

70. Koivisto T, Vanninen R, Hurskainen H, et al: Outcomes of early endovascular versus surgical treatment of ruptured cerebral aneurysms. A prospective randomized study. Stroke 31:2369–2377, 2000.

71. Konishi Y, Maemura E, Shiota M, et al: Treatment of vasospasm by balloon angioplasty: experimental studies and clinical experiences. J Neurol Res 14:273–281, 1992.

72. Kumar R, Wijdicks EFM, Brown RD Jr, et al: Isolated angiitis of the CNS presenting as subarachnoid haemorrhage. J Neurol Neurosurg Psychiatry 62:649–651, 1997.

73. Lennihan L, Mayer SA, Fink ME, et al: Effect of hypervolemic therapy on cerebral blood flow after subarachnoid hemorrhage: a randomized controlled trial. Stroke 31:383–391, 2000.

74. Le Roux PD, Dailey AT, Newell DW, et al: Emergent aneurysm clipping without angiography in the moribund patient with intracerebral hemorrhage: the use of infusion computed tomography scans. Neurosurgery 33:189–197, 1993.

75. Levy ML, Rabb CH, Zelman V, et al: Cardiac performance enhancement from dobutamine in patients refractory to hypovolumic therapy for cerebral vasospasm. J Neurosurg 79:494–499, 1993.

76. Linn FH, Rinkel GJ, Algra A, et al: Incidence of subarachnoid hemorrhage: role of region, year, and rate of computed tomography: a meta-analysis. Stroke 27:625–629, 1996.

77. Linn FH, Wijdicks EFM, van der Graaf Y, et al: Prospective study of sentinel headache in aneurysmal subarachnoid haemorrhage. Lancet 344:590–593, 1994.

78. Linskey ME, Horton JA, Rao GR, et al: Fatal rupture of the intracranial carotid artery during transluminal angioplasty for vasospasm induced by subarachnoid hemorrhage. Case report. J Neurosurg 74:985–990, 1991.

79. Mavaddat N, Sahakian BJ, Hutchinson PJ, et al: Cognition following subarachnoid hemorrhage from anterior communicating artery aneurysm: relation to timing of surgery. J Neurosurg 91:402–407, 1999.

80. Mayer SA, Fink ME, Homma S, et al: Cardiac injury associated with neurogenic pulmonary edema following subarachnoid hemorrhage. Neurology 44:815–820, 1994.

81. Mayer SA, Solomon RA, Fink ME, et al: Effect of 5% albumin solution on sodium balance and blood volume after subarachnoid hemorrhage. Neurosurgery 42:759–767, 1998.

82. McIver JI, Friedman JA, Wijdicks EFM, et al: Preoperative ventriculostomy is not associated with increased risk of rebleeding following aneurysmal subarachnoid hemorrhage. J Neurosurg 97:1042–1044, 2002.

83. Miller JA, Dacey RG Jr, Diringer MN: Safety of hypertensive hypervolemic therapy with phenylephrine in the treatment of delayed ischemic deficits after subarachnoid hemorrhage. Stroke 26:2260–2266, 1995.

84. Millikan CH: Cerebral vasospasm and ruptured intracranial aneurysm. Arch Neurol 32:433–449, 1975.

85. Mori T, Katayama Y, Kawamata T, et al: Improved efficiency of hypervolemic therapy with inhibition of natriuresis by fludrocortisone in patients with aneurysmal subarachnoid hemorrhage. J Neurosurg 91:947–952, 1999.

86. Nichols DA: Endovascular treatment of the acutely ruptured intracranial aneurysm (editorial). J Neurosurg 79:1–2, 1993.

87. Nichols DA, Meyer FB, Piepgras DG, et al: Endovascular treatment of intracranial aneurysms. Mayo Clin Proc 69:272–285, 1994.

88. Nonaka Y, Kusumoto M, Mori K, et al: Pure acute subdural haematoma without subarachnoid haemorrhage caused by rupture of internal carotid artery aneurysm. Acta Neurochir 142:941–944, 2000.

89. Oder W, Dal Bianco P, Kollegger H, et al: Spontaneous subarachnoid hemorrhage. Prognostic factors for social readjustment. Scand J Rehabil Med 22:85–91, 1990.

90. Öhman J: Hypertension as a risk factor for epilepsy after aneurysmal subarachnoid hemorrhage and surgery. Neurosurgery 27:578–581, 1990.

91. Öhman J, Heiskanen O: Effect of nimodipine on the outcome of patients after aneurysmal subarachnoid hemorrhage and surgery. J Neurosurg 69:683–686, 1988.

92. Oliveira-Filho J, Ezzeddine MA, Segal AZ, et al: Fever in subarachnoid hemorrhage: relationship to vasospasm and outcome. *Neurology* 56:1299–1304, 2001.

93. Oropello JM, Weiner L, Benjamin E: Hypertensive, hypervolemic, hemodilutional therapy for aneurysmal subarachnoid hemorrhage. Is it efficacious? No. *Crit Care Clin* 12:709–730, 1996.

94. Petruk KC, West M, Mohr G, et al: Nimodipine treatment in poor-grade aneurysm patients. Results of a multicenter double-blind placebo-controlled trial. *J Neurosurg* 68:505–517, 1988.

95. Pfausler B, Belcl R, Metzler R, et al: Terson's syndrome in spontaneous subarachnoid hemorrhage: a prospective study in 60 consecutive patients. *J Neurosurg* 85:392–394, 1996.

96. Philippon J, Grob R, Dagreou F, et al: Prevention of vasospasm in subarachnoid haemorrhage. A controlled study with nimodipine. *Acta Neurochir (Wien)* 82:110–114, 1986.

97. Pickard JD, Murray GD, Illingworth R, et al: Effect of oral nimodipine on cerebral infarction and outcome after subarachnoid haemorrhage: British Aneurysm Nimodipine Trial. *BMJ* 298:636–642, 1989.

98. Piepgras DG, Khurana VG, Whisnant JP: Ruptured giant intracranial aneurysms. Part II. A retrospective analysis of timing and outcome of surgical treatment. *J Neurosurg* 88:430–435, 1998.

99. Polin RS, Coenen VA, Hansen CA, et al: Efficacy of transluminal angioplasty for the management of symptomatic cerebral vasospasm following aneurysmal subarachnoid hemorrhage. *J Neurosurg* 92:284–290, 2000.

100. Powell J, Kitchen N, Heslin J, et al: Psychosocial outcomes at three and nine months after good neurological recovery from aneurysmal subarachnoid haemorrhage: predictors and prognosis. *J Neurol Neurosurg Psychiatry* 72:772–781, 2002.

101. Rabinstein AA, Pichelmann MA, Friedman JA, et al. Symptomatic vasospasm and outcome following aneurysmal subarachnoid hemorrhage: surgical repair versus endovascular coil occlusion (submitted).

102. Rinkel GJ, van Gijn J, Wijdicks EFM: Subarachnoid hemorrhage without detectable aneurysm. A review of the causes. *Stroke* 24:1403–1409, 1993.

103. Rinkel GJ, Wijdicks EFM, Hasan D, et al: Outcome in patients with subarachnoid haemorrhage and negative angiography according to pattern of haemorrhage on computed tomography. *Lancet* 338:964–968, 1991.

104. Rinkel GJ, Wijdicks EFM, Vermeulen M, et al: The clinical course of perimesencephalic nonaneurysmal subarachnoid hemorrhage. *Ann Neurol* 29:463–468, 1991.

105. Roos Y: Antifibrinolytic treatment in subarachnoid hemorrhage: a randomized placebo-controlled trial. STAR Study Group. *Neurology* 54:77–82, 2000.

106. Rordorf G, Koroshetz WJ, Copen WA, et al: Diffusion- and perfusion-weighted imaging in vasospasm after subarachnoid hemorrhage. *Stroke* 30:599–605, 1999.

107. Rosenwasser RH, Armonda RA, Thomas JE, et al: Therapeutic modalities for the management of cerebral vasospasm: timing of endovascular options. *Neurosurgery* 44:975–979, 1999.

108. Saito I, Asano T, Sano K, et al: Neuroprotective effect of an antioxidant, ebselen, in patients with delayed neurological deficits after aneurysmal subarachnoid hemorrhage. *Neurosurgery* 42:269–277, 1998.

109. Säveland H, Brandt L: Which are the major determinants for outcome in aneurysmal subarachnoid hemorrhage? A prospective total management study from a strictly unselected series. *Acta Neurol Scand* 90:245–250, 1994.

110. Schievink WI: Genetics of intracranial aneurysms. *Neurosurgery* 40:651–662, 1997.

111. Schievink WI: Spontaneous dissection of the carotid and vertebral arteries. *N Engl J Med* 344:898–906, 2001.

112. Schievink WI, Wijdicks EFM: Pretruncal subarachnoid hemorrhage: an anatomically correct description of the perimesencephalic subarachnoid hemorrhage. *Stroke* 28:2572, 1997.

113. Schievink WI, Wijdicks EFM: Origin of pretruncal nonaneurysmal subarachnoid hemorrhage: Ruptured vein, perforating artery, or intramural hematoma? *Mayo Clin Proc* 75:1169–1173, 2000.

114. Schievink WI, Wijdicks EFM, Meyer FB, et al: Spontaneous intracranial hypotension mimicking aneurysmal subarachnoid hemorrhage. *Neurosurgery* 48:513–516, 2001.

115. Schievink WI, Wijdicks EFM, Parisi JE, et al: Sudden death from aneurysmal subarachnoid hemorrhage. *Neurology* 45:871–874, 1995.

116. Schievink WI, Wijdicks EFM, Piepgras DG, et al: Perimesencephalic subarachnoid hemorrhage. Additional perspectives from four cases. *Stroke* 25:1507–1511, 1994.

117. Schievink WI, Wijdicks EFM, Piepgras DG, et al: The poor prognosis of ruptured intracranial aneurysms of the posterior circulation. *J Neurosurg* 82:791–795, 1995.

118. Schievink WI, Wijdicks EFM, Spetzler RF: Diffuse vasospasm after pretruncal nonaneurysmal subarachnoid hemorrhage. *AJNR Am J Neuroradiol* 21:521–523, 2000.

119. Sheehan JP, Polin RS, Sheehan JM, et al: Factors associated with hydrocephalus after aneurysmal subarachnoid hemorrhage. *Neurosurgery* 45:1120–1127, 1999.

120. Shimoda M, Oda S, Shibata M, et al: Results of early surgical evacuation of packed intraventricular hemorrhage from aneurysm rupture in patients with poor-grade subarachnoid hemorrhage. *J Neurosurg* 91:408–414, 1999.

121. Smoker WRK: The neuroradiology of aneurysmal subarachnoid hemorrhage. *Semin Neurol* 4:315–342, 1984.

122. Suzuki M, Otawara Y, Doi M, et al: Neurological grades of patients with poor-grade subarachnoid hemorrhage improve after short-term pretreatment. *Neurosurgery* 47:1098–1104, 2000.

123. Tang-Wai DF, Phan TG, Wijdicks EFM: Hypertensive encephalopathy presenting with thunderclap headache. *Headache* 41:198–200, 2001.

124. Terada T, Okuno T, Hayashi S, et al: A case of vessel perforation during interventional neuroradiological procedure. Operative findings of the perforated vessel. *Surg Neurol* 40:241–244, 1993.

125. Tokuda Y, Inagawa T, Katoh Y, et al: Intracerebral hematoma in patients with ruptured cerebral aneurysms. *Surg Neurol* 43:272–277, 1995.

126. Toyota BD: The efficacy of an abbreviated course of nimodipine in patients with good-grade aneurysmal subarachnoid hemorrhage. *J Neurosurg* 90:203–206, 1999.

127. Treggiari-Venzi MM, Suter PM, Romand JA: Review of medical prevention of vasospasm after aneurysmal subarachnoid hemorrhage: a problem of neurointensive care. *Neurosurgery* 48:249–261, 2001.

128. Tsutsumi K, Ueki K, Morita A, et al: Risk of aneurysm recurrence in patients with clipped cerebral aneurysms: results of long-term follow-up angiography. *Stroke* 32:1191–1194, 2001.

129. Tsutsumi K, Ueki K, Usui M, et al: Risk of recurrent subarachnoid hemorrhage after complete obliteration of cerebral aneurysms. *Stroke* 29:2511–2513, 1998.

130. van der Jagt M, Hasan D, Bijvoet HW, et al: Validity of prediction of the site of ruptured intracranial aneurysms with CT. *Neurology* 52:34–39, 1999.

131. van der Wee N, Rinkel GJ, Hasan D, et al: Detection of subarachnoid haemorrhage on early CT: Is lumbar puncture still needed after a negative scan? *J Neurol Neurosurg Psychiatry* 58:357–359, 1995.

132. van Gijn J, Hijdra A, Wijdicks EFM, et al: Acute hydrocephalus after aneurysmal subarachnoid hemorrhage. *J Neurosurg* 63:355–362, 1985.

133. van Gijn J, Rinkel GJ: Subarachnoid haemorrhage: diagnosis, causes and management. *Brain* 124:249–278, 2001.

134. van Gijn J, van Dongen KJ, Vermeulen M, et al: Peri-mesencephalic hemorrhage: a nonaneurysmal and benign form of subarachnoid hemorrhage. *Neurology* 35:493–497, 1985.

135. Vanninen R, Koivisto T, Saari T, et al: Ruptured intracranial aneurysms: acute endovascular treatment with electrolytically detachable coils—a prospective randomized study. *Radiology* 211:325–336, 1999.

136. Velthuis BK, Rinkel GJ, Ramos LM, et al: Perimesencephalic hemorrhage. Exclusion of vertebrobasilar aneurysms with CT angiography. *Stroke* 30:1103–1109, 1999.

137. Velthuis BK, van Leeuwen MS, Witkamp TD, et al: Surgical anatomy of the cerebral arteries in patients with subarachnoid hemorrhage: comparison of computerized tomography angiography and digital subtraction angiography. *J Neurosurg* 95:206–212, 2001.

138. Vermeulen M, Lindsay KW, Murray GD, et al: Antifibrinolytic treatment in subarachnoid hemorrhage. *N Engl J Med* 311:432–437, 1984.

139. Vermeulen M, van Gijn J, Hijdra A, et al: Causes of acute deterioration in patients with a ruptured intracranial aneurysm. A prospective study with serial CT scanning. *J Neurosurg* 60:935–939, 1984.

140. Viñuela F, Duckwiler G, Mawad M: Guglielmi detachable coil embolization of acute intracranial aneurysm: perioperative anatomical and clinical outcome in 403 patients. *J Neurosurg* 86:475–482, 1997.

141. Wijdicks EFM: Worst-case scenario: management in poor-grade aneurysmal subarachnoid hemorrhage. *Cerebrovasc Dis* 5:163–169, 1995.

142. Wijdicks EFM, Hasan D, Lindsay KW, et al: Short-term tranexamic acid treatment in aneurysmal subarachnoid hemorrhage. *Stroke* 20:1674–1679, 1989.

143. Wijdicks EFM, Kerkhoff H, van Gijn J: Long-term follow-up of 71 patients with thunderclap headache mimicking subarachnoid haemorrhage. *Lancet* 2:68–70, 1988.

144. Wijdicks EFM, Schievink WI: Perimesencephalic nonaneurysmal subarachnoid hemorrhage: first hint of a cause? *Neurology* 49:634–636, 1997.

145. Wijdicks EFM, Schievink WI, Miller GM: MR imaging in pretruncal nonaneurysmal subarachnoid hemorrhage: Is it worthwhile? *Stroke* 29:2514–2516, 1998.

146. Wijdicks EFM, Schievink WI, Miller GM: Pretruncal nonaneurysmal subarachnoid hemorrhage. *Mayo Clin Proc* 73:745–752, 1998.

147. Wijdicks EFM, VanDongen KJ, Van Gijn J, et al: Enlargement of the third ventricle and hyponatraemia in aneurysmal subarachnoid haemorrhage. *J Neurol Neurosurg Psychiatry* 51:516–520, 1988.

148. Wijdicks EFM, Vermeulen M, Murray GD, et al: The effects of treating hypertension following aneurysmal subarachnoid hemorrhage. *Clin Neurol Neurosurg* 92:111–117, 1990.

149. Wijdicks EFM, Vermeulen M, ten Haaf JA, et al: Volume depletion and natriuresis in patients with a ruptured intracranial aneurysm. *Ann Neurol* 18:211–216, 1985.

150. Wijdicks EFM, Vermeulen M, van Brummelen P, et al: The effect of fludrocortisone acetate on plasma volume and natriuresis in patients with aneurysmal subarachnoid hemorrhage. *Clin Neurol Neurosurg* 90:209–214, 1988.

151. Winn HR, Almaani WS, Berga SL, et al: The long-term outcome in patients with multiple aneurysms. Incidence of late hemorrhage and implications for treatment of incidental aneurysms. *J Neurosurg* 59:642–651, 1983.

152. Young N, Dorsch NW, Kingston RJ: Pitfalls in the use of spiral CT for identification of intracranial aneurysms. *Neuroradiology* 41:93–99, 1999.

153. Young N, Dorsch NW, Kingston RJ, et al: Intracranial aneurysms: evaluation in 200 patients with spiral CT angiography. *Eur Radiol* 11:123–130, 2001.

154. Zouaoui A, Sahel M, Marro B, et al: Three-dimensional computed tomographic angiography in detection of cerebral aneurysms in acute subarachnoid hemorrhage. *Neurosurgery* 41:125–130, 1997.

13

Ganglionic and Lobar Hemorrhages

Ganglionic and lobar hemorrhages account for a considerable proportion of admissions to the neurologic intensive care unit. Each type of cerebral hematoma has different characteristics, and they may be related to the risk of deterioration. Patients with expanding lobar hemorrhages with shift may be sent directly to the operating room. In most other patients, medical management is preferred and touches on nearly all aspects of critical care neurology.[19,20,42,46,61] Treatment decisions that are apposite include management of herniation and increased intracranial pressure, management of uncontrolled hypertension and coagulopathy, and, in certain cases, repair of arteriovenous malformations. These hemorrhages have the potential to enlarge in at least one-third of patients; therefore, virtually every patient with a putaminal or lobar hemorrhage needs close monitoring in the neurologic intensive care unit, at least in the first 24 hours.

CLINICAL RECOGNITION

The clinical hallmark of a spontaneous cerebral hemorrhage is rapid unfolding of a focal neurologic deficit, vomiting, and then fluctuating alertness.[25]

The neurologic manifestations of intracranial hematoma depend on the localization of the hematoma. Patients with frontal lobe hematoma are markedly disoriented in time and space, and many are abulic (from the Greek *abulia*, indecision). Patients with abulia be-

come diverted when asked to perform a simple task or to recall a recent major event in the world. They lack any initiative and truncate their conversation with a simple "yes," "no," or "I don't know," and these answers require a disproportionately long time.

Patients with hematomas in the dominant parietal lobe display abnormalities in naming, reading, writing, calculations, finger identification, and left–right distinction. In contrast, patients with hematomas in the nondominant parietal lobe largely experience neglect of the opposite body half and constructional difficulties. Neglect of a hemiparesis may be associated with visually based naming errors and difficulty with writing, particularly omission of letters. Occipital hematomas may be manifested by visual hallucinations and bright colors, but homonymous hemianopia often remains the sole clinical finding on examination.

Ganglionic hemorrhages involve the striatum or thalamus. The striatum is divided into the putamen and the caudate nucleus. Putaminal hemorrhages in the dominant hemisphere appear with aphasia and marked hemiparesis of arm and leg and in the nondominant hemisphere, as expected, with additional neglect. Language disorders in putaminal hemorrhage could be a nonfluent motor-type aphasia. However, fluent Wernicke-type aphasia with literal and verbal paraphasic errors and neologisms may occur if it extends to the posterior temporal region.[54]

Hemorrhage into the caudate nucleus is uncommon, as is its clinical presentation.[83,88]

Many patients are confused, often after acute headache and vomiting. Other patients may manifest amnesia (with thalamic extension) and abulia. It is less frequently associated with hemiparesis and is expected only when the hemorrhage extends to the internal capsule. Other unusual findings have included Horner's syndrome and vertical gaze palsy,[83] and all these confound its clinical recognition. Findings on CT scan often seem a chance discovery.

Hemorrhages in the thalamus produce eye movement abnormalities, such as downward gaze, skew deviation, and limited abduction of both eyes, simulating a sixth nerve palsy, and prominent loss of pinprick sensation. Hemiparesis occurs with paramedian extension. The pattern of anosognosia and visual spatial neglect in the nondominant thalamus and aphasia in the dominant thalamus holds.[55] This type of aphasia is notable for mutism evolving into verbose jargon speech with relatively retained perception, understanding, and repetition. In patients who have extension of the thalamic hemorrhage into the striatum, verbal output may be less impressive, and hypophonia and dysarthria may predominate. Sentences offered for repetition are at times restated in a different manner.

As a rule, consciousness is impaired in lobar and putaminal hemorrhages when mass effect occurs. However, putaminal hemorrhages (more than 60 cm^3 on CT scan) may also disconnect the diencephalon from the ascending reticular activating system[77] by direct destruction (Chapter 9). Obstructive hydrocephalus from ventricular extension of a deep-seated hematoma or compression of the foramen of Monro is often difficult to implicate as a potential mechanism for stupor. Enlargement of the hematoma must be suspected in patients who lapse into deeper stages of coma and certainly in patients with an underlying coagulopathy or recent use of anticoagulants or thrombolytic agents.[94] It is not uncommon to find a major discrepancy between clinical examination and initial CT scan. Repeat CT scan often uncovers massive enlargement.

Seizures have been reported, with an incidence of approximately 30% in lobar hemorrhages but a much lower incidence (5%) in ganglionic hemorrhages that spare the cortex. Seizures occur close to the presentation of hemorrhage or in the next 3 days, and late-onset seizures are rare.[21,90]

NEUROIMAGING AND LABORATORY TESTS

Computed tomography scan in putaminal hemorrhage usually demonstrates a very localized hemorrhage into the putamen (Fig. 13–1A), but the hemorrhage may dissect into the anterior or posterior limb of the internal capsule.[91] When the hematoma further enlarges, putaminal hemorrhage may enter the ventricular system or extend into the thalamus.

Caudate hemorrhage (Fig. 13–1B) may be difficult to detect because the intraventricular extension may be most visible, often with some ventricular enlargement, disguising the true source of the hematoma. Hemorrhages originating in the thalamus (Fig. 13–1C) are often small but may expand into the adjacent internal capsule or corona radiata or further extend vertically, destroying the hypothalamus and midbrain (Fig. 13–1D).

Both putaminal and thalamic hemorrhages may expand in the first 12 hours after the ictus. The volume may enlarge 20% to 100% from baseline.[7,11,15,33,52]

Computed tomography scans should be read carefully, with attention directed to estimation of the volume of the clot, possible hydrocephalus, septum pellucidum and pineal shift, and intraventricular extension.

The volume of the hematoma can be measured[10] (for details, see Chapter 12). A total volume of 60 cm^3 together with a Glasgow coma scale score of less than 8 seems to define a cutoff point that indicates a poor prognosis.

The assessment of horizontal displacement of the septum pellucidum or pineal gland is relevant because the degree of various stages of drowsiness is correlated with the degree of horizontal displacement of the pineal gland.[76] Shift of these CT landmarks can be used to monitor progression of mass effect.

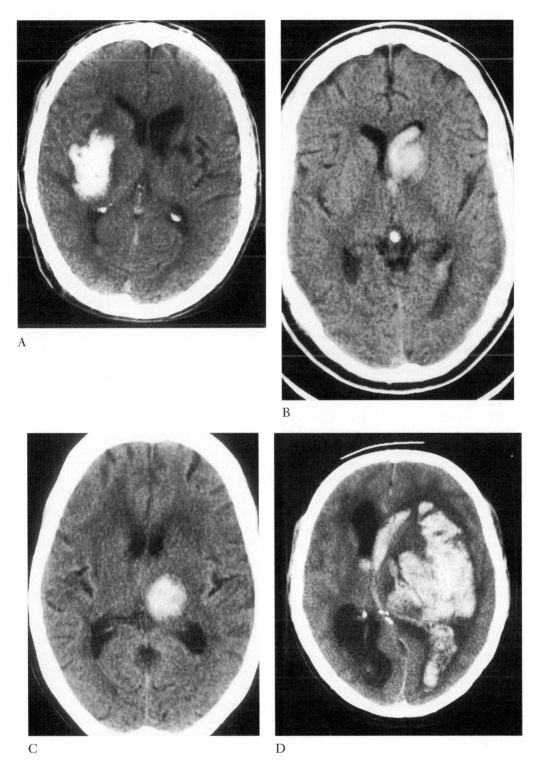

Figure 13–1. (*A*) Typical intracerebral hematoma localized in the putamen. (*B*) Typical caudate hemorrhage on computed tomography scan. (*C*) Typical thalamic hemorrhage on computed tomography scan. (*D*) Destructive ganglionic hemorrhage with rupture into the ventricular system, enlarging it dramatically, and extension into the diencephalon.

Hydrocephalus due to acute hemoventricle may occur in 40% of patients (for grading, see Chapter 12), or unilateral enlargement may occur from obstruction at the foramen of Monro. Although hemorrhagic dilatation of the fourth ventricle is a predictor of poor outcome,[81] this finding is often associated with a large intracranial hemorrhage that in itself predicts poor outcome.

Lobar hematomas are more common in younger patients, and underlying structural causes are more probable. Long-standing hypertension should therefore not be easily accepted as the cause.[12] In sylvian fissure and anterior interhemispheric hematomas, an anterior cerebral or middle cerebral artery aneurysm should be excluded by cerebral angiography. A thalamic hematoma, usually accompanied by some evidence of blood in the basal cistern, may be due to a posterior cerebral artery aneurysm.[16] Peripheral dense hematomas with irregular borders are highly suggestive of amyloid angiopathy in elderly patients.[45] Patients with lobar hematomas may have an underlying arteriovenous malformation or cavernous angioma. Simultaneous multiple hemorrhages should point to previous use of anticoagulants[50] or thrombolytic agents,[94] toxoplasma infestation,[92] disseminated intravascular coagulation,[96] or metastatic disease[69] (Fig. 13–2), but they may occur in uncontrolled hypertension.[59] A blood-fluid interface into the hematoma predicts an acquired (e.g., leukemia, idiopathic thrombocytopenic purpura, hemophilia) or drug-related (e.g., warfarin, heparin, thrombolytic agents) bleeding disorder (Fig. 13–3).

Magnetic resonance imaging with magnetic resonance angiography is a useful additional test that may demonstrate metastasis, occult vascular malformations, occasional previous hemorrhages associated with amyloid angiopathy, or cerebral venous thrombosis, all conditions beyond the detection of CT. The changes with use of different sequences are summarized in Table 13–1.[57] The earliest sign, that of peripheral deoxygenation, is a rim of hypointensity on T2-weighted spin-echo images surrounding the hematoma.[4,57] Gradient-echo MRI may demonstrate additional asympto-

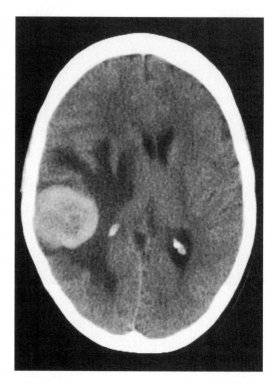

Figure 13–2. Finger-like edema and lobar hematoma in metastatic breast carcinoma.

matic petechial or small-volume hemorrhages of different ages, suggesting cerebral amyloid angiopathy[37] or leukoencephalopathy.[36] Although uncommon, lobar hematomas may in fact be hemorrhagic cerebral infarcts associated with cerebral venous thrombosis (see Chapter 15). Patients with a lobar hematoma into a primary tumor or metastasis may have an additional surrounding mass or edema (Fig. 13–2), but MRI is much more sensitive in separating tumor density from clot. Magnetic resonance imaging may document a meningioma which can easily be disguised as a lobar hematoma on CT scan.[75]

The diagnostic value of cerebral angiography for underlying vascular abnormalities has been reviewed.[101] Many of the studies are limited because selection criteria are unclear. The yield of arteriovenous malformations or aneurysms depends on the site of hemorrhage, a history of hypertension (or persistent hypertension 2 weeks after admission), and age.

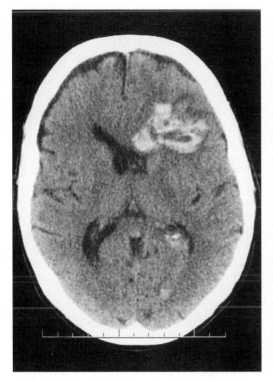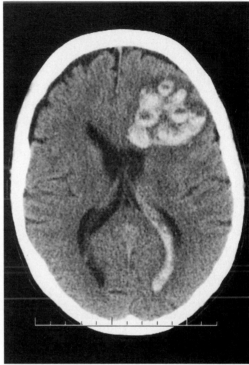

Figure 13–3. (*Left* and *right*) Anticoagulation-associated lobar hematoma. Note multiple fluid levels. *Source:* Ecker RD, Wijdicks EFM: Footprints of coagulopathy. *J Neurol Neurosurg Psychiatry* 73:534, 2002. By permission.

Normotensive patients with a hemorrhage in the putamen or thalamus who are younger than 45 years may have an underlying vascular lesion (50% occurrence). The detection rate drops to 7% in similar patients older than 45 years. However, yield from cerebral angiography in chronically hypertensive patients with ganglionic hemorrhages is very low.[101] The yield in patients with primary intraventricular hemorrhage varies from 30% to 75%.

Table 13–1. Magnetic Resonance Imaging Signal Features of Hyperacute Hemorrhage*

	Center	Periphery	Surrounding Rim	Acute Evolution
T2WI	Isointense to hyperintense, heterogeneous, larger than SWI	Hypointense, smaller than SWI	Hyperintense	Slower progressive enlargement of hypointense periphery toward center
T1WI	Isointense to hypointense, heterogeneous	Isointense	Hypointense	Hypointense rim enlargement
Interpretation	Oxyhemoglobin dominant	Deoxyhemoglobin dominant	Vasogenic edema	Progressive increase in concentration of deoxyhemoglobin from periphery toward center

SWI, susceptibility-weighted imaging; T1WI, T1-weighted imaging; T2WI, T2-weighted imaging.
*Less than 5 hours old.
Source: Linfante I, Llinas RH, Caplan LR, et al: MRI features of intracerebral hemorrhage within 2 hours from symptom onset. *Stroke* 30:2263–2267, 1999. By permission of the American Heart Association.

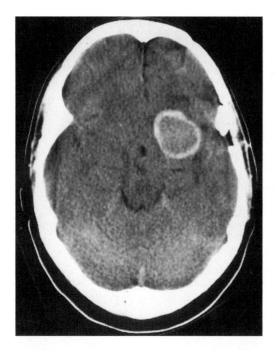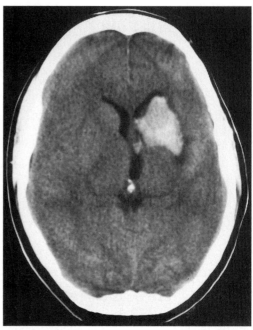

Figure 13–4. (*Left* and *right*) Computed tomography scans demonstrating putaminal caudate hemorrhage associated with giant middle cerebral artery aneurysm.

Cerebral angiography is probably not warranted in patients with a typical putaminal or thalamic hemorrhage and long-standing hypertension. Putaminal hemorrhages are seldom associated with cerebral aneurysms but when present are virtually always visible on CT scans (Fig. 13–4). Cerebral angiography is warranted in patients with a lobar hematoma, but the cause may remain unknown in 40% of patients.[44] Repeat angiography may be needed as a follow-up study when cerebral angiography yields negative results in a patient with a lobar hematoma. It is possible that the mass effect of a hematoma obscures a small arteriovenous malformation. Repeat angiography detected four arteriovenous malformations in 22 patients with initially negative cerebral angiograms (Fig. 13–5).[44]

Laboratory evaluation should include, in addition to routine hematologic survey and smear and chemistry group, other specific tests pertaining to possible causes (Table 13–2).

In patients with prior hypertension, chest radiography with measurement of cardiac ratio, electrocardiography, and urinalysis with quantification of proteinuria are required. They can be supplemented in younger patients by abdominal CT and vanillylmandelic acid analysis to screen for pheochromocytoma. Toxicologic screening for cocaine use should be considered in appropriate circumstances.

FIRST STEPS IN MANAGEMENT

Initial management in ganglionic and lobar cerebral hemorrhages is summarized in Table 13–3. If consciousness has decreased to a level at which protective laryngeal reflexes are lost, endotracheal intubation should follow. Mechanical ventilation with a combination of intermittent mandatory ventilation mode and pressure support is usually sufficient, because most patients retain the ability to trigger the ventilator.

Anticoagulation-related lobar or putaminal hematoma should be immediately reversed with two units of fresh frozen plasma and vit-

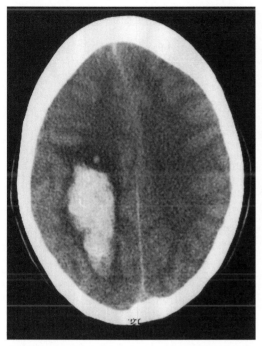

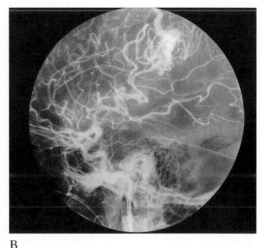

B

A

Figure 13–5. (*A*) Computed tomography image and (*B*) cerebral angiogram showing arteriovenous malformation in recent lobar hematoma.

amin K. The prolonged effect of oral anticoagulation often requires frequent repeated doses. A difficult situation arises if an intracerebral hematoma appears in a patient anticoagulated for a prosthetic valve or a patient who has atrial fibrillation with prior systemic embolization. However, in these clinical dilem-

Table 13–2. Laboratory Tests in Spontaneous Intracerebral Hematoma

---

Complete white cell count, platelet count, blood smear, sedimentation rate
Activated partial thromboplastin time, international normalized ratio
Aspartate transaminase, alkaline phosphatase
VDRL test
Fibrinogen and fibrinogen split products
Transthoracic echocardiography and serial blood cultures (optional)
Human immunodeficiency virus serology (optional)
Drug screen (optional)
Hemoglobin electrophoresis (optional)

VDRL, Venereal Disease Research Laboratories.

mas, it appears that discontinuation of warfarin for a week in a patient with an intracranial hematoma very rarely leads to valve failure or immediate systemic embolization. In a study of 26 patients with intracerebral hematomas or anticoagulation for metallic valves, discontinuation of 2 days to 3 months (median, 8 days) was safe.[95] Brief interruption of anticoagulation was also without complications in 9 high-risk patients (defined as having the following criteria: cage-ball valve, atrial fibrillation, mitral valve position, and enlarged chambers on echocardiogram). Resumption of anticoagulation using orally administered warfarin only was equally safe, without rebleeding. A recent extension of this study in 141 patients showed that the risk of recurrent transient ischemic attack or stroke was 2.9% (95% confidence limit of 0% to 8%) in patients with prosthetic valves, 2.6% (0% to 7.6%) in patients with atrial fibrillation and stroke, and 4.8% (0% to 13.6%) in patients with prior recurrent transient ischemic

Table 13–3. Initial Management in Ganglionic and Lobar Hemorrhages

Airway management	Correct hypoxemia with nasal O_2 catheter, 3 L/minute
	Intubate and add pressure support or initiate in combination with IMV of 8/minute
	Increase IMV to 15 when hyperventilation is indicated
Fluid management	2 L of 0.9% NaCl
	Add 3% NaCl or mannitol, 1 g/kg, when shift appears on CT scan and patient deteriorates rapidly
Blood pressure management	Avoid antihypertensive medication
	Consider enalapril, 1.25–5 mg IV q6h; labetalol, 20–40 mg IV; or esmolol, 500 μg/kg IV if MAP is persistently > 130 mm Hg
Nutrition	Enteral feeding after day 2
ICP management	Place ICP monitor when patient is comatose (aim at CPP of > 60 mm Hg)
	Evacuate hematoma if patient is stuporous and has lobar hematoma with shift
Specific measures	DVT prophylaxis with pneumatic devices
	Fresh frozen plasma (2 packets), vitamin K, 1–2 mg IV, or protamine sulfate, 1 mg/100 U of heparin, to reverse anticoagulation. Autoplex 25–100 U/kg rate 2–10 mL/min and 10 mg of vitamin K if rapidly deteriorating
	Fosphenytoin loading 20 mg/kg in lobar hematomas and in patients with documented increased ICP
	No corticosteroids

CPP, cerebral perfusion pressure; CT, computed tomography; DVT, deep venous thrombosis; ICP, intracranial pressure; IMV, intermittent mandatory ventilation; IV, intravenously; MAP, mean arterial pressure.

attacks.[68] Anticoagulation was discontinued in this series of patients with cerebral hemorrhage and withheld for a median of 10 days, and the patients received fresh frozen plasma and vitamin K.

Reversal of anticoagulation with fresh frozen plasma has some disadvantages. Although fresh frozen plasma is readily available, there is serious concern about the length of time to complete reversal, which is delayed by the limited infusion rate of large volumes of plasma and the time required for thawing. Alternatively, an activated prothrombin complex concentrate (Autoplex, Feiba) can be used if available. This concentrate carries the risk of thromboembolization. It should be considered in a patient with CT-documented enlargement and clinical deterioration (Autoplex: 25 to 100 U/kg; rate, 2 to 10 mL/minute). It must be followed by intravenous administration of 10 mg of vitamin K and careful attention to the decrease in the international normalized ratio.[9,13,14,32] Whether rapid reversal halts continued deterioration from enlargement is not known. A blood clot may grow despite normalization of the international normalized ratio (Fig. 13–6).

Intracranial hematomas in patients with myocardial infarction associated with recent use of thrombolytic agents require reversal of heparin (often similarly given to reduce the risk of reocclusion of coronary or pulmonary arteries) with protamine sulfate (1 mg/100 U of heparin), 10 units of cryoprecipitate, and approximately 2 units of fresh frozen plasma.

Fluid management should focus on reduction of free water intake, and most patients are best managed with 2 L of isotonic saline. Patients with hematomas of large volume and evidence of rapid clinical deterioration can be additionally treated with 50 mL of hypertonic saline 3% (infused in 10 minutes) or mannitol, 1 g/kg in a bolus, to reduce intracranial pressure.

Many patients have greatly increased mean arterial blood pressure, and treatment may cause marked reduction of cerebral perfusion pressure. (One should be reminded here that chronic hypertension leads to a change in the autoregulation curve, with a shift to the right; Chapter 9.) Patients with significant and persistent increases in blood pressure may be treated cautiously. Patients with intracerebral hematoma from long-standing hypertension are best managed with a bolus of esmolol or, preferably, angiotensin-converting enzyme inhibitors, which have the added advantage of dilating cerebral blood vessels in chronically hypertensive patients (Chapter 8).

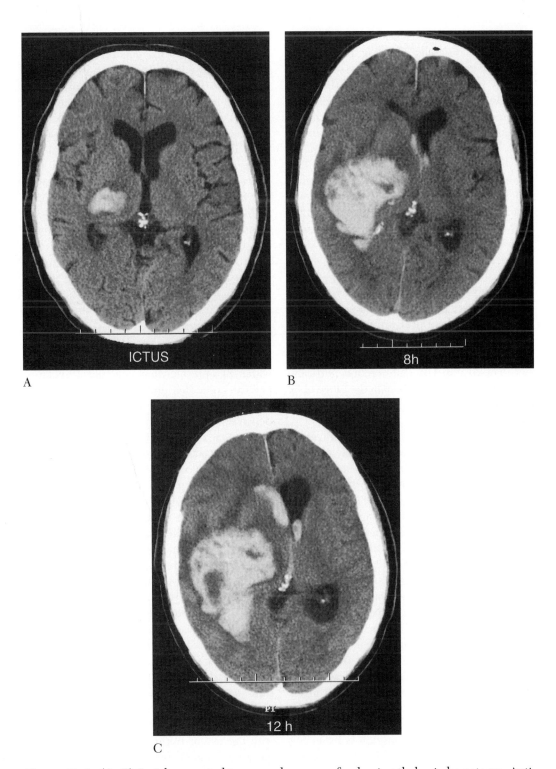

Figure 13–6. (*A–C*) Serial computed tomography scans of enlarging thalamic hematoma. Anticoagulation was rapidly corrected, and the international normalized ratio was 1.4. Note enlargement between time periods.

The control of hypertension may reduce re-bleeding or continuing bleeding, but very few data are known. Conversely, aggressive lowering may change the cerebral blood flow, particularly in the tissue surrounding the clot. An important study using single-photon emission computed tomography documentation in patients an average of 12 hours after onset did not show any reduction in cerebral blood flow, but because the data were obtained in a small series of patients with small hematomas hours after onset, the findings were inconclusive.[71]

The management of comatose patients with deep-seated hematomas not eligible for evacuation could benefit from monitoring of intracranial pressure with fiber-optic devices.[78] It could substantially facilitate management of blood pressure. With intracranial pressure and mean arterial blood pressure values, cerebral perfusion pressure can be calculated and titrated. Intracranial pressure should remain less than 20 mm Hg, and cerebral perfusion pressure ideally must remain in the range of 60 to 80 mm Hg to provide adequate cerebral blood flow.

The use of corticosteroids is discouraged. A randomized study of dexamethasone administered for 2 weeks in intracranial hemorrhage found no reduction in mortality.[70] In this study, many patients died from systemic complications tentatively linked to unnecessarily prolonged (up to 3 weeks) treatment with corticosteroids. In an elderly population, corticosteroids may also rapidly induce nonketotic hyperglycemia, certainly when osmotic agents, which may contribute to dehydration, are used. It is possible that high doses of corticosteroids (e.g., methylprednisolone) for only a brief period can be effective in these patients, but current data are not available. A small pilot study that used high-dose methylprednisolone within 12 hours was without demonstrable effect but also without major complications (Wijdicks EFM, unpublished observations).

Using antiepileptic medication is balancing risks. A generalized tonic-clonic seizure can result in marked hypoxemia from a direct effect on respiratory drive and from aspiration and in a risk of cardiac arrhythmias. On the other hand, the adverse effects are uncommon. A hypersensitivity syndrome occurs in 1 of 5000 patients, usually 2 to 4 weeks after administration begins. Fever, rash, and a morbilliform (measles-like) eruption, often with hepatitis, may occur that occasionally is fatal. Other side effects of phenytoin within weeks of use are agranulocytosis, severe thrombocytopenia, and interstitial nephritis. The *purple glove syndrome* with intravenous use (most often with infusion in small hand veins) is the most dramatic and may lead to amputation. This syndrome is characterized by a swollen, purple, and extremely painful hand caused by vasoconstriction and the beginning of a compartment syndrome. Elderly patients with underlying vascular disease and patients who cannot communicate early signs of pain during infusion may be at risk.

Thus, antiepileptic medication probably can be used more selectively. In lobar hematomas, with a 30% prevalence of generalized seizures, one can argue that prophylaxis with phenytoin (e.g., 3 weeks) is justified.[8,21,53,90] The incidence of seizures in putaminal hemorrhage is so low that exposure to antiepileptic drugs is probably an added risk and expense. In patients with clearly documented generalized tonic-clonic seizures, phenytoin is indicated for an arbitrary period of 1 month. In patients with poorly compliant brain tissue and frequent increases in intracranial pressure with any type of stimulation, intravenous loading with (fos)phenytoin is probably justified, but antiepileptic administration should be discontinued if intracranial pressure has returned to normal or more stable levels.

Primary surgical intervention in lobar or ganglionic hemorrhages[5,41] is practiced in only a few institutions in the United States[51] but is widely used in Japan.[34,48] In two randomized trials, no significant differences in outcome between surgical and medical management were found.[46,61] Stereotactic aspiration of the clot with the use of fibrinolytic drugs (urokinase) has been proposed, but comparative studies are not available.[43,47,49] Patients with a large intracranial hematoma (e.g., volume of 30 to 60 cm³) or temporal lobe hematoma may particularly benefit from early surgery, possibly because of the increased risk of secondary deterioration from enlargement, but this treatment should ideally be compared with the best medical management, including monitoring and control of intracranial pressure.

Lobar hematomas associated with arteriovenous malformations require neurosurgical evaluation. The risk of fatal recurrent hemorrhage during the same admission is very low (< 1%), and surgical repair or other interventions (intravascular occlusion, stereotactic radiosurgery) can be carefully planned. The annual rebleeding risk is 15% to 20% in some studies. Deep venous drainage emerged as a strong risk factor for recurrent hemorrhage.[58] Arteriovenous malformations are usually graded (I to V) (Table 13–4), and the grade predicts postoperative morbidity and mortality. In the Barrow Neurological Institute experience, permanent major neurologic deficit was absent in grades I to III but 22% in grade IV and 17% in grade V arteriovenous malformation.[39] Surgical excision is preferred in grade I arteriovenous malformation; perioperative mortality is low. Radiosurgery or combined therapies are reserved for other grades. Which

Table 13–4. Spetzler-Martin Grading System for Arteriovenous Malformations

Variable	Score*
Size of arteriovenous malformation†	
Small (< 3 cm)	1
Medium (3–6 cm)	2
Large (> 6 cm)	3
Eloquence of adjacent brain‡	
No	0
Yes	1
Patterns of venous drainage§	
Superficial only	0
Deep	1

*Score of 1 equals grade I, score of 2 equals grade II, etc.
†Greatest diameter on magnetic resonance imaging, cerebral angiography, or computed tomography scan.
‡Eloquent or functionally important areas are sensory-motor, language, visual cortex, diencephalon, internal capsule, brain stem, and peduncles or deep nuclei of the cerebellum.
§Deep venous drainage and deep perforating arterial feeders.
Source: From Martin NA, Vinters HV: Arteriovenous malformations. In Carter LP, Spetzler RF (eds): *Neurovascular Surgery.* New York, McGraw-Hill, 1995, pp 875–903. By permission of the publisher.

approach is most satisfactory is decided by the neurosurgeon and is not further discussed here. Superb reviews of the subject have recently been published.[2,26,65]

DETERIORATION: CAUSES AND MANAGEMENT

The condition of approximately 30% of patients with lobar and ganglionic hemorrhages deteriorates to a more significant neurologic deficit.[60] In our series, one of four patients with a lobar hemorrhage had deterioration, which was more common in those with certain CT characteristics such as a hematoma larger than 60 cm^3, any shift of the septum pellucidum, effacement of the contralateral ambient cistern, and widening of the temporal horn.[28] Worsening in the degree of hemiparesis and decrease in the level of alertness are most common, and in others, a new neurologic deficit, such as speech and language difficulties, may become apparent. Pupil dilatation on the side of the hematoma indicates uncal herniation in a temporal lobe hematoma or extension of the thalamic hemorrhage to the midbrain.

In the first 12 to 24 hours, enlargement of the hematoma is the cause of deterioration. Patients with superficially located lobar hematomas from amyloid angiopathy are at comparatively low risk of deterioration, as are patients with a hematoma of small CT volume (≤ 30 cm^3). Further growth of the hematoma is typically associated with a 50% to 75% risk of mortality within 1 month (Fig. 13–7). Mortality in patients whose condition is deteriorating is the sum of systemic complications, progression to brain death, and, increasingly, withdrawal of support instigated by advance directives or family requests in elderly patients with catastrophic hypertensive hemorrhage.

The most comprehensive study on enlargement of intracerebral hematoma (from Niigata University in Japan) included 627 patients with serial CT scans (30 minutes after arrival and follow-up within 24 hours). Major risk factors for enlargement of hematoma (more than 50% or an increase of 20 cm^3) included daily heavy

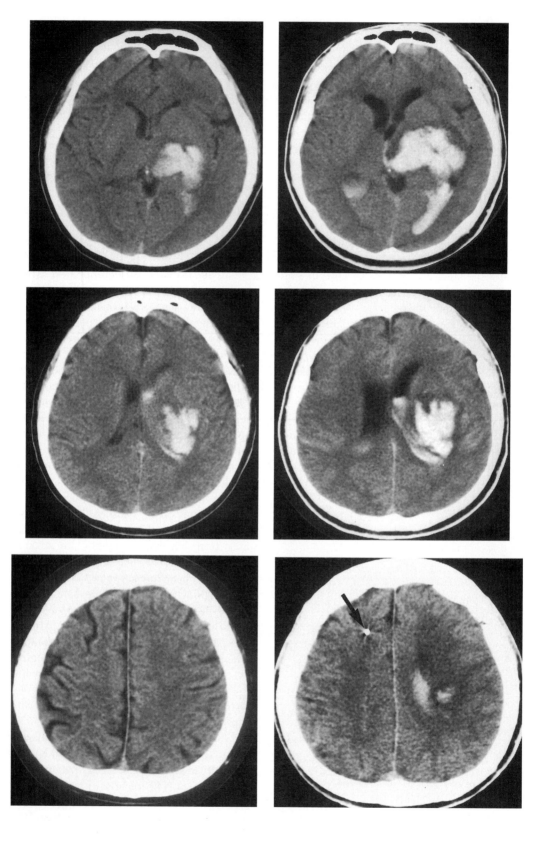

Figure 13–7. Enlargement of thalamic hemorrhage with dissection of intraparenchymal hemorrhage into the ventricular system. Note intracranial pressure monitor (*arrow*).

◄ _____

alcohol consumption, large hematoma, impaired consciousness on admission, low level of fibrinogen, and a short time between onset and admission.[33]

Considerable CT volume of the clot (> 60 cm³) is one of the most important predictors of clinical neurologic deterioration, and the risk of further deterioration from enlargement of the hematoma is increased.[33] Patients with an irregularly shaped hematoma (possibly from active bleeding at multiple sites within the parenchyma), are also at risk. In our study, deterioration in lobar hematoma also increases in patients who have a reduced Glasgow coma scale score at presentation and in patients with early CT evidence of mass effect and shift.[27] A massive increase suggestive of rebleeding may occur and is associated with sudden deterioration, rapidly resulting in brain death or persistent coma.[93]

Anticoagulation-related hemorrhages are significantly larger, often progress in size, and have a worse outcome.[82] Outcome in thrombolysis-associated hemorrhages is particularly poor. Expansion of the hematoma associated with thrombolysis may be dramatic, with virtually no time to successfully intervene medically or surgically.

Deterioration can be explained not only by enlargement of the hematoma but also by development of edema surrounding the hematoma (Fig. 13–8), obstructive hydrocephalus, and systemic metabolic factors.[60,100] Cerebral edema surrounding intracerebral hemorrhage is not due to cerebral damage but is a result of disruption of the blood-brain barrier from lysed red blood cells. Influx of iron or prothrombin has been implicated.[97,98] Mass effect from edema may occur up to the second or third week but remains an uncommon course.[100]

Acute hydrocephalus is a possible cause for deterioration, and when it is documented by serial CT scan, ventriculostomy can be considered as a diagnostic procedure. Patients who

present in coma from intracranial hemorrhage with ventricular hemorrhage and dilatation seldom benefit from ventriculostomy, although it often seems the only rational option.[1] Ventriculostomy may be beneficial in patients with documented deterioration and enlarging hydrocephalus who have a comparatively small obstructing thalamic or caudate hemorrhage, but published experience is limited to only a few well-documented cases.

Treatment of patients with massive intraventricular hemorrhage and cast formation, particularly in caudate or thalamic hemorrhages, is difficult. Results of a preliminary study using intraventricular urokinase were promising because of clearing of parts of the ventricle, but a dramatic resolution of the clot was not observed.[84] This therapy is not recommended outside a well-designed study protocol.

Patients in deteriorating clinical condition need to be intubated and supported by mechanical ventilation. The fluid management protocol should not change, because these patients need adequate intravascular volume. Fluid restriction in an attempt to reduce edema formation in these patients with deterioration is potentially harmful if the use of osmotic agents is anticipated, and the combination can lead to rapid dehydration if effective at all.

Surgical evacuation is pursued after deterioration, particularly if no effect is seen after a bolus of 2 g of mannitol. All randomized trials (six completed controlled trials at the time of this writing) found no evidence of improved outcome in surgically treated patients.[22,23,40,63,72,73] The most recent trial testing the feasibility and safety of very early (within 4 hours of the ictus) surgical removal of ganglionic hemorrhages found an increased incidence of early rebleeding despite good attempts at hemostasis with bipolar coagulation and absorbable gelatin sponge (Gelfoam).[63] However, the lit-

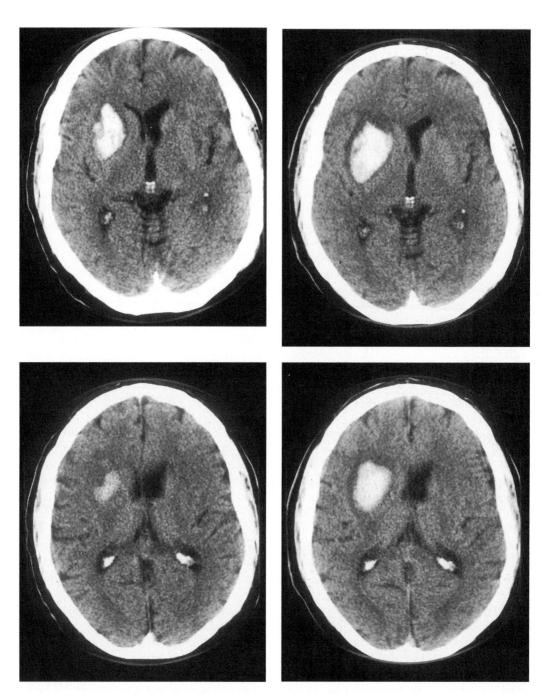

Figure 13–8. Computed tomography scans showing putaminal hemorrhage. (*Left*) Circumscribed moderate-sized putaminal hemorrhage with obliteration of the frontal horn. (*Right*) Repeat scan after worsening in level of consciousness shows enlargement of the hematoma, perihematoma edema, and complete effacement of the frontal horn.

erature consists of a heterogeneous mix of different techniques in different hemorrhages in patients with different prior states of health, and therefore comparison is quite difficult.

Alternative therapeutic options are liquefaction of the hematoma with urokinase through a catheter placed inside the clot[62,89] and endoscopic evacuation,[5] but these procedures have not been established as standard and have not consistently demonstrated major improvement over medical management in ganglionic-type hemorrhages.

Surgical evacuation in putaminal hemorrhage is often the only option to prevent further progression to brain death, but the procedure should be considered lifesaving, with often a dismal quality of life.[46]

The options in lobar hematomas are clearly different. A particularly difficult clinical situation is a fluctuating level of consciousness in a patient with a moderate-sized hematoma and some shift but superficial localization in the frontal or temporal lobe. The threshold for evacuation should probably be low. Indeed, these hematomas are comparatively easy to evacuate, and it may be too intimidating to wait for the patient's condition to deteriorate (Fig. 13–9). Nonetheless, in some instances we have been able to manage patients medically and have asked neurosurgeons to evacuate these hematomas after deterioration to localization of pain stimuli from following commands or when increasing brain shift on CT scans is present.

Emergency craniotomy in patients with hematomas was to no avail when comatose patients presented with absent pontomesencephalic reflexes (pupil, cornea, oculocephalic) and extensor posturing. In our series with pre-

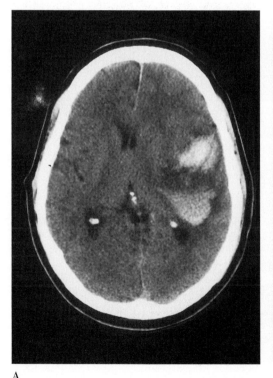 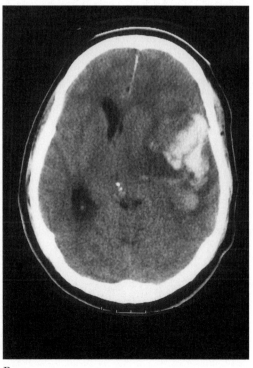

A   B

Figure 13–9. Temporal lobe hematoma. (A) Midline shift and compression of the lateral ventricle. (B) Computed tomography scan several hours later (at the time of clinical deterioration) shows a marked increase in shift with early contralateral hydrocephalus.

dominantly younger patients and hematomas in the right hemisphere, functional independence was a possible outcome in approximately 20% of patients who had these reflexes preserved before surgery. Therefore, massive hematomas producing brain tissue shift and features of herniation on CT scans were not incompatible with functional recovery.[74] Patients should improve quickly after evacuation, and some in a very dramatic fashion, with reappearance of pupil reflexes. Failure to improve could represent rebleeding in the operating bed (Fig. 13–10).

OUTCOME

Spontaneous intracerebral hematomas may constitute a diverse group in terms of prognosis. Most data originate from stroke data reg-

istries, but the findings have not been confirmed in an independent new series of patients.[19,30,42,79,85,86] Nonetheless, simple rules may apply. Mortality has been significantly increased in patients with a hematoma volume of 40 cm^3, displacement of the pineal gland,[27] stupor, and hyperglycemia.[31] Others found that patients with large intraventricular volumes, fever of any cause,[80] hydrocephalus,[18,67,87] increased systolic blood pressure, gaze palsy, neurologic deterioration after admission, and need for mechanical ventilation[38] had a poor outcome.[66,85,86,99] Acute hydrocephalus in putaminal hemorrhage predicts 30-day mortality.[67]

Early mortality from intracranial hemorrhage in hospital-based series is approximately 20%, in-hospital mortality 1 month from onset adds 10%, and mortality figures after 2 years may add an additional 20%, for a total mortality of 50%

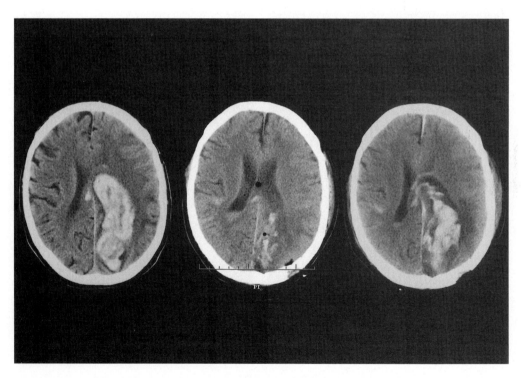

Figure 13–10. Rebleeding after evacuation of lobar hematoma. Immediate CT scan hours after return from operating room showed near-total evacuation. CT scan on second postoperative day after failure to fully awaken showed rebleeding in operative bed.

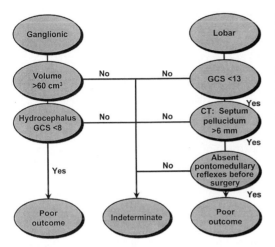

Figure 13–11. Algorithm of outcome in lobar and ganglionic intracranial hemorrhages. CT, computed tomography; GCS, Glasgow coma scale score. Poor outcome: severe disability or death, vegetative state. Indeterminate: Any statement would be a premature conclusion.

from neurologic causes and systemic complications from a persistent neurologic deficit.

Recurrence of hemorrhage in patients with ganglionic hemorrhage is clearly related to poor subsequent control of blood pressure.[3,6,29,35,56,64,79] The risk seems low with diastolic control of less than 90 mm Hg.[79]

Survivors do relatively well, and independent survival has been reported in 50% to 70% of patients after 1 year.[17,24] Early predictive factors for a significant handicap are virtually unknown. In many patients, marked improvement in motor function can be expected within 1 month. Patients who leave the neurologic intensive care unit comatose but weaned from the ventilator and who show no clinical signs of improvement probably have no chance of independent recovery, although improvement to severe disability may be observed in the following month. An algorithm of outcome is shown in Figure 13–11.

CONCLUSIONS

- Medical management includes correction of possible coagulopathy (prothrombin complex concentrate, fresh frozen plasma, vitamin K), control of increased intracranial pressure (3% hypertonic saline or mannitol, 1 g/kg), cautious use of antihypertensive agents and antiepileptic drugs for 2 to 3 weeks in lobar hematoma only.
- Surgical intervention is indicated for marked clinical deterioration refractory to treatment and persistently increased intracranial pressure. Early surgical intervention in superficial frontal lobe or temporal lobe hematoma with shift is indicated.
- Emergency surgery for lobar hematomas in patients whose condition is worsening is to no avail if the pontomesencephalic reflexes are absent before surgery. If they are present, good outcome is still possible in approximately 20% of patients despite signs of herniation.

REFERENCES

1. Adams RE, Diringer MN: Response to external ventricular drainage in spontaneous intracerebral hemorrhage with hydrocephalus. *Neurology* 50:519–523, 1998.
2. Al-Shahi R, Warlow C: A systematic review of the frequency and prognosis of arteriovenous malformations of the brain in adults. *Brain* 124:1900–1926, 2001.
3. Arakawa S, Saku Y, Ibayashi S, et al: Blood pressure control and recurrence of hypertensive brain hemorrhage. *Stroke* 29:1806–1809, 1998.

4. Atlas SW, Thulborn KR: MR detection of hyperacute parenchymal hemorrhage of the brain. *AJNR Am J Neuroradiol* 19:1471–1477, 1998.
5. Auer LM, Deinsberger W, Niederkorn K, et al: Endoscopic surgery versus medical treatment for spontaneous intracerebral hematoma: a randomized study. *J Neurosurg* 70:530–535, 1989.
6. Bae H, Jeong D, Doh J, et al: Recurrence of bleeding in patients with hypertensive intracerebral hemorrhage. *Cerebrovasc Dis* 9:102–108, 1999.
7. Bae HG, Lee KS, Yun IG, et al: Rapid expansion of

hypertensive intracerebral hemorrhage. *Neurosurgery* 31:35–41, 1992.

8. Berger AR, Lipton RB, Lesser ML, et al: Early seizures following intracerebral hemorrhage: implications for therapy. *Neurology* 38:1363–1365, 1988.

9. Boulis NM, Bobek MP, Schmaier A, et al: Use of factor IX complex in warfarin-related intracranial hemorrhage. *Neurosurgery* 45:1113–1118, 1999.

10. Broderick JP, Brott TG, Duldner JE, et al: Volume of intracerebral hemorrhage. A powerful and easy-to-use predictor of 30-day mortality. *Stroke* 24:987–993, 1993.

11. Brott T, Broderick J, Kothari R, et al: Early hemorrhage growth in patients with intracerebral hemorrhage. *Stroke* 28:1–5, 1997.

12. Brott T, Thalinger K, Hertzberg V: Hypertension as a risk factor for spontaneous intracerebral hemorrhage. *Stroke* 17:1078–1083, 1986.

13. Butler AC, Tait RC: Management of oral anticoagulant-induced intracranial haemorrhage. *Blood Rev* 12:35–44, 1998.

14. Cartmill M, Dolan G, Byrne JL, et al: Prothrombin complex concentrate for oral anticoagulant reversal in neurosurgical emergencies. *Br J Neurosurg* 14:458–461, 2000.

15. Chen ST, Chen SD, Hsu CY, et al: Progression of hypertensive intracerebral hemorrhage. *Neurology* 39:1509–1514, 1989.

16. Crum BA, Wijdicks EFM: Thalamic hematoma from a ruptured posterior cerebral artery aneurysm. *Cerebrovasc Dis* 10:475–477, 2000.

17. Daverat P, Castel JP, Dartigues JF, et al: Death and functional outcome after spontaneous intracerebral hemorrhage. A prospective study of 166 cases using multivariate analysis. *Stroke* 22:1–6, 1991.

18. Diringer MN, Edwards DF, Zazulia AR: Hydrocephalus: a previously unrecognized predictor of poor outcome from supratentorial intracerebral hemorrhage. *Stroke* 29:1352–1357, 1998.

19. Dixon AA, Holness RO, Howes WJ, et al: Spontaneous intracerebral haemorrhage: an analysis of factors affecting prognosis. *Can J Neurol Sci* 12:267–271, 1985.

20. Duff TA, Ayeni S, Levin AB, et al: Nonsurgical management of spontaneous intracerebral hematoma. *Neurosurgery* 9:387–393, 1981.

21. Faught E, Peters D, Bartolucci A, et al: Seizures after primary intracerebral hemorrhage. *Neurology* 39:1089–1093, 1989.

22. Fayad PB, Awad IA: Surgery for intracerebral hemorrhage. *Neurology* 51 Suppl 3:S69–S73, 1998.

23. Fernandes HM, Mendelow AD: Spontaneous intracerebral haemorrhage: a surgical dilemma. *Br J Neurosurg* 13:389–394, 1999.

24. Fieschi C, Carolei A, Fiorelli M, et al: Changing prognosis of primary intracerebral hemorrhage: results of a clinical and computed tomographic follow-up study of 104 patients. *Stroke* 19:192–195, 1988.

25. Fisher CM: Clinical syndromes in cerebral hemorrhage. In Fields WS (ed): *Pathogenesis and Treatment of Cerebrovascular Disease*. Springfield, Illinois: Charles C Thomas, 1961, pp 318–342.

26. Fleetwood IG, Steinberg GK: Arteriovenous malformations. *Lancet* 359:863–873, 2002.

27. Flemming KD, Wijdicks EFM, Li H: Can we predict poor outcome at presentation in patients with lobar hemorrhage? *Cerebrovasc Dis* 11:183–189, 2001.

28. Flemming KD, Wijdicks EFM, St Louis EK, et al: Predicting deterioration in patients with lobar haemorrhages. *J Neurol Neurosurg Psychiatry* 66:600–605, 1999.

29. Fogelholm R, Avikainen S, Murros K: Prognostic value and determinants of first-day mean arterial pressure in spontaneous supratentorial intracerebral hemorrhage. *Stroke* 28:1396–1400, 1997.

30. Fogelholm R, Nuutila M, Vuorela AL: Primary intracerebral haemorrhage in the Jyvaskyla region, central Finland, 1985–89: incidence, case fatality rate, and functional outcome. *J Neurol Neurosurg Psychiatry* 55:546–552, 1992.

31. Franke CL, van Swieten JC, Algra A, et al: Prognostic factors in patients with intracerebral haematoma. *J Neurol Neurosurg Psychiatry* 55:653–657, 1992.

32. Fredriksson K, Norrving B, Stromblad LG: Emergency reversal of anticoagulation after intracerebral hemorrhage. *Stroke* 23:972–977, 1992.

33. Fujii Y, Takeuchi S, Sasaki O, et al: Multivariate analysis of predictors of hematoma enlargement in spontaneous intracerebral hemorrhage. *Stroke* 29:1160–1166, 1998.

34. Fujitsu K, Muramoto M, Ikeda Y, et al: Indications for surgical treatment of putaminal hemorrhage. Comparative study based on serial CT and time-course analysis. *J Neurosurg* 73:518–525, 1990.

35. Gonzalez-Duarte A, Cantu C, Ruiz-Sandoval JL, et al: Recurrent primary cerebral hemorrhage: frequency, mechanisms, and prognosis. *Stroke* 29:1802–1805, 1998.

36. Greenberg SM: Cerebral amyloid angiopathy and vessel dysfunction. *Cerebrovasc Dis* 13 Suppl 2:42–47, 2002.

37. Greenberg SM, O'Donnell HC, Schaefer PW, et al: MRI detection of new hemorrhages: potential marker of progression in cerebral amyloid angiopathy. *Neurology* 53:1135–1138, 1999.

38. Gujjar AR, Deibert E, Manno EM, et al: Mechanical ventilation for ischemic stroke and intracerebral hemorrhage: indications, timing, and outcome. *Neurology* 51:447–451, 1998.

39. Hamilton MG, Spetzler RF: The prospective application of a grading system for arteriovenous malformations. *Neurosurgery* 34:2–6, 1994.

40. Hankey GJ, Hon C: Surgery for primary intracerebral hemorrhage: Is it safe and effective? A systematic review of case series and randomized trials. *Stroke* 28:2126–2132, 1997.

41. Heiskanen O: Treatment of spontaneous intracerebral and intracerebellar hemorrhages. *Stroke* 24 Suppl:I94–I95, 1993.

42. Helweg-Larsen S, Sommer W, Strange P, et al: Prognosis for patients treated conservatively for spontaneous intracerebral hematomas. *Stroke* 15:1045–1048, 1984.

43. Higgins AC, Nashold BS Jr: Stereotactic evacuation of large intracerebral hematoma. *Appl Neurophysiol* 43:96–103, 1980.

44. Hino A, Fujimoto M, Yamaki T, et al: Value of repeat angiography in patients with spontaneous subcortical hemorrhage. *Stroke* 29:2517–2521, 1998.

45. Ishihara T, Takahashi M, Yokota T, et al: The significance of cerebrovascular amyloid in the aetiology of superficial (lobar) cerebral haemorrhage and its incidence in the elderly population. *J Pathol* 165:229–234, 1991.

46. Juvela S, Heiskanen O, Poranen A, et al: The treatment of spontaneous intracerebral hemorrhage. A prospective randomized trial of surgical and conservative treatment. *J Neurosurg* 70:755–758, 1989.

47. Kandel EI, Peresedov VV: Stereotaxic evacuation of spontaneous intracerebral hematomas. *J Neurosurg* 62:206–213, 1985.

48. Kaneko M, Tanaka K, Shimada T, et al: Long-term evaluation of ultra-early operation for hypertensive intracerebral hemorrhage in 100 cases. *J Neurosurg* 58:838–842, 1983.

49. Kanno T, Nagata J, Nonomura K, et al: New approaches in the treatment of hypertensive intracerebral hemorrhage. *Stroke* 24 Suppl:I96–I100, 1993.

50. Kase CS, Robinson RK, Stein RW, et al: Anticoagulant-related intracerebral hemorrhage. *Neurology* 35:943–948, 1985.

51. Kaufman HH: Treatment of deep spontaneous intracerebral hematomas. A review. *Stroke* 24 Suppl: I101–I106, 1993.

52. Kelley RE, Berger JR, Scheinberg P, et al: Active bleeding in hypertensive intracerebral hemorrhage: computed tomography. *Neurology* 32:852–856, 1982.

53. Kilpatrick CJ, Davis SM, Tress BM, et al: Epileptic seizures in acute stroke. *Arch Neurol* 47:157–160, 1990.

54. Kreisler A, Godefroy O, Delmaire C, et al: The anatomy of aphasia revisited. *Neurology* 54:1117–1123, 2000.

55. Kumral E, Kocaer T, Ertubey NO, et al: Thalamic hemorrhage. A prospective study of 100 patients. *Stroke* 26:964–970, 1995.

56. Lee KS, Bae HG, Yun IG: Recurrent intracerebral hemorrhage due to hypertension. *Neurosurgery* 26:586–590, 1990.

57. Linfante I, Llinas RH, Caplan LR, et al: MRI features of intracerebral hemorrhage within 2 hours from symptom onset. *Stroke* 30:2263–2267, 1999.

58. Mattle HP, Schroth G, Seiler RW: Dilemmas in the management of patients with arteriovenous malformations. *J Neurol* 247:917–928, 2000.

59. Mauriõ J, Saposnik G, Lepera S, et al: Multiple simultaneous intracerebral hemorrhages: clinical features and outcome. *Arch Neurol* 58:629–632, 2001.

60. Mayer SA, Sacco RL, Shi T, et al: Neurologic deterioration in noncomatose patients with supratentorial intracerebral hemorrhage. *Neurology* 44:1379–1384, 1994.

61. McKissock W, Richardson A, Taylor J: Primary intracerebral hemorrhage: a controlled trial of surgical and conservative treatment in 180 unselected cases. *Lancet* 2:221–226, 1961.

62. Montes JM, Wong JH, Fayad PB, et al: Stereotactic computed tomographic-guided aspiration and thrombolysis of intracerebral hematoma: protocol and preliminary experience. *Stroke* 31:834–840, 2000.

63. Morgenstern LB, Demchuk AM, Kim DH, et al: Rebleeding leads to poor outcome in ultra-early craniotomy for intracerebral hemorrhage. *Neurology* 45:1294–1299, 2001.

64. Neau JP, Ingrand P, Couderq C, et al: Recurrent intracerebral hemorrhage. *Neurology* 49:106–113, 1997.

65. Ogilvy CS, Stieg PE, Awad I, et al: Recommendations for the management of intracranial arteriovenous malformations: a statement for healthcare professionals from a special writing group of the Stroke Council, American Stroke Association. *Stroke* 32: 1458–1471, 2001.

66. Passero S, Ulivelli M, Reale F: Primary intraventricular haemorrhage in adults. *Acta Neurol Scand* 105:115–119, 2002.

67. Phan TG, Koh M, Vierkant RA, et al: Hydrocephalus is a determinant of early mortality in putaminal hemorrhage. *Stroke* 31:2157–2162, 2000.

68. Phan TG, Koh M, Wijdicks EFM: Safety of discontinuation of anticoagulation in patients with intracranial hemorrhage at high thromboembolic risk. *Arch Neurol* 57:1710–1713, 2000.

69. Posner JB: *Neurologic Complications of Cancer*. Philadelphia, FA Davis Company, 1995.

70. Poungvarin N, Bhoopat W, Viriyavejakul A, et al: Effects of dexamethasone in primary supratentorial intracerebral hemorrhage. *N Engl J Med* 316:1229–1233, 1987.

71. Powers WJ, Zazulia AR, Videen TO, et al: Autoregulation of cerebral blood flow surrounding acute (6 to 22 hours) intracerebral hemorrhage. *Neurology* 57:18–24, 2001.

72. Prasad K, Browman G, Srivastava A, et al: Surgery in primary supratentorial intracerebral hematoma: a meta-analysis of randomized trials. *Acta Neurol Scand* 95:103–110, 1997.

73. Qureshi AI, Tuhrim S, Broderick JP, et al: Spontaneous intracerebral hemorrhage. *N Engl J Med* 344: 1450–1460, 2001.

74. Rabinstein AA, Atkinson JL, Wijdicks EFM: Emergency craniotomy in patients worsening due to expanded cerebral hematoma: To what purpose? *Neurology* 58:1325–1326, 2002.

75. Rabinstein AA, Wijdicks EFM, Fulgham JR: Meningioma disguised as cerebral hematoma. *Neurology* 58:146, 2002.

76. Ropper AH: Lateral displacement of the brain and level of consciousness in patients with an acute hemispheral mass. *N Engl J Med* 314:953–958, 1986.

77. Ropper AH, Gress DR: Computerized tomography and clinical features of large cerebral hemorrhages. *Cerebrovasc Dis* 1:38–42, 1991.

78. Ropper AH, King RB: Intracranial pressure monitoring in comatose patients with cerebral hemorrhage. *Arch Neurol* 41:725–728, 1984.

79. Rosenow F, Hojer C, Meyer-Lohmann C, et al: Spontaneous intracerebral hemorrhage. Prognostic factors in 896 cases. *Acta Neurol Scand* 96:174–182, 1997.

80. Schwarz S, Hafner K, Aschoff A, et al: Incidence and prognostic significance of fever following intracerebral hemorrhage. *Neurology* 54:354–361, 2000.

81. Shapiro SA, Campbell RL, Scully T: Hemorrhagic dilation of the fourth ventricle: an ominous predictor. *J Neurosurg* 80:805–809, 1994.

82. Sjöblom L, Hårdemark H-G, Lindgren A, et al: Management and prognostic features of intracerebral hemorrhage during anticoagulant therapy: a Swedish multicenter study. *Stroke* 32:2567–2574, 2001.

83. Stein RW, Kase CS, Hier DB, et al: Caudate hemorrhage. *Neurology* 34:1549–1554, 1984.

84. Todo T, Usui M, Takakura K: Treatment of severe intraventricular hemorrhage by intraventricular infusion of urokinase. *J Neurosurg* 74:81–86, 1991.

85. Tuhrim S, Dambrosia JN, Price TR, et al: Prediction of intracerebral hemorrhage survival. *Ann Neurol* 24:258–263, 1988.

86. Tuhrim S, Horowitz DR, Sacher M, et al: Validation and comparison of models predicting survival following intracerebral hemorrhage. *Crit Care Med* 23:950–954, 1995.

87. Tuhrim S, Horowitz DR, Sacher M, et al: Volume of ventricular blood is an important determinant of outcome in supratentorial intracerebral hemorrhage. *Crit Care Med* 27:617–621, 1999.

88. Waga S, Fujimoto K, Okada M, et al: Caudate hemorrhage. *Neurosurgery* 18:445–450, 1986.

89. Wagner KR, Xi G, Hua Y, et al: Ultra-early clot aspiration after lysis with tissue plasminogen activator in a porcine model of intracerebral hemorrhage: edema reduction and blood-brain barrier protection. *J Neurosurg* 90:491–498, 1999.

90. Weisberg LA, Shamsnia M, Elliott D: Seizures caused by nontraumatic parenchymal brain hemorrhages. *Neurology* 41:1197–1199, 1991.

91. Weisberg LA, Stazio A, Elliott D, et al: Putaminal hemorrhage: clinical-computed tomographic correlations. *Neuroradiology* 32:200–206, 1990.

92. Wijdicks EFM, Borleffs JC, Hoepelman AI, et al: Fatal disseminated hemorrhagic toxoplasmic encephalitis as the initial manifestation of AIDS. *Ann Neurol* 29:683–686, 1991.

93. Wijdicks EFM, Fulgham JR: Acute fatal deterioration in putaminal hemorrhage. *Stroke* 26:1953–1955, 1995.

94. Wijdicks EFM, Jack CR Jr: Intracerebral hemorrhage after fibrinolytic therapy for acute myocardial infarction. *Stroke* 24:554–557, 1993.

95. Wijdicks EFM, Schievink WI, Brown RD, et al: The dilemma of discontinuation of anticoagulation therapy for patients with intracranial hemorrhage and mechanical heart valves. *Neurosurgery* 42:769–773, 1998.

96. Wijdicks EFM, Silbert PL, Jack CR, et al: Subcortical hemorrhage in disseminated intravascular coagulation associated with sepsis. *AJNR Am J Neuroradiol* 15:763–765, 1994.

97. Xi G, Hua Y, Bhasin RR, et al: Mechanisms of edema formation after intracerebral hemorrhage: effects of extravasated red blood cells on blood flow and blood-brain barrier integrity. *Stroke* 32:2932–2938, 2001.

98. Xi G, Wagner KR, Keep RF, et al: Role of blood clot formation on early edema development after experimental intracerebral hemorrhage. *Stroke* 29:2580–2586, 1998.

99. Young WB, Lee KP, Pessin MS, et al: Prognostic significance of ventricular blood in supratentorial hemorrhage: a volumetric study. *Neurology* 40:616–619, 1990.

100. Zazulia AR, Diringer MN, Derdeyn CP, et al: Progression of mass effect after intracerebral hemorrhage. *Stroke* 30:1167–1173, 1999.

101. Zhu XL, Chan MS, Poon WS: Spontaneous intracranial hemorrhage: Which patients need diagnostic cerebral angiography? A prospective study of 206 cases and review of the literature. *Stroke* 28:1406–1409, 1997.

14

Cerebellum and Brain Stem Hemorrhages

Parenchymal hemorrhage in brain structures that make up the posterior fossa poses a unique circumstance. The small confines of this compartment surrounded by a taut tentorium border leave little room for a cerebellar hemorrhage. Interruption of cerebrospinal fluid circulation quickly follows.

Hemorrhages into the cerebellum and brain stem are by all means critical neurologic disorders that require immediate action. In fact, hemorrhage into the cerebellum is a neurosurgical emergency. Deterioration can be rapid in many of these wakeful patients. The decision is often either to evacuate the clot or, alternatively, to place a ventricular drain to manage acute hydrocephalus.

Pontine hemorrhages, which are uncommon, are highly destructive if due to hypertension but have considerably better prospects if due to underlying vascular malformations.

This chapter focuses on the neurologic critical care of patients with cerebellar hemorrhages, indications for suboccipital craniotomy, and a brief discussion of specific management problems with hemorrhages in the pons and medulla oblongata.

CLINICAL RECOGNITION

Cerebellar hemorrhages are difficult to diagnose. The delay in diagnosis may be due to imperfect clinical judgment or atypical manifestations. Cerebellar hemorrhage usually appears suddenly, often during sedentary activity or sleep. The most consistent signs in cerebellar hemorrhage are an acute sense of vertigo, sudden onset of appendicular ataxia, dysarthria, and vomiting.[9,12,14,26] The imbalance can be striking, and commonly patients are struggling to stand and need the assistance of two persons. Headache may have the characteristics of a thunderclap headache or rapidly build up to a profound occipital or holocephalic headache. Orthostatic headache may be prominent and conceal other signs.[4] Loss of consciousness is common and 10% to 20% of the patients remain stuporous or comatose.[9,12,14,25]

Cranial nerve deficits are invariably present. Nystagmus is typically horizontal rotary but may additionally change in direction or become up-beat. Gaze palsy to the side of the lesion is often found, but in patients with marked obstructive hydrocephalus, vertical gaze palsy may become more apparent. Many types of eye movement disorders have been reported, including ocular bobbing and skew deviation. Ipsilateral facial palsy is fairly common when compression of the brain stem occurs. However, the presenting triad of ipsilateral facial palsy, gaze preference, and limb ataxia is uncommon.[32,40]

Patients with brain stem compression have marked impairment of consciousness, bilateral miosis, and sluggish or absent oculocephalic responses. Fairly typical are breathing abnormalities, varying from hyperventilation to episodes of shallow breathing or apnea. Most patients in this stage of brain stem compression also have brief runs of bradycardia. Compression of the brain stem may result in increased vagal sensitivity and bradycardia, which may be observed during tracheal suctioning but may also be elicited with gentle pressure on the orbit. Surges of systolic hypertension (> 200 mm Hg) due to brain stem compression are associated with dysfunction of the sympathic projections but are not necessarily coupled with bradycardia.[40] When present, these signs indicate significant brain stem distortion, and evacuation of the hematoma becomes critical for survival.

Loss of brain stem reflexes may be imminent, although patients with rapid deterioration still have preserved corneal reflexes and gag reflex on tracheal suctioning despite flaccid tetraplegia with sporadic extensor posturing. Outcome can be surprisingly good after rapid evacuation of the hematoma.

Midbrain hemorrhages are uncommon but may cause significant mass effect. As expected, third and fourth nerve palsies are common,[22] but when the hemorrhage is situated in the rostral midbrain tegmentum, Parinaud's syndrome (upgaze palsy, large pupils with absent pupil response to light but preservation of convergence and lid retraction) may be present.[36] Drowsiness is noted in 50% of the patients but soon resolves. Outcome is invariably good, and stay in the neurologic intensive care unit is usually overnight. In two-thirds of cases, the cause is unknown or is tentatively linked to long-standing hypertension.

Spontaneous hemorrhage into the pons justifies admission to the NICU for mechanical ventilation and supportive therapy. The destruction is often more catastrophic than that in patients with cerebellar hematoma. Pontine hemorrhages are likely to be massive from rupture of the distal midpontine perforating branches of the basilar artery and to occupy the entire pons or force their way into the ventricles. Patients are instantly comatose, have pinpoint but light-responsive pupils and no oculocephalic responses, and display vigorous extensor responses.[13,20] Ocular bobbing (fast downward disconjugate jerks with much slower return to midposition) is virtually diagnostic.[29] Oculovestibular testing using ice water injection may bring on bilateral internuclear ophthalmoplegia or loss of horizontal gaze in comatose patients. Agonal breathing, such as brief gasping or marked hypoventilation, often necessitates mechanical ventilation. In addition, there is almost immediate significant pharyngeal and tongue weakness causing obstructive pooling of secretions. Many patients with large pontine hemorrhages become hyperthermic, and more than one-third have temperatures exceeding 40°C and sweat profusely.[16,29] Massive shivering may occur that may suggest seizures to novices. In these patients, death is expected within 24 hours of the event, but unfortunately patients may stabilize not to awaken from coma. It should be differentiated from a locked-in syndrome if the hemorrhage remains confined to the basis pontis, but it is not common. Localization in the unilateral pons or tegmentum alone causes lesser degrees of impairment of consciousness, dysarthria, ataxic hemiparesis, crossed sensory loss, internuclear ophthalmoplegia, oculomotor palsy, and ipsilateral facial weakness.[8] Visual hallucinations have been noted, and the content of these hallucinations may include very graphic descriptions of landscapes and objects as if patients were in a dream. These hallucinations have not been satisfactorily explained but could be due to a lesion in the reticular formation localized in the tegmentum of the pons.[29]

A very uncommon type of brain stem hemorrhage is primary medullary hemorrhage.[2] Vertigo and headache are often followed by progressive hemiparesis. Hiccups may occur. Recognized presenting signs are nystagmus, palatal weakness, hypoglossal palsy, cerebellar ataxia, and limb weakness—combinations of the classic descriptions of lateral and medial medullary syndromes.

NEUROIMAGING AND LABORATORY TESTS

Cerebellar hematoma can be localized in the hemisphere or vermis (Fig. 14–1). Neuroimaging in posterior fossa hemorrhages is important

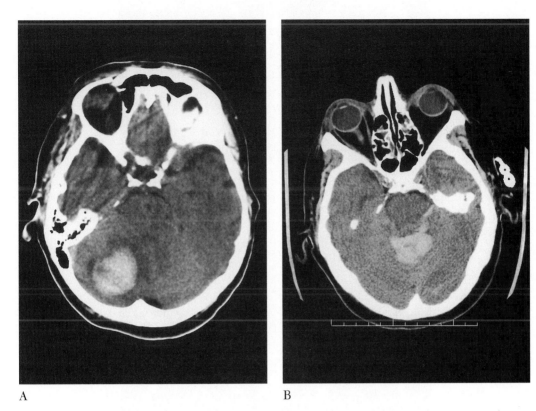

A   B

Figure 14–1. Types of cerebellar hematoma. (A) Hemisphere. (B) Vermis.

because it can classify patients at potential risk for further deterioration. In major textbooks, the size of the hematoma has traditionally been measured by using the diameter in axial cross section in centimeters and converting to true measurements. A diameter of 3 cm or more has been noted as a critical value—without much validation—to decide on evacuation.

Cerebellar hematomas, well visualized on CT scans, typically compress and distort surrounding structures. The fourth ventricle is partly or completely effaced, and there is early evidence of obstructive hydrocephalus, with enlargement of the temporal horns, dilatation of the third ventricle, and subependymal effusions surrounding the lateral ventricles and frontal horns. Less commonly, a cerebellar hematoma is small and only mildly displaces or distorts the fourth ventricle without obstructive hydrocephalus.

Important neuroradiologic signs of upward herniation are compression of the ambient cisterns and upward displacement of the vermis

into the tentorial notch, and the posterior portion of the cistern surrounding the pineal gland changes from a diamond shape into a more blunted triangular shape[31] (Fig. 14–2). These abnormalities have become known as signs of a *tight posterior fossa*[47] and, rightly so, have influenced clinical management. Complete obliteration of the quadrigeminal cistern predicts poor outcome despite surgical evacuation, whereas in partial obliteration, the predictive value is less clear.[42] Primary vermian hemorrhage or extension to the vermis is less common, but, due to its proximity with the brainstem, indicates a high probability of further deterioration.[40]

On CT scans, therefore, the features of cerebellar hematoma that should be assessed are size, hydrocephalus, and, particularly, mass effect and degree of upward herniation.

In patients with a pontine hemorrhage, CT scans often show massive destruction (Fig. 14–3A). Four types of pontine hemorrhage

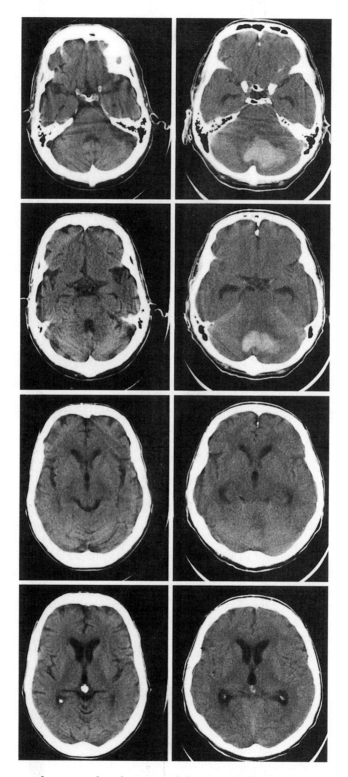

Figure 14–2. Computed tomographic changes with large cerebellar hematoma. (*Left column*) Normal appearance for comparison. (*Right column*) Typical features of a tight posterior fossa showing upward herniation: "toothy smile" appearance becomes "toothless frown" (from compression of the quadrigeminal cistern), diamond-shaped peritectal fluid space becomes squared-off and more triangular, fourth ventricle and prepontine cisterns disappear, and temporal horns are enlarged.[31]

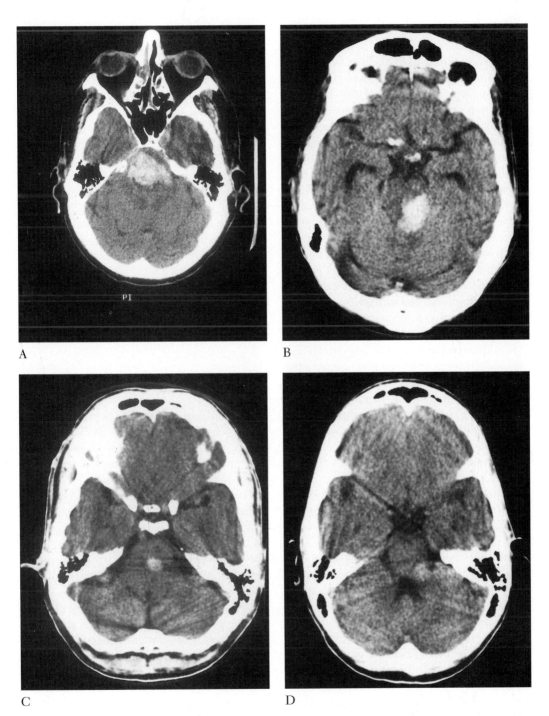

Figure 14–3. Types of pontine hemorrhages. (A) Large, destructive pontine hemorrhage (massive type). (B) Pontine hemorrhage sparing a large part of the basis pontis. (C) Basal tegmental type. (D) Unilateral tegmental type.

have been described on CT scan. They can be classified as massive pontine, basal tegmental, bilateral tegmental, and small unilateral pontine hemorrhages.[5,24,48] Massive hemorrhages with complete destruction of the basis and tegmentum pontis are most frequent, almost invariably with intraventricular blood and prominent early hydrocephalus. Bilateral segmental hematoma with sparing of the basis pontis is less common (Fig. 14–3). The basal tegmental type is an elliptical hematoma at the junction between the basis pontis and the tegmentum along with some extension to the cerebellar peduncle and rupture into the fourth ventricle (Fig. 14–3C). A unilateral tegmental hemorrhage, with exclusive localization in one part of the tegmentum, often with a very small volume, has virtually no extension to the basis pontis or intraventricular rupture (Fig. 14–3D).

It is important to recognize whether the hematoma crosses over the midline, because this signifies a much worse prognosis than that in patients with unilateral tegmental hemorrhage.[5] Intraventricular blood or extension into the cerebellum has less prognostic value than the actual length of the hematoma.

Magnetic resonance imaging (including images with gadolinium) becomes an important study in survivors of pontine and cerebellar hemorrhages. The sensitivity for detection of underlying primary tumor, metastasis, and vascular malformations is good.

The overwhelming majority of cerebellar hemorrhages are due to a ruptured superior cerebellar artery branch from hypertension-induced lipohyalinosis. A dural arteriovenous fistula can be considered if the hematoma is comparatively small and near the fourth ventricle, and this justifies cerebral angiography.[37] It is important to consider hemorrhage into a metastasis, a not infrequently defining manifestation of widespread cancer. Remote hemorrhages in the cerebellum following craniotomy are discussed in Chapter 28.

Laboratory studies in patients with cerebellar hematoma should include complete blood cell count and smear, platelet count, prothrombin time, and partial thromboplastin time. In our hospital-based series, 25% of the patients with cerebellar hematomas were anticoagulated, 75% of them beyond therapeutic range.[40]

Involvement of other target organs from long-standing hypertension may be present and should be evaluated. Renal function tests; full urinalysis, including measurement of total protein, if present; electrocardiography or echocardiography; and grading of atherosclerotic changes of the fundus should be done. Results of liver function tests, which may indicate early evidence for a coagulopathy, must be known at admission; if they are abnormal, abdominal ultrasonography or CT of the liver is indicated. Optional tests include toxicology screen (for amphetamine and cocaine), human immunodeficiency virus testing, coagulation profile (fibrin degradation products, deficiency in factors 8 and 9), and hemoglobin electrophoresis if sickle cell disease is suspected.

FIRST STEPS IN MANAGEMENT

In 40% of cases, cerebellar hematoma would have to be evacuated immediately.[11,17,25] In others, monitoring in the neurologic intensive care unit is imperative, because deterioration can occur in minutes and sometimes abruptly.

The initial steps in management are shown in Table 14–1. Airway management and endotracheal intubation in patients with progressive impairment of consciousness have a high priority because some patients may have unsuspected apnea. In others, marked hypoxemia occurs from aspiration during the ictus. Most patients can breathe spontaneously with pressure support of 5 cm H_2O, which is equivalent to a T-piece. Intermittent mandatory ventilation mode (beginning at 10 breaths/minute; tidal volume of 500 to 700 mL) can be added if gas exchange remains insufficient or apnea continues. Fluid management is important, and dehydration, if present, should be corrected. Swelling is inevitable and may cause irreversible brain stem compression in those with a so-called tight posterior fossa. However, it is not certain whether the amount of swelling can be reduced by marked free water restric-

Table 14-1. Initial Management of Cerebellar Hematoma

Airway management	Intubation for hypoxemic or apneic episodes; intermittent mandatory ventilation or T-piece
Fluid management	2 L of 0.9% NaCl Mannitol, 1 g/kg bolus, in patients with tight posterior fossa on CT scans
Blood pressure	Labetalol, 20–40 mg IV, for persistent hypertension (mean arterial pressure > 130 mm Hg)
Cardiac arrhythmia	Sinus bradycardia: atropine, 0.5–2.0 mg IV Sinus tachycardia: fluid bolus, 500 mL of 0.9% NaCl or 250 mL of albumin 5%
Surgical management	Surgical evacuation (hematoma size > 3 cm, obliterated 4th ventricle, or collapsed quadrigeminal cistern on CT) Ventriculostomy for hydrocephalus
Prophylactic measures	Deep venous thrombosis prophylaxis with intermittent pneumatic devices Stress ulcer prophylaxis with pantoprazole 40 mg IV in patients receiving mechanical ventilation

CT, computed tomography.

tion. A bolus of mannitol, 1 g/kg, can be given en route to the operating room and can be repeated. Anticoagulation should be reversed with fresh frozen plasma and vitamin K (10 mg) given intravenously, or prothrombin complex concentrate should be administered (Chapter 13). Some neurosurgeons administer dexamethasone in a loading dose of 10 mg followed by 4 mg every 4 hours when craniotomy is anticipated, and this may further reduce edema in the tight compartment of the posterior fossa.

Increases in blood pressure are treated only when persistently high. In most patients, however, hypertension is a manifestation of the Cushing response, a compensatory mechanism that should not be touched.

Bradycardia is often a sign of brain stem compression. When it is associated with a decrease in blood pressure and when bradycardia occurs in runs, atropine (0.5 to 2 mg intravenously) should be considered. Tachycardia, however, may be related to dehydration, and fluid challenge should be considered first (Table 14–1).

Decompressive suboccipital craniotomy is indicated in any patient with signs of upward herniation on CT images, frequent episodes of bradycardia, less than localization to pain as a best motor response, or significant cranial nerve dysfunction. It is unclear whether size alone should prompt surgical evacuation. Most neurosurgeons favor craniotomy for hemispheric hematomas and vermian hematomas larger than 3 cm, but mass effect (for example, obliteration of the 4th ventricle) and decreased level of alertness are probably more meaningful clues than absolute size of the hematoma.[35] A recently completed protocol in 50 consecutively treated patients with cerebellar hematoma found that 43% of patients with a completely effaced 4th ventricle deteriorated before transfer to the neurosurgical unit.[16] In patients with small hematomas (clot diameter less than 3 cm on CT scan) who have open ambient and quadrigeminal cisterns but significant hydrocephalus with a clinical history of progressive drowsiness after a fairly lucid interval, ventriculostomy alone can be considered. In our series, this occurred in only 10% of patients, and suboccipital craniotomy followed soon after.[40] Medical management is probably the most reasonable choice in pa-

Table 14-2. Initial Management of Brain Stem Hemorrhage

Airway management	Endotracheal intubation; intermittent mandatory or assist-control mode of ventilation
Fluid management	2 L of 0.9% NaCl; increase amount in hyperthermia to 1 L per 1°C increase in temperature
Blood pressure	Labetalol, 20–40 mg IV, for persisting hypertension (mean arterial pressure > 130 mm Hg)
Nutrition	Enteral feeding; gastrostomy after day 7
Prophylactic measures	Deep venous thrombosis prophylaxis with intermittent-compression devices; stress ulcer prophylaxis with pantoprazole (40 mg IV)

tients with maximal or nearly maximal level of consciousness, no cranial nerve deficits, and a small hematoma without any major mass effect on CT scan. However, patients with marked cerebellar atrophy—as seen in chronic alcoholics—may tolerate hematomas of limited size, and treatment of withdrawal delirium is a bigger concern.

The management of patients with spontaneous brain stem hemorrhages is largely supportive. Stereotactic removal has been advocated, and impressive results have been reported.[3,6,19] The architecture of the pons is quite delicate, but with stereotactic aspiration, good-to-fair recovery has been claimed in 65% of 20 patients with limited pontine hemorrhages (5 to 10 mL in volume). Outcome in patients with larger hematomas (more than 10 mL) was poor and no better than that in a matched medically treated group.[38] Surgical intervention becomes a very important issue in patients with limited hematomas, particularly if additional magnetic resonance images demonstrate a cavernous angioma or cryptic arteriovenous malformation located near the fourth ventricle. In patients with subependymal or tegmental localization of the hematoma, surgical removal through the vermis has resulted in good outcomes.[19] Recurrent hemorrhage is a major concern.[23] Although timing is uncertain, surgery is elective in most patients and most likely eliminates further risk of hemorrhage.

The almost universally large size of the brain stem hemorrhage destroys respiratory control and mandates mechanical ventilation. It is important to set the ventilator on an assist-control or intermittent mandatory ventilation mode, because patients with markedly impaired ventilatory drive cannot breathe spontaneously. Patients with a pontine hemorrhage may have aspirated during the catastrophic ictus, and a large alveolar-arterial oxygen ratio may necessitate increasing positive end-expiratory pressure ventilation and high FIO_2. There is no physiologic rationale to hyperventilate beyond the mild respiratory acidosis associated with mechanical ventilation.

Hyperthermia has been noted in patients with pontine hemorrhages, and fluid intake could become insufficient (Fig. 14–4). Cooling is indicated in patients with increased temperatures often exceeding 40°C.

Blood pressures are markedly increased in patients with pontine hemorrhages. It is rea-

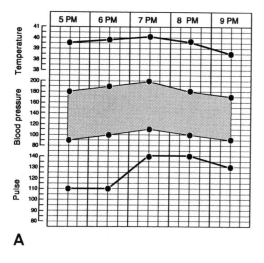

A

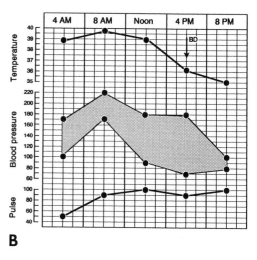

B

Figure 14–4. Time course of temperature, pulse, and blood pressure (*A*) on admission in a patient with a pontine hemorrhage and (*B*) in a patient with pontine hemorrhage extending to the midbrain at time of loss of all brainstem reflexes (BD, brain death [*arrow*]). (From Wijdicks and St Louis.[50] By permission of the American Academy of Neurology.)

sonable to mute marked elevations in mean arterial blood pressure, but in many patients, the increases are brief, disappearing within 24 hours. Extension of the lesion from edema may produce complete loss of brain stem function. A change from hypertension to hypotension in patients with a large pontine hemorrhage and a sudden decrease in temperature to a subnormal level are ominous signs. Dopamine may be needed to support blood pressure. As expected, diabetes insipidus is absent in patients with primary brain stem lesions.

Protection of the gastric mucosa in pontine hemorrhage with antacids and histamine$_2$-blockers is important. In a series of fatal cases of pontine hemorrhage, gastrointestinal bleeding was found within 1 week in one-third of the patients.[29] Nutrition is postponed in patients with spontaneous pontine hemorrhage because swallowing mechanisms are impaired. Gastroparesis is likely in these patients, who additionally may have marked central autonomic dysfunction. Enteral feeding can be started on the second or third day after admission, and possible recovery of swallowing can be awaited during the first week. Percutaneous endoscopic gastrostomy is mandatory in patients with pontine hemorrhage who have an impaired swallowing mechanism and who are expected to require long-term care (Chapter 7).

For recovery to occur, a change for the better must be signaled by improvement in motor score on the Glasgow coma scale or in brain stem function in the first 5 to 7 days after the ictus. In patients without any change after 1 week, the rationale for continuing supportive care, which includes tracheostomy and percutaneous endoscopic gastrostomy, must be discussed with the family.

Patients with small (usually) tegmental hemorrhages often have an underlying cavernous malformation. Recurrence is expected. In a series of 100 patients from the Barrow Neurological Institute, the median interval between hemorrhages was 12 months.[33] The calculated repeat hemorrhage rate was 30% per person per year. Surgical resection is recommended for lesions abutting the pial surface.[54] Deep-seated lesions may be treated with stereotactic radiosurgery, but no proof exists that it reduces the rate of hemorrhage.[18]

DETERIORATION: CAUSES AND MANAGEMENT

Further deterioration in patients with cerebellar hematoma can be predicted with certainty. The odds are higher when systolic blood pressure at admission is uncontrolled and higher than 200 mm Hg, corneal reflexes are abnormal, and oculocephalic reflexes are impaired. These signs reflect brain stem distortion but a fragile balance. Neurologic deterioration also is likely in patients with vermian hemorrhage or hemispheric hemorrhage tracking into the vermis and in patients with early hydrocephalus on the initial CT scan. Risk of further clinical deterioration is low in patients without brain stem distortion, upward herniation, or, particularly, distortion of the fourth ventricle.[40]

Most patients with a cerebellar hematoma have deterioration from direct brain stem compression rather than hydrocephalus.[1,45,46] The clinical features are progressive limitation and loss of upward gaze and deepening coma. Pupils become asymmetrical in size and, soon after, pinpoint. Spontaneous hyperventilation with considerable respiratory alkalosis often occurs at the same time as marked deterioration in consciousness. Often, blood pressure increases with widening of the pulse pressure, and we have found this a helpful clinical sign of early deterioration. Bradycardia may be absent when vagal traffic, as a compensatory response, is interrupted by medullary compression and ischemia. The clinicopathologic correlate of upward herniation should be subject to criticism. Whether a consistently recognizable pattern exists has been questioned after a careful autopsy report.[7] In addition, the relation with ventriculostomy remains of doubtful causality. Of 52 patients with upward herniation noted in the literature, only 25% had ventriculostomy, but not all patients deteriorated minutes after placement.[7] However, emergency evacuation is indicated because the opportunity for survival is lost with unnecessary delay. Evacuation of the hematoma together with ventriculostomy is a reasonable consideration if the ventricles are enlarged on the initial CT scan, but the benefit is derived from relieving brain stem compression.

Deterioration from hydrocephalus alone may occur in patients with cerebellar hematoma, usually in those with only marginal compression of the fourth ventricle, and presents with a much more gradual clinical course.[27] Computed tomography scanning confirms further enlargement of the lateral horns, shows bulging of the third ventricles, and, on lower CT scan slices, clearly visualizes the temporal horns. These patients gradually become more drowsy, new neurologic signs or symptoms seldom develop, and they are unable to protect the airway. The opening pressure is increased at the time of insertion of the ventricular drain, and several days of CSF drainage are required. A permanent ventriculoperitoneal drain is considered after 7–10 days. Ventricular drains should be removed when the cerebrospinal fluid has been clear and there is no obstructive clot in the third or fourth ventricle but also when the production of cerebrospinal fluid is minimal and clamping has not resulted in an upsurge of intracranial pressure.

Placement of a ventricular catheter in patients with a pontine hemorrhage and an enlarged ventricular system but without a clinical history of deterioration is rarely useful. Most patients with a massive pontine hemorrhage with an acute enlargement of the ventricular system present with clinical symptoms related to the pontine damage itself, not to hydrocephalus.

Patients with massive pontine hemorrhages may have progression to loss of all brain stem function on the day of admission.[30] Many patients, however, continue to trigger the ventilator and do not become candidates for organ donation. Confirmatory tests are useless in this situation because blood flow to the brain may be preserved, certainly initially. In addition, electroencephalographic findings are expected to be abnormal but not isoelectric. In these patients, theta or delta activity may occur with sporadic alpha activity but without reactivity to light or pain stimuli. Primary brain stem death is highly uncommon. We have extended our observation time to 24 hours. Loss of all brain function occurs from the development of massive obstructive hydrocephalus.

OUTCOME

Mortality in hemorrhages of posterior fossa structures is considerable. In addition, because most published data are from large medical centers with the most experience in treatment and probably also the best outcomes, the risk of fatal outcome most likely is underreported. Nonetheless, salvage is possible in patients with cerebellar hematomas, resulting in a very acceptable functional state.

Predictive factors for poor outcome in cerebellar hemorrhage have not been studied prospectively. Patients of any age with loss of many brain stem functions may do surprisingly well after evacuation of the hematoma. In patients with less dramatic presentations, the prospects of independent recovery with preservation of gait are good.[25] However, suboccipital craniotomy may be a futile surgical intervention. It is not known whether a dividing line exists between potential for functional outcome and remaining in a crippled state. Absent corneal reflexes, acute hydrocephalus, and absent oculocephalic responses predict a poor outcome, but reversal of this desperate clinical state has been documented in exceptional cases.[41] In addition, neurosurgeons are biased toward younger patients and reluctant to consider surgical intervention in patients older than 70 years with clots of more than 3 cm in diameter on CT scans.[51] The degree of brain stem damage is important, and a recent study documented that T2 changes in the brain stem on postoperative magnetic resonance imaging were correlated with poor outcome.[52] The timing of surgery in relation to the clinical signs of brain stem compression remains unknown. A study of 16 comatose patients with dilated pupils, compression of perimesencephalic cis-

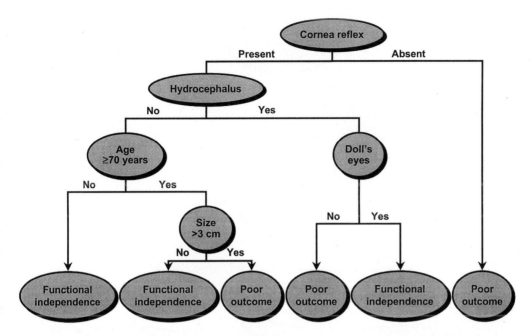

Figure 14–5. Outcome predictors in cerebellar hematoma. Poor outcome: severe disability or death, vegetative state. Functional independence: no assistance needed, minor handicap may remain.

terns, and hydrocephalus who were operated on within hours of admission found that all had poor outcomes.[53] In another study, patients with a cerebellar hematoma and a Glasgow coma scale score of 5 or less and compressed quadrigeminal cistern on CT scan did not fare well, but the number of patients was small.[42]

Upward herniation on CT scan (often also directly related to the total volume of the clot in cerebellar parenchyma) is a poor prognostic sign, but evacuation of the hematoma should nevertheless still be seriously considered. Coma alone should not be considered a reason to withdraw support or reduce the level of support, but some disagree.[25,44] Outcome in cerebellar hematoma is shown in Figure 14–5. The decision whether to surgically intervene could be guided by these clinical and neuroimaging variables. Recurrence of a cerebellar hematoma is a possibility, but usually in patients with poorly controlled hypertension.[49]

The outcome in patients with pontine hemorrhage, coma within hours of onset, and horizontal extension (more than 2 cm on CT) is invariably poor.[24] We found no survivors in patients presenting with hyperthermia, extension to the thalamus, intraventricular hemorrhage, and acute hydrocephalus on the admission CT scan.[50] Surgically treated patients with large pontine hematomas have a better chance of survival but very likely at the expense of devastating disability due to diplopia and ataxia.[43] Lack of the N20 component on somatosensory evoked potentials has predicted poor outcome in pontine hemorrhage. In a preliminary study, preservation of one or both cortical somatosensory evoked potentials signified a chance for good recovery, even in a patient with a hemorrhage that crossed the midline of the pons.[10] Patients with small lateral tegmental pontine hemorrhages do very well with medical management[15,39] but need further evaluation for underlying vascular lesions and possibly surgery.[21,28,34] The first episode of hemorrhage in patients with brain stem vascular malformations is usually benign. As alluded to earlier, MRI should be routinely obtained to search for a vascular anomaly. Outcome predictors in pontine hemorrhage are shown in Figure 14–6.

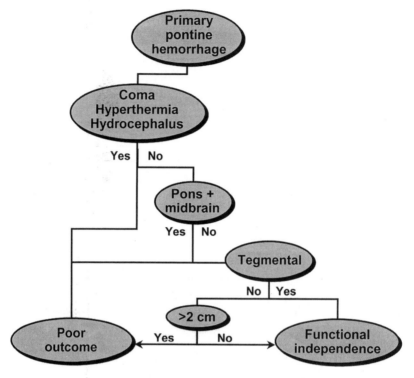

Figure 14–6. Outcome predictors in primary pontine hemorrhage. Poor outcome: severe disability or death, vegetative state. Functional independence: no assistance needed, minor handicap may remain.

CONCLUSIONS

- The CT scan signs in cerebellar hemorrhages are disappearance of the fourth ventricle, compression of ambient and quadrigeminal cisterns, and squaring off of the peritectal cistern, features most often seen in hematomas larger than 3 cm.
- Suboccipital decompressive craniotomy is the mainstay of management for large cerebellar hematomas.
- Management of cerebellar hematoma includes elective intubation in patients with rapid impairment of consciousness, mannitol in patients with computed tomographic evidence of tight posterior fossa, and labetalol intravenously for blood pressure control. Runs of bradycardia can be countered with atropine.
- Suboccipital craniotomy in comatose patients with cerebellar hemorrhage and loss of some brain stem reflexes may still result in independent recovery, but this is less likely when corneal reflexes are absent.
- Primary pontine hemorrhages carry a high mortality, often in patients with hyperthermia at presentation, intraventricular hematoma, and extension to midbrain and thalamus.
- In patients with a small localized hemorrhage, magnetic resonance imaging studies are needed to demonstrate a possible arteriovenous malformation that can be successfully removed surgically.

REFERENCES

1. Aoki N, Mizuguchi K: Expanding intracerebellar hematoma: a possible clinicopathological entity. *Neurosurgery* 18:94–96, 1986.
2. Barinagarrementeria F, Cantú C: Primary medullary hemorrhage. Report of four cases and review of the literature. *Stroke* 25:1684–1687, 1994.
3. Beatty RM, Zervas NT: Stereotactic aspiration of a brain stem hematoma. *Neurosurgery* 13:204–207, 1983.
4. Chen WT, Fuh JL, Lu SR, et al: Cerebellar hemorrhage presenting as orthostatic headache: two case reports. *Neurology* 53:1887–1888.
5. Chung CS, Park CH: Primary pontine hemorrhage: a new CT classification. *Neurology* 42:830–834, 1992.
6. Colak A, Bertan V, Benli K, et al: Pontine hematoma. A report of three surgically treated cases. *Zentralbl Neurochir* 52:33–36, 1991.
7. Cuneo RA, Caronna JJ, Pitts L, et al: Upward transtentorial herniation: seven cases and a literature review. *Arch Neurol* 36:618–623, 1979.
8. Del-Brutto OH, Noboa CA, Barinagarrementeria F: Lateral pontine hemorrhage: reappraisal of benign cases. *Stroke* 18:954–956, 1987.
9. Dunne JW, Chakera T, Kermode S: Cerebellar haemorrhage—diagnosis and treatment: a study of 75 consecutive cases. *Q J Med* 64:739–754, 1987.
10. Ferbert A, Buchner H, Brückmann H: Brainstem auditory evoked potentials and somatosensory evoked potentials in pontine haemorrhage. Correlations with clinical and CT findings. *Brain* 113:49–63, 1990.
11. Firsching R, Huber M, Frowein RA: Cerebellar haemorrhage: management and prognosis. *Neurosurg Rev* 14:191–194, 1991.
12. Freeman RE, Onofrio BM, Okazaki H, et al: Spontaneous intracerebellar hemorrhage. Diagnosis and surgical treatment. *Neurology* 23:84–90, 1973.
13. Goto N, Kaneko M, Hosaka Y, et al: Primary pontine hemorrhage: clinicopathological correlations. *Stroke* 11:84–90, 1980.
14. Guillermain P, Lena G, Reynier Y, et al: Hématomes intracérébelleux spontanés de l'adulte. 44 cas. *Rev Neurol (Paris)* 146:478–483, 1990.
15. Iwasaki Y, Kinoshita M: Lateral pontine hemorrhage: atypical clinical manifestations and good outcome. *Comput Med Imaging Graph* 12:371–373, 1988.
16. Kirollos RW, Tyagi AK, Ross SA, et al: Management of spontaneous cerebellar hematomas: a prospective treatment protocol. *Neurosurgery* 49:1378–1386, 2001.
17. Kobayashi S, Sato A, Kageyama Y, et al: Treatment of hypertensive cerebellar hemorrhage—surgical or conservative management? *Neurosurgery* 34:246–250, 1994.
18. Kondziolka D, Lunsford LD, Flickinger JC, et al: Reduction of hemorrhage risk after stereotactic radiosurgery for cavernous malformations. *J Neurosurg* 83:825–831, 1995.
19. Konovalov AN, Spallone A, Makhmudov UB, et al: Surgical management of hematomas of the brain stem. *J Neurosurg* 73:181–186, 1990.
20. Kushner MJ, Bressman SB: The clinical manifestations of pontine hemorrhage. *Neurology* 35:637–643, 1985.
21. Lancman M, Norscini J, Mesropian H, et al: Tegmental pontine hemorrhages: clinical features and prognostic factors. *Can J Neurol Sci* 19:236–238, 1992.
22. Link MJ, Bartleson JD, Forbes G, et al: Spontaneous midbrain hemorrhage: report of seven new cases. *Surg Neurol* 39:58–65, 1993.
23. Maraire JN, Awad IA: Intracranial cavernous malformations: lesion behavior and management strategies. *Neurosurgery* 37:591–605, 1995.
24. Masiyama S, Niizuma H, Suzuki J: Pontine haemorrhage: a clinical analysis of 26 cases. *J Neurol Neurosurg Psychiatry* 48:658–662, 1985.
25. Mathew P, Teasdale G, Bannan A, et al: Neurosurgical management of cerebellar haematoma and infarct. *J Neurol Neurosurg Psychiatry* 59:287–292, 1995.
26. Melamed N, Satya-Murti S: Cerebellar hemorrhage. A review and reappraisal of benign cases. *Arch Neurol* 41:425–428, 1984.
27. Mezzadri JJ, Otero JM, Ottino CA: Management of 50 spontaneous cerebellar haemorrhages. Importance of obstructive hydrocephalus. *Acta Neurochir (Wien)* 122:39–44, 1993.
28. Murata Y, Yamaguchi S, Kajikawa H, et al: Relationship between the clinical manifestations, computed tomographic findings and the outcome in 80 patients with primary pontine hemorrhage. *J Neurol Sci* 167:107–111, 1999.
29. Nakajima K: Clinicopathological study of pontine hemorrhage. *Stroke* 14:485–493, 1983.
30. Ogata J, Imakita M, Yutani C, et al: Primary brainstem death: a clinico-pathological study. *J Neurol Neurosurg Psychiatry* 51:646–650, 1988.
31. Osborn AG, Heaston DK, Wing SD: Diagnosis of ascending transtentorial herniation by cranial computed tomography. *AJR Am J Roentgenol* 130:755–760, 1978.
32. Ott KH, Kase CS, Ojemann RG, et al: Cerebellar hemorrhage: diagnosis and treatment. A review of 56 cases. *Arch Neurol* 31:160–167, 1974.
33. Porter RW, Detwiler PW, Spetzler RF, et al: Cavernous malformations of the brainstem: experience with 100 patients. *J Neurosurg* 90:50–58, 1999.
34. Rabinstein AA, Tisch SH, McClelland RL, et al: Cause is the main predictor of outcome in patients with pontine hemorrhage (submitted for publication).
35. Salvati M, Cervoni L, Raco A, et al: Spontaneous cerebellar hemorrhage: clinical remarks on 50 cases. *Surg Neurol* 55:156–161, 2001.
36. Sand JJ, Biller J, Corbett JJ, et al: Partial dorsal mesencephalic hemorrhages: report of three cases. *Neurology* 36:529–533, 1986.
37. Satoh K, Satomi J, Nakajima N, et al: Cerebellar hemorrhage caused by dural arteriovenous fistula: a review of five cases. *J Neurosurg* 94:422–426, 2001.

38. Shitamichi M, Nakamura J, Sasaki T, et al: Computed tomography guided stereotactic aspiration of pontine hemorrhages. *Stereotact Funct Neurosurg* 54–55:453–456, 1990.

39. Shuaib A: Benign brainstem hemorrhage. *Can J Neurol Sci* 18:356–357, 1991.

40. St Louis EK, Wijdicks EFM, Li H: Predicting neurologic deterioration in patients with cerebellar hematomas. *Neurology* 51:1364–1369, 1998.

41. St Louis EK, Wijdicks EFM, Li H, et al: Predictors of poor outcome in patients with a spontaneous cerebellar hematoma. *Can J Neurol Sci* 27:32–36, 2000.

42. Taneda M, Hayakawa T, Mogami H: Primary cerebellar hemorrhage. Quadrigeminal cistern obliteration on CT scans as a predictor of outcome. *J Neurosurg* 67:545–552, 1987.

43. Teasell R, Foley N, Doherty T, et al: Clinical characteristics of patients with brainstem strokes admitted to a rehabilitation unit. *Arch Phys Med Rehabil* 83:1013–1016, 2002.

44. van der Hoop RG, Vermeulen M, van Gijn J: Cerebellar hemorrhage: diagnosis and treatment. *Surg Neurol* 29:6–10, 1988.

45. van Loon J, Van Calenbergh F, Goffin J, et al: Controversies in the management of spontaneous cerebellar haemorrhage. A consecutive series of 49 cases and review of the literature. *Acta Neurochir (Wien)* 122:187–193, 1993.

46. Waidhauser E, Hamburger C, Marguth F: Neurosurgical management of cerebellar hemorrhage. *Neurosurg Rev* 13:211–217, 1990.

47. Weisberg LA: Acute cerebellar hemorrhage and CT evidence of tight posterior fossa. *Neurology* 36:858–860, 1986.

48. Weisberg LA: Primary pontine haemorrhage: clinical and computed tomographic correlations. *J Neurol Neurosurg Psychiatry* 49:346–352, 1986.

49. Wijdicks EFM: Recurrent cerebellar hematomas (letter to the editor). *Stroke* 26:2198, 1995.

50. Wijdicks EFM, St Louis EK: Clinical profiles predictive of outcome in pontine hemorrhage. *Neurology* 49:1342–1346, 1997.

51. Wijdicks EFM, St Louis EK, Atkinson JD, et al: Clinician's biases toward surgery in cerebellar hematomas: an analysis of decision-making in 94 patients. *Cerebrovasc Dis* 10:93–96, 2000.

52. Yanaka K, Meguro K, Fujita K, et al: Postoperative brainstem high intensity is correlated with poor outcomes for patients with spontaneous cerebellar hemorrhage. *Neurosurgery* 45:1323–1327, 1999.

53. Yanaka K, Meguro K, Fujita K, et al: Immediate surgery reduces mortality in deeply comatose patients with spontaneous cerebellar hemorrhage. *Neurol Med Chir (Tokyo)* 40:295–299, 2000.

54. Zimmerman RS, Spetzler RF, Lee KS, et al: Cavernous malformations of the brain stem. *J Neurosurg* 75:32–39, 1991.

15

Cerebral Venous Thrombosis

Cerebral venous thrombosis may lead to venous hypertension and hemorrhagic infarction. Its presentation commonly confuses clinicians, who may consider more exotic causes when confronted with a young person with a sudden hemorrhagic mass. However, the diagnosis of cerebral venous thrombosis has been greatly aided by MRI and magnetic resonance venography.

It can be estimated that fewer than 10% of patients with cerebral venous thrombosis will need neurologic intensive care during the course of the disease. Reasons for admission to the NICU include the development of hemorrhagic infarction, seizures, and other life-threatening complications in patients with a hypercoagulable state, such as pulmonary embolus or arterial occlusion. Patients are less commonly admitted to the NICU with obstruction at the cavernous sinus which results in painful ophthalmoplegia, which involves the third, fourth, fifth (first two divisions), and sixth cranial nerves. Most challenging are management difficulties in association with increased intracranial pressure due to a culmination of bilateral cerebral infarctions and edema. Thrombus formation in the cerebral venous system may result in a cascade of clinical problems, and early aggressive treatment (anticoagulation or endovascular therapy) may prevent serious disability and death.

CLINICAL RECOGNITION

Knowledge of the anatomical ramifications of the larger veins is needed to understand the propagation of clot. Most of the cortical veins drain into the superior sagittal sinus, which follows the falx cerebri. The inferior sagittal sinus follows the ventral side of the falx and drains into the straight sinus. Both transverse sinuses are located at the tentorium cerebelli. The superior sagittal sinus, straight sinus, and both transverse sinuses form a confluence called the "torcular Herophili." The anatomy of the cerebral venous system, including important anastomosis, is shown in Figure 15–1.

The typical sequence of events in cerebral venous thrombosis is dilatation of the venous and capillary bed, gradual progression of interstitial edema, disruption of veins, and formation of hematomas[75] (Fig. 15–2). Cytotoxic edema, however, may occur early; some animal studies, in fact, suggest that cytotoxic edema is followed by vasogenic edema and that treatment with tissue plasminogen activator may partially resolve cytotoxic edema.[57] Generally, the venous system is most commonly obstructed at the superior sagittal sinus, with a possible extension to the cortical veins, leading to hemorrhagic cerebral infarction. Obstruction at the level of the deep internal cerebral veins may result in hemorrhagic infarction of the thalami or caudate heads.

The defining characteristics of cerebral venous thrombosis include profound headache, papilledema, and, in more severe cases, seizures and localizing findings. Patients with cerebral venous thrombosis (most often, the superior sagittal sinus) invariably complain of a persistent headache of new onset. The headache is dull but intense and bilateral. Movements of the head, sneezing, and coughing may

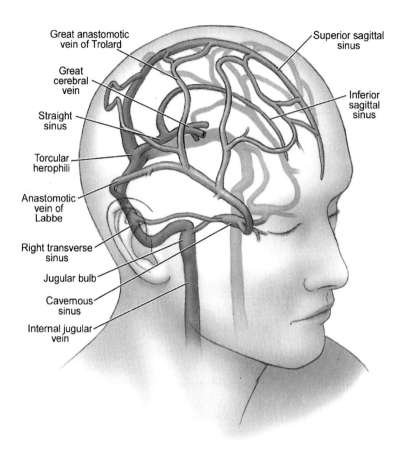

Figure 15–1. Anatomy of the cerebral venous system.

be aggravating, but the headache can also be instantaneous in onset, mimicking a thunderclap type of headache. If the headache becomes worse when the patient bends forward and suddenly exacerbates with a sharp throb of pain after sneezing, an underlying sinusitis must be suspected, although septic sagittal sinus thrombosis is very uncommon.

Papilledema is an important clinical finding and may be manifested by obscurations. These typical blackouts last only seconds, are often in one eye, and may be either spontaneous or elicited by change in posture. In a few instances, pressure on the globe by the examiner may bring them on. When papilledema is subtle, it is detected only by disappearance of the venous pulsation. Disk elevation, blurring of disk margins, and dilated and tortuous veins occur in fewer than half the patients with the di-

agnosis of sagittal sinus thrombosis.[11] Visual loss may ensue in long-standing papilledema, but visual blurring may occur early when retinal exudate extends to the macula. Diplopia in a horizontal plane may occur as a result of an associated sixth nerve palsy. In patients with unilateral transverse sinus thrombosis alone, compression of the contralateral jugular vein may cause unilateral facial venous engorgement (Crowe's test), but the diagnostic value of this test is uncertain.

Patients with sagittal sinus thrombosis may become confused and may exhibit bizarre behavior but also nonspecific signs such as progressive anorexia and forgetfulness.[13,34] However, localizing deficits, such as hemiparesis, aphasia, abnormal visual fields, and anosognosia, likely denote the development of venous cerebral infarction.

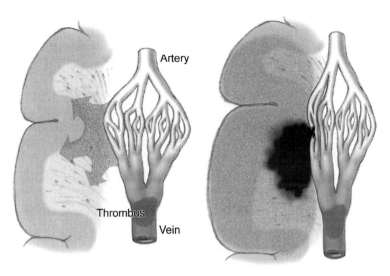

Figure 15–2. Edema and hemorrhagic infarction. (Modified from Yuh et al.[75] By permission of the American Society of Neuroradiology.)

Because initially small cortical areas are involved, seizures are focal, and presenting generalized tonic-clonic seizures are less common. Seizures are often isolated events and may not herald further progression into status epilepticus. A focal seizure may result in hemiparesis of several hours' duration (Todd's paresis) and may not indicate permanent infarction of the brain.

Progression into coma may be caused by diffuse cerebral edema or bilateral cerebral, often hemorrhagic, infarctions. The volume of one hemorrhagic infarct, however, may predominate over the other and may cause mass effect with marked brain shift. Diffuse massive brain edema occurs rarely, and the outcome is often hopeless despite aggressive measures to reduce edema.

Venous infarction in both thalami may produce marked fluctuations in arousal and substantial memory deficits later. Other clinical signs of bilateral hemorrhagic thalamic infarcts are delirium, abulia, dyscalculia, confabulation, and atypical transcortical sensory aphasia with impaired naming and comprehension but preserved fluency and repetition.[6,34] Unusual presenting symptoms are acute micrographia and hypophonia from venous infarction in both thalami, the putamen, and the caudate nucleus.[47]

Isolated multiple cranial nerve palsy (III, VII, VIII) has recently been reported in patients with unilateral occlusion of the transverse-sigmoid sinus. This unusual presentation has been explained by venous congestion of the ventral pontine and lateral medullary veins.[42]

NEUROIMAGING AND LABORATORY TESTS

Cerebral venous sinus thrombosis is often without an identifiable precipitating trigger, and the results of a battery of diagnostic tests could be unrevealing. A comprehensive investigation of potential causes is expensive, time-consuming, and negative in 20% of the patients, including those with 2-year follow-up, in whom an underlying disorder, if present, should have become apparent.[11] The therapeutic consequences of a once-detected thrombophilia are quite important.

Major causes for cerebral sinus thrombosis are all stages of pregnancy (but more likely the puerperium) and use of oral contraceptives.[46] Other causes are coagulation disorders, connective tissue disorders, cancer[54] or chemotherapeutic treatment,[38] nephrotic syndrome, bacteremia or disseminated intravascular coagulation, and conditions of extreme dehydration. Local invasion of the sagittal sinus by metastatic disease should be considered in patients with metastatic carcinoma. Behçet's disease, Crohn's disease, ulcerative colitis, and acquired immunodeficiency syndrome may appear with cerebral venous thrombosis and should all be considered.[20,39] One group of investigators reported that approximately 40% of a large series of patients had an underlying systemic disease.[53] Damage to the jugular vein from trauma to or surgical procedures involving the neck is a well-recognized cause. In several patients, cerebral venous thrombosis has been reported after placement of a jugular vein catheter for parenteral nutrition[58] or perioperative monitoring or after placement of pacemaker wires.[27,32,43]

Superior sagittal sinus thrombosis has been reported in at least 12 patients after nonpenetrating head injury.[36] The mechanism in head injury remains unresolved. No studies are available to prove the theory that thromboplastin, which is present in large quantities in the brain after injury, alters blood coagulation.

Rare causes for cerebral venous thrombosis are dural arteriovenous fistula[24] and antifibrinolytic agents.[1] Table 15–1 summarizes a complete evaluation schedule. Cerebral venous thrombosis may be the first defining disorder in patients with a hypercoagulable state. More likely, recurrent spontaneous abortions, recurrent deep vein thrombosis, pulmonary embolism at a young age, and arterial occlusions at uncommon sites may have been earlier indicators of a coagulation abnormality.[2,40,61,71] Congenital thrombophilias, such as protein S deficiency,[31] anticardiolipin antibodies,[12] activated protein C resistance, hyperhomocystinemia, and increased levels of factors VIII and XI, should be investigated. Both a heterozygous and a homozygous state for factor V Leiden and a 20210A sequence variation of the prothrombin gene have been associated with cerebral venous thrombosis in sporadic cases and in up to 9% of patients in larger series.[8,9,56,61] Although inherited coagulopathy accounts for a minority of occurrences of cerebral venous thrombosis, a study from Germany found that the incidence

Table 15–1. Laboratory Studies in Patients with Cerebral Venous Thrombosis

Blood smear, platelet count, differential count
Antithrombin III, protein C, and protein S
Heparin cofactor II
Plasma fibrinogen
Lupus anticoagulant
Anticardiolipin antibodies
Plasma homocysteine
Hemoglobin electrophoresis
Urinalysis with quantification of protein and
　determination of hemosiderin
Coombs' test, rheumatoid factor, antineutrophil
　cytoplasmic autoantibody, antinuclear antibody
Drug screen
Computed tomography scan of chest or abdomen, or
　both
Optional
　Human immunodeficiency virus
　Colonoscopy
　Skin and conjunctiva biopsy
　Blood cultures
　Bone marrow
　Hematology consultation
　Rheumatology consultation
　Otorhinolaryngology consultation

approached 40%.[65] Simultaneous occurrence of factor V Leiden and the 20210A genotype of the prothrombin gene has also been reported in one patient,[44] and in another patient with a lateral and sagittal sinus thrombosis, protein C deficiency, and mastoiditis.[55] Both examples emphasize a comprehensive search into underlying thrombophilia.

Magnetic resonance imaging and magnetic resonance angiography have become the standard imaging tests and have reduced the need for conventional cerebral angiography.[51,62,74] The combination of spin-echo T2-weighted sequences[66] and two-dimensional time of flight (2DTOF) probably is the most sensitive technique. The 2DTOF images may better visualize the deeper venous structures; spin-echo sequences clearly image the parenchymal lesions but also differentiate a thrombus from an artifact. The T1 images may demonstrate the lack of flow void in the sinuses, and the T2 images may show abnormal periventricular and thalamic signals that most likely represent increased interstitial edema or may show an intracerebral hematoma with surrounding edema. The thrombus is initially isointense on T1-weighted and hypointense on T2-weighted images but 1 to 2 weeks after onset becomes hyperintense in both images. An example of cerebral venous thrombosis on MRI is shown in Figure 15–3.

Magnetic resonance venography (2DTOF) is useful in the diagnosis and assessment of the propagation of cerebral sinus thrombosis. However, hypoplastic nondominant transverse sinuses (commonly left) may appear as an artifactual flow gap, a finding that should not be interpreted as thrombosis without clear clinical features[4] (Fig. 15–4A). In addition, not all veins are identified on current 2DTOF sequences. Using 2DTOF technology, one study in 100 normal controls found the inferior sagittal sinus in only 52%, occipital sinus in 10%, vein of Rosenthal in 91%, vein of Trolard in 37%, and vein of Labbé in 91% on the right and 96% on the left.[4] An example of the diagnostic capability of magnetic resonance venography is shown in Figure 15–4B.

Diffusion-weighted imaging with echoplanar imaging has been studied more recently.[74] Diffusion-weighted MRI may discriminate between vasogenic and cytotoxic edema, but it is not clear whether this distinction contributes to prognosis.[15,50] Cytotoxic edema is a common radiologic finding early in the course of cerebral venous thrombosis.[28] Decreased apparent diffusion coefficient values suggest cellular edema, and increased values suggest vasogenic edema. However, in a small study, reduced apparent diffusion coefficient values did not correlate with later development of infarction.[22]

Computed tomography scanning is inferior to MRI in sensitivity, and findings are normal in 50% of patients,[3,33,49] but it may nevertheless show hemorrhagic cerebral infarction, decreased ventricular size as a consequence of diffuse edema, or compression of the ventricles from swelling in the thalamus. Diffuse edema may be difficult to appreciate in young patients, whose sulci often are poorly visualized on CT scans. The "empty triangle sign" (thrombosis in the sagittal or straight sinus) after contrast administration is not often present but remains a classic CT imaging sign.[68] The cord sign (hyperdense superficial lesion that may represent a thrombosed cortical vein) may be seen as well, usually close to the bone structures (Fig. 15–5).

Cerebral angiography is not necessary if MRI and magnetic resonance angiography have demonstrated cerebral venous sinus thrombosis. Cerebral angiography with careful studies of the venous phase remains important in patients with a high clinical likelihood of thrombosis and equivocal MRI findings, but the procedure has become more important in

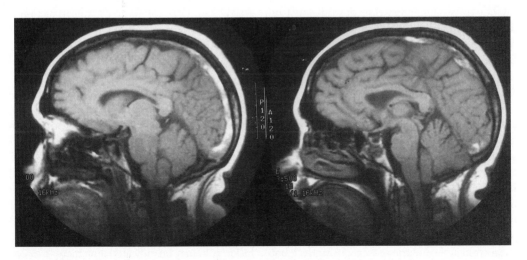

Figure 15–3. Magnetic resonance images of the brain showing clot in superior sagittal sinus thrombosis.

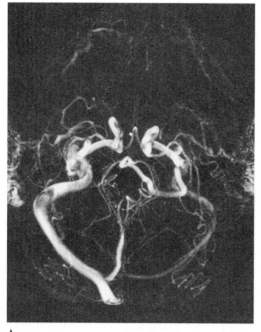

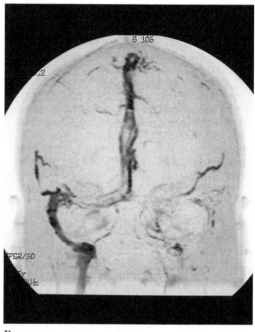

A   B

Figure 15–4. Magnetic resonance venography. (*A*) Hypoplastic transverse sinus with a flow gap mimicking transverse sinus thrombosis (often the length of the flow gap is one-third the length of the ipsilateral sinus). (*B*) Extensive clot in the superior sagittal sinus and both transverse sinuses but with partial recanalization. No flow in the left transverse sinus.

patients for whom neuroradiologic intervention is considered.

Examination of the cerebrospinal fluid could exclude an inflammatory disorder but must be deferred in patients with progression to hemorrhagic infarction and brain shift. The cerebrospinal fluid pressure is typically abnormal and often increased, with values of more than 200 mm H_2O.

Transcranial Doppler ultrasonography has shown a fairly typical pattern of a prominent venous signal with a high amplitude bilaterally. Insonation uses the transtemporal and transorbital approaches (Chapter 11), and the basal vein of Rosenthal is insonated posteriorly.[69,72] Normal mean venous values are 11 ± 2 cm/second in the deep middle cerebral vein, 10 ± 2 cm/second in the basal vein of Rosenthal, and 27 ± 17 cm/second in the anterior cavernous sinus,[69] but they are highly variable. It may also show increased drainage to cavernous sinus and deep cerebral veins, flow reversal in basal veins, and reversed flow in transverse sinus.[65] It may be a useful device for monitoring the effect of anticoagulation (Fig. 15–6), and early reduction of velocities or normalization within 90 days indicates favorable outcome.[64]

FIRST STEPS IN MANAGEMENT

Initial management in patients with cerebral venous thrombosis is largely supportive with prompt anticoagulation (Table 15–2).

Most patients can adequately protect the airway, and endotracheal intubation is indicated only for those with developing cerebral edema. Patients with cerebral venous thrombosis are at risk for pulmonary embolism, and a ventilation-perfusion scan may be indicated if an increased alveolar-arterial gradient and hypoxemia intervene.

Fluid intake is important because it is pos-

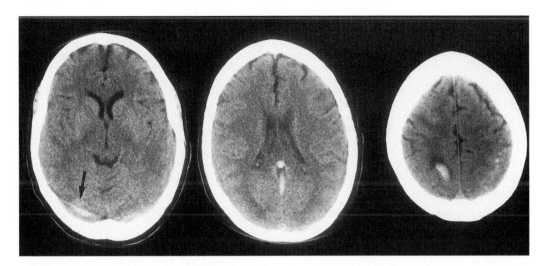

Figure 15–5. Computed tomography scans of hemorrhagic infarction associated with cerebral venous thrombosis and the cord sign (*arrow*).

sible that dehydration may increase the risk of further clot extension. Certainly, patients with an infectious trigger for cerebral venous thrombosis should receive a fluid bolus with albumin 5% or increased intake of crystalloids to ensure adequate fluid status. The danger of fluid overload is of much less concern in these patients, who are often young and previously healthy.

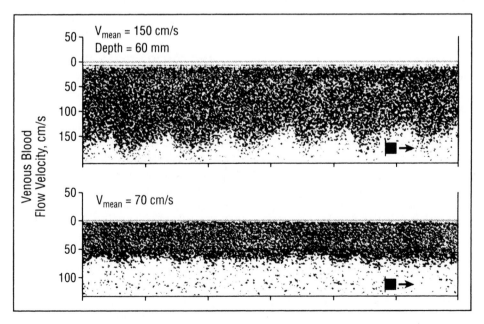

Figure 15–6. Venous transcranial Doppler ultrasonography reveals mean venous blood flow velocities (V_{mean}) of 150 cm/second (*top*) that decreased to a plateau of about 70 cm/second within 4 days of anticoagulation therapy (*bottom*). *Arrows* indicate flow away from the probe. (From Valdueza et al.[69] By permission of the American Medical Association.)

Table 15–2. Initial Management in Cerebral Venous Thrombosis

Airway management	Intubation for progressive drowsiness
	Ventilation-perfusion scan if increased alveolar-arterial gradient and hypoxemia
Fluid management	Rapid hydration with albumin 5%
	Fluid intake, 3 L of 0.9% NaCl
Intracranial pressure management	Propofol (up to 5 mg/kg/h infusion) in diffuse cerebral edema or infarction when increased ICP
	Hyperventilation to P_{CO_2} of 30 mm Hg
Specific treatment	Heparin, 10,000-U infusion, activated partial thromboplastin time two times control
	Thrombolysis or snare catheter disruption if medical management fails
	Fenestration can be considered if papilledema is present

ICP, intracranial pressure.

Anticoagulation is the standard therapy in any patient with cerebral venous thrombosis. In patients with CT evidence of either cerebral ischemia or hemorrhagic conversion of the infarcts, heparin remains indicated. In a randomized trial of anticoagulation in cerebral venous thrombosis, outcome also improved in patients with intracranial hematomas.[23] Overall outcome in anticoagulated patients was significantly better than that in the placebo group. In two retrospective studies of patients with moderate-sized hematomas, anticoagulation was not associated with increased hemorrhage volume, neurologic deterioration, or worse outcome. Both studies suggested that deterioration from intracerebral hematoma was related more to untreated progression of the disease than to worsening by anticoagulation.[26,73]

Heparin administration begins with an infusion of 10,000 units, and the dose is adjusted to achieve an activated partial thromboplastin time that is two times the control value. A weight-based nomogram can also be considered to rapidly achieve full anticoagulation (Chapter 8). Warfarin administration can begin after approximately 5 days of observation. A recent trial concluded that low-molecular-weight heparin followed by warfarin for 3 months did not result in a statistically significant improvement or worsening from placebo results. In this study, 50% of 59 patients had CT or MRI documented cerebral hemorrhage.[18]

Prophylactic administration of antiepileptic medication is hardly justified in adults because of the low incidence of seizures (10% to 15%), most of which are focal.

Corticosteroids are administered only to patients in whom cerebral venous thrombosis is a first manifestation of a collagen vascular disease, Behçet's disease, Crohn's disease, or sarcoidosis. In others, corticosteroids are of no demonstrated benefit in reducing cerebral edema.

Patients with marked papilledema are best treated with repeat lumbar punctures, but fenestration of the optic nerve may be needed to reduce the risk of visual loss; surgical complications are few.[5] Serial perimetry may reveal an enlarging blind spot that may guide the decision to proceed.

DETERIORATION: CAUSES AND MANAGEMENT

Clinical neurologic deterioration is probably a consequence of further thrombosis in the venous system. An altered state of consciousness indicates extension of the thrombosis into the tributary cortical veins. An increase in sagittal sinus pressure may result in the formation of hemorrhagic infarction, often bilaterally in the parietal lobes, and an increase in capillary filtration, causing cerebral edema.

Clinical experience with deterioration in cerebral venous thrombosis is small, because most patients remain relatively stable despite development of cerebral infarction. In addition, hemorrhagic cerebral infarcts may be located in the occipital lobes and may not produce a significant mass effect. Monitoring of these patients with serial CT scans is necessary. Deterioration from an enlarging hematoma

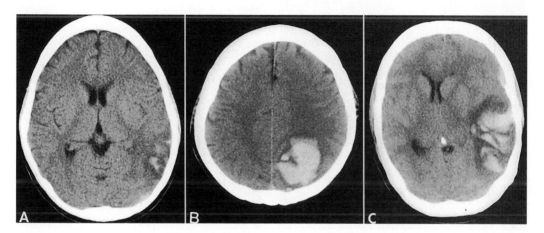

Figure 15–7. Three types of hemorrhagic infarcts and hematoma in cerebral venous thrombosis. (*A*) Small hemorrhages. (*B*) Large parietal lobe hematoma without significant mass effect. (*C*) Large parietal lobe hematoma with swelling and significant shift of midline structures.

with progressive brain stem compression may have to be treated with a craniotomy to evacuate the hematoma. Examples of intracranial hematoma associated with cerebral venous thrombosis are shown in Figure 15–7.

When deterioration occurs despite aggressive use of intravenous heparin, an attempt to lyse the clot with thrombolytic agents is reasonable.[7,41] This practice with an invasive technique is controversial and may not be more beneficial than anticoagulation alone. The bulk of the evidence is drawn from small case studies with different end points (recanalization or clinical improvement). To complicate matters further, patients have recovered from coma with medical management alone.

The timing of endovascular thrombolysis is unresolved. There is some consensus that this treatment should be considered second-line in a patient with deterioration from clot propagation despite adequate intravenous heparinization or use of low-molecular-weight heparin. Inadequate heparinization may be implicated in some patients. Current data on endovascular thrombolysis may be biased toward less severe cases, and in some reports, it is unclear whether the effects of intravenous heparin have been properly evaluated.[48] Worsening intracerebral hematoma in patients treated with urokinase or tPA infusion has been reported in

some series but not in others.[30,37,63] Management remains complex and time-consuming, and complete lysis of a substantial clot may take days.

Endovascular intervention has been successful in a large proportion of patients, including those with pretreatment hemorrhagic infarcts, with lysis of the clot and significant neurologic improvement.[37] A catheter is inserted via puncture of the jugular vein or through the transfemoral route, advanced to the transverse sinus, and, if possible, advanced to the superior sagittal sinus or placed at the torcular Herophili.[25,37,67] tPA is usually infused at 1 mg/min for several hours. Heparin infusion should continue at the regular dose. If no intracranial blood is demonstrated on CT scan after tPA infusion for 12 hours and lysis is still incomplete, the catheter should be repositioned and the procedure continued until complete lysis is achieved.

Several major concerns remain, including treatment in patients with hemorrhagic infarcts, the exact time window, and whether tPA infusion needs to be repeated after a failed or partially failed first attempt. Thrombolysis may seem less successful if the disorder has been present for days, but recanalization can be achieved in patients who had had symptoms for weeks.[37]

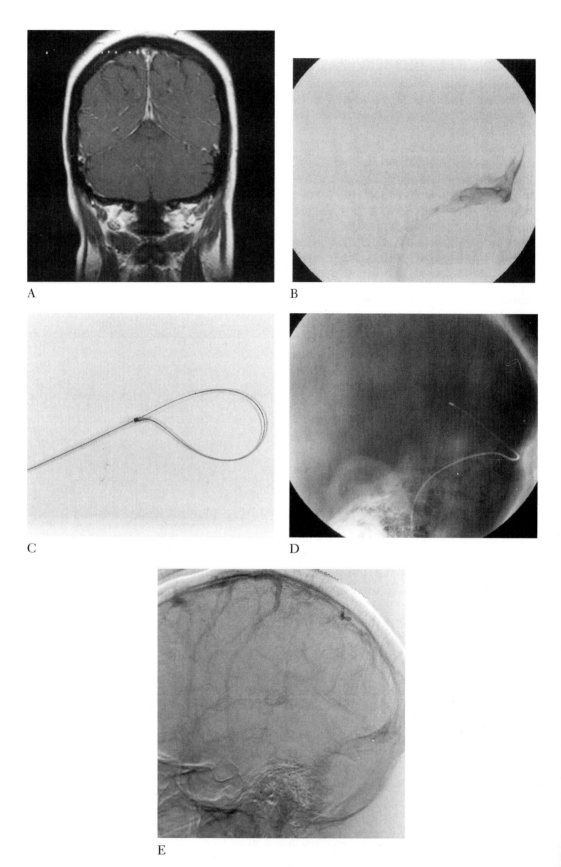

A

B

C

D

E

264

Figure 15–8. Mechanical disruption of intracranial thrombus. (*A*) Coronal gadolinium-enhanced, T1-weighted image in a 35-year-old woman with ulcerative colitis and headache, nausea, and vomiting reveals extensive thrombus and lack of normal enhancement within the superior sagittal, straight, and transverse sinuses. (*B*) Digital subtraction venogram demonstrates extensive filling defect, representing thrombus, within the left transverse sinus and the superior sagittal sinus at the torcula. (*C*) Microsnare used for transvenous clot fragmentation. (*D*) Lateral projection of the skull shows the microsnare within the superior sagittal sinus and a microcatheter (used for thrombolytic infusion) within the straight sinus. (*E*) Venous phase of digital subtraction angiogram after mechanical clot fragmentation and infusion of thrombolytic agent demonstrates flow within the straight, superior sagittal, transverse, and sigmoid sinuses. The sinuses are somewhat irregular, and a small amount of residual thrombus remains within them. (Courtesy of Drs. G. P. Sinson, L. Bagley, and R. Hurst.)

Another option is mechanical disruption of the clot by use of a microsnare or rheolytic thrombectomy catheter. Early experience is promising. Microsnare catheter disruption may seem less cumbersome, and in the initial experience from the University of Pennsylvania School of Medicine, microsnare maceration in two patients with thrombus refractory to urokinase infusion resulted in patency[52] (Fig. 15–8). Another device, the rheolytic thrombectomy catheter, has been used in other disorders, such as occlusion of coronary and peripheral arteries. High-pressure saline jets macerate the thrombus, which is then aspirated into the catheter. Major limitations for use in cerebral venous thrombosis are bulky size, difficult navigation, and inability to advance beyond Galen's vein.[14,21,59]

Patients with progressive cerebral edema become progressively drowsy, fail to localize pain, and cannot protect the airway. After endotracheal intubation and mechanical ventilation, hyperventilation (PCO_2 of approximately 30 mm Hg) can be tried. Patients with multiple hemorrhagic infarcts or progressive cerebral edema may not be successfully treated with osmotic agents. The blood-brain barrier may be defective at several locations, and an osmotic agent may be drawn into the brain with the theoretical potential for further worsening. Treatment of increased intracranial pressure should be guided by values obtained by fiberoptic monitoring. Propofol infusion (1 to 5 mg/kg per hour) may be a very useful alternative way to treat intracranial pressure, but experience is limited.

As a last resort, cerebral blood flow can be reduced by barbiturates if propofol fails to reduce intracranial pressure. Barbiturate coma can effectively reduce intracranial pressure in this situation. A report of successful management in two patients by administration of high doses of pentobarbital has been published,[35] but there is very little recent experience. Barbiturate coma can be continued for at least 1 week, and improvement on CT scans or MRI may guide timing of tapering the barbiturate dose.

Patients with cerebral venous thrombosis may have sudden deterioration from pulmonary emboli. This was noted in 11% of 203 patients reported in the literature, with a 95% mortality.[19] Emboli may originate from the thrombosed jugular veins rather than, for example, from deep venous thrombosis associated with immobilization.

OUTCOME

Because the disorder is infrequent, series of patients with cerebral venous thrombosis have been small, and the prognosis may be determined by underlying disease. Cerebral sinus thrombosis is caused by direct destruction and invasion of malignant cells in some patients; in others, cerebral venous thrombosis is related to coagulopathy from hematologic malignant disease or infection. A recent review from Memorial Sloan-Kettering Cancer Center documented a 0.3% incidence of cerebral sinus thrombosis in cancer patients seen in consultation.[54] Notable features were involvement of multiple veins, more than one contributing factor, such as dural metastasis and antiestrogen therapy, but good clinical neurologic recovery with anticoagulation.

In a review of 103 cases reported in the literature before anticoagulation was recommended, only 14 of 66 patients (21%) with complete sagittal sinus thrombosis survived. Outcome was significantly better in patients with only partial occlusion. Early diagnosis (and thus treatment) appears to influence outcome, and mortality decreases when the diagnosis is made within 1 week of symptoms.[60]

In a series of patients after the introduction of anticoagulation who were usually treated with heparin, outcome was considerably better, with a mortality of 10% but persistent neurologic deficits in approximately 20% of the patients.[2] Coma at presentation or its development during hospitalization, seizures, or underlying disease has no effect on short-term outcome, and thus these features should not preclude any type of therapeutic intervention. Morbidity in cerebral venous thrombosis can be devastating and may include akinetic mutism, blindness from optic atrophy, and ataxia.[53] Bilateral thalamic infarcts may cause marked memory impairment and hypersomnia, but improvement has been reported.[29] Long-term cognitive impairment seems prevalent, with nearly half the patients not returning to the workforce.[16]

Long-term outcome is most likely worse in patients with coma (Glasgow coma scale score < 8) and involvement of superior sagittal and straight sinuses on magnetic resonance venography or angiography, but recovery can be observed in exceptional cases.[10,17] Another follow-up study (77 patients) emphasized good recovery in 86% and a very low (4%) incidence of epilepsy, but altered consciousness was an infrequent presentation.[53] Recurrent seizures usually appeared within 1 year, not unexpectedly more often in patients who presented with seizures. Long-term antiepileptic therapy (> 1 year) is not indicated. An outcome algorithm is shown in Figure 15–9.

When evaluation for possible causes of cerebral venous thrombosis has been repeatedly negative and the cerebral venous system has recanalized and no other systemic clotting sites have appeared on MRI, administration of warfarin could be discontinued. Some investigators have continued anticoagulation for 12 months when venous occlusion was still detectable on MRI at follow-up. Recurrence is unusual, affecting fewer than 10% of patients without underlying systemic illness.[53] Long-term follow-up in patients with specific congenital thrombophilia is not available, but one study of cerebral venous thrombosis and factor V Leiden mutation suggested an increased risk of pulmonary emboli and deep venous thrombosis but not cerebral venous thrombosis.[45] Recurrence of puerperal thrombosis has not been reported, most likely because patients

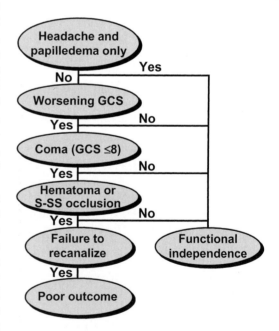

Figure 15–9. Outcome algorithm for cerebral venous thrombosis. GCS, Glasgow coma scale score; S-SS, sagittal-straight sinus. Functional independence: no assistance needed, minor handicap may remain. Poor outcome: severe disability or death, vegetative state.

have been advised against future pregnancies. However, pregnancies in 12 patients with a history of cerebral venous thrombosis not related to pregnancy were without complications.[53] One patient with prior puerperal thrombosis

treated with heparin for 3 weeks before delivery and anticoagulation for 3 months postpartum did not have a relapse.[70] Coverage with low-molecular-weight heparin around the time of delivery seems an appropriate measure.

CONCLUSIONS

- MRI and magnetic resonance venography remain the preferred diagnostic tests. Cerebral angiography should be performed if thrombolysis is considered.
- Management consists of rehydration, rapid anticoagulation with heparin to an activated partial thromboplastin time of two times the control value, and control of intracranial pressure in comatose patients.
- Intravenous administration of heparin should be continued in patients with hemorrhagic infarcts or hematomas without mass effect.
- Increased intracranial pressure can be controlled by hyperventilation (diffuse edema or bilateral cerebral infarcts), propofol, or barbiturates.
- Pulmonary emboli should be considered as a cause of deterioration.

REFERENCES

1. Achiron A, Gornish M, Melamed E: Cerebral sinus thrombosis as a potential hazard of antifibrinolytic treatment in menorrhagia. *Stroke* 21:817–819, 1990.
2. Ameri A, Bousser MG: Cerebral venous thrombosis. *Neurol Clin* 10:87–111, 1992.
3. Anxionnat R, Blanchet B, Dormont D, et al: Present status of computerized tomography and angiography in the diagnosis of cerebral thrombophlebitis cavernous sinus thrombosis excluded. *J Neuroradiol* 21:59–71, 1994.
4. Ayanzen RH, Bird CR, Keller PJ, et al: Cerebral MR venography: normal anatomy and potential diagnostic pitfalls. *AJNR Am J Neuroradiol* 21:74–78, 2000.
5. Banta JT, Farris BK: Pseudotumor cerebri and optic nerve sheath decompression. *Ophthalmology* 107:1907–1912, 2000.
6. Baumgartner RW, Landis T: Venous thalamic infarction. *Cerebrovasc Dis* 2:353–358, 1992.
7. Benamer HT, Bone I: Cerebral venous thrombosis: Anticoagulants or thrombolytic therapy? *J Neurol Neurosurg Psychiatry* 69:427–430, 2000.
8. Biousse V, Conard J, Brouzes C, et al: Frequency of the 20210 G → A mutation in the 3'-untranslated region of the prothrombin gene in 35 cases of cerebral venous thrombosis. *Stroke* 29:1398–1400, 1998.
9. Bloem BR, van Putten MJ, van der Meer FJ, et al: Superior sagittal sinus thrombosis in a patient heterozygous for the novel 20210 A allele of the prothrombin gene. *Thromb Haemost* 79:235, 1998.
10. Bousser MG: Cerebral venous thrombosis: diagnosis and management. *J Neurol* 247:252–258, 2000.
11. Bousser MG, Chiras J, Bories J, et al: Cerebral venous thrombosis—a review of 38 cases. *Stroke* 16:199–213, 1985.
12. Carhuapoma JR, Mitsias P, Levine SR: Cerebral venous thrombosis and anticardiolipin antibodies. *Stroke* 28:2363–2369, 1997.
13. Case records of the Massachusetts General Hospital. *N Engl J Med* 346:1651–1658, 2002.
14. Chow K, Gobin YP, Saver J, et al: Endovascular treatment of dural sinus thrombosis with rheolytic thrombectomy and intra-arterial thrombolysis. *Stroke* 31:1420–1425, 2000.
15. Chu K, Kang D-W, Yoon B-W, et al: Diffusion-weighted magnetic resonance in cerebral venous thrombosis. *Arch Neurol* 58:1569–1576, 2001
16. de Bruijn SF, Budde M, Teunisse S, et al: Long-term outcome of cognition and functional health after cerebral venous sinus thrombosis. *Neurology* 54:1687–1689, 2000.
17. de Bruijn SF, de Haan RJ, Stam J: Clinical features and prognostic factors of cerebral venous sinus thrombosis in a prospective series of 59 patients. For The Cerebral Venous Sinus Thrombosis Study Group. *J Neurol Neurosurg Psychiatry* 70:105–108, 2001.
18. de Bruijn SF, Stam J: Randomized, placebo-controlled trial of anticoagulant treatment with low-molecular-weight heparin for cerebral sinus thrombosis. *Stroke* 30:484–488, 1999.
19. Diaz JM, Schiffman JS, Urban ES, et al: Superior sagittal sinus thrombosis and pulmonary embolism: a syndrome rediscovered. *Acta Neurol Scand* 86:390–396, 1992.
20. Doberson MJ, Kleinschmidt-DeMasters BK: Superior

sagittal sinus thrombosis in a patient with acquired immunodeficiency syndrome. *Arch Pathol Lab Med* 118: 844–846, 1994.

21. Dowd CF, Malek AM, Phatouros CC, et al: Application of a rheolytic thrombectomy device in the treatment of dural sinus thrombosis: a new technique. *AJNR Am J Neuroradiol* 20:568–570, 1999.

22. Ducreux D, Oppenheim C, Vandamme X, et al: Diffusion-weighted imaging patterns of brain damage associated with cerebral venous thrombosis. *AJNR Am J Neuroradiol* 22:261–268, 2001.

23. Einhaupl KM, Villringer A, Meister W, et al: Heparin treatment in sinus venous thrombosis. *Lancet* 338: 597–600, 1991.

24. Enevoldson TP, Russell RW: Cerebral venous thrombosis: New causes for an old syndrome? *Q J Med* 77: 1255–1275, 1990.

25. Eskridge JM, Wessbecher FW: Thrombolysis for superior sagittal sinus thrombosis. *J Vasc Interv Radiol* 2:89–93, 1991.

26. Fink JN, McAuley DL: Safety of anticoagulation for cerebral venous thrombosis associated with intracerebral hematoma. *Neurology* 57:1138–1139, 2001.

27. Floyd WL, Mahaley MS: Cerebral dural venous sinus thrombosis following cardiac pacemaker implantation. *Arch Intern Med* 124:368–372, 1969.

28. Forbes KP, Pipe JG, Heiserman JE: Evidence for cytotoxic edema in the pathogenesis of cerebral venous infarction. *AJNR Am J Neuroradiol* 22:450–455, 2001.

29. Forsting M, Krieger D, Seier U, et al: Reversible bilateral thalamic lesions caused by primary internal cerebral vein thrombosis: a case report. *J Neurol* 236: 484–486, 1989.

30. Frey JL, Muro GJ, McDougall CG, et al: Cerebral venous thrombosis: combined intrathrombus rtPA and intravenous heparin. *Stroke* 30:489–494, 1999.

31. Galan HL, McDowell AB, Johnson PR, et al: Puerperal cerebral venous thrombosis associated with decreased free protein S: a case report. *J Reprod Med* 40:859–862, 1995.

32. Girard DE, Reuler JB, Mayer BS, et al: Cerebral venous sinus thrombosis due to indwelling transvenous pacemaker catheter. *Arch Neurol* 37:113–114, 1980.

33. Goldberg AL, Rosenbaum AE, Wang H, et al: Computed tomography of dural sinus thrombosis. *J Comput Assist Tomogr* 10:16–20, 1986.

34. Haley EC Jr, Brashear HR, Barth JT, et al: Deep cerebral venous thrombosis. Clinical, neuroradiological, and neuropsychological correlates. *Arch Neurol* 46: 337–340, 1989.

35. Hanley DF, Feldman E, Borel CO, et al: Treatment of sagittal sinus thrombosis associated with cerebral hemorrhage and intracranial hypertension. *Stroke* 19: 903–909, 1988.

36. Hesselbrock R, Sawaya R, Tomsick T, et al: Superior sagittal sinus thrombosis after closed head injury. *Neurosurgery* 16:825–828, 1985.

37. Horowitz M, Purdy P, Unwin H, et al: Treatment of

dural sinus thrombosis using selective catheterization and urokinase. *Ann Neurol* 38:58–67, 1995.

38. Hotton KM, Khorsand M, Hank JA, et al: A phase Ib/II trial of granulocyte-macrophage-colony stimulating factor and interleukin-2 for renal cell carcinoma patients with pulmonary metastases: a case of fatal central nervous system thrombosis. *Cancer* 88:1892–1901, 2000.

39. Imai WK, Everhart FR Jr, Sanders JM Jr: Cerebral venous sinus thrombosis: report of a case and review of the literature. *Pediatrics* 70:965–970, 1982.

40. Kalbag RM, Woolf AL: Thrombosis and thrombophlebitis of cerebral veins and dural sinuses. In Vinken PJ, Bruyn GW (eds): *Handbook of Clinical Neurology*. Vol 12. Amsterdam: North-Holland Publishing Company, 1972, pp 422–446.

41. Kim SY, Suh JH: Direct endovascular thrombolytic therapy for dural sinus thrombosis: infusion of alteplase. *AJNR Am J Neuroradiol* 18:639–645, 1997.

42. Kuehnen J, Schwartz A, Neff W, et al: Cranial nerve syndrome in thrombosis of the transverse/sigmoid sinuses. *Brain* 121:381–388, 1998.

43. Larkey D, Williams CR, Fanning J, et al: Fatal superior sagittal sinus thrombosis associated with internal jugular vein catheterization. *Am J Obstet Gynecol* 169: 1612–1614, 1993.

44. Liu XY, Gabig TG, Bang NU: Combined heterozygosity of factor V Leiden and the G20210A prothrombin gene mutation in a patient with cerebral cortical vein thrombosis. *Am J Hematol* 64:226–228, 2000.

45. Ludemann P, Nabavi DG, Junker R, et al: Factor V Leiden mutation is a risk factor for cerebral venous thrombosis: a case-control study of 55 patients. *Stroke* 29:2507–2510, 1998.

46. Martinelli I, Sacchi E, Landi G, et al: High risk of cerebral-vein thrombosis in carriers of a prothrombin-gene mutation and in users of oral contraceptives. *N Engl J Med* 338:1793–1797, 1998.

47. Murray BJ, Llinas R, Caplan LR, et al: Cerebral deep venous thrombosis presenting as acute micrographia and hypophonia. *Neurology* 54:751–753, 2000.

48. Novak Z, Coldwell DM, Brega KE: Selective infusion of urokinase and thrombectomy in the treatment of acute cerebral sinus thrombosis. *AJNR Am J Neuroradiol* 21:143–145, 2000.

49. Nussel F, Huber P: High resolution computed tomography of superior sagittal sinus–thrombosis and abnormalities. *Neuroradiology* 31:307–311, 1989.

50. Peeters E, Stadnik T, Bissay F, et al: Diffusion-weighted MR imaging of an acute venous stroke: case report. *AJNR Am J Neuroradiol* 22:1949–1952, 2001.

51. Perkin GD: Cerebral venous thrombosis: developments in imaging and treatment (editorial). *J Neurol Neurosurg Psychiatry* 59:1–3, 1995.

52. Philips MF, Bagley LJ, Sinson GP, et al: Endovascular thrombolysis for symptomatic cerebral venous thrombosis. *J Neurosurg* 90:65–71, 1999.

53. Preter M, Tzourio C, Ameri A, et al: Long-term prog-

nosis in cerebral venous thrombosis: follow-up of 77 patients. *Stroke* 27:243–246, 1996.

54. Raizer JJ, DeAngelis LM: Cerebral sinus thrombosis diagnosed by MRI and MR venography in cancer patients. *Neurology* 54:1222–1226, 2000.

55. Ram B, Meiklejohn DJ, Nunez DA, et al: Combined risk factors contributing to cerebral venous thrombosis in a young woman. *J Laryngol Otol* 115:307–310, 2001.

56. Reuner KH, Ruf A, Grau A, et al: Prothrombin gene G20210 → A transition is a risk factor for cerebral venous thrombosis. *Stroke* 29:1765–1769, 1998.

57. Rother J, Waggie K, van Bruggen N, et al: Experimental cerebral venous thrombosis: evaluation using magnetic resonance imaging. *J Cereb Blood Flow Metab* 16:1353–1361, 1996.

58. Saxena VK, Heilpern J, Murphy SF: Pseudotumor cerebri. A complication of parenteral hyperalimentation. *JAMA* 235:2124, 1976.

59. Scarrow AM, Williams RL, Jungreis CA, et al: Removal of a thrombus from the sigmoid and transverse sinuses with a rheolytic thrombectomy catheter. *AJNR Am J Neuroradiol* 20:1467–1469, 1999.

60. Schell CL, Rathe RJ: Superior sagittal sinus thrombosis. Still a killer. *West J Med* 149:304–307, 1988.

61. Seligsohn U, Lubetsky A: Genetic susceptibility to venous thrombosis. *N Engl J Med* 344:1222–1231, 2001.

62. Selim M, Fink J, Linfante I, et al: Diagnosis of cerebral venous thrombosis with echo-planar T2-weighted magnetic resonance imaging. *Arch Neurol* 59:1021–1026, 2002.

63. Spearman MP, Jungreis CA, Wehner JJ, et al: Endovascular thrombolysis in deep cerebral venous thrombosis. *AJNR Am J Neuroradiol* 18:502–506, 1997.

64. Stolz E, Gerriets T, Bodeker RH, et al: Intracranial venous hemodynamics is a factor related to a favorable outcome in cerebral venous thrombosis. *Stroke* 33:1645–1650, 2002.

65. Stolz E, Kemkes-Matthes B, Potzsch B, et al: Screening for thrombophilic risk factors among 25 German patients with cerebral venous thrombosis. *Acta Neurol Scand* 102:31–36, 2000.

66. Sze G, Simmons B, Krol G, et al: Dural sinus thrombosis: verification with spin-echo techniques. *AJNR Am J Neuroradiol* 9:679–686, 1988.

67. Tsai FY, Higashida RT, Matovich V, et al: Acute thrombosis of the intracranial dural sinus: direct thrombolytic treatment. *AJNR Am J Neuroradiol* 13:1137–1141, 1992.

68. Ulmer JL, Elster AD: Physiologic mechanisms underlying the delayed delta sign. *AJNR Am J Neuroradiol* 12:647–650, 1991.

69. Valdueza JM, Hoffmann O, Weih M, et al: Monitoring of venous hemodynamics in patients with cerebral venous thrombosis by transcranial Doppler ultrasound. *Arch Neurol* 56:229–234, 1999.

70. van der Stege JG, Engelen MJ, van Eyck J: Uncomplicated pregnancy and puerperium after puerperal cerebral venous thrombosis. *Eur J Obstet Gynecol Reprod Biol* 71:99–100, 1997.

71. Villringer A, Bousser M-G, Einhäupl KM: Cerebral sinus venous thrombosis. In Hacke W, Hanley DF, Einhäupl KM, et al (eds): *Neurocritical Care*. Berlin: Springer-Verlag, 1994, pp 654–660.

72. Wardlaw JM, Vaughan GT, Steers AJ, et al: Transcranial Doppler ultrasound findings in cerebral venous sinus thrombosis. Case report. *J Neurosurg* 80:332–335, 1994.

73. Wingerchuk DM, Wijdicks EFM, Fulgham JR: Cerebral venous thrombosis complicated by hemorrhagic infarction: factors affecting the initiation and safety of anticoagulation. *Cerebrovasc Dis* 8:25–30, 1998.

74. Yoshikawa T, Abe O, Tsuchiya K, et al: Diffusion-weighted magnetic resonance imaging of dural sinus thrombosis. *Neuroradiology* 44:481–488, 2002.

75. Yuh WT, Simonson TM, Wang AM, et al: Venous sinus occlusive disease: MR findings. *AJNR Am J Neuroradiol* 15:309–316, 1994.

16

Acute Middle Cerebral Artery Occlusion

In terms of severity and proclivity for clinical deterioration, a large hemispheric stroke due to occlusion of the main arterial tributary is generally recognized as one of the major neurologic critical illnesses. The arterial occlusion may involve the stem or one of the larger branches of the middle cerebral artery (MCA).

Although many neurologists are appreciably complacent about therapeutic interventions in patients with a massive stroke in whom expectations for functional recovery seem low, aggressive management in selected patients may result in a very reasonable outcome. This may include use of thrombolytic agents in patients with hypoperfused but viable tissue. In others, decompressive craniotomy or induction of hypothermia in massive cerebral swelling may be required in appropriate circumstances.

Absolute admission criteria to the NICU are early CT scan abnormalities (e.g., hyperdense MCA sign and sulcal effacement), seizures at presentation, cardiac arrhythmia or new electrocardiographic abnormality, possible failure to adequately protect the upper airway, or evidence of pulmonary aspiration.

CLINICAL RECOGNITION

The distinguishing clinical findings of a large infarct in the territory of the MCA are hemianopia, facial palsy with a marked asymmetrical grimacing to pain, hemiplegia of the arm with less significant hemiparesis of the leg,

hemianesthesia, and preferential direction of the eyes and head toward the side of the involved hemisphere. Involvement of the upper division of the MCA produces aphasia when the infarction is located in the dominant hemisphere and results in unilateral neglect when it is located in the nondominant hemisphere. Failure of the patient to recognize the paralyzed left body parts may result in a long delay before the stroke is discovered. Occasionally, patients fall and are not able to stand up from the floor. In others, a compartment syndrome with rhabdomyolysis from prolonged muscle compression may appear.

Patients may appear indifferent and inert from frontal lobe or caudate nucleus involvement.[33] Lack of concern (anosodiaphoria) is more common in nondominant lesions. However, the level of consciousness is normal unless swelling supervenes. Elderly patients can become less alert from dehydration alone, which can easily occur if they are unable to signal thirst. Other triggers for dehydration—a fairly constant observation during the initial encounter—are diuretics and poor oral fluid intake.[69] Other causes of drowsiness are marked hypoxemia due to aspiration and seizures at presentation. Seizures are infrequent in patients with a large ischemic stroke; if they occur, they are usually observed within days of presentation and are focal.[63] Complex partial seizures and progression of a single generalized tonic-clonic seizure to status epilepticus are not common. Brief loss of consciousness is very unusual but may implicate a cardiac source for stroke (e.g., transient atrial fibrillation with marked hypotension). Delirium or agitated confusion can decrease the level of consciousness and seems more frequent in patients with right hemispheric lesions. However, a patient with newly developing agitation soon after admission may, in fact, have a drug- or alcohol-withdrawal syndrome. (The potential causes of delirium have been further described in Chapter 4.)

Patients with a dominant MCA territory stroke usually have profound aphasia and may vocalize only single, distorted words. Comprehension is significantly impaired. Improvement to a less profound aphasia with some recovery of comprehension and grammatical order is possible in the first week.

In a nondominant large hemispheric stroke, spatial neglect is the major clinical feature. Denial of hemiplegia (anosognosia), flat affect, speech without much modulation in intonation (aprosody), and motor impersistence may be observed. Bilateral ptosis is typical in large nondominant hemispheric infarcts.[2] It is an underrecognized sign, mistaken for drowsiness. We and others have noted bilateral complete ptosis as the first sign of imminent herniation, preceding pupillary dilation in some patients (Fig. 16–1). In others, ptosis improved with resolving edema on CT scan.

Eye deviation indicates involvement of a large territory, is more frequent in patients with right-sided infarcts of the brain, and possibly is also related to neglect of the left side of the body. However, the volume of infarcted tissue is larger in patients with a conjugate eye deviation associated with an infarct in the left hemisphere.[65] Homonymous hemianopia is invariably present, and an asymmetrical blink re-

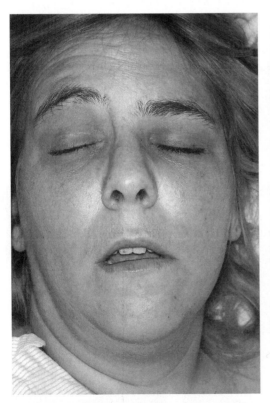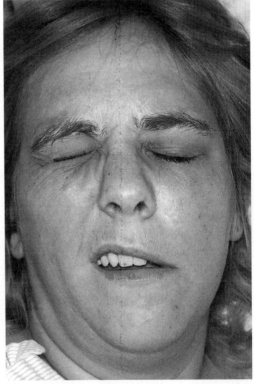

Figure 16–1. Patient with acute right-sided carotid occlusion and bilateral ptosis. Note asymmetric eyelid closure and facial asymmetry. Hours after this photo was taken, patient fatally deteriorated from massive cerebral edema unresponsive to decompressive craniotomy and hypothermia.

sponse is usually elicited by a rapidly approaching hand. Pupils are usually equal in size. New pupillary asymmetry and a blunted pupillary light response when observed together with drowsiness must be considered important early signs of brain swelling.[53] Unilateral miosis from Horner's syndrome due to damage to the sympathetic terminals in the carotid sheath may be evident and could indicate an acute carotid occlusion or dissection.[29,39] Additional involvement of lower cranial nerves (IX, X, XII) in patients with an acute ischemic stroke should also point to possible carotid dissection. Carotid dissection is almost certain when Horner's syndrome and tongue paresis with deviation to the involved side on protrusion are found. Displacement of the parapharyngeal space close to the internal carotid artery may compress these cranial nerves.[38,55,64]

Asymmetrical facial grimacing spontaneously or to pain can involve all facial muscles and is responsible for a muted corneal reflex. The gag reflex is diminished. The tongue can be markedly involved as well and may rest virtually frozen in the mouth. This could place these patients at considerable risk of aspiration.

Hemiplegia of the upper limb involves complete hypotonic paralysis with some preservation of shoulder shrug. The lower limb is relatively preserved but usually equally affected with large territorial infarction and when it involves the perforating arteries to the internal capsule. Withdrawal to pinprick is diminished.

NEUROIMAGING AND LABORATORY TESTS

In patients with a complete MCA territory infarct, CT scan often shows early subtle abnormalities. As early as several hours after the event, CT findings are effacement of sulci, loss of distinction of the caudate nucleus and lentiform nucleus, and loss of the insular ribbon. The hyperdense MCA sign, which represents the obstructing clot, is a distinctive feature in many patients with occlusion of the MCA stem[66] (Figs. 16–2 and 16–3). When CT scanning is performed within the first 2 hours, it is present in approximately 50% of patients with an occlusion of the MCA trunk.

The CT scan in patients with acute MCA territory infarct can be further categorized by determining the size of the infarct, degree of swelling, and hemorrhagic conversion. An early sizable hypodensity on CT scan predicts the further development of cerebral edema. Different intervals of ictus to CT scan may define different CT predictors for swelling. The likelihood of progressive cerebral edema is 85% if

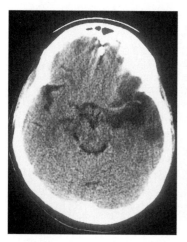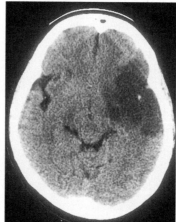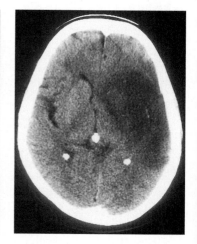

Figure 16–2. Computed tomography scans showing hyperintense middle cerebral artery sign within brain parenchyma hypodense from infarction. Also shown is the dot sign (middle image).

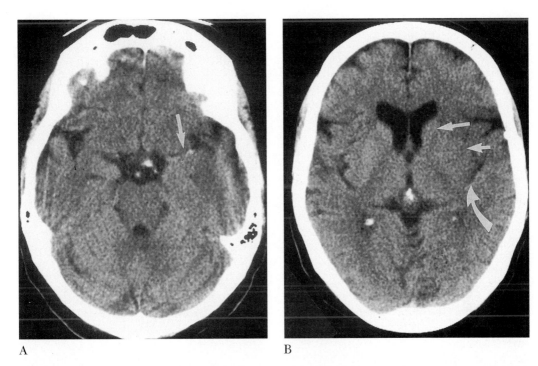

Figure 16–3. Early signs of infarction in computed tomography scans 3 hours after ictus. (*A*) Hyperdense middle cerebral artery sign (*arrow*). (*B*) Caudate nucleus definition (*long arrow*), insular ribbon and lentiform nucleus (*short arrow*), and sylvian fissure (*curved arrow*) are less apparent.

a CT scan performed within 5 hours after onset shows a hypodensity that involves more than 50% of the MCA territory.[31,68] The probability of deterioration is more than 70% when a CT scan done within 24 hours shows at least a combination of hyperdense MCA signs and sulcal effacement.[36] In addition, a significantly higher incidence of hemorrhagic conversion (approximately 70%) is expected in patients with early hypodensity, but many patients do deteriorate clinically.[6]

Follow-up CT scanning within 3 days shows the characteristic triangular shape of the hypodensity, and mass effect may become more apparent with compression of the frontal horn. Patients with a large infarct in the MCA territory may have some scattered petechial hemorrhages, indicating hemorrhagic conversion. The clinical significance of hemorrhagic infarction is uncertain, and MRI studies have found that the phenomenon is more common and often underrecognized by CT scans.

Magnetic resonance imaging is more sensitive in assessment of acute hemispheric infarction. Diffusion-weighted imaging may be very useful in determination of the extent of ischemic injury. Increased signal intensity due to reduction in the apparent diffusion coefficient of water is a marker of tissue loss. Perfusion-weighted images may be complementary, but use in practice is not defined. Preliminary studies have suggested that when a perfusion-weighted lesion exceeds a diffusion-weighted lesion (PWI–DWI mismatch), an ischemic penumbra is present that could be salvaged by thrombolysis. On the other hand, a matching pattern may potentially defer thrombolysis.[45] These techniques, when further evidence of their promise is developed, are quite important but are not readily accessible on a timely basis, not even in large institutions.

Magnetic resonance imaging may show small, scattered infarcts within the MCA territory, a sign of early recanalization. The clinical

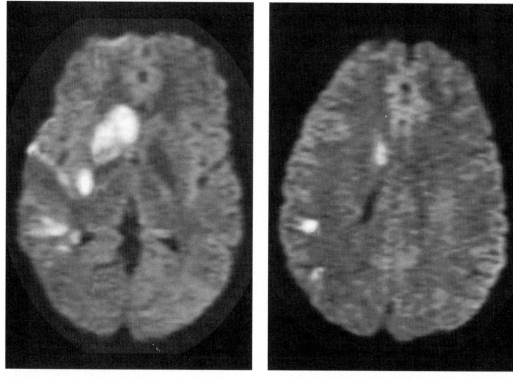

Figure 16–4. Diffusion-weighted images showing scattered abnormalities in a patient with "rapidly shrinking deficit."

correlate frequently is rapid improvement, often to only a fraction of the initial deficit (Fig. 16–4). When carotid dissection is considered, magnetic resonance angiography can be helpful. If carotid dissection has resulted in an occlusion, typical flame-like tapering is seen (Fig. 16–5). The sensitivity for detection of dissection in the carotid system by MRI is approximately 80%.[42,77]

Computed tomography angiography may be a helpful test, because one study found "carotid T occlusion" highly predictive of swelling.[32] These occlusions stagnate flow in the M_1 and A_1 segments and prevent cross-flow to the ischemic MCA territory.

Xenon CT blood flow studies have been published and could be useful. Xenon-enhanced CT documentation of severely reduced cerebral blood flow (mean flow less than 15 mL/100 g/minute) predicted future brain edema but only when the test was performed within 6 hours.[14] The validity of this technique used in combination with CT angiography may be comparable to that of diffusion-weighted imaging.[3] Cerebral blood flow can be rapidly quantified and may also estimate affected volume. Reversible cerebral blood flow was estimated at 7 to 30 mL/100 g per minute, and within this range, patients could still benefit from thrombolytic therapy.[28] Thus, MRI techniques, CT angiography, and xenon CT may become useful imaging determinants of viable tissue and predict swelling. Their value for clinical practice is currently under study.

Transcranial Doppler ultrasonography can demonstrate acute MCA occlusion, and the correlation with cerebral angiography is good. The most characteristic findings of acute MCA occlusion on ultrasonography are lack of flow in this segment and increased velocities in the

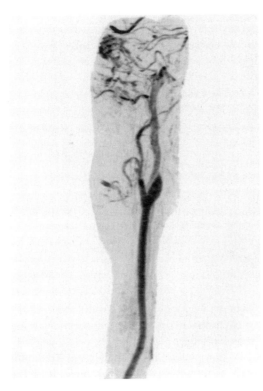

Figure 16–5. Magnetic resonance angiogram showing typical flame-like tapering in carotid dissection.

insonated ipsilateral arteries of the anterior and posterior circulation. The sensitivity for detection of MCA occlusion is 79%, and the specificity is 100%. Transcranial Doppler ultrasonography has potential value in detection of carotid dissections[10] (see Chapter 11 for technique) and in assessing patency after successful intra-arterial thrombolysis.

Evaluation in patients with a large hemispheric infarction must include transesophageal echocardiography. This study is important not only to demonstrate a potential cardiac source or severe disease of the ascending aortic arch but also to provide important information about left ventricular function.

Early cerebral angiography is performed in patients with a large hemispheric stroke who are candidates for intra-arterial thrombolysis (Chapter 8). Later, if a stroke has been estab-

lished, cerebral angiography should be considered if a marked improvement in neurologic function is observed in the following days and ultrasonography of the carotid indicates occlusive carotid artery disease.

The most essential laboratory tests in these patients besides routine hematologic and chemistry studies are a full profile of coagulation abnormalities, blood smear, serial electrocardiography, serum creatine kinase, and troponin (particularly in those with a history of insulin-dependent diabetes, who may have a silent myocardial infarct that triggered a cardioembolic stroke). Blood cultures for 3 consecutive days are indicated when the suspicion of bacterial endocarditis is high. In elderly patients, it is important to determine the ratio of blood urea nitrogen to creatinine. A ratio of 25 or more indicates dehydration.

FIRST STEPS IN MANAGEMENT

The management of patients with large hemispheric ischemia focuses on two main issues: adequate stabilization of a patient with a sudden major deficit and thrombolysis (Table 16–1).

Airway management is important, but many patients do not need endotracheal intubation for airway control. Oxygenation can be secured by 3 L of oxygen through nasal prongs. Elective intubation must be performed in patients who are unable to cough forcefully, are barely localizing to pain, or are stuporous and scheduled to undergo a long catheterization procedure with thrombolysis. Early intubation followed by mechanical ventilation is certainly indicated in patients with poor oxygenation and chest radiographic evidence of aspiration and at times indicated in patients with a series of seizures treated with repeated doses of benzodiazepines.

There is reasonable evidence that increased core body temperature increases ischemia-induced lactate accumulation and has a deleterious effect. Body temperature has been associated with initial stroke severity and mortality, suggesting a causal relationship.[50] Although

Table 16–1. Initial Management in Acute Middle Cerebral Artery Occlusion

Airway	Intubate in patients with early swelling and impaired cough; T piece with pressure support or IMV setting
	3 L of O_2 by nasal prongs
Fluid management	Isotonic saline, 2 L daily
	Rehydrate with 500 mL of saline or albumin
Blood pressure management	No antihypertensive agents unless MAP > 120 mm Hg
Nutrition	Early nutrition preferred
	Pantoprazole, 40 mg intravenously daily if mechanical ventilation or history of gastric ulcers
ICP management	Fiber-optic ICP monitoring in comatose patients with a motor response less than localization to pain and CT confirmation of swelling
	Mannitol bolus of 1 g/kg if increased ICP documented
	Consider decompressive craniotomy in a rapidly deteriorating patient
Specific treatment	Consider intravenous tPA (0.9 mg/kg, 90 mg maximum, 10% as bolus and 90% in 1-hour infusion) when ≤ 3 hr from ictus; consider intra-arterial tPA when 3–6 hours from ictus (if no contraindications)

APTT, activated partial thromboplastin time; CT, computed tomography; ICP, intracranial pressure; IMV, intermittent mandatory ventilation; MAP, mean arterial pressure; tPA, tissue plasminogen activator.

the benefit of fever reduction in any patient with any type of stroke is clinically unproven, core temperature probably should initially be maintained at a point between 36°C and 37°C. Cooling blankets and acetaminophen in high doses (up to 4000 mg/day) may be needed, but two randomized trials found only very little reduction in temperature with these high doses.[13,26]

Patients with a major hemispheric stroke tend to be in a hypovolemic state and display marginal blood pressure readings when seen in the emergency department or the NICU. Hypotension from hypovolemia is often manifested by low systolic blood pressure for age and mild sinus tachycardia but also by an orthostatic pulse increase of 10 to 20 beats/minute. Hypovolemia is almost always incurred during transport if adequate amounts of fluid—beyond an intravenous drip to keep an open venous access—are not provided. A bolus of fluid with 500 mL of saline or albumin is important to correct this volume deficit. Blood pressure could be marginal because of very poor cardiac output from comorbid ischemic cardiomyopathy. If systolic blood pressure remains less than 110 mm Hg despite adequate volume loading, cardiac output can be markedly improved by intermittent administration of dobutamine (2.5 to 10 μg/kg per minute for 48 hours). It could be ineffective in

patients who recently received a β-blocker; in such instances, peripheral vascular resistance may increase.

Maintenance fluid management in patients with acute hemispheric stroke includes 3 L of crystalloids such as isotonic saline. One may consider discontinuing administration of any diuretic agent for 24 hours. Glucose-containing fluids should be avoided, and blood glucose should be closely monitored in the first 2 days of admission and aggressively lowered to strict normoglycemia (glucose 70–100 mL/dL). Hyperglycemia is very often stress-related (values up to 200 mmol/L) and resolves spontaneously. Progression to nonketotic hyperglycemic coma (values up to 1000 mmol/L) is rare and, if present, is associated with marked dehydration.

Hypertension must be left alone in the first 24 hours after hemispheric stroke. Patients may have a marked hypertensive response after stroke, but it is seldom sustained.

Nutrition should not be deferred in patients with a large hemispheric stroke. Pantoprazole is indicated in patients with a history of gastric ulcers or prior use of nonsteroidal anti-inflammatory drugs and in any patient on a mechanical ventilator.

Anticoagulation with heparin in patients with a large hemispheric stroke[9] is problematic because of a true risk of significant hemorrhagic conversion of infarct. However, in one study of massive cerebral infarcts and swelling, hemorrhagic conversion developed in only 4 of 32 fully anticoagulated patients without significant deterioration.[52] Absolute indications are atrial fibrillation, clinical suspicion of myocardial infarction, and a large akinetic segment revealed by echocardiography.[76] In this category of patients, the risk of reembolization has been reported to be up to 21% in the first 3 weeks in patients with any type of acute cardioembolic infarction when anticoagulation is deferred. In patients treated with anticoagulation, recurrences are reduced to less than 3%. This reduction probably is more significant in patients with acute myocardial infarction or with atrial fibrillation and rapid ventricular response. Overcoagulation should be avoided, and the goal should be an activated partial thromboplastin time of 1.5 to 2 times control. If no embolic source is evident, it may be prudent to defer intravenous heparin for several days to reduce hemorrhagic conversion in the first days, a complication that commonly evolves into a massive hematoma with cerebral herniation.

Patients seen within 3 hours after the ictus probably should receive intravenous tissue plasminogen activator (see Chapter 8). Intravenous thrombolysis may also be considered in patients with carotid artery dissection and distal emboli. Initial concerns of extension of intramural hematoma or arterial rupture have not been substantiated in treated patients with a carotid dissection.[1,12] In other patients with acute hemispheric ischemia, the clinician is faced with the logistic problems of intra-arterial thrombolysis that can be successfully performed only within 6 hours. The use of intra-arterial thrombolysis is attractive in MCA stem occlusion and can be very successful, but it takes time to set up a fully staffed neuroradiology suite. Patients seen 3 hours after the event should be considered eligible for intra-arterial thrombolysis, with 1 hour allowed for transport and catheterization. The catheter is advanced by Seldinger techniques, placed inside the clot, and gradually advanced until the clot is dissolved (see also Chapter 8). The MCA perforating branches are visualized first, and then the entire MCA territory is opened (Fig. 16–6). After thrombolysis, the femoral sheath should remain in place to reduce the development of hematoma, but heparinization should be continued.

DETERIORATION: CAUSES AND MANAGEMENT

Deterioration in patients with a large hemispheric stroke most often is caused by brain swelling. Brain swelling occurs, invariably of some degree in patients with complete MCA territory occlusion, usually after a 2- to 7-day interval (median, 4 days).[53,56,60,72]

The pathophysiology of brain edema is complex and may have different explanations. The most striking effect probably is due to reperfusion of already irreversibly damaged brain and could be more common after thrombolytic therapy.[54] The formation of brain edema due to flooding of the infarcted territory may also be facilitated by the generation of reactive oxidants triggered after oxygen is provided to these ischemic parts. The delayed cerebral swelling is more difficult to explain. Cellular edema occurs from influx of water and sodium into the cells (cytotoxic edema phase), and osmotically active particles in the brain (e.g., *myo*-inositol) may contribute. Impairment of the blood–brain barrier follows later, adding more edema (vasogenic edema phase).

Severe new-onset unilateral headache or vomiting may precede progressive drowsiness in patients with brain swelling.[53] As mentioned earlier, an important initial clinical sign of brain swelling is the development of anisocoria (2 mm or more)[53] and bilateral ptosis.[2] Very often, a Cheyne-Stokes breathing pattern changes into sustained hyperventilation,[48] but periodic breathing may follow when coma deepens and must prompt endotracheal intubation and mechanical ventilation. A unilateral fixed, dilated pupil may be observed early, but small and constricted but reactive pupils from downward diencephalic displacement are more common.

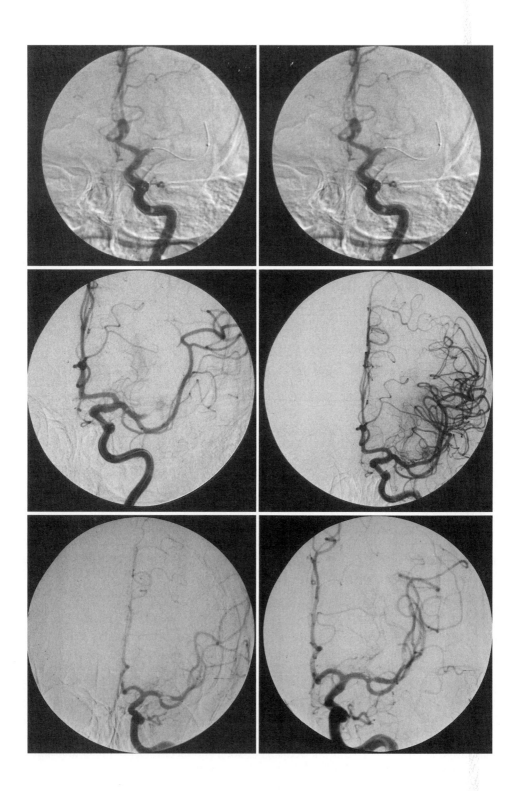

Figure 16–6. Three common clinical courses after intra-arterial thrombolysis in patients with acute middle cerebral artery occlusive disease. All patients had global aphasia and a dense hemiparesis at presentation and received urokinase within 3 hours after the ictus. (*Top row*) Failure to recanalize proximal (M1) occlusion by injection of urokinase through side holes of catheter inside clot. No clinical improvement. Note that the catheter has passed through the clot, which has a jelly-like consistency. (*Middle row*) Successful recanalization of M2 branch of the middle cerebral artery but no clinical improvement. (*Bottom row*) Successful lysis of a proximal (left M2) intraluminal clot, with significant improvement in distal flow and flow in penetrating branches. Patient had an immediate full recovery. We have not yet seen dramatic improvement after urokinase infusion in any patient with a persistent clot. Note that the middle cerebral artery is divided into segments. The M1 segment (sphenoidal) ends in a bifurcation (insular segment) consisting of an inferior branch and a superior branch (the M2 segment).

◄─────────────────────────────

The clinical course usually gradually worsens in most patients over days. However, drowsiness from brain swelling can be transient, and the level of consciousness can improve. Resolution of brain swelling can be documented by serial CT scanning (Fig. 16–7). In other patients, CT scan may show a massive expanding, swollen infarct (Fig. 16–8). This type of rapidly developing edema, termed "'malignant' middle cerebral artery territory infarction,"[17] is much less common than reported.[72]

Measurement of intracranial pressure is important in patients with deterioration from swelling because its value may predict the success of intervention. In two series of patients, persistently increased intracranial pressure (> 15 mm Hg) predicted death.[53] However, in many patients with early deterioration to stupor, intracranial pressure is normal or mildly increased.[15] Clinical deterioration is caused by progressive brain stem distortion both horizontally and vertically, and these pressure differences

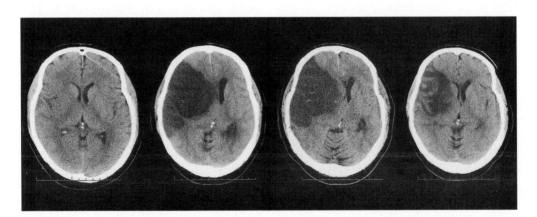

Figure 16–7. Serial computed tomography scans showing the evolution of a middle cerebral artery infarct with brain swelling. From left to right: Admission scan shows effacement of sulci in the entire middle cerebral artery territory of the dominant hemisphere. The lentiform nucleus is effaced. Several days later, a large swollen ischemic mass has developed, with compression of the frontal horn and shift of the septum pellucidum and pineal gland. The posterior horn has enlarged substantially. Without any surgical intervention, marked reduction of the swelling followed. The patient had only brief periods of decreased level of consciousness but continued to localize to pain, occasionally followed commands, and protected his airway. At his last scan, he was alert but had major neglect and flaccid hemiplegia.

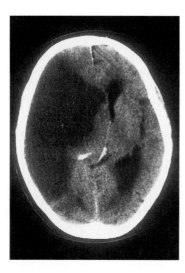

Figure 16–8. Computed tomography image of brain swelling in patient with occlusion of the middle cerebral artery. Massive hypodensity with shift of septum pellucidum and pineal gland, and contralateral hydrocephalus. (From Wijdicks.[71] By permission of Mayo Foundation for Medical Education and Research.)

may not be measured by a peripherally located parenchymal monitor.[56] More likely, the swollen hemisphere grows like a tumor mass, with some increase in intracranial pressure but much more displacement of the upper brain stem.

Management of cerebral edema in patients with unilateral swelling in a large portion of the hemisphere is very difficult and often fails. Corticosteroids have been ineffective in controlling cerebral edema.[49,62] This result is expected, because their membrane stabilizing effect would not influence the cytotoxic edema phase. Osmotic agents are the first line of treatment, and the effect of mannitol should be observed first. Mannitol is administered as a bolus of 1 g/kg, and if no measurable effect is seen, a second intravenous dose of 2 g/kg is tried to reduce intracranial pressure. We have seen dramatic reversal of the uncal syndrome with mannitol and hyperventilation in brain edema associated with acute hemispheric infarction.[73] Lack of response to mannitol, often noted in more advanced stages of herniation,[35] and further clinical deterioration can be fol-

lowed by decompressive surgery if no major comorbid condition exists and the patient is comparatively young.

We place an intracranial pressure monitor when patients with swelling from a large MCA stroke become too drowsy to protect the airway and need intubation. Intracranial pressure monitoring should be continued for 5 days, because the pressure may gradually rise within this interval. Increased intracranial pressure should be countered with mannitol administration. If deterioration continues and CT scans document further mass effect, the patient's next of kin is offered the choice of decompressive craniotomy. The timing of craniotomy with duraplasty is unresolved, but it is reasonable to proceed when mannitol fails to control intracranial pressure or, more commonly, when the patient's condition deteriorates to withdrawal to pain or new pupil abnormalities emerge. In addition, a ventriculostomy drain can be placed if significant contralateral hydrocephalus is present. If family members refuse decompressive craniotomy, a regimen of moderate hypothermia (33°-34°C) can be instituted.

Moderate hypothermia has received considerable interest as a treatment modality. However, the evidence for reducing infarct size is much more compelling than that for treatment of cerebral swelling. Hypothermia could possibly suppress a glutamate flux and intraneuronal calcium mobilization, elements of excitotoxic neuronal damage. It may also decrease metabolic rate and the development of lactic acidosis. Experimental studies have consistently shown not only reduction in infarct volume but also continued neuroprotection after discontinuation of hypothermia even several hours after surgical occlusion of the MCA.[34,75] Clinical trials of moderate hypothermia in massive hemispheric infarcts are in progress. Moderate hypothermia can be achieved by surface cooling (Fig. 16–9A) or invasive devices (Fig. 16–9B). The patient is positioned between two cooling blankets. The cooling blankets are set at 4.0°C initially and then adjusted to a core temperature of 33°-34°C. It may take up to 6 hours to reach this goal (range, 4 to 8 hours).[30] The process can be supplemented by alcohol rubbing and ice wa-

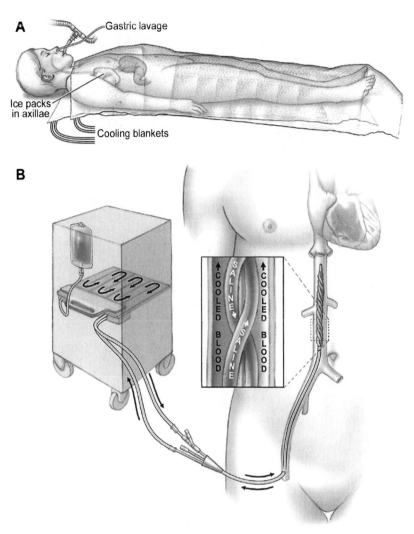

Figure 16–9. Methods of cooling. (*A*) Surface cooling with adjunctive measures. (*B*) Closed cooled saline circuit for invasive cooling.

ter gastric lavage and by intravenous infusion of cold fluids.[24,57] Complications have included reduced platelet count and cold-induced pancreatic failure, evidenced by increased serum amylase concentration; but with this level of core temperature, life-threatening cardiac arrhythmias have rarely occurred.[24,30]

Another option is placement of a closed saline infusion loop after insertion of a probe into the vena cava or subclavian vein. Invasive cooling devices that have been introduced in the market all use a similar principle of core cooling. Maximal cooling rates of 5°C to 8°C/hour have been claimed. Studies are under way to address its therapeutic application. Preliminary results suggest that this device may greatly facilitate the management of hypothermia. Shivering can be treated with meperidine or propofol. A neuromuscular blocking agent is usually not needed. Intercurrent infections, particularly pneumonia, and hemorrhagic conversion of the infarct increase temperature significantly, and maintaining hypothermia becomes much more difficult.

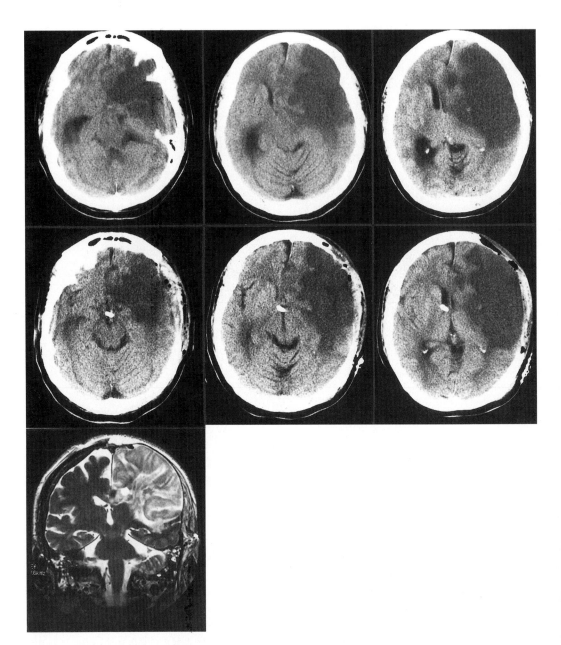

Figure 16–10. Serial computed tomography scans showing decompressive craniotomy with ventriculostomy. Note the significant decrease in ventricle size, reduction in the size of the contralateral temporal horn, decompression of the midbrain and resolution of uncal herniation, marked reduction in pineal shift, and reopening of the third ventricle and quadrigeminal cistern. A magnetic resonance image (coronal view) 2 days later shows virtually no horizontal (falx is in midline) or vertical shift (left and right red nuclei are at the same level and not tilted downward).

Decompressive surgery has been mostly successful in patients with ischemic stroke in the nondominant hemisphere, including those with progression to coma and a fixed, dilated pupil[11,22,23,51] (Fig. 16–10). There is presumptive evidence that salvaged patients do well despite a fixed hemiparesis, and many return to their previous intellectual level.[8] The experience, largely from Germany, in more than 60 surgically treated patients suggests that mortality is substantially decreased, but one of four patients has severe disability.[52] Early decompressive hemicraniotomy (arbitrarily defined as surgery before the first signs of herniation) has been advocated by some, but good results can also be explained by a favorable natural history.[58,70] No patients have remained in a persistent vegetative state. Concerns about major morbidity in survivors have been voiced, and the functional outcome in elderly patients is marginal. One study found severe disability even in patients older than 55 years.[19] Decompressive surgery must be limited to a large parieto-occipital craniotomy with removal of the bony flap and opening of the dura but without removal of infarcted tissue and closing with cadaver dura[71] or other material (Figs. 16–11 and 16–12). The bone flap is stored at −70°C.

Alternative therapies include a preemptive approach with repeated mannitol infusions in patients at very high risk (hypodensity involving more than 50% of the MCA territory on CT, hyperdense MCA sign, and sulcal effacement). Hypertonic saline (10%) may be effective when mannitol fails.[59] A recent important study in Sprague-Dawley rats suggested that albumin therapy virtually eliminated brain swelling.[4] Albumin (2 g/kg) may reduce cerebral swelling by increasing the oncotic pressure of plasma without affecting osmolality because of the high molecular weight of plasma. It may be used when mannitol fails and possibly before hypothermia or decompressive craniotomy.

A protocol for management in cerebral swelling is shown in Table 16–2.

Another neurologic cause for deterioration in patients with hemispheric stroke is hemorrhagic conversion of the infarct. The mecha-nism of development of an intracerebral hematoma in a large territory infarct is unresolved, but development of a large intracranial hematoma has tentatively been linked to excessive prolongation of activated partial thromboplastin time and surges in blood pressure. Early arterial recanalization would appear more likely as a possible explanation, but it was not confirmed in a study of four patients.[43]

It has been clearly established that most patients do not have clinical deterioration.[18,20,21,44] This can be explained by either petechial hemorrhage or small hematomas without significant mass effect (Fig. 16–13). Patients with hemorrhagic conversion of infarcts are best managed by reduction of the intensity of anticoagulation to borderline anticoagulation. Certainly, in patients with excessive activated partial thromboplastin time values, it is more prudent to hold heparin for 1 or 2 days. Studies of hemorrhagic infarction during heparinization, although retrospective, convincingly showed that this approach is safe.[46,47,67]

Clinical worsening is much more prevalent and often devastating in patients with large hematomas (Fig. 16–13). This uncommon cause of deterioration occurs in patients irrespective of anticoagulation. In a large study of hemorrhagic transformation of ischemic stroke, a massive hematoma developed in 1 of 65 patients.[67] Clinical deterioration may be gradual at first and usually during the day after admission. Often, large hemorrhagic infarcts are centrally located and may produce a diencephalic herniation syndrome. The progression may be gradual and involves development of small midposition pupils, Cheyne-Stokes breathing, and hypertonia in previously flaccid limbs evolving to pathologic flexion responses. Progression in many patients halts at this midbrain stage of central herniation, and they do not recover. Surgical removal of the clot is often a last resort, but many patients do poorly.

Seizures and status epilepticus are uncommon causes for deterioration.[16,27] Periodic lateralized epileptiform discharges are more commonly seen on electroencephalograms in patients with large ischemic strokes but are sel-

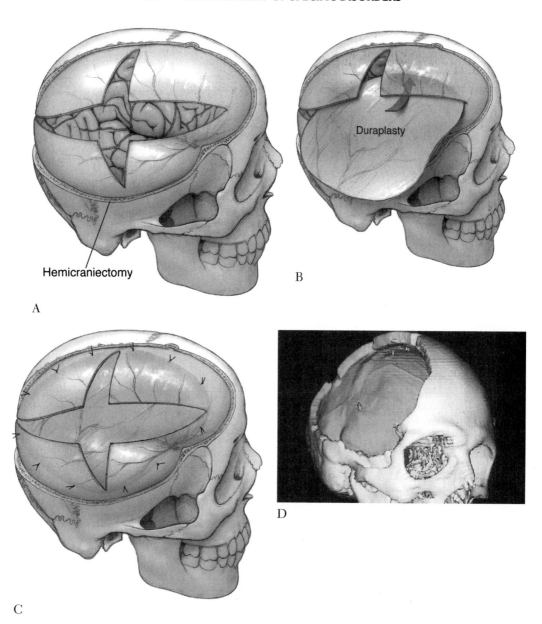

Figure 16–11. Hemicraniectomy. (*A*) After removal of bone flap, limited dural incision. (*B*) Duraplasty expands the intracranial vault. (*C*) Ample room is left for the infarcted brain to swell. (*D*) Bone window of 3D reconstructed computed tomogram showing the extent of the skull removal. (From Wijdicks.[71] By permission of Mayo Foundation for Medical Education and Research.)

dom accompanied by clinical manifestations. These findings should not be interpreted as signs of subclinical seizures or nonconvulsant status epilepticus or lead to aggressive treatment with antiepileptic medication. These discharges, however, may predict later seizures, and in a patient with a single seizure, intravenous loading with phenytoin should be con-

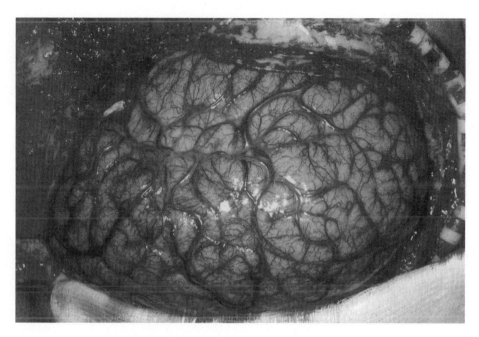

Figure 16–12. Intraoperative image of swollen, infarcted, hyperemic brain after decompressive craniotomy. The wide dura removal is evident, and the opening was later closed with bovine pericardium.

sidered. Focal seizures can become notoriously difficult to treat and may need repeated use of benzodiazepines or devalproex sodium (Chapter 24).

Because of comorbidity and poor general health, patients with large hemispheric infarcts may have deterioration from systemic causes. Congestive heart failure may worsen rapidly with pulmonary edema, sometimes because of iatrogenic fluid loading or inadequate diuretic therapy. Almost half the patients who need mechanical ventilation have poor gas exchange from significant pulmonary edema associated with poor diastolic cardiac function rather than from "neurogenic" pulmonary edema.[74]

Similarly, cardiac arrhythmias emerge in patients with a large hemispheric stroke, and this may be the only reason for monitoring in the NICU. Rapid atrial fibrillation is more common in elderly patients but not exclusively in patients with coexisting cardiac disease. Significant arrhythmias, including ventricular tachycardia and series of ventricular ectopic beats, can be observed after hemispheric infarcts.[40] Recognition

and treatment of the most common cardiac arrhythmias are discussed in Chapter 30.

Sudden death after a large territory hemispheric stroke may have its origin in a saddle pulmonary embolus. In our series of 30 pa-

Table 16–2. Treatment Options for Cerebral Swelling in Hemispheric Infarction

Maintain adequate hydration but restrict free water

Assess the effect of mannitol 20%, 1 g/kg

If mannitol is unsuccessful, use infusion of 75 mL of 10% saline

If hypertonic saline therapy is unsuccessful, consider decompressive hemicraniotomy

If decompressive hemicraniotomy is refused or unsuccessful, begin hypothermia therapy, reducing core body temperature to 33°C–34°C by using cooling blankets or cooling devices, gastric lavage with ice water, and alcohol rubbing

Treat shivering with propofol (up to 3–5 mg/kg per hour) or meperidine (0.35 mg/kg at a rate of 0.5 mg per minute) as needed

Monitor serum amylase, activated partial thromboplastin time, platelet count, and troponin daily during hypothermia

Continue hypothermia for 3 days and rewarm, ideally increasing temperature 1°C every 6 hours

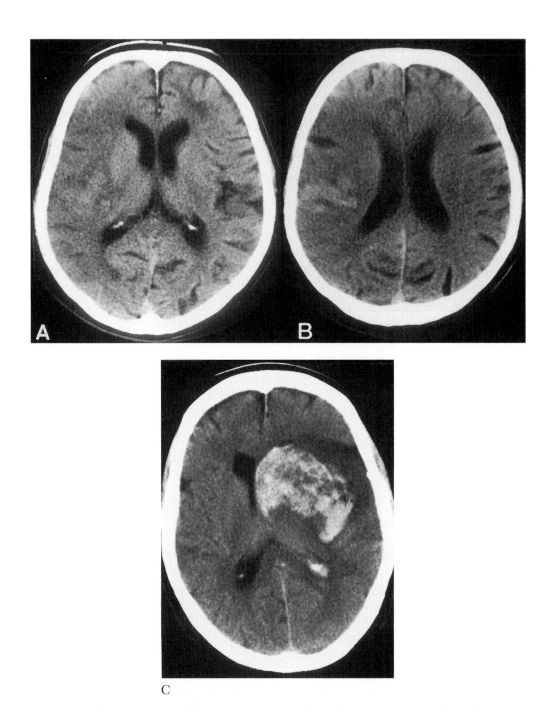

Figure 16–13. Two extremes of hemorrhagic conversion after a complete middle cerebral artery territory infarct. (*A* and *B*) Computed tomography images of petechial hemorrhagic infarction. (*C*) Hemorrhagic conversion producing a hemorrhagic mass.

tients with pulmonary emboli after stroke, pulmonary embolism defied antemortem detection in half the cases, and in 1 of 3 patients, it was associated with deep venous thrombosis in the paralyzed leg (see Chapter 29).

OUTCOME

Although less appreciated in the NICU because of a bias toward the more severe cases, the clinical course in patients with a large hemispheric infarct is commonly a very gradual improvement. Few patients have unexpectedly rapid recovery ("spectacular shrinking deficit"). The interval is within 24 hours and in many patients within 4 hours[37] (Fig. 16–4). This phenomenon may be seen in patients with a cardioembolic source, arterial dissection, and intraluminal clot formation. Outcome is good in most patients, but recurrence, this time with a persistent deficit, may unfortunately occur.

Mortality is high in patients with a large ischemic stroke.[5,7,17,72] When acute stroke occurs in patients with acute myocardial infarction, cardiac arrhythmias may contribute to early mortality.[61] Treatment of neurologic (control of intracranial pressure) and medical (infection control, prophylactic anticoagulation, supportive cardiac care) complications can be expected to substantially decrease mortality. Unrelenting cerebral swelling is a common cause of early death.[5,17,61] Brain swelling may halt and improvement may follow.[41,48,72] These two entirely different clinical courses cannot be predicted at onset, but a recent study of 201 patients found fatal brain edema in those with more than 50% hypodensity on CT scans and involvement of other vascular territories.[25] The effect of age on swelling is uncertain; we found that clinical deterioration from swelling is less frequent, although poorly tolerated, in patients younger than 45 years.[72]

Mortality is high in patients who need mechanical ventilation. In a study of 24 patients with acute MCA territory stroke who eventually needed ventilatory support, only 5 patients survived. We and others found that outcome is particularly poor (80% to 100% mortality) in patients with CT scan evidence of swelling and a need for mechanical ventilation.[17,74] It is unclear whether decompressive surgery, at this juncture, improves survival. Independent outcome is possible in surviving patients who needed prolonged ventilatory assistance and tracheostomy.

Patients who remain in a coma for at least 1 week after a large ischemic stroke generally remain severely disabled and are often in need of nursing home placement.

Whether patients reach an independent functional level depends on location, size, and comorbid condition. Intensive rehabilitation to improve walking, to optimize independence in daily living by significant adjustments in the home and at work, and to support psychologic stress and depression is imperative for any survivor of a large hemispheric stroke. An outcome algorithm is shown in Figure 16–14.

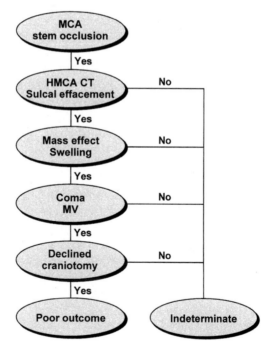

Figure 16–14. Outcome algorithm in acute middle cerebral artery (MCA) occlusion. HMCA CT, hyperdense MCA sign on computed tomography; MV, mechanical ventilation. Poor outcome: severe disability or death, vegetative state. Indeterminate: any statement would be a premature conclusion.

CONCLUSIONS

- Deterioration in patients with MCA occlusion consists of brain swelling, cerebral hematoma from hemorrhagic conversion or pulmonary edema due to aspiration or fluid overload.
- Clinical features of brain swelling after acute ischemic hemispheric infarction are drowsiness, bilateral ptosis, pupillary asymmetry, and, less commonly, unilateral fixed pupil.
- Early hypodensity on CT scans that involves 50% or more of the MCA territory predicts brain swelling and hemorrhagic conversion.
- Primary control of brain swelling must be with mannitol or hypertonic saline, but only if intracranial pressure is elevated. Decompressive surgery or hypothermia should be considered.
- Mechanical ventilation is often needed in patients with brain swelling, seizures, or pulmonary edema. Survival is reduced.

REFERENCES

1. Arnold M, Nedeltchev K, Sturzenegger M, et al: Thrombolysis in patients with acute stroke caused by cervical artery dissection. *Arch Neurol* 59:549–553, 2002.
2. Averbuch-Heller L, Leigh RJ, Mermelstein V, et al: Ptosis in patients with hemispheric strokes. *Neurology* 58:620–624, 2002.
3. Barber PA, Darby DG, Desmond PM, et al: Identification of major ischemic change. Diffusion-weighted imaging versus computed tomography. *Stroke* 30:2059–2065, 1999.
4. Belayev L, Liu Y, Zhao W, et al: Human albumin therapy of acute ischemic stroke: marked neuroprotective efficacy at moderate doses and with a broad therapeutic window. *Stroke* 32:553–560, 2001.
5. Bounds JV, Wiebers DO, Whisnant JP, et al: Mechanisms and timing of deaths from cerebral infarction. *Stroke* 12:474–477, 1981.
6. Bozzao L, Angeloni U, Bastianello S, et al: Early angiographic and CT findings in patients with hemorrhagic infarction in the distribution of the middle cerebral artery. *AJNR Am J Neuroradiol* 12:1115–1121, 1991.
7. Caronna JJ, Levy DE: Clinical predictors of outcome in ischemic stroke. *Neurol Clin* 1:103–117, 1983.
8. Carter BS, Ogilvy CS, Candia GJ, et al: One-year outcome after decompressive surgery for massive nondominant hemispheric infarction. *Neurosurgery* 40:1168–1175, 1997.
9. Chamorro A, Vila N, Saiz A, et al: Early anticoagulation after large cerebral embolic infarction: a safety study. *Neurology* 45:861–865, 1995.
10. de Bray JM, Lhouste P, Dubas F, et al: Ultrasonic features of extracranial carotid dissections: 47 cases studied by angiography. *J Ultrasound Med* 13:659–664, 1994.
11. Delashaw JB, Broaddus WC, Kassell NF, et al: Treatment of right hemispheric cerebral infarction by hemicraniectomy. *Stroke* 21:874–881, 1990.
12. Derex L, Nighoghossian N, Turjman F, et al: Intravenous tPA in acute ischemic stroke related to internal carotid artery dissection. *Neurology* 54:2159–2161, 2000.
13. Dippel DW, van Breda EJ, van Gemert HM, et al: Effect of paracetamol (acetaminophen) on body temperature in acute ischemic stroke: a double-blind, randomized phase II clinical trial. *Stroke* 32:1607–1612, 2001.
14. Firlik AD, Yonas H, Kaufmann AM, et al: Relationship between cerebral blood flow and the development of swelling and life-threatening herniation in acute ischemic stroke. *J Neurosurg* 89:243–249, 1998.
15. Frank JI: Large hemispheric infarction, deterioration, and intracranial pressure. *Neurology* 45:1286–1290, 1995.
16. Giroud M, Gras P, Fayolle H, et al: Early seizures after acute stroke: a study of 1,640 cases. *Epilepsia* 35:959–964, 1994.
17. Hacke W, Schwab S, Horn M, et al: 'Malignant' middle cerebral artery territory infarction. Clinical course and prognostic signs. *Arch Neurol* 53:309–315, 1996.
18. Hart RG, Easton JD: Hemorrhagic infarcts. *Stroke* 17:586–589, 1986.
19. Holtkamp M, Buchheim K, Unterberg A, et al: Hemicraniectomy in elderly patients with space occupying media infarction: improved survival but poor functional outcome. *J Neurol Neurosurg Psychiatry* 70:226–228, 2001.
20. Hornig CR, Bauer T, Simon C, et al: Hemorrhagic transformation in cardioembolic cerebral infarction. *Stroke* 24:465–468, 1993.
21. Hornig CR, Dorndorf W, Agnoli AL: Hemorrhagic cerebral infarction—a prospective study. *Stroke* 17:179–185, 1986.
22. Ivamoto HS, Numoto M, Donaghy RM: Surgical decompression for cerebral and cerebellar infarcts. *Stroke* 5:365–370, 1974.
23. Kalia KK, Yonas H: An aggressive approach to massive middle cerebral artery infarction. *Arch Neurol* 50:1293–1297, 1993.

24. Kammersgaard LP, Rasmussen BH, Jorgensen HS, et al: Feasibility and safety of inducing modest hypothermia in awake patients with acute stroke through surface cooling: a case-control study: the Copenhagen Stroke Study. *Stroke* 31:2251–2256, 2000.

25. Kasner SE, Demchuk AM, Berrouschot J, et al: Predictors of fatal brain edema in massive hemispheric ischemic stroke. *Stroke* 32:2117–2123, 2001.

26. Kasner SE, Wein T, Piriyawat P, et al: Acetaminophen for altering body temperature in acute stroke: a randomized clinical trial. *Stroke* 33:130–135, 2002.

27. Kilpatrick CJ, Davis SM, Hopper JL, et al: Early seizures after acute stroke. Risk of late seizures. *Arch Neurol* 49:509–511, 1992.

28. Kilpatrick MM, Yonas H, Goldstein S, et al: CT-based assessment of acute stroke: CT, CT angiography, and xenon-enhanced CT cerebral blood flow. *Stroke* 32:2543–2549, 2001.

29. Klossek JM, Neau JP, Vandenmarq P, et al: Unilateral lower cranial nerve palsies due to spontaneous internal carotid artery dissection. *Ann Otol Rhinol Laryngol* 103:413–415, 1994.

30. Krieger DW, De Georgia MA, Abou-Chebl A, et al: Cooling for acute ischemic brain damage (COOL AID): an open pilot study of induced hypothermia in acute ischemic stroke. *Stroke* 32:1847–1854, 2001.

31. Krieger DW, Demchuk AM, Kasner SE, et al: Early clinical and radiological predictors of fatal brain swelling in ischemic stroke. *Stroke* 30:287–292, 1999.

32. Kucinski T, Koch C, Grzyska U, et al: The predictive value of early CT and angiography for fatal hemispheric swelling in acute stroke. *AJNR Am J Neuroradiol* 19:839–846, 1998.

33. Kumral E, Evyapan D, Balkir K. Acute caudate vascular lesions. *Stroke* 30:100–108, 1999.

34. Maier CM, Sun GH, Kunis D, et al: Delayed induction and long-term effects of mild hypothermia in a focal model of transient cerebral ischemia: neurological outcome and infarct size. *J Neurosurg* 94:90–96, 2001.

35. Manno EM, Adams RE, Derdeyn CP, et al: The effects of mannitol on cerebral edema after large hemispheric cerebral infarct. *Neurology* 52:583–587, 1999.

36. Manno E, Fulgham JR, Wijdicks EFM: Coexisting hyperdense MCA sign and sulcal effacement on CT scan predicts deterioration from brain swelling *Mayo Clin Proc* 2003 (in press).

37. Minematsu K, Yamaguchi T, Omae T: 'Spectacular shrinking deficit': rapid recovery from a major hemispheric syndrome by migration of an embolus. *Neurology* 42:157–162, 1992.

38. Mokri B, Schievink WI, Olsen KD, et al: Spontaneous dissection of the cervical internal carotid artery. Presentation with lower cranial nerve palsies. *Arch Otolaryngol Head Neck Surg* 118:431–435, 1992.

39. Mokri B, Sundt TM Jr, Houser OW, et al: Spontaneous dissection of the cervical internal carotid artery. *Ann Neurol* 19:126–138, 1986.

40. Myers MG, Norris JW, Hachinski VC, et al: Cardiac sequelae of acute stroke. *Stroke* 13:838–842, 1982.

41. Ng LK, Nimmannitya J: Massive cerebral infarction with severe brain swelling: a clinicopathological study. *Stroke* 1:158–163, 1970.

42. Nguyen Bui L, Brant-Zawadzki M, Verghese P, et al: Magnetic resonance angiography of cervicocranial dissection. *Stroke* 24:126–131, 1993.

43. Ogata J, Yutani C, Imakita M, et al: Hemorrhagic infarct of the brain without a reopening of the occluded arteries in cardioembolic stroke. *Stroke* 20:876–883, 1989.

44. Okada Y, Yamaguchi T, Minematsu K, et al: Hemorrhagic transformation in cerebral embolism. *Stroke* 20:598–603, 1989.

45. Parsons MW, Barber PA, Chalk J, et al: Diffusion- and perfusion-weighted MRI response to thrombolysis in stroke. *Ann Neurol* 51:28–37, 2002.

46. Pessin MS, Estol CJ, Lafranchise F, et al: Safety of anticoagulation after hemorrhagic infarction. *Neurology* 43:1298–1303, 1993.

47. Pessin MS, Teal PA, Caplan LR: Hemorrhagic infarction: Guilt by association? *AJNR Am J Neuroradiol* 12:1123–1126, 1991.

48. Plum F: Brain swelling and edema in cerebral vascular disease. *Res Publ Assoc Res Nerv Ment Dis* 41:318–348, 1966.

49. Qizilbash N, Lewington SL, Lopez-Arrieta JM: Corticosteroids for acute ischaemic stroke. *Cochrane Database Syst Rev* 2:2000.

50. Reith J, Jørgensen HS, Pedersen PM, et al: Body temperature in acute stroke: relation to stroke severity, infarct size, mortality, and outcome. *Lancet* 347:422–425, 1996.

51. Rengachary SS, Batnitzky S, Morantz RA, et al: Hemicraniectomy for acute massive cerebral infarction. *Neurosurgery* 8:321–328, 1981.

52. Rieke K, Schwab S, Krieger D, et al: Decompressive surgery in space-occupying hemispheric infarction: results of an open, prospective trial. *Crit Care Med* 23:1576–1587, 1995.

53. Ropper AH, Shafran B: Brain edema after stroke. Clinical syndrome and intracranial pressure. *Arch Neurol* 41:26–29, 1984.

54. Rudolf J, Grond M, Stenzel C, et al: Incidence of space-occupying brain edema following systemic thrombolysis of acute supratentorial ischemia. *Cerebrovasc Dis* 8:166–171, 1998.

55. Schievink WI: Spontaneous dissection of the carotid and vertebral arteries. *N Engl J Med* 344:898–906, 2001.

56. Schwab S, Aschoff A, Spranger M, et al: The value of intracranial pressure monitoring in acute hemispheric stroke. *Neurology* 47:393–398, 1996.

57. Schwab S, Schwarz S, Spranger M, et al: Moderate hypothermia in the treatment of patients with severe middle cerebral artery infarction. *Stroke* 29:2461–2466, 1998.

58. Schwab S, Steiner T, Aschoff A, et al: Early hemicraniectomy in patients with complete middle cerebral artery infarction. *Stroke* 29:1888–1893, 1998.

59. Schwarz S, Georgiadis D, Aschoff A, et al: Effects of hypertonic (10%) saline in patients with raised intracranial pressure after stroke. *Stroke* 33:136–140, 2002.

60. Shaw C-M, Alvord EC Jr, Berry RG: Swelling of the brain following ischemic infarction with arterial occlusion. *Arch Neurol* 1:161–177, 1959.

61. Silver FL, Norris JW, Lewis AJ, et al: Early mortality following stroke: a prospective review. *Stroke* 15:492–496, 1984.

62. Slivka AP, Murphy EJ: High-dose methylprednisolone treatment in experimental focal cerebral ischemia. *Exp Neurol* 167:166–172, 2001.

63. So EL, Annegers JF, Hauser WA, et al: Population-based study of seizure disorders after cerebral infarction. *Neurology* 46:350–355, 1996.

64. Sturzenegger M, Huber P: Cranial nerve palsies in spontaneous carotid artery dissection. *J Neurol Neurosurg Psychiatry* 56:1191–1199, 1993.

65. Tijssen CC, van Gisbergen JA, Schulte BP: Conjugate eye deviation: side, site, and size of the hemispheric lesion. *Neurology* 41:846–850, 1991.

66. Tomsick TA, Brott TG, Chambers AA, et al: Hyperdense middle cerebral artery sign on CT: efficacy in detecting middle cerebral artery thrombosis. *AJNR Am J Neuroradiol* 11:473–477, 1990.

67. Toni D, Fiorelli M, Bastianello S, et al: Hemorrhagic transformation of brain infarct: predictability in the first 5 hours from stroke onset and influence on clinical outcome. *Neurology* 46:341–345, 1996.

68. von Kummer R, Meyding-Lamadé U, Forsting M, et al: Sensitivity and prognostic value of early CT in occlusion of the middle cerebral artery trunk. *AJNR Am J Neuroradiol* 15:9–15, 1994.

69. Weinberg AD, Minaker KL: Dehydration. Evaluation and management in older adults. Council on Scientific Affairs, American Medical Association. *JAMA* 274:1552–1556, 1995.

70. Wijdicks EFM: Hemicraniotomy in massive hemispheric stroke: a stark perspective on a radical procedure. *Can J Neurol Sci* 27:271–273, 2000.

71. Wijdicks EFM: Management of massive hemispheric cerebral infarct: Is there a ray of hope? *Mayo Clin Proc* 75:945–952, 2000.

72. Wijdicks EFM, Diringer MN: Middle cerebral artery territory infarction and early brain swelling: progression and effect of age on outcome. *Mayo Clin Proc* 73:829–836, 1998.

73. Wijdicks EFM, Schievink WI, McGough PF: Dramatic reversal of the uncal syndrome and brain edema from infarction in the middle cerebral artery territory. *Cerebrovasc Dis* 7:349–352, 1997.

74. Wijdicks EFM, Scott JP: Causes and outcome of mechanical ventilation in patients with hemispheric ischemic stroke. *Mayo Clin Proc* 72:210–213, 1997.

75. Yanamoto H, Nagata I, Niitsu Y, et al: Prolonged mild hypothermia therapy protects the brain against permanent focal ischemia. *Stroke* 32:232–239, 2001.

76. Yatsu FM, Hart RG, Mohr JP, et al: Anticoagulation of embolic strokes of cardiac origin: an update. *Neurology* 38:314–316, 1988.

77. Zuber M, Meary E, Meder JF, et al: Magnetic resonance imaging and dynamic CT scan in cervical artery dissections. *Stroke* 25:576–581, 1994.

17

Acute Basilar Artery Occlusion

Acute occlusion of the basilar artery can be such a devastating neurologic illness that any therapeutic intervention with a more or less remote potential to reverse outcome seems justified. Progress has been made in improving care, and a potential breakthrough could be the use of intra-arterial infusion of a thrombolytic drug, a therapy that has been successful even 12 hours after the first signs and symptoms.[27,30,68,71]

Patients with acute occlusion of the basilar artery may have rapid deterioration to coma and then often need to be intubated. The need for mechanical ventilation in this disorder marks a very poor prognosis, and if no endovascular intervention is available or considered, death from propagating clot may follow. In other patients, progression of brain stem dysfunction has not yet occurred or the neurologic deficit is limited. Patients in both categories are admitted with some frequency to the NICU. When they arrive early, management ranges from blood pressure augmentation to lysis or fragmentation of the thrombus by advancement of an intra-arterial catheter.

CLINICAL RECOGNITION

Acute vertebrobasilar occlusive disease leads to several major clinical presentations, each of which can progress to loss of virtually all brain stem function. Each of these syndromes has become known in the neurologic lexicon by a colorful name—*locked-in syndrome, top-of-*

the-basilar syndrome—or by its French or German eponym. These syndromes are characterized by partial involvement of the brain stem.[4,10,11,66] Artery-to-artery embolus from atheromatous disease of the vertebral artery or ascending aortic arch or an embolus from a cardiac source or a vertebral artery dissection can be implicated. The sites of occlusion are shown in Figure 17–1.

Acute basilar artery occlusion results in median and paramedian pontine infarction. The most consistent signs and symptoms are altered consciousness from involvement of reticular formation in the tegmentum, ataxic or pseudobulbar speech, horizontal gaze palsy, ocular bobbing, facial diplegia, dysphagia, and profound tetraplegia that is notably asymmetrical in degree of motor weakness. Uncontrollably crazy laughter (*fou rire prodromique*) may occur and can be a presenting symptom.[21]

The eye findings in basilar artery occlusion are often impressive (Table 17–1): (*1*) a lesion of the medial longitudinal fasciculus that produces an internuclear ophthalmoplegia consisting of abnormal ipsilateral adduction and more profound nystagmus in the abducting eye, (*2*) one and one-half syndrome, consisting of one immobile eye in the horizontal plane and preservation of abduction alone in the other eye, (*3*) ocular bobbing, a type of vertical nystagmus that is a frequent finding in patients with extensive pontine infarction and is recognized by brisk conjugate downward eye movement followed by slow correction to baseline midposition, (*4*) bilateral ptosis due to involve-

Table 17–1. Brain Stem Syndromes with Eye Findings

Eponym	Level	Key Signs and Symptoms
Weber	M	Ipsilateral oculomotor paralysis with alternating hemiplegia
Benedikt	M	Oculomotor paralysis
		Crossed hemiparesis with tremor
Nothnagel-Claude	M	Oculomotor paresis with alternating ataxia
Parinaud	M	Paralysis of upward gaze
		Paresis of convergence
Koerber-Salus-Elschnig	M	Retractory nystagmus
		Vertical gaze palsy
		Pupillary abnormalities
Millard-Gubler	P	Nuclear seventh nerve palsy with crossed hemiparesis
Foville	P	Conjugate lateral gaze paralysis
		Ipsilateral nuclear palsy of the seventh nerve
		Crossed hemiparesis
Raymond-Cestan	P	Abducens nerve paralysis with contralateral hemiparesis
Wallenberg	Me	Horner's syndrome
		Absent corneal reflex
		Lateropulsion of saccadic eye movements
		Nystagmus
		Dysphagia
		Crossed sensory loss (may spare face, arm)

M, mesencephalon; Me, medulla oblongata; P, pons.

ment of the sympathetic fibers in the pontine tegmentum, or unilateral ptosis due to infarction of the third nerve nucleus, and (5) a fairly common skew deviation, with eyes positioned out of their normal vertical axis (Fig. 17–2).

When hemiparesis occurs, the most affected side may alternate from left to right in the first hours. In the extreme form, patients may have hemiparesis for a few hours, resolution, and then newly appearing hemiparesis on the opposite side, return of the initial hemiparesis, and eventually quite rapid progression to significant paresis of all four limbs. The fluctuation of signs and symptoms may be related to position change, and the virtual disappearance of symptoms in the supine or Trendelenburg position has been tentatively linked to an improvement in perfusion pressure in a slow-flow system. Hemiplegia falsely suggesting hemispheric involvement can be present in 40% of patients seen early in the course of the disorder. Initial occlusion of the paramedian penetrating arteries may produce hemiparesis and horizontal gaze palsy in association with normal speech, swallowing, and level of consciousness (Foville's syndrome). The course of basilar artery occlusion is often rapidly pro-

gressive. In a large series of patients seen early for thrombolytic intervention, only a few had a deficit at maximal onset.[22]

Breathing becomes clearly irregular in many patients, coughing is very weak, and when the tegmentum is infarcted, sustained hyperventilation may occur. In patients with more extensive infarction of the pons, a cluster type of breathing pattern may develop, consisting of brief episodes with respiratory rates of 4 per minute, occasionally with superimposed gasps, all causing marginal gas exchange. Frequent episodes of apnea or labored breathing from inability to protect the upper airway develop in most patients, and either condition should prompt immediate intubation and often further assistance with mechanical ventilation. Untreated, many patients become comatose, with bilateral unequal fixed pupils and extensor posturing. Terminal hyperthermia with temperatures reaching 42°C may occur.[36]

In complete occlusion of the basilar artery, the basis pontis may be destroyed but the rostral tegmentum can be spared and level of consciousness is intact. In this so-called locked-in syndrome, patients are stuck in a motionless state, and communication is possible only by

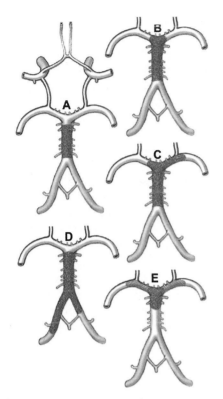

Figure 17–1. Sites of basilar artery occlusion. Most likely as deduced from clinicopathologic correlation, (*A*) a thrombus occludes the paramedian or short circumferential branch, with possible further extension into the basilar artery (*B*), posterior cerebral artery (*C*), or vertebral artery (*D*). An embolus or thrombus may also lodge at the tip of the basilar artery (*E*), occluding supply to the thalamus, cerebral peduncle, and temporal and occipital lobes. (Modified from Kubik and Adams.[36] By permission of Oxford University Press.)

vertical eye movements and blinking. These patients can feel, hear, and reason. In any patient "comatose" from presumed acute basilar artery occlusion on arrival in the NICU, one must eliminate the possibility of locked-in syndrome immediately by asking the patient to look up and blink on command. Failure of the examiner to test for these responses may obviously cause unimaginable stress to the patient. Patients may hear any conversation (including discussion of withdrawal of support) and have

to bear repetitive pain stimuli but cannot respond. In many patients, locked-in syndrome is not complete, and some motor function is preserved, including jaw opening and hand signaling. In other patients, consciousness is impaired from involvement of both thalami or extension to the tegmentum, and responses are not consistent.

Top-of-the-basilar artery syndrome is a constellation of signs and symptoms caused by an obstructing distal embolus. The strategic location of the clot at the juncture of the basilar artery with the posterior cerebral arteries and thalamic perforations produces, besides infarction in the mesencephalon, a fairly extensive area of infarction in thalamic nuclei, medial temporal lobes, and occipital lobes. At presentation, patients have an impaired, fluctuating level of consciousness from infarction of the bilateral paramedian rostral brain stem or the bithalamic nuclei.

Typically, patients prefer to sleep most of the day, and response to questions is sluggish. Visual hallucinations, which may include vivid colors, tend to occur at twilight and could be due to occipital lobe ischemia or brain stem involvement (peduncular hallucinations). Cortical blindness is unusual, but in some patients, brief episodes of sudden blindness have forewarned of basilar artery occlusion. As noted earlier, besides initial quadriplegia and dysarthria, findings often involve neuro-ophthalmologic signs, including pupillary abnormalities (pupils are poorly reactive and small), ptosis, third nerve

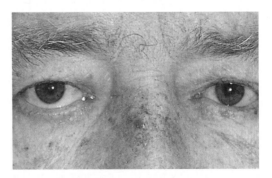

Figure 17–2. Patient with pontine infarction and typical skew deviation.

palsy, vertical or horizontal gaze abnormalities, skew deviation, and convergence nystagmus.

Brief extensor spasms—so-called tonic fits[36,54]—are occasionally mistaken for seizures. These movements may be bizarre, including flapping, repetitive twitching, rhythmic shaking as in a chill, and head jerking with opisthotonos.[54] More often, they are myorhythmias involving facial musculature. Myoclonus or athetoid movements have been associated with thalamic infarcts. Palatal myoclonus, usually seen at a later stage, produces a nagging clicking sound.

Acute basilar artery occlusion may have its origin in vertebral artery dissection. The general physical examination of patients with a vertebral dissection should focus on predisposing conditions, although most dissections are spontaneous. Stigmata of Marfan's disease[55] (dilated aortic root, joint laxity, and floppy mitral valve) and Ehlers-Danlos syndrome (easily bruising skin, hypermobile joints, and prolapse of mitral and tricuspid valves) should be recognized.

Patients with vertebral artery dissection may present with severe neck pain and almost instantaneous brain stem findings. Although usually severe and intense, headache can be mild and may not even be present, further clouding recognition. Most patients with vertebral artery dissection present with cerebellar symptoms (appendicular ataxia) or symptoms involving the lateral medulla oblongata (Horner's syndrome, horizontal-rotatory nystagmus directed away from the site of the lesion, ataxia, and crossed hemianesthesia).[26] Sensory involvement may be less traditional, with ipsilateral lower face, contralateral leg, and trunk hypalgesia or spinothalamic sensory loss (pinprick and temperature) at a midthoracic level. This sensory level may falsely suggest a thoracic hemicord lesion. The explanation is involvement of the far lateral spinothalamic fibers, sparing face and arm.[49] Dissection may be due to trauma, and other signs of traumatic brain injury may be absent.[31] Sudden deterioration in level of consciousness may occur on the same day, quickly followed by brain stem signs.[31]

Vertebral artery dissection may be associated with cerebellar infarction in young patients.[2,40,59,70,73] Neck manipulation from chiropractic therapy[43,57] neck extension due to shampooing (beauty parlor stroke syndrome), drinking ("bottoms up"), and polytrauma[6] have been particularly noted in young persons. Neck pain may be the only sign.[35] Although the relationship between chiropractic manipulation and vertebral artery dissection has been reported, the risk has not been appropriately defined in prospective studies.[57] Some patients may have sought a chiropractor for neck pain due to dissection. "Bone setters" in certain ethnic populations may apply vigorous neck manipulation.[53]

Dissection of the basilar artery is very uncommon, is more likely to occur in young patients, and is manifested by clinical symptoms of pontine infarction.[56] Dissection through the wall in the intradural, intracranial portion of the vertebral artery may lead to subarachnoid hemorrhage.[29]

NEUROIMAGING AND LABORATORY TESTS

Computed tomography scanning is the initial study, but in any lesion in the posterior fossa, it is significantly limited by degradation associated with bony artifacts. Often, CT scanning demonstrates scattered hypodensities in cerebellar vascular territories in patients with massive pontine infarcts. In others, hypodensities on CT scan may be noted in the occipital lobe and thalamus, indicating a more distal basilar artery occlusion (Fig. 17–3).

A hyperdense basilar artery indicative of a clot is virtually diagnostic if no intra-arterial density changes are seen in the supraclinoid portions of the carotid arteries,[61] and this CT sign can be demonstrated at least 6 hours after onset[25] (Fig. 17–3). The predictive value of the hyperdense basilar artery sign for outcome is not certain, because full recovery has been reported in patients with this sign.[25] A CT scan may show subarachnoid hemorrhage in patients with dissection through the entire wall,

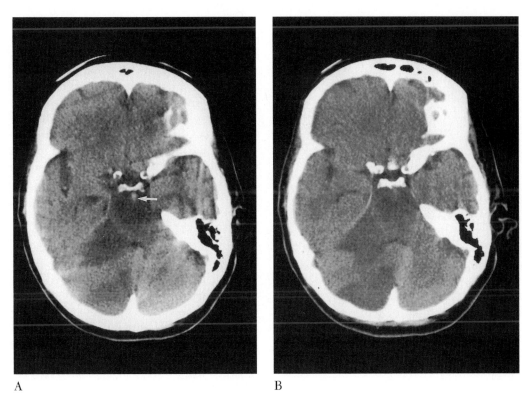

A   B

Figure 17–3. Computed tomography images showing (*A*) characteristic hyperdense basilar artery sign (*arrow*) and (*B*) scattered infarcts in the cerebellum and pons.

predominantly in the basal cisterns but often with significant blood casts in the ventricles.[58]

Magnetic resonance imaging confirms the diagnosis of acute basilar artery occlusion.[5,62] Magnetic resonance imaging not only delineates the area of pontine infarction (Fig. 17–4) but also may demonstrate absent flow in the basilar artery or a double lumen diagnostic of a dissection.[33] Magnetic resonance imaging can demonstrate abnormalities at the base of the pons, usually increased signal intensities on T2-weighted images, but findings can be normal as early as 12 hours after the episode, limiting its use in the early stage.[5,41] Magnetic resonance imaging fluid-attenuated inversion recovery (FLAIR) or diffusion-weighted sequences may be more useful to demonstrate early ischemic changes (Fig. 17–5). Magnetic resonance angiography may not be a perfect study in the detection of vertebral dissection,[38] tends to overestimate vertebrobasilar occlusive disease, and may falsely show lack

of flow in a patent but severely narrowed lumen. Two-dimensional time-of-flight magnetic resonance angiography is reasonably accurate (sensitivity, 100%; specificity, 75% to 90%) in documenting occlusive disease in the basilar artery but less so in the vertebral artery.[3]

Transcranial Doppler ultrasonography may complement magnetic resonance angiography, but the suboccipital probe usually cannot insonate the far distal portion of the basilar artery. Computed tomography angiography may be quite helpful, but we believe it makes better sense to proceed with a selective cerebral angiogram when patients present early and have a limited deficit or deficit in flux.[12] With the arrival of intra-arterial thrombolytic therapy, cerebral angiography is performed more often and earlier.[8,71,74]

Cerebral angiography may demonstrate partial or complete occlusion of the basilar artery.[1,47] Most clots in the basilar artery are

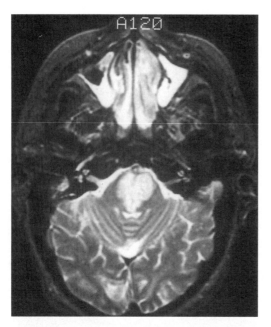

Figure 17–4. Massive pontine infarct on magnetic resonance image.

located in the middle or distal segments and often at the branching points. A proximal clot usually implies a trajectory from the confluence of the vertebral arteries to the branching of the anterior inferior cerebellar artery. A midbasilar clot is located between the anterior inferior and superior cerebellar arteries, and the remaining clots are designated distal clots. The distributions—proximal, middle, and distal— are, respectively, 45%, 35%, and 20%.[50] A typical pearl or string sign, double-contrast appearance, or sausage-like swelling strongly suggests vertebral dissection.

Assessment of collateral flow on cerebral angiography is important. One study suggested that lack of contralateral flow contributes to poor outcome despite recanalization of the basilar artery by thrombolysis.[48] Conversely, good collateral circulation (e.g., retrograde carotid artery to basilar artery channeled through prominent posterior communicating arteries) has been associated with good functional survival with basilar artery occlusion.[7]

Laboratory evaluation should include transesophageal echocardiography and studies of coagulation in young patients to exclude coagulopathy from increased factor VIII; tests to detect deficiency of antithrombin III and proteins C and S; specific tests for the antiphospholipid syndrome, such as IgG or (less important and nonspecific) IgM antiphospholipid antibodies, Coombs' test, antinuclear antibodies, VDRL, activated partial thromboplastin time and prothrombin time, lupus anticoagulant, plasma homocysteine, and a blood smear.

FIRST STEPS IN MANAGEMENT

Management in acute basilar artery occlusion is becoming much more invasive and aggressive (Table 17–2). Recent studies have clearly defined the potential of thrombolytic therapy.[13,22,50,71,74] If intra-arterial infusion of thrombolytic agents is possible, cerebral angiography could be the preferred initial approach. First, cerebral angiography maps out the extent of occlusion and collateral rescue, and use of thrombolytic agents can be deferred in patients with early recanalization. Second, in some patients, mechanical fragmentation alone may be successful. However, comparative studies of different modes of therapy are not available, and therapeutic results remain anecdotal. Moreover, experience has been largely limited to use of urokinase, production of which was recently suspended by the United States Food and Drug Administration.[67] Large doses of thrombolytic agents may increase the risk of intracranial hematoma. In a series of 66 patients, fatal pontine hemorrhage developed in two patients after successful recanalization, but massive doses were required to achieve clot lysis.[22]

The decision to proceed with thrombolytic therapy still remains difficult because fatal intracranial hemorrhage may occur in 10% and inability to reopen the occlusion in approximately 40%, and poor results are expected in patients who are comatose. Nonetheless, outcome in acute basilar artery occlusion is often devastating, and family members should be informed about the natural course and the possible opportunity to reverse it with throm-

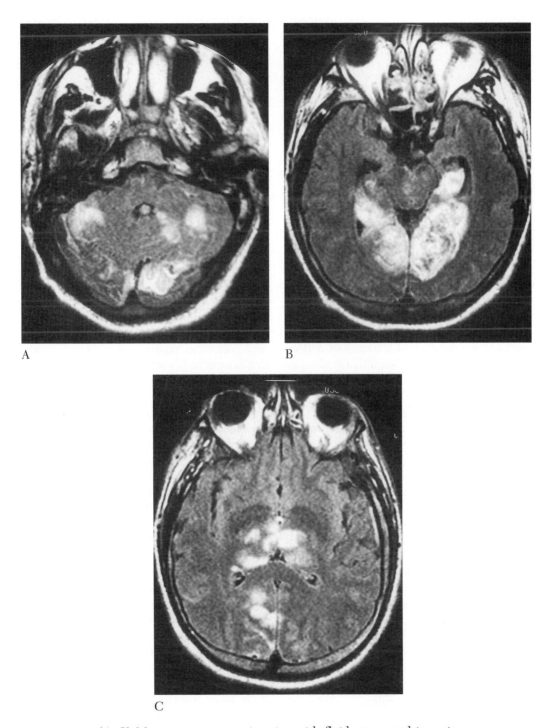

Figure 17–5. (*A–C*) Magnetic resonance imaging with fluid-attenuated inversion recovery sequence showing scattered cerebellar infarcts, mesencephalon, mesial temporal lobe, thalamus, and occipital lobes typical of top-of-the-basilar syndrome.

Table 17–2. Initial Management in Acute Basilar Artery Occlusion

Airway management	Intubation for apnea or frequent stridor from tongue observation
	Glycopyrrolate, 2 mg b.i.d., to reduce secretions
Fluid management	Maintenance with 3 L of 0.9% NaCl
Blood pressure	Flat body position
management	Blood pressure augmentation with dopamine, 10–40 μg/kg per minute to mean arterial pressure of 110–130 mm Hg, can be considered
Nutrition	Nasogastric tube feeding is withheld for 24 hours; formal swallowing evaluation
	Percutaneous endoscopic gastrostomy is considered in patients with massive brain stem stroke
Specific therapy	Intra-arterially, tissue plasminogen activator, 1.5–15 mg/hour), or reteplase, 0.1–1.0 U/hour
	Tissue plasminogen activator, maximum of 90 mg IV (if intra-arterial thrombolysis is not possible), 10% in bolus and 90% in 1-hour infusion

bolytic agents. Within the wide spectrum of presentations, we generally do not consider cerebral angiography and thrombolytic therapy in apneic patients who are mechanically ventilated and have lost virtually all brain stem reflexes or in patients who have marked fluctuation in clinical signs and tend to improve considerably. Absence of tetraparesis and no alterations in consciousness probably also justify a more conservative approach.[50] Only a few case reports have noted dramatic awakening from coma with angiographically proven recanalization[27,28,45] but in a larger experience in treated comatose patients with acute basilar artery occlusion, mortality was high (of 12 patients, 10 died, 6 of whom had basilar artery recanalization).[30] Little experience is reported in patients with locked-in syndrome who had successful opening of the basilar artery after thrombolytic treatment. In our unit, recanalization of the basilar artery resulted in no measurable neurologic deficit in two patients with locked-in syndrome, but we did not have the opportunity to reproduce this feat.[72] Early infarction noted on CT or MRI should not be interpreted as low probability of success with thrombolytic agents, nor is the interval of 12 hours considered a strict contraindication. We and others have been successful in reversing neurologic deficit in patients with limited MRI abnormalities.[18,71] We have considered thrombolysis in a patient with fluctuating signs but sudden worsening of symptoms. Experience remains limited.

Intra-arterial thrombolysis is performed by infusion of tissue plasminogen activator (1.5 to 15 mg/hour) or reteplase (Retavase) (0.1 to 1.0

U/hour) into a catheter advanced into the clot;[13] angiography is repeated at 30-minute intervals (Fig. 17–6). Before the procedure, patients need immediate treatment with a bolus of heparin (2000 U plus 500 U/hour for 2 hours). Activated partial thromboplastin time should be monitored regularly, with a goal of two times the control value. The femoral sheath must be left in place to reduce the postprocedural risk of hematoma at the puncture site. The femoral sheath usually can be removed the next day. Magnetic resonance imaging should be performed the next day. Scattered infarcts in the cerebellum or pons may account for any remaining clinical symptoms in patients with recanalization but may also appear in clinically asymptomatic patients. For patients with limited deficits seen 12 hours after initial presentation or if an interventional neuroradiologist is unavailable, an intravenous infusion of alteplase (Activase), 0.9 mg/kg (maximum, 90 mg), should be administered (10% as bolus and 90% of total dose in a 1-hour infusion).

Patients who return to the NICU after thrombolysis need further supportive measures. Airway management and endotracheal intubation are initiated if apneic episodes exist or if progressive drowsiness results in an inability to protect the airway. Death from sudden apnea has been reported, including in patients with a unilateral brain stem infarct.[37] Marked swallowing difficulties and difficulty in clearing secretions can be managed with glycopyrrolate to reduce secretions. In patients with a massive pontine infarct and no clinical change in 1 to 2 weeks, one should proceed with a tracheostomy if the patient or family members support further management despite expectations of poor outcome.

Blood pressure needs to be carefully controlled and may be abnormal in both directions. Acute basilar artery occlusion is often associated with long-standing hypertension and cardiovascular disease, and hypertension may become difficult to control soon after the ictus. In other patients, blood pressure may be bordering on hypotension. Fluctuations in motor weakness can be linked to hypotension and may disappear with increasing blood pressure with low doses of vasopressors. One may find marginal ventricular function in some of these patients with acute basilar artery occlusion, with a decreased ejection fraction on echocardiography.

These patients are probably best treated flat or in Trendelenburg's position in the first 24 hours. Administration of diuretic and antihypertensive agents is discontinued. Blood pressure may be increased by use of dopamine, 10 to 40 μg/kg, with titration to a mean arterial blood pressure of 110 to 130 mm Hg. The use of dopamine, however, is at the expense of ventricular irritability (predominantly premature ventricular contractions) and an increase in heart rate. Invasive monitoring is not absolutely required in these patients. Inotropic treatment can be continued for a few days, and then the dose should be tapered. At that time, the clinical outcome should become clear, and further management decisions should be based on the severity of the clinical deficit.

The management of blood pressure may be different and more prudent, however, in patients with acute vertebral artery dissection. In patients with a typical history of vertebral dissection or angiographic confirmation, control of blood pressure possibly needs to be more aggressive. Whether normalization of blood pressure reduces the risk of extension of the dissection to a larger segment or dissection through the entire wall is not known. In fact, progression of the dissection when monitored by repeated angiography is seldom seen.[34] The ideal blood pressure in patients with vertebral artery dissection has not been established, but one may want to attempt to attain normal mean arterial blood pressure values of 90 to 100 mm Hg.

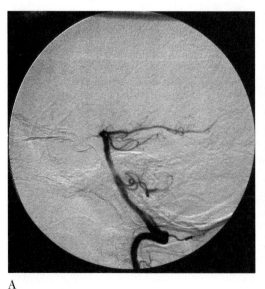
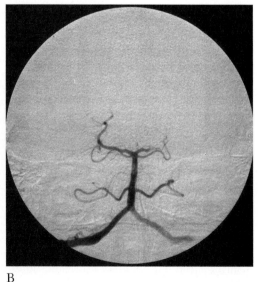

A   B

Figure 17–6. Digital subtraction angiographic series. (*A*) Nonocclusive and (*B*) occlusive thrombi in the mid-basilar artery distal to the origins of the anterior inferior cerebellar arteries and in the left posterior cerebral artery.

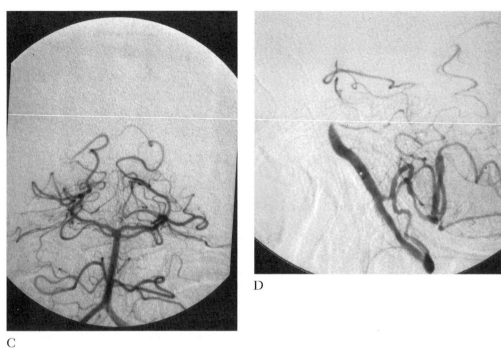

C

D

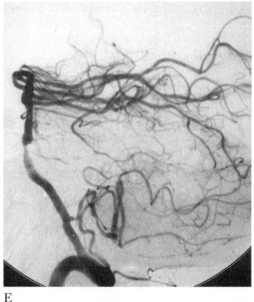

E

Figure 17–6. (*Continued*) (*C*) Dissolution of the thrombus in the basilar artery and restoration of flow of the distal left posterior cerebral artery after thrombolysis. The patient remained dysarthric, but left hemiparesis and an internuclear ophthalmoplegia resolved completely. (*D*) In another patient, occlusive thrombus in the proximal basilar artery was accompanied by some collateral reconstitution. (*E*) Complete opening was achieved, but a significant basilar artery stenosis remained. The patient made a complete recovery.

One should be particularly alert to vertebral artery dissection associated with a lateral medullary infarct (Wallenberg's syndrome), which may be associated with dysautonomia, supine hypotension, and significant bradycardia.[32]

Normal maintenance fluids with 0.9% sodium chloride suffice. In stable patients, swallowing should be assessed before liquid foods are administered orally. In patients with massive pontine infarction and mechanical ventilation, it is reasonable to proceed with percutaneous endoscopic gastrostomy.

Intravenous heparin has been a common treatment in acute basilar occlusion (activated partial thromboplastin time of 1.5 to 2 times control). However, whether heparin is effective in patients with acute basilar artery occlusion and major neurologic deficits is very doubtful, and often deterioration continues in most patients despite adequate anticoagulation.[73] It is important that a therapeutic level be achieved promptly, and a weight-based nomogram should be used to calculate the dose (Chapter 8). The weight-based nomogram has a tendency to exceed the partial thromboplastin time value, but in a patient with a deteriorating basilar artery occlusion, it is probably less troublesome than inadequate anticoagulation. Survivors with a mild neurologic deficit and high-grade stenosis of the basilar trunk of the artery can be treated with warfarin, but management should be readdressed if marked ataxia is observed at the first attempts of mobilization from bed rest.

DETERIORATION: CAUSES AND MANAGEMENT

A maximal deficit is present on the first day of admission in approximately one-third of the patients.[19] In another third, deterioration from further outgrowth of the clot results in successive occlusion of perforating arteries originating from the basilar artery. Many patients devastated by occlusion of the basilar artery remain in coma with retention of some brain stem reflexes. Acute basilar artery occlusion rarely results in complete loss of brain stem reflexes, and some function of the medulla oblongata often remains (Chapter 34).

An unfortunate cause of secondary deterioration is reocclusion after recanalization by thrombolysis. Patients with significant remaining stenosis of the basilar artery and possibly patients with small or absent posterior communicating arteries are at risk. We have been administering the intravenous antiplatelet drug abciximab (ReoPro) in such instances. Successful improvement after reocclusion in at least one patient has been reported,[69] but with our very limited experience, we have not yet noted substantial clinical improvement.

Pontine hemorrhage may occur and is immediately devastating. As expected, it is most common after use of intra-arterial thrombolytic agents. Only survival in a disabled state has been reported, and most patients die. Remote hemorrhages in the cerebellum, however, can be small and clinically irrelevant.[71]

Whether a remaining significant stenosis of the basilar artery should be followed by balloon angioplasty to reduce the chance of reocclusion after thrombolysis is unresolved.[44,65] Dilatation of the basilar artery may reduce the risk of future occlusion of that artery, and clots may pass into the smaller branches with less damage. The potential for artery-to-artery embolization is not likely to be reduced. The potential for damage to the multiple perforations also remains considerable. Reconstructive surgery of the vertebrobasilar territory is very controversial in this situation and is limited to patients with posture-related transient ischemic attacks.

Most earlier experience with stent-assisted angioplasty was in elective cases, but recently 3 periprocedural deaths and 1 delayed death among 11 patients were described.[39] Endovascular stenting of an acutely thrombosed basilar artery after thrombolysis that resulted in good patency was recently reported. The risks of placement and choice of stent are unclear.[51]

Patients with vertebral artery dissection rarely have deterioration, and in most the event is monophasic. Patients with dissection and recurrent transient ischemic attacks in the posterior circulation can be successfully treated with balloon occlusion of the vertebral artery if sufficient collateral circulation is present. This usually implies retrograde flow from the contralateral vertebral artery to the ipsilateral posterior inferior cerebellar artery.[24,42]

OUTCOME

Persistent coma after the onset of acute basilar artery occlusion strongly predicts poor outcome.[17,18] Outcome is particularly poor in patients with acute basilar occlusion who remain comatose and are supported by mechanical ventilation. Of 25 comatose patients with acute basilar occlusion and mechanical ventilation, none had any improvement in neurologic function in the next 2 to 3 weeks.[72] Weaning from the ventilator and spontaneous breathing through a T-tube circuit were possible in patients intubated for airway protection. In eight patients, apneic episodes prompted intubation, and all had progression within 24 to 48 hours to locked-in syndrome or lost most brain stem reflexes. Most comatose patients with basilar occlusion and the need for mechanical ventilation died after withdrawal of support at the request of family members; in others, fatal aspiration pneumonitis or cardiac arrest in association with acute myocardial infarction intervened.[72]

Mortality remains high in patients with acute basilar artery occlusion, but a favorable outcome is possible in some patients with limited neurologic deficits.[7,9,16,20] Patients with limited infarcts in the pons may have a reasonable functional outcome, although diplopia may be a major handicap. If infarction remains limited to the lateral medulla, long-term outcome is good and recurrent strokes in the posterior circulation are uncommon.[46] Patients with top-of-the-basilar syndrome may be severely disabled from a memory deficit caused by bilateral thalamic involvement.

Long-term outcome in vertebral dissection has not been studied, but in patients with cervical artery dissection, the risk of recurrence is 1% and is greater in younger patients.[60] In most patients, brain stem stroke is a single event, and follow-up by magnetic resonance angiography shows complete resolution of the dissection within 3 months.[52,60]

Patients with locked-in syndrome from brain stem infarction have a high mortality. A review of the literature noted 67% mortality in 117 patients.[23] Long-term survival from locked-in syndrome is possible, even beyond a decade after the onset, but only with superb and continuously dedicated nursing care. Recovery from complete locked-in syndrome is very unusual; however, recovery to a more functional state has been reported. It is impossible to predict which patients with locked-in syndrome will improve. They may have gradual improvement, over a period of months, regaining some muscle strength, but the ultimate result is marked pseudobulbar palsy with spastic tetraparesis. In addition, many patients die of intercurrent pulmonary infection. In contrast, patients in incomplete locked-in syndrome with spared oropharyngeal function and some element of motor function may improve considerably despite MRI documentation of pontine infarction.

There is no incentive to maintain a high level of aggressive management in comatose, ventilated patients with MRI-demonstrated massive pontine infarction. Life-prolonging procedures, such as cardiac resuscitation, tracheostomy, and percutaneous endoscopic gastrostomy, are futile.

In summary, good outcome from acute basilar artery occlusion is possible in patients with limited clinical deficits and certain cerebral angiographic criteria, such as short segmental occlusions, distal clot, and good collateral supply.[7,14,15,63] Outcome does not seem to be noticeably influenced by time (more than or less than 6 hours) between intra-arterial thrombolysis and recanalization.[64] Their clinical course is usually recognized by slowly progressive deficits and often by marked fluctuation, whereas in patients with poor outcome, the maximal neurologic deficit often arrives rapidly. An outcome algorithm is shown in Figure 17–7.

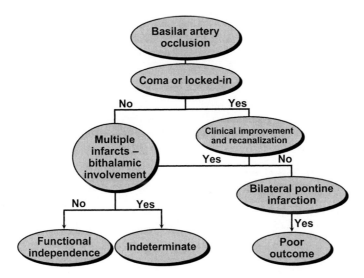

Figure 17–7. Outcome algorithm in acute basilar artery occlusion. Functional independence: no assistance needed, minor handicap may remain. Indeterminate: any statement would be a premature conclusion. Poor outcome: severe disability or death, vegetative state.

CONCLUSIONS

- Intra-arterial thrombolysis should be considered in patients with acute basilar artery occlusion seen within 12 hours.
- Tissue plasminogen activator, 90 mg intravenous dose in 1 hour (10% in bolus, 90% by infusion), should be considered if intra-arterial thrombolysis is not available.
- Standard management includes heparin (activated partial thromboplastin time 1.5 to 2 times the control value). In patients with hypotension, consider further blood pressure support with flat body position and dopamine, 10 to 40 μg/kg per hour (to achieve a mean arterial pressure 110 to 130 mm Hg).
- Mechanical ventilation for apneic episodes, persistent coma for 1 week, and MRI showing entire pontine infarction carry a very poor prognosis.
- Good outcome can be expected in patients with a slowly progressive clinical course, limited neurologic deficits, short segmental abnormalities, and good collateral flow on cerebral angiography.

REFERENCES

1. Archer CR, Horenstein S: Basilar artery occlusion: clinical and radiological correlation. *Stroke* 8:383–390, 1977.
2. Barinagarrementeria F, Amaya LE, Cantu C: Causes and mechanisms of cerebellar infarction in young patients. *Stroke* 28:2400–2404, 1997.
3. Bhadelia RA, Bengoa F, Gesner L, et al: Efficacy of MR angiography in the detection and characterization of occlusive disease in the vertebrobasilar system. *J Comput Assist Tomogr* 25:458–465, 2001.
4. Biemond A: Thrombosis of the basilar artery and the vascularization of the brain stem. *Brain* 74:300–317, 1951.
5. Biller J, Yuh WT, Mitchell GW, et al: Early diagnosis of basilar artery occlusion using magnetic resonance imaging. *Stroke* 19:297–306, 1988.
6. Blacker D, Wijdicks EFM: Stroke after polytrauma: clinical characteristics and mechanisms in 14 patients (abstract). *Ann Neurol* Suppl 1:S28, 2002.
7. Brandt T, Pessin MS, Kwan ES, et al: Survival with basilar artery occlusion. *Cerebrovasc Dis* 5:182–187, 1995.

8. Brückmann H, Ferbert A, del Zoppo GJ, et al: Acute vertebral-basilar thrombosis. Angiologic-clinical comparison and therapeutic implications. *Acta Radiol Suppl* 369:38–42, 1986.

9. Caplan LR: Occlusion of the vertebral or basilar artery. Follow up analysis of some patients with benign outcome. *Stroke* 10:277–282, 1979.

10. Caplan LR: Vertebrobasilar embolism. *Clin Exp Neurol* 28:1–22, 1991.

11. Caplan LR: *Posterior Circulation Disease: Clinical Findings, Diagnosis, and Management.* Cambridge, MA: Blackwell Science, 1996.

12. Caplan LR, Rosenbaum AE: Role of cerebral angiography in vertebrobasilar occlusive disease. *J Neurol Neurosurg Psychiatry* 38:601–612, 1975.

13. Cross DT III, Derdeyn CP, Moran CJ: Bleeding complications after basilar artery fibrinolysis with tissue plasminogen activator. *AJNR Am J Neuroradiol* 22:521–525, 2001.

14. Cross DT III, Moran CJ, Akins PT, et al: Relationship between clot location and outcome after basilar artery thrombolysis. *AJNR Am J Neuroradiol* 18:1221–1228, 1997.

15. Cross DT III, Moran CJ, Akins PT, et al: Collateral circulation and outcome after basilar artery thrombolysis. *AJNR Am J Neuroradiol* 19:1557–1563, 1998.

16. De la Vega F, Phan TG, Wijdicks EFM: Long-term outcome of basilar artery occlusion confirmed by magnetic resonance angiography (abstract). *Neurology* 56 Suppl 3:A289, 2001.

17. Devuyst G, Bogousslavsky J, Meuli R, et al: Stroke or transient ischemic attacks with basilar artery stenosis or occlusion: clinical patterns and outcome. *Arch Neurol* 59:567–573, 2002.

18. du Mesnil de Rochemont R, Neumann-Haefelin T, Berkefeld J, et al: Magnetic resonance imaging in basilar artery occlusion. *Arch Neurol* 59:398–402, 2002.

19. Ferbert A, Brückmann H, Drummen R: Clinical features of proven basilar artery occlusion. *Stroke* 21:1135–1142, 1990.

20. Glass TA, Hennessey PM, Pazdera L, et al: Outcome at 30 days in the New England Medical Center Posterior Circulation Registry. *Arch Neurol* 59:369–376, 2002.

21. Gondim FAA, Parks BJ, Cruz-Flores S: "Fou rire prodromique" as the presentation of pontine ischaemia secondary to vertebrobasilar stenosis. *J Neurol Neurosurg Psychiatry* 71:802–804, 2001.

22. Hacke W, Zeumer H, Ferbert A, et al: Intra-arterial thrombolytic therapy improves outcome in patients with acute vertebrobasilar occlusive disease. *Stroke* 19:1216–1222, 1988.

23. Haig AJ, Katz RT, Sahgal V: Mortality and complications of the locked-in syndrome. *Arch Phys Med Rehabil* 68:24–27, 1987.

24. Halbach VV, Higashida RT, Dowd CF, et al: Endovascular treatment of vertebral artery dissections and pseudoaneurysms. *J Neurosurg* 79:183–191, 1993.

25. Harrington T, Roche J: The dense basilar artery as a sign of basilar territory infarction. *Australas Radiol* 37:375–378, 1993.

26. Hart RG: Vertebral artery dissection. *Neurology* 38:987–989, 1988.

27. Hayashi J, Oguma F, Miyamura H, et al: Direct thrombolytic revascularization of the occluded basilar artery. *Cardiovasc Surg* 1:547–549, 1993.

28. Herderscheê D, Limburg M, Hijdra A, et al: Recombinant tissue plasminogen activator in two patients with basilar artery occlusion. *J Neurol Neurosurg Psychiatry* 54:71–73, 1991.

29. Hosoda K, Fujita S, Kawaguchi T, et al: Spontaneous dissecting aneurysms of the basilar artery presenting with a subarachnoid hemorrhage. Report of two cases. *J Neurosurg* 75:628–633, 1991.

30. Huemer M, Niederwieser V, Ladurner G: Thrombolytic treatment for acute occlusion of the basilar artery. *J Neurol Neurosurg Psychiatry* 58:227–228, 1995.

31. Iwase H, Kobayashi M, Kurata A, et al: Clinically unidentified dissection of vertebral artery as a cause of cerebellar infarction. *Stroke* 32:1422–1424, 2001.

32. Khurana RK: Autonomic dysfunction in pontomedullary stroke (abstract). *Ann Neurol* 12:86, 1982.

33. Kitanaka C, Tanaka J, Kuwahara M, et al: Magnetic resonance imaging study of intracranial vertebrobasilar artery dissection. *Stroke* 25:571–575, 1994.

34. Kitanaka C, Tanaka J, Kuwahara M, et al: Nonsurgical treatment of unruptured intracranial vertebral artery dissection with serial follow-up angiography. *J Neurosurg* 80:667–674, 1994.

35. Krespi Y, Gurol ME, Coban O, et al: Vertebral artery dissection presenting with isolated neck pain. *J Neuroimaging* 12:179–182, 2002.

36. Kubik CS, Adams RD: Occlusion of the basilar artery—a clinical and pathological study. *Brain* 69:73–121, 1946.

37. Levin BE, Margolis G: Acute failure of automatic respirations secondary to a unilateral brainstem infarct. *Ann Neurol* 1:583–586, 1977.

38. Levy C, Laissy JP, Raveau V, et al: Carotid and vertebral artery dissections: three-dimensional time-of-flight MR angiography and MR imaging versus conventional angiography. *Radiology* 190:97–103, 1994.

39. Levy EI, Horowitz MB, Koebbe CJ, et al: Transluminal stent-assisted angioplasty of the intracranial vertebrobasilar system for medically refractory, posterior circulation ischemia: early results. *Neurosurgery* 48:1215–1221, 2001.

40. Malm J, Kristensen B, Carlberg B, et al: Clinical features and prognosis in young adults with infratentorial infarcts. *Cerebrovasc Dis* 9:282–289, 1999.

41. Martinez HR, Elizondo G, Herrera J, et al: Basilar artery thrombosis diagnosed by MR imaging. *AJNR Am J Neuroradiol* 10 Suppl 5:81, 1989.

42. McCormick GF, Halbach VV: Recurrent ischemic events in two patients with painless vertebral artery dissection. *Stroke* 24:598–602, 1993.

43. Mueller S, Sahs AL: Brain stem dysfunction related to cervical manipulation. Report of three cases. *Neurology* 26:547–550, 1976.

44. Nakayama T, Tanaka K, Kaneko M, et al: Thrombolysis and angioplasty for acute occlusion of intracranial vertebrobasilar arteries. Report of three cases. *J Neurosurg* 88:919–922, 1998.

45. Nenci GG, Gresele P, Taramelli M, et al: Thrombolytic therapy for thromboembolism of vertebrobasilar artery. *Angiology* 34:561–571, 1983.

46. Norrving B, Cronqvist S: Lateral medullary infarction: prognosis in an unselected series. *Neurology* 41:244–248, 1991.

47. Pessin MS, Gorelick PB, Kwan ES, et al: Basilar artery stenosis: middle and distal segments. *Neurology* 37:1742–1746, 1987.

48. Pfeiffer G, Thayssen G, Arlt A, et al: Vertebrobasilar occlusion: outcome with and without local intra-arterial fibrinolysis. In Hacke W, del Zoppe GJ, Hirschberg M (eds): *Thrombolytic Therapy in Acute Ischemic Stroke.* New York, Springer, 1991, pp 216–220.

49. Phan TG, Wijdicks EFM: A sensory level on the trunk and sparing the face from vertebral artery dissection: How much more subtle can we get? (Letter to the editor.) *J Neurol Neurosurg Psychiatry* 66:691–692, 1999.

50. Phan TG, Wijdicks EFM: Intra-arterial thrombolysis for vertebrobasilar circulation ischemia. *Crit Care Clin* 15:719–742, 1999.

51. Phatouros CC, Higashida RT, Malek AM, et al: Endovascular stenting of an acutely thrombosed basilar artery: technical case report and review of the literature. *Neurosurgery* 44:667–673, 1999.

52. Pozzati E, Padovani R, Fabrizi A, et al: Benign arterial dissections of the posterior circulation. *J Neurosurg* 75:69–72, 1991.

53. Quintana JG, Drew EC, Richtsmeier TE, et al: Vertebral artery dissection and stroke following neck manipulation by Native American healer. *Neurology* 58:1434–1435, 2002.

54. Ropper AH: 'Convulsions' in basilar artery occlusion. *Neurology* 38:1500–1501, 1988.

55. Rose BS, Pretorius DL: Dissecting basilar artery aneurysm in Marfan syndrome: case report. *AJNR Am J Neuroradiol* 12:503–504, 1991.

56. Ross GJ, Ferraro F, DeRiggi L, et al: Spontaneous healing of basilar artery dissection: MR findings. *J Comput Assist Tomogr* 18:292–294, 1994.

57. Rothwell DM, Bondy SJ, Williams JI: Chiropractic manipulation and stroke: a population-based case-control study. *Stroke* 32:1054–1060, 2001.

58. Sasaki O, Ogawa H, Koike T, et al: A clinicopathological study of dissecting aneurysms of the intracranial vertebral artery. *J Neurosurg* 75:874–882, 1991.

59. Schievink WI: Spontaneous dissection of the carotid and vertebral arteries. *N Engl J Med* 344:898–906, 2001.

60. Schievink WI, Mokri B, O'Fallon WM: Recurrent spontaneous cervical-artery dissection. *N Engl J Med* 330:393–397, 1994.

61. Schuknecht B, Ratzka M, Hofmann E: The "dense artery sign"—major cerebral artery thromboembolism demonstrated by computed tomography. *Neuroradiology* 32:98–103, 1990.

62. Schwaighofer BW, Klein MV, Lyden PD, et al: MR imaging of vertebrobasilar vascular disease. *J Comput Assist Tomogr* 14:895–904, 1990.

63. Schwarz S, Egelhof T, Schwab S, et al: Basilar artery embolism. Clinical syndrome and neuroradiologic patterns in patients without permanent occlusion of the basilar artery. *Neurology* 49:1346–1352, 1997.

64. Sliwka U, Mull M, Stelzer A, et al: Long-term follow-up of patients after intraarterial thrombolytic therapy of acute vertebrobasilar artery occlusion. *Cerebrovasc Dis* 12:214–219, 2001.

65. Terada T, Higashida RT, Halbach VV, et al: Transluminal angioplasty for arteriosclerotic disease of the distal vertebral and basilar arteries. *J Neurol Neurosurg Psychiatry* 60:377–381, 1996.

66. Terada T, Yokote H, Tsuura M, et al: Tissue plasminogen activator thrombolysis and transluminal angioplasty in the treatment of basilar artery thrombosis: case report. *Surg Neurol* 41:358–361, 1994.

67. United States Food and Drug Administration: Letter to Healthcare Providers. Washington, DC, Food and Drug Administration, January 25, 1999.

68. Vonofakos D, Marcu H, Hacker H: CT diagnosis of basilar artery occlusion. *AJNR Am J Neuroradiol* 4:525–528, 1983.

69. Wallace RC, Furlan AJ, Moliterno DJ, et al: Basilar artery rethrombosis: successful treatment with platelet glycoprotein IIB/IIIA receptor inhibitor. *AJNR Am J Neuroradiol* 18:1257–1260, 1997.

70. Weintraub MI: Beauty parlor stroke syndrome: report of five cases. *JAMA* 269:2085–2086, 1993.

71. Wijdicks EFM, Nichols DA, Thielen KR, et al: Intra-arterial thrombolysis in acute basilar artery thromboembolism: the initial Mayo Clinic experience. *Mayo Clin Proc* 72:1005–1013, 1997.

72. Wijdicks EFM, Scott JP: Outcome in patients with acute basilar artery occlusion requiring mechanical ventilation. *Stroke* 27:1301–1303, 1996.

73. Youl BD, Coutellier A, Dubois B, et al: Three cases of spontaneous extracranial vertebral artery dissection. *Stroke* 21:618–625, 1990.

74. Zeumer H, Freitag HJ, Grzyska U, et al: Local intraarterial fibrinolysis in acute vertebrobasilar occlusion. Technical developments and recent results. *Neuroradiology* 31:336–340, 1989.

18

Cerebellar Infarct

Cerebellar infarction accounts for only 1% of all patients with ischemic stroke but is more common in younger patients, probably because of vertebral artery dissection.[25] Cerebellar infarction can be isolated or coexist with brain stem, thalamic, or cortical infarcts.[23] However, cerebellar infarcts may become of greater relevance when swollen tissue produces a mass effect. Usually within 3 days, signs of swelling overshadow vertigo and ataxia. Mass effect develops more frequently in patients with full territorial cerebellar infarcts, although only half have clinical deterioration.[22] Clinical deterioration may be particularly more frequent in patients with a posterior inferior cerebellar artery (PICA) occlusion or superior cerebellar artery (SCA) occlusion and in those with infarcts confined to the medial vermian hemispheric branches of these arteries.[11,17,20] Involvement of the anterior inferior cerebellar artery (AICA) is much less associated with mass effect.[22] The initial phase of cerebellar infarction is punctuated by clinical signs from cerebellar dysfunction, and practical knowledge is needed to recognize the subsequent stage of brain stem compression or ventricular obstruction.

Different clinical stages of deterioration could prompt neurosurgical intervention to remove the necrotic tissue or to place a ventriculostomy tube. There are some similarities in clinical course with cerebellar hematoma (Chapter 14), but swelling after infarction of the cerebellum is more protracted.

One must implicitly assume that early recognition of deterioration in cerebellar stroke can-

not be guaranteed in a neurologic ward, and not much should stand in the way to admit these patients for observation.

CLINICAL RECOGNITION

The clinical spectrum of cerebellar infarction has been investigated in much detail, largely in the seminal papers of Amarenco et al.[1–4] Some background is necessary. The arterial topography is depicted in Figure 18–1. Three main arteries supply the cerebellum: the PICA, which arises from the vertebral artery and supplies the caudal part of the cerebellar hemisphere and vermis; the AICA, originating from the basilar artery and supplying a small area of the anterior and medial cerebellum, including the middle cerebellar peduncle and flocculus on the lower posterior border of the cerebellum; and the SCA, which originates from the distal basilar artery close to the posterior cerebral artery and supplies the rostral half of the cerebellar hemisphere and vermis as well as the dentate nucleus.[1,28] Other infarcts may involve territories between two major arterial territories (junctional infarcts).[6] Swelling is less common in these types.[6] Multiple cerebellar infarcts may occur.[14,30] Most likely, a single large PICA providing branches to both cerebellar hemispheres is occluded.[14,30]

Patients with a cerebellar infarct in the PICA territory complain of severe vertigo, headache, nausea, vomiting, and unsteadiness of gait with dysarthria.[5,7,10,16,17] Hiccups may emerge and can be extremely invalidating. Patients with a

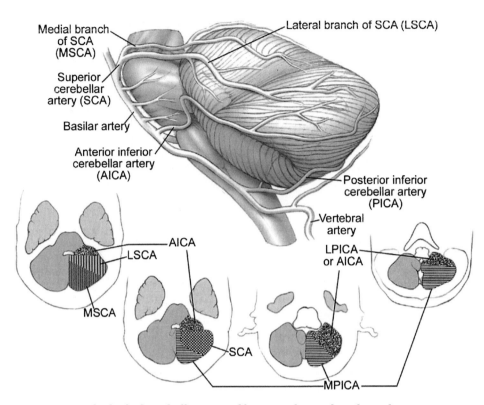

Figure 18–1. Vascular bed of cerebellum. Serial horizontal cuts identify single territories. LPICA, lateral branch of posterior inferior cerebellar artery; MPICA, medial branch of posterior inferior cerebellar artery. (Modified from Amarenco.[1] By permission of the American Academy of Neurology.)

PICA infarct (approximately 30% of cases) may have lateral medullary syndrome, or Wallenberg's syndrome, consisting of Horner's syndrome, weakness of the vocal cords or tongue, ataxia, unilateral facial analgesia, and contralateral analgesia in the trunk and limbs.

In patients with an AICA infarct, acute vertigo may develop and can be followed by acute deafness, tinnitus, peripheral facial palsy, hemiataxia, and thermoanalgesia. However, AICA infarcts can also produce more isolated cerebellar signs.

Infarction of the SCA predominantly produces dysarthria and ataxia, and although it may superficially mimic a lacunar syndrome, it is typically recognized by ipsilateral dysmetria, choreiform movements, Horner's syndrome, and crossed thermoanalgesia with palsy of the trochlear nerve. Bilateral infarcts in the SCA

territory may appear, pointing to the presence of an embolus in the distal basilar artery. Only complete involvement of these territories can lead to brain stem compression, which is uncommon.[31] The clinical syndromes of infarction in the distribution of the cerebellar arteries are summarized in Table 18–1.

NEUROIMAGING AND LABORATORY TESTS

The typical occurrence of a cerebellar infarct may not be recognized clinically. In addition, hypodensity indicating infarction may not be visible on the initial CT scan, and the appearance of distinctive hypodensity in the cerebellar hemisphere on CT scans may be delayed up to a few days ("stroke somewhere, stroke nowhere,

Table 18–1. Clinical Syndromes of Infarction in the Distribution of the Cerebellar Arteries

Arterial Territory	Structures Affected	Clinical Manifestations
Posterior inferior cerebellar artery	Restiform body, inferior surface of cerebellar hemisphere	Limb ataxia, gait ataxia
	Descending tract and nucleus of fifth nerve	Facial hypesthesia to pain and temperature
	Nucleus ambiguus	Palatal weakness, decreased gag reflex, dysphonia (vocal cord paresis)
	Descending sympathetic tract	Horner's syndrome
	Spinothalamic tract	Hypesthesia to pain and temperature of limbs and trunk
	Vestibular nuclei	Vertigo, nystagmus
Anterior inferior cerebellar artery	Brachium pontis, inferior surface of cerebellar hemisphere	Limb ataxia, gait ataxia
	Descending sympathetic tract	Horner's syndrome
	Cochlear nucleus	Deafness
	Intrapontine course of seventh nerve	Facial paralysis
	Trigeminal nuclei (descending tract and main sensory tract)	Facial hypesthesia
	Spinothalamic tract	Hypesthesia to pain and temperature of limbs and trunk
	Vestibular nuclei	Vertigo, nystagmus
Superior cerebellar artery	Brachium pontis, superior surface of cerebellar hemisphere (including vermis), dentate nucleus	Limb ataxia, gait ataxia
	Brachium conjunctivum (uncertain)	Choreiform dyskinesia
	Descending sympathetic tract	Horner's syndrome
	Spinothalamic tract	Hypesthesia to pain and temperature of limbs and trunk
	Pontine tectum	Trochlear nerve palsy

Source: Modified from Kase CS: Cerebellar infarction. *Heart Dis Stroke* 3:38–45, 1994. By permission of the American Heart Association.

stroke in the cerebellum").[22] Moreover, the specificity of a single CT scan is poor, and space-occupying lesions, including metastasis or abscess, may underlie the hypodensity. When cerebellar infarction appears, it is an ill-defined area of decreased density and can obliterate or distort the fourth ventricle. Disappearance of the quadrigeminal and ambient cisterns is a prominent CT scan indicator of cerebellar infarction but also of swelling and herniation. Another important feature of CT scanning is obstructive hydrocephalus. Hydrocephalus is evidenced on CT scans by enlargement of the temporal horns followed by enlargement of the lateral and third ventricles. Obstructive hydrocephalus sometimes becomes more apparent on serial CT scans; therefore, it is useful to repeat CT scanning with specific attention to deformity or disappearance of the fourth ventricle and further enlargement of the third and lateral ventricles. Hemorrhagic conversion is more common in larger infarcts and anticoagulated patients and may be associated with later dete-

rioration.[22] When an initially negative CT scan is obtained, 1 mm slices of the posterior fossa can be considered, but MRI and magnetic resonance angiography have the major advantages of localizing the lesion, delineating the extent of infarction and presence of swelling (Fig. 18–2), and documenting occlusion in the posterior circulation. Dissection of the vertebral artery can be found in any type of cerebellar infarct but, as expected, more frequently in PICA infarcts. Magnetic resonance angiography can be diagnostic and should be the initial test.

Examination of the cerebrospinal fluid is contraindicated. However, in a hectic emergency room, lumbar puncture may already have been performed. Typically, this occurs in patients with prominent initial severe headache that masks the cerebellar findings and with "normal" CT findings. Lumbar puncture could cause marked compartmental shifts and tonsillar herniation resulting in sudden death, but there is little documentation to support this commonly stated assertion.

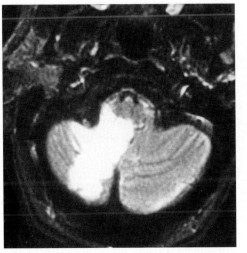

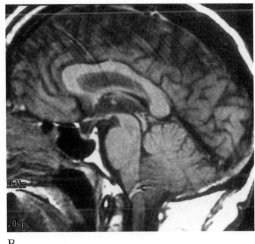

A

B

Figure 18–2. (*A,B*) Posterior inferior cerebellar artery distribution infarct (cerebellum, peduncle, pons) on magnetic resonance image with bowing of the brain stem from compression.

Further laboratory tests are tailored toward possible causes of cerebellar infarction. In a series of 115 patients with cerebellar infarcts, Amarenco et al.[3] found that 35% had a cardiac source of emboli. Transesophageal echocardiography should be performed to document an important cardioembolic source, as evidenced by markedly akinetic segments or intramural clots, or to grade atherosclerotic aortic arch disease.

FIRST STEPS IN MANAGEMENT

The decision to admit patients to the neurologic intensive care unit depends sometimes on the degree of arousal but more often on evidence of a mass effect on the initial CT scan. Airway management is important, and many patients require intubation for airway protection because of inability to maintain an open airway from drowsiness or from reduced oropharyngeal function.

It is well advised to restrict free water intake in the first 24 hours. Fluid intake can be more liberal if no swelling intervenes, but it is prudent to reduce fluid intake only to match sensible loss and urine output. No studies support

the use of hyperventilation, osmotic diuresis, or corticosteroids as preventive measures.

Intravenous administration of heparin must be started immediately, because cerebellar infarcts can be the first manifestation of a propagating clot in the basilar artery. Heparin may also reduce recurrence of embolization from a cardioembolic source. Heparin is particularly germane in patients who have atrial fibrillation and in patients with a recent myocardial infarct or ventricular failure. Generally, the risk of clinically relevant hemorrhagic conversion in the cerebellar infarct is low, and, if present, often only petechial hemorrhages appear on CT scans.[8] Even if deterioration occurs, it may be due to larger volumes of infarction and swelling rather than to expanding hematoma.[22] Cerebellar hemorrhagic infarction most commonly occurs in infarcts involving the SCA territory.[22] Routine follow-up CT scan may discover hemorrhagic conversion without much evidence of clinical worsening.[8]

Patients with concomitant brain stem infarction may have hiccups that can be difficult to manage. These hiccups not only are annoying and tiresome but also can significantly increase the risk of aspiration. Baclofen in a starting dose of 10 mg orally four times a day may substantially relieve hiccups and should be the drug of choice.[24] The dose of baclofen can be increased to 60 mg a day orally. Alternative choices are chlorpromazine, 25 to 50 mg intravenously in fractional injections over 30 minutes and then 50 to 60 mg per day orally; metoclopramide, 10 mg intravenously and then 10 to 40 mg orally; haloperidol, 2 mg intramuscularly every 4 to 8 hours; and valproic acid, 5 mg/kg four times a day.

Progressive swelling in patients with cerebellar infarcts can be associated with brief episodes of sinus bradycardia, but usually they can be left alone. If these episodes of bradycardia are associated with marked hypotension (systolic blood pressure of < 90 mm Hg), atropine (0.5 to 2.0 mg intravenously) should be administered. Patients who have marked hypertension as part of a Cushing response possibly should not be treated unless hypertension persists at high values (mean arterial pressure > 130 mm Hg).

Nutrition can be started only after swallowing mechanisms have been assessed. Typically, a nasogastric tube must be placed, also when patients are vomiting profusely.

The initial management of cerebellar infarct is summarized in Table 18–2.

DETERIORATION: CAUSES AND MANAGEMENT

The clinical course in patients admitted to the neurologic intensive care unit may evolve along three possible clinical scenarios. The mechanism of deterioration in a patient with a cerebellar infarct is direct compression of the brain stem, development of obstructive hydrocephalus, or progression of concurrent brain stem infarction. First, patients may be alert at presentation and exhibit cerebellar symptoms and signs that seem to stabilize in the first days but are succeeded by later rapid deterioration in level of consciousness. Progressive compression of the brain stem from swelling of the infarcted tissue is the most probable explanation in these patients. Second, patients may develop fluctuating responsiveness without progressive brain stem symptoms. Most often, CT scans show early enlargement of the ventricular system from obstruction at the level of the fourth ventricle. Third, and an almost invariably hopeless situation, patients become comatose within hours of the first initial symptoms. It is likely that this clinical course is most often observed in patients with additional extensive brain stem infarction. Pinpoint pupils, loss of oculocephalic reflexes, and ocular bobbing are present. Clearly distinguishing these mechanisms on clinical grounds alone remains difficult, particularly in patients with an impaired level of consciousness due to swelling. (Autopsy may not be revealing either. In a postmortem study of 16 patients with space-occupying cerebellar infarcts, tetraplegia correlated strongly with massive paramedian pontine infarction rather than with compression.[1] In another autopsy study, however, only a few structural changes in the brain stem were found in

Table 18–2. Initial Management of Cerebellar Infarct

Airway management	Intubate if hypoxemia, bulbar dysfunction, or progressive drowsiness
	T piece with pressure support only or IMV
Fluid management	2 L of 0.9% NaCl; avoid free water intake
Blood pressure management	No treatment of hypertension unless persistent mean arterial pressure ≥ 130 mm Hg
Nutrition	Assess swallowing mechanism and place nasogastric tube
Specific treatment	Heparin intravenously (activated partial thromboplastin time twice control value)
	Baclofen for hiccups (10 mg q6h)
	Ventriculostomy if progressive hydrocephalus but no expanding effect on the brain stem
	Suboccipital decompressive craniotomy if further neurologic deterioration from brain stem compression

IMV, intermittent mandatory ventilation.

patients who died of space-occupying cerebellar infarcts.[29])

Compression of the brain stem can be at the midbrain level in patients who have ascending (upward) transtentorial herniation and at the medullary level in patients with descending tonsillar herniation.

Upward cerebellar transtentorial herniation has some distinguishing features. Upward herniation may have more distinct signs of progressive drowsiness, hyperventilation, paralysis of upward gaze from pretectal compression, and development of unreactive pinpoint pupils and brisk oculocephalic responses. The distinction between upward transtentorial herniation and rapid development of acute hydrocephalus, however, can be very difficult, and both can be present at the same time. These clinical features can be accompanied by radiologic progression that begins with fourth ventricle deformity and continues to fourth ventricle shift, obstructive hydrocephalus, brain stem deformity, and effacement of the basal cisterns. Upward cerebellar transtentorial herniation has been linked to ventriculostomy,[18] but this dramatic development is not commonly seen, if at all.

Descending tonsillar herniation can be recognized by increasing neck stiffness (occasionally with a tendency toward opisthotonos), development of cardiac arrhythmias (usually bradycardia), and ataxic respiration (leading to frequent apneic episodes). Other symptoms of brain stem compression are gaze deviation in the horizontal plane, ipsilateral hemiparesis (from compression of the contralateral pyramid against the clivus),[15] and development of bilateral Babinski responses.[11] Signs that particularly localize brain stem compression are peripheral facial nerve palsy and loss of corneal reflexes. Eventually, further herniation produces extensor responses, oculocephalic responses disappear, and apnea occurs.

The management of cerebellar infarcts remains suboccipital craniotomy with resection of necrotic material[9] (Fig. 18–3). Ventriculostomy alone has been proposed as a temporary measure, but many neurosurgeons agree that suboccipital craniotomy should be offered in deteriorating patients to relieve brain stem compression. Ventriculostomy is reasonable if deterioration can be clearly attributed only to obstructive hydrocephalus.[12,32] The typical development in

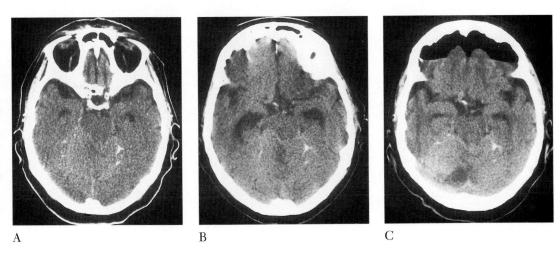

A   B   C

Figure 18–3. Progressive clinical deterioration in a patient with cerebellar infarct and swelling. (A) Brain stem compression and disappearance of fourth ventricle (note indentation of brain stem). (B) Brain stem compression with developing hydrocephalus. (C) After decompressive surgery, ambient cistern is partially open and bifrontal air appears associated with surgery in the sitting position.

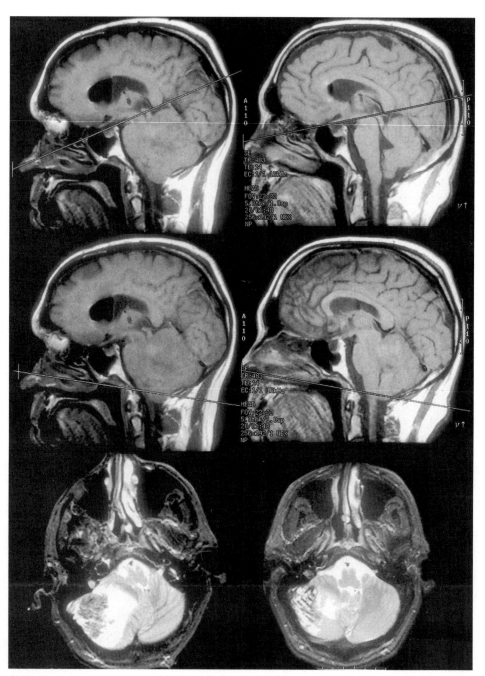

A

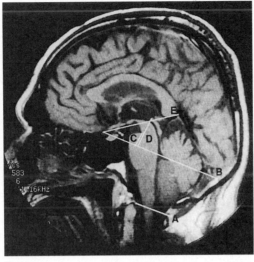

B

Figure 18–4. (*A*) Serial magnetic resonance images. Left image series shows massive cerebellar infarct with obstruction of the fourth ventricle and upward and downward herniation. The radiographic landmarks show upward displacement of the iter and tonsillar herniation with spontaneous resolution. Right image series shows resolution without craniotomy. (*B*) Magnetic resonance reference lines are added to assess shifts in the posterior fossa. Brain stem displacement or tonsillar descent can be appreciated by use of three reference lines on a sagittal magnetic resonance image. Twining's line (**B**) extends from the anterior tuberculum sellae to the internal occipital protuberance. In this image, **C** represents the line to the pontomesencephalic junction and **D** the line to the aqueduct. The incisural line (**E**) connects the anterior tuberculum sellae to the confluence of the straight sinus, great cerebral vein, and inferior sagittal sinus. The iter (tip of the aqueduct) is exactly on this line. The foramen magnum line (**A**) extends from the inferior tip of the clivus to the posterior tip of the foramen magnum. (*B* from Koh et al.[22] By permission of the American Heart Association.)

these patients is marked impairment of consciousness associated with enlargement of the ventricles, evolving sub-ependymal effusions surrounding the frontal horns, and disappearance of the fourth ventricle but with retained visualization of the ambient cisterns. Compression of the brain stem and simultaneously developing hydrocephalus in patients with cerebellar softening can rarely be managed conservatively. If acute hydrocephalus progresses on CT images, clinical deterioration soon follows, and improvement is commonly dramatic after decompression and ventriculostomy. The decision to proceed with suboccipital craniotomy to decompress the posterior fossa should not be made solely on the basis of CT or MRI findings. We have docu-

mented significant compression on MRI but virtually no impairment of consciousness after ventriculostomy (Fig. 18–4) and spontaneous resolution.[34] In addition, vertical displacement on MRI did not correlate with clinical presentation[22] or deterioration. This result suggests mechanism of deterioration is more likely due to lateral compression or anterior bowing with hydrocephalus.[22]

OUTCOME

Poor surgical outcome after craniotomy can be expected in patients older than 60 years, patients with brain stem signs at presentation, and patients in a late clinical stage, defined as coma with extensor posturing and recurrent cardiac arrhythmias, at the time of admission.[13] Nonetheless, in one study of patients with cerebellar infarcts, 40% of comatose patients had good recovery after decompressive surgery. Again, some patients with cerebellar infarcts can improve with conservative treatment alone. In a series of 11 patients with large cerebellar infarcts (8 with CT scan evidence of hydrocephalus), 5 were treated with ventriculostomy and 6 with supportive care alone. One patient died of progressive brain stem infarction, and the others had a good to fair outcome.[20]

The long-term outcome in patients with surgical treatment of expanding cerebellar infarcts has been studied only sparingly. Dysphagia and ataxia may remain significant handicaps. Patients with persistent dysphagia may benefit from cricopharyngeal myotomy, but recovery may not occur until after 3 years.[26] Many patients are able to function independently at home with only mild, nondisabling instability of gait, although some have transient ischemic attacks in the posterior circulation in the following years.[21] Patients with acute bilateral cerebellar infarcts (AICA[27] or PICA) also have the possibility of a good recovery. Two studies using more comprehensive measures of func-

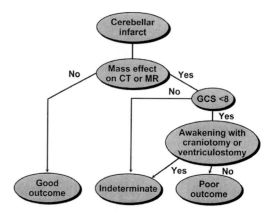

Figure 18–5. Outcome algorithm for cerebellar infarction. CT, computed tomography; GCS, Glasgow coma scale score; MR, magnetic resonance imaging. Good outcome: no assistance needed, minor handicap may remain. Indeterminate: any statement would be a premature conclusion. Poor outcome: severe disability or death, vegetative state.

tional independence found a less favorable outcome in patients with SCA occlusion.[19,33] Involvement of the dentate nucleus or superior cerebellar peduncle has been implicated. An outcome prediction algorithm is shown in Figure 18–5.

CONCLUSIONS

- Important CT scan criteria for the diagnosis of cerebellar swelling are hypodensity with obliteration of the fourth ventricle, brain stem deformity, obstructive hydrocephalus, and obliteration of the ambient cistern. MRI findings of brain stem displacement do not predict deterioration.
- Patients with PICA infarcts have a 30% risk of further deterioration from swelling.
- Symptoms of brain stem compression are from descending tonsillar herniation (gaze deviation in the horizontal plane, disappearing corneal reflexes, bilateral Babinski responses) or from ascending transtentorial herniation (drowsiness, paralysis of upward gaze, pinpoint pupils).
- Definitive management of cerebellar infarcts remains suboccipital craniotomy in patients with deterioration or who fail to improve. Ventriculostomy is considered only if deterioration is from obstructive hydrocephalus alone.

REFERENCES

1. Amarenco P: The spectrum of cerebellar infarctions. *Neurology* 41:973–979, 1991.
2. Amarenco P, Hauw JJ, Gautier JC: Arterial pathology in cerebellar infarction. *Stroke* 21:1299–1305, 1990.
3. Amarenco P, Lévy C, Cohen A, et al: Causes and mechanisms of territorial and nonterritorial cerebellar infarcts in 115 consecutive patients. *Stroke* 25:105–112, 1994.
4. Amarenco P, Roullet E, Hommel M, et al: Infarction in the territory of the medial branch of the posterior inferior cerebellar artery. *J Neurol Neurosurg Psychiatry* 53:731–735, 1990.
5. Barth A, Bogousslavsky J, Regli F: The clinical and topographic spectrum of cerebellar infarcts: a clinical-magnetic resonance imaging corrrelation study. *Ann Neurol* 33:451–456, 1993.
6. Canaple S, Bogousslavsky J: Multiple large and small cerebellar infarcts. *J Neurol Neurosurg Psychiatry* 66:739–745, 1999.
7. Chaves CJ, Caplan LR, Chung CS, et al: Cerebellar infarcts in the New England Medical Center Posterior Circulation Stroke Registry. *Neurology* 44:1385–1390, 1994.
8. Chaves CJ, Pessin MS, Caplan LR, et al: Cerebellar hemorrhagic infarction. *Neurology* 46:346–349, 1996.
9. Chen HJ, Lee TC, Wei CP: Treatment of cerebellar infarction by decompressive suboccipital craniectomy. *Stroke* 23:957–961, 1992.
10. Feely MP: Cerebellar infarction. *Neurosurgery* 4:7–11, 1979.
11. Hornig CR, Rust DS, Busse O, et al: Space-occupying cerebellar infarction. Clinical course and prognosis. *Stroke* 25:372–374, 1994.
12. Horwitz NH, Ludolph C: Acute obstructive hydrocephalus caused by cerebellar infarction. Treatment alternatives. *Surg Neurol* 20:13–19, 1983.
13. Jauss M, Krieger D, Hornig C, et al: Surgical and medical management of patients with massive cerebellar infarctions: results of the German-Austrian Cerebellar Infarction Study. *J Neurol* 246:257–264, 1999.
14. Kang DW, Lee SH, Bae HJ, et al: Acute bilateral cerebellar infarcts in the territory of posterior inferior cerebellar artery. *Neurology* 55:582–584, 2000.
15. Kanis KB, Ropper AH, Adelman LS: Homolateral hemiparesis as an early sign of cerebellar mass effect. *Neurology* 44:2194–2197, 1994.
16. Kase CS: Cerebellar infarction. *Heart Dis Stroke* 3: 38–45, 1994.
17. Kase CS, Norrving B, Levine SR, et al: Cerebellar infarction. Clinical and anatomic observations in 66 cases. *Stroke* 24:76–83, 1993.
18. Kase CS, Wolf PA: Cerebellar infarction: upward transtentorial herniation after ventriculostomy (letter to the editor). *Stroke* 24:1096–1098, 1993.
19. Kelly PJ, Stein J, Shafqat S, et al: Functional recovery after rehabilitation for cerebellar stroke. *Stroke* 32: 530–534, 2001.
20. Khan M, Polyzoidis KS, Adegbite AB, et al: Massive cerebellar infarction: "conservative" management. *Stroke* 14:745–751, 1983.
21. Klugkist H, McCarthy J: Surgical treatment of space-occupying cerebellar infarctions—4 1/2 years post-operative follow-up. *Neurosurg Rev* 14:17–22, 1991.
22. Koh MG, Phan TG, Atkinson JL, et al: Neuroimaging in deteriorating patients with cerebellar infarcts and mass effect. *Stroke* 31:2062–2067, 2000.
23. Kumral E, Bayulkem G, Akyol A, et al: Mesencephalic and associated posterior circulation infarcts. *Stroke* 33:2224–2231, 2002.
24. Launois S, Bizec JL, Whitelaw WA, et al: Hiccup in adults: an overview. *Eur Respir J* 6:563–575, 1993.
25. Malm J, Kristensen B, Carlberg B, et al: Clinical features and prognosis in young adults with infratentorial infarcts. *Cerebrovasc Dis* 9:282–289, 1999.
26. Perie S, Wajeman S, Vivant R, et al: Swallowing difficulties for cerebellar stroke may recover beyond three years. *Am J Otolaryngol* 20:314–317, 1999.
27. Roquer J, Lorenzo JL, Pou A: The anterior inferior cerebellar artery infarcts: a clinical-magnetic resonance imaging study. *Acta Neurol Scand* 97:225–230, 1998.
28. Savoiardo M, Bracchi M, Passerini A, et al: The vascular territories in the cerebellum and brainstem: CT and MR study. *AJNR Am J Neuroradiol* 8:199–209, 1987.
29. Scotti G, Spinnler H, Sterzi R, et al: Cerebellar softening. *Ann Neurol* 8:133–140, 1980.
30. Sorenson EJ, Wijdicks EFM, Thielen KR, et al: Acute bilateral infarcts of the posterior inferior cerebellar artery. *J Neuroimaging* 7:250–251, 1997.
31. Stangel M, Stapf C, Marx P: Presentation and prognosis of bilateral infarcts in the territory of the superior cerebellar artery. *Cerebrovasc Dis* 9:328–333, 1999.
32. Taneda M, Ozaki K, Wakayama A, et al: Cerebellar infarction with obstructive hydrocephalus. *J Neurosurg* 57:83–91, 1982.
33. Tohgi H, Takahashi S, Chiba K, et al: Cerebellar infarction. Clinical and neuroimaging analysis in 293 patients. The Tohoku Cerebellar Infarction Study Group. *Stroke* 24:1697–1701, 1993.
34. Wijdicks EFM, Maus TP, Piepgras DG: Cerebellar swelling and massive brain stem distortion: spontaneous resolution documented by MRI. *J Neurol Neurosurg Psychiatry* 65:400–401, 1998.

19

Acute Bacterial Meningitis

Community-acquired acute bacterial meningitis remains a potentially devastating neurologic disorder prone to fatal outcome. Not only is meningitis at times difficult to control, but, in some patients, pathogens (*Neisseria meningitidis*) continue to pose a threat to close contacts. Overall survival has improved, but major risks for persistent neurologic sequelae remain, predominantly from complications or late recognition and delayed initiation of antibiotic therapy.[20,28]

Some introductory remarks on epidemiology are appropriate. Acute bacterial meningitis can be community-acquired or nosocomial, and the circumstances are different (Table 19–1). Many patients have otogenic meningitis or had surgery for cholesteatoma causing chronic otitis.[5] In neurosurgical patients, penetrating injury, foreign bodies, placement of ventricular catheters, and instrumentation of the spine are the main potential triggers. The risk of acute bacterial meningitis is considerable in patients with wounds inflicted by high-velocity missiles. Cerebrospinal fluid leaks followed by bacterial meningitis are uncommon (3%) and not always prevented by antibiotic prophylaxis.[62]

In 30% to 50% of adults, bacterial meningitis is caused by *Streptococcus pneumoniae*. In another 10% to 15% each, *Escherichia coli*, *N. meningitidis*, and *Staphylococcus* species can be implicated. Less common organisms, including *Listeria monocytogenes* and *Pseudomonas aeruginosa*, are found in the remaining patients with acute bacterial meningitis. *L. monocytogenes* has been a major cause of bacterial meningitis in renal transplant recipients but also is seen in acquired immunodeficiency syndrome and in debilitated patients with alcohol abuse and diabetes.[7,31,40] *L. monocytogenes* may be on the rise as a cause of bacterial meningitis because of the increase in organ transplantation and advanced age. In a review from an urban center in Canada, it was the second most common pathogen after *S. pneumoniae*.[36] Human immunodeficiency virus infection is a major risk factor for *Listeria* infection, increasing the odds substantially.[38,42] The distribution of organisms causing acute bacterial meningitis in adults is summarized in Figure 19–1. Gram-negative bacilli include *E. coli*, *P. aeruginosa*, *Klebsiella pneumoniae*, and *Acinetobacter*. Streptococci include groups A, B, and G, *viridans*, *bovis*, and other species. Vaccines have greatly reduced *Haemophilus influenzae* type b in children to 5 years of age, at least in the United States, and it has not been replaced by other types. *H. influenzae* is now most commonly detected in adults, although its prevalence is low.[54]

The pathologic inflammatory cascade induced by bacterial meningitis is very complicated and mostly unresolved. Operative factors that may be avenues for new therapies include reactive oxygen (e.g., superoxide), nitrogen (e.g., nitric oxide and peroxynitrite), and matrix metalloproteinases. Matrix metalloproteinases are endopeptidases induced by tumor necrosis factor; they degrade extracellular matrix and open the blood–brain barrier.[47,58] Eventually this leads to disruption of the blood–brain barrier, brain edema, and neuronal damage due to vasculitis.[39,56]

Table 19–1. Predisposing Factors for Acute Bacterial Meningitis

Community-acquired	Nosocomial
Diabetes mellitus	Ventriculostomy
Liver cirrhosis or alcoholism	Endocarditis due to
Chronic otitis media	*Staphylococcus*
Prior head injury or	Immunosuppression in
craniotomy	recipients of
Gunshot wounds	transplants

Because of the complexity of acute bacterial meningitis and possible systemic involvement, very few patients with the disease are properly managed and monitored on wards. Admitted to the NICU often are patients lapsing into coma or patients with early complications (such as seizures or brain edema), associated pulmonary infection, or an uncertain clinical diagnosis.

CLINICAL RECOGNITION

The clinical features of acute bacterial meningitis have a very recognizable pattern. A history of myalgias, ear pain, sore throat, joint stiffness, and fatigue occurring several days before major clinical deterioration is often ob-

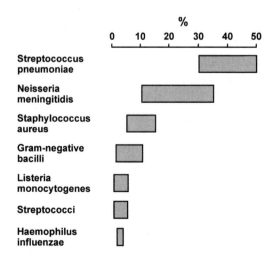

Figure 19–1. Distribution of causes of bacterial meningitis.

tained. Fever and vomiting are the most constant early signs, present in more than three-fourths of the patients, without much variation between age groups. Headache, often described as bursting and splitting, is severe enough to overcome the most commonly prescribed medications. Altered consciousness is characteristic but may vary from delirium to drowsiness and stupor. Therefore, an acute confusional state in a febrile elderly patient should always raise the possibility of acute bacterial meningitis, and symptoms should not be assumed to have resulted from a trivial pneumonia or urinary tract infection.[6] In contrast, diagnosing acute bacterial meningitis in a fully alert patient is exceptional.

Neck stiffness, an important sign, is obscured in patients who are comatose. In patients who are drowsy and stuporous, testing of neck stiffness by neck flexion or passive extension of the knees with the hips flexed at 90° (Kernig's sign) results in pain, opening of the eyes, a verbal response, and occasional combative behavior. Brudzinski's sign may be useful as well: neck flexion results in flexion of the knees and hips. The diagnostic validity of these tests is quite poor, and they do not identify most patients with meningitis.[59]

Papilledema in the early stages is unusual but may point to an evolving sagittal sinus thrombosis or progressive brain edema. Papilledema is most likely to be observed in a comatose patient with a fulminant clinical course.

Cranial nerves are generally not affected in patients with acute bacterial meningitis, but if they are (most commonly oculomotor nerves III, IV, and VI), tuberculosis, syphilis, or carcinomatous meningitis should be considered.

Focal or generalized tonic-clonic seizures should raise the suspicion of extension of bacterial meningitis to the parenchyma. Persistent generalized or focal seizures may also be seen in patients with subdural empyema, a disorder associated with sinusitis or mastoiditis that not only strongly resembles acute bacterial meningitis but also may be documented only by magnetic resonance imaging.

Systemic manifestations of acute bacterial meningitis may occur but do not predict a specific cause. Shock arises more frequently in meningitis from *N. meningitidis* or *S. aureus*. However, any fulminant acute bacterial meningitis may result in hypovolemic shock from dehydration, sometimes provoked by rigorous fluid restriction in an erroneous attempt to treat brain edema.[51] Rashes are not specific for any cause, nor is there any characteristic distribution. Petechiae and erythematous rashes may be seen in Rocky Mountain spotted fever, West Nile fever, and echovirus 9 infection (Chapter 21). A maculopapular rash, however, may suggest acute bacterial meningitis caused by *S. pneumoniae* or *S. aureus*. A limited petechial rash may occur in *S. aureus* meningitis or *N. meningitidis* meningitis and in any type of viral meningitis. In addition, hemorrhagic lesions, including circumscribed, raised petechial hemorrhages, subconjunctival

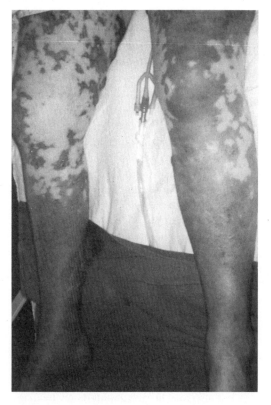

Figure 19–2. Characteristic purpura associated with *N. meningitidis* meningitis.

hemorrhages, purpura with a geographic border (Fig. 19–2), and lesions evolving into bullae, have traditionally been linked to *N. meningitidis* meningitis and are typically associated with shock.

Differentiation of postneurosurgical chemical meningitis from bacterial meningitis on the basis of clinical and CSF data is very difficult. A review of 70 patients suggested a very low probability when wound infection, new focal findings, coma, new-onset seizures, temperature exceeding 39.4°C, rhinorrhea, and otorrhea were all absent. Whether antibiotic therapy can be withheld in these patients is very debatable.[9,23]

Certain organisms are expected to be more frequent in particular circumstances[7,18,37,40] (Table 19–2). Gram-negative bacilli meningitis (*Pseudomonas* and *E. coli*) should be considered in neutropenic patients after treatment with neoplastic agents and in patients with hematologic malignant disease. Bacterial meningitis in immunocompromised patients is often a more severe manifestation of *S. pneumoniae* or could be caused by *L. monocytogenes*. With the reemergence of *Mycobacterium tuberculosis*, extrapulmonary manifestations may become prevalent in human immunodeficiency virus-infected patients and intravenous drug abusers.[13]

Clinical manifestations of tuberculous meningitis can be quite different, with a more gradual course of evolution, vague general feeling of malaise, and comparably less frequent neck stiffness (up to 30%).[45] Behavioral change, low-grade fever, and cranial nerve deficits (III, IV, VI, VIII) are observed significantly more often. Chest radiography may be helpful, and miliary lesions have been found in 25% to 50% of patients.

Aseptic meningitis can be considered when CSF lymphocytic pleocytosis is not associated with an isolated organism, particularly in patients with recent administration of drugs. Well-known drugs are intravenous gamma globulin, ibuprofen, carbamazepine, sulindac, trimethoprim-sulfamethoxazole, muromonab-CD3, and isoniazid. Symptoms usually resolve within days after discontinuation.[14]

Table 19-2. Causes of Bacterial Meningitis

Clinical Situation	Highly Probable Organism
Otitis media, mastoiditis, sinusitis	Streptococcus pneumoniae, Haemophilus influenzae
Pneumonia	S. pneumoniae, Neisseria meningitidis
Endocarditis	Staphylococcus aureus, S. pneumoniae
Asplenism	S. pneumoniae
	H. influenzae
	N. meningitidis
Alcoholism	S. pneumoniae
	Listeria monocytogenes
Cerebrospinal fluid shunt	Staphylococcus epidermidis
Penetrating trauma	S. aureus
Intravenous drug abuse	S. aureus
Immunosuppression, acquired immunodeficiency syndrome, and transplantation	L. monocytogenes
	Pseudomonas aeruginosa
	Escherichia coli

See also references 7, 18, 37, and 40.

NEUROIMAGING AND LABORATORY TESTS

Acute bacterial meningitis is diagnosed by examination of the CSF.[32] Turbid CSF often confirms the initial diagnosis. Conversely, crystal-clear CSF decreases the probability of acute bacterial meningitis, since only a few hundred leukocytes are necessary to reduce CSF clarity. Cerebrospinal fluid with a high viscosity or early clotting indicates very high protein content. Cerebrospinal fluid opening pressures are often increased (200 to 500 mm H_2O) in acute bacterial meningitis. The characteristic CSF profile in bacterial meningitis is a markedly increased cell count (10 to 10,000 leukocytes/mm^3, with more than 80% neutrophils), but may be much less very early in the illness or in immunocompromised patients. In patients with a marginal increase in the total number of cells, differentiation from viral meningitis becomes virtually impossible and a second sample of CSF is needed 8 to 24 hours later. Typical CSF findings in tuberculous meningitis are pleocytosis with a lymphocytic predominance, a greatly increased protein level (about 200 mg/dL), and a markedly reduced glucose value. Smears are often negative, and only cultures identify the organism.

A traumatic lumbar puncture may increase the leukocyte count. The true leukocyte count can be estimated by subtracting 1 leukocyte for every 700 erythrocytes. The CSF glucose concentration is normally 70% of the serum glucose value and in acute bacterial meningitis may be normal or decreased. Any ratio of CSF to serum that is less than 0.50 indicates a decrease in glucose concentration. (A decreased glucose ratio may be less reliable in patients who have had a recent infusion of glucose-containing fluids, and 2 hours are required for equilibration.) Protein values are usually more than 100 mg/dL and may be less discriminating between viral and bacterial meningitides. An unconfirmed study in children suggested that urine reagent strips may be helpful in the initial assessment of bacterial meningitis.[44] Normal CSF was differentiated from infected CSF by use of semiquantitative measurements of glucose, protein, and leukocytes; specificity was 100% and sensitivity 97%. The test, if results are replicated, may indeed be useful during the wait for laboratory results, which can easily require 45 to 60 minutes.

An essential diagnostic procedure is a Gram stain of the first uncentrifuged CSF sample. Gram-positive staining may suggest specific organisms (lancet-shaped indicate *S. pneumoniae*, rods indicate *L. monocytogenes*, and cocci in clusters indicate *Staphylococcus*). Gram-negative bacilli often point to *Klebsiella, P. aeruginosa,* or *E. coli.* Gram-negative diplococci indicate *N. meningitidis*; one must be certain, however, that there is no technical error, possibly caused by delayed processing of the CSF or by faulty use of the dye material, that falsely suggests *Neisseria* species in patients with streptococcal meningitis (and may unnecessarily cause an upsetting alert). The recent development of a polymerase chain reaction has facilitated recognition of *Neisseria,* but its sensitivity is not yet known[16,48] and it is not commercially available in the United States.

Cultures of CSF coupled with blood cultures remain the standard for evaluation of suspected acute bacterial meningitis. However, 2 days may be required for classification of the responsible species. In one study of bacterial meningitis, positive identification in blood cultures was 79% for *H. influenzae,* 56% for *S. pneumoniae,* 33% for *N. meningitidis,* 29% for β-hemolytic streptococcus meningitis, and only 17% for *S. aureus* meningitis.

Other diagnostic tests are readily available. Latex particle agglutination, which may rapidly test for bacterial antigens, has a specificity in CSF of 95% in *H. influenzae* and 50% in *S. pneumoniae* but only 30% in *N. meningitidis.* Measurement of C-reactive protein for differentiation between viral and bacterial meningitides, particularly in patients partially treated with oral antibiotics, is not very reliable in adults. The Limulus amebocyte lysate assay detects gram-negative endotoxin with a sensitivity of almost 100% but a specificity of about 90%.[21]

At the time of admission to the neurologic intensive care unit, it is reasonable to perform a baseline CT scan in every patient with acute bacterial meningitis despite the low yield. Computed tomography scan may unexpectedly demonstrate a subdural empyema or epidural abscess, either of which can clinically mimic acute bacterial meningitis. An otherwise normal CT scan of the brain should be additionally scrutinized for sinusitis or mastoiditis, which requires additional bone windows.

Computed tomography scanning is definitely indicated in patients without improvement after appropriate antibiotic treatment. Cerebral edema, an indication of poor prognosis, is occasionally seen. Resistance to antibiotic therapy seems a probable explanation in some of these unfortunate patients. Computed tomography scan is also indicated in patients with marked decrease in level of consciousness, papilledema, or neurologic findings indicating a parenchymal lesion. A prospective study of 301 adults with "suspected" meningitis (limited in applicability because most patients had a normal level of consciousness and only nine pathogens were isolated, three of which were bacterial) suggested that very few patients (2%) had a mass effect on CT. Computed tomography scanning had a higher yield of abnormal findings in patients who were older than 60 years, were in an immunocompromised state, had a history of seizures, had focal signs and a prior central nervous system lesion, and had reduction in level of consciousness.[34]

Antibiotics must be administered intravenously before transport to the CT scanner. Antibiotic treatment affects CSF cultures but not significantly so if the specimen is obtained within 2 hours after antibiotic administration. When samples were obtained 4 to 12 hours after administration of antibiotics, CSF cultures were positive in approximately 50% of the patients.[60] In addition, as noted earlier, the latex particle agglutination test can be helpful when a significant delay between antibiotic administration and CSF examination has occurred.

Magnetic resonance imaging is more sensitive in diagnosing possible complications of bacterial meningitis, such as subdural effusions, cerebritis or abscess, cerebral sinus thrombosis, early hydrocephalus (most commonly in patients with tuberculous meningitis), and cerebral infarcts. Pyogenic ventriculitis can be documented by magnetic resonance imaging, preferably in infections caused by gram-negative organisms and *Staphylococcus.* The magnetic resonance characteristics include irregularly contoured sedimentary material in the posterior horns and a bright signal on diffusion-weighted sequences.[25]

FIRST STEPS IN MANAGEMENT

The initial management in patients with acute bacterial meningitis is shown in Table 19–3.

Respiratory isolation precaution is indicated only for patients in whom the possibility of N. meningitidis infection is very high and is continued for the first 24 hours of treatment. For all other patients, no specific measures other than hand-washing for 2 minutes are necessary.

Patients with acute bacterial meningitis are almost invariably dehydrated from vomiting and fever. Adequate fluid replacement should be established with at least 3 L of isotonic saline. Free water administration should be avoided because it aggravates hyponatremia in some patients. Hyponatremia is frequently seen and has traditionally been attributed to the syndrome of inappropriate antidiuretic hormone, although this mechanism has recently been questioned (see Chapter 31). The clinical manifestations of hyponatremia are mild in most cases and seldom affect the level of consciousness. A rapid decrease in plasma sodium may, however, decrease the threshold of seizures. Mild free water restriction is the treatment of choice in hyponatremia associated with bacterial meningitis, but the electrolyte abnormality is self-limiting in most instances.

Any patient with acute severe bacterial meningitis should have cannulation of the radial artery for display of intra-arterial blood pressure and a large-bore, peripherally placed intravenous catheter for administration of fluids and antibiotics. Hemodynamic monitoring with a centrally placed venous catheter is not indicated except in patients with shock associated with meningococcal meningitis.

Hemodynamic management in patients with endotoxic septic shock is complex. Septic shock is recognized by hypotension, clammy skin, and poor perfusion of the kidneys, evidenced by oliguria. When hemodynamic variables are available, patients are found to have an increase in cardiac output associated with tachycardia and decreased systemic vascular resistance and an increase in oxygen uptake (see Chapter 10). Blood lactate concentration, an important marker, is increased. Treatment is volume infusion with albumin 5% to attain pulmonary artery wedge pressures of 12 to 14 mm Hg and blood transfusions to increase the hematocrit to 35% to ensure oxygen-carrying capacity.

Empirical antibiotic coverage generally includes a cephalosporin (cefotaxime or ceftriaxone), and definitive treatment should be adjusted when cultures and sensitivities become known.[12,33,50] The minimal inhibitory concentration for each of the antibiotics is shown in Table 19–4. The addition of vancomycin is strongly recommended for coverage of penicillin-resistant pneumococci strains (Table 19–3), particularly in geographic areas where it is more prevalent. The recommended antibiotic dosages for each of the pathogens is shown in Table 19–5. The time between admission to the emergency department and the first antibiotic dose should be within hours. An-

Table 19–3. Initial Management in Patients with Acute Bacterial Meningitis

Fluid management	3 L of isotonic saline; fluid restriction to 50 mL/hour in severe hyponatremia (plasma sodium ≤ 125 mmol/L)
Antibiotic treatment	Cefotaxime, 8–12 g/day intravenously (IV) in divided doses every 4 hours, or ceftriaxone 2–4 g/day in divided doses every 12 hours Vancomycin, 2 g/day in divided doses every 12 hours Ampicillin, 12 g/day in divided doses every 4 hours, in immunosuppressed patients and those older than 50 years
Adjuvant therapy	Dexamethasone, 0.6 mg/kg per day in 4 divided doses for 4 days (in fulminant course); consider adding rifampin, 600 mg orally
Preventive measures	Subcutaneous heparin for prophylaxis of deep venous thrombosis

Table 19–4. Minimal Inhibitory Concentration Breakpoints for Antimicrobial Agents Used to Treat *Streptococcus pneumoniae* Infections (μg/mL)

Antimicrobial Agent	Susceptible	NONSUSCEPTIBLE Intermediate	Resistant
Penicillin	≤ 0.06	0.1–1.0	≥ 2.0
Ceftriaxone	≤ 0.5	1.0	≥ 2.0
Cefotaxime	≤ 0.5	1.0	≥ 2.0
Cefepime	≤ 0.5	1.0	≥ 2.0
Vancomycin	≤ 1.0	—	—
Rifampin	≤ 1.0	2.0	≥ 4.0
Chloramphenicol	≤ 4.0	—	≥ 8.0
Imipenem	≤ 0.12	0.25–0.5	≥ 1.0
Meropenem°	≤ 0.12	≥ 0.25	—

°Susceptibility interpretive criteria have not yet been established by the National Committee for Clinical Laboratory Standards.
Data from National Committee for Clinical Laboratory Standards: *Methods for Dilution Antimicrobial Susceptibility Tests for Bacteria That Grow Aerobically: Approved Standard.* 4th ed, NCCLS Document M7-A4. Wayne, PA, National Committee for Clinical Laboratory Standards, 1997.

tibiotics should always be administered if a major delay in CT scanning is anticipated and CSF examination has to be deferred. A blood culture before the first dose of antibiotics is advised. Chemoprophylaxis is given to household contacts of patients admitted with *N. meningitidis* meningitis and to health care workers who have intimate contact with respiratory secretions (Table 19–6). The prophylactic effect may be minimal if the drug is given 14 days after onset.[53]

In adults, the use of corticosteroids is highly debatable, certainly when administration is 24 hours after onset of the illness.[27] Corticosteroids may reduce inflammation and reduce crossing of the antibiotic over the blood–brain barrier. On a cellular level, they may mute the inflammatory response by reducing cytokines (e.g., interleukin-1β), reducing expression of adhesion molecules, and lessening alteration of the blood–brain barrier by reducing matrix metalloproteinases.[47,58] On the other hand, dexamethasone in randomized studies has reduced mortality and hearing loss in children with meningitis from *H. influenzae*.[2,30,35,41] Its effect in adults with bacterial meningitis

Table 19–5. Treatment of Bacterial Meningitis After Identification of the Infecting Organism

Streptococcus pneumoniae	Penicillin G, 20–24 million U/day IV (in divided doses q4h),° or cefotaxime, 8–12 g/day IV (in divided doses q4h)
Neisseria meningitidis	Penicillin G, 20–24 million U/day IV (in divided doses q4h), or ampicillin, 12 g/day IV (in divided doses q4h)
Staphylococcus aureus	Vancomycin (methicillin-resistant), 2 g/day IV (in divided doses q12h), or nafcillin (methicillin-sensitive), 8–12 g/day IV (in divided doses q4h)
Enterobacter	Cefotaxime, 8–12 g/day (in divided doses q4h), or ceftriaxone, 2–4 g/day (q12h)
Haemophilus influenzae	Cefotaxime, 8–12 g/day (in divided doses q4h)
Pseudomonas aeruginosa	Ceftazidime, 6 g/day (in divided doses q8h)
Listeria monocytogenes	Ampicillin, 12 g/day (in divided doses q4h)
Mycobacterium tuberculosis[†]	Isoniazid (start at 5 mg/kg per day PO)
	Rifampin (start at 10 mg/kg per day PO)
	Pyrazinamide, 15–30 mg/kg per day PO
	Consider adding ethambutol, 15 mg/kg per day PO, if resistance is suspected

IV, intravenously; PO, by mouth.
°Consider continuous infusion.
[†]Treatment for 6 months.

Table 19–6. Schedule for Administering Chemoprophylaxis Against Meningococcal Disease

Drug and Age Group	Dosage*
Rifampin[†]	
Children < 1 month	5 mg/kg of body weight every 12 hours for 2 days
Children ≥ 1 month	10 mg/kg every 12 hours for 2 days
Adults	600 mg every 12 hours for 2 days
Ciprofloxacin[‡]	
Children	—
Adults	500 mg in a single dose
Ceftriaxone	
Children < 15 years	125 mg in a single intramuscular dose
Children ≥ 15 years and adults	250 mg in a single intramuscular dose

*The drug is administered orally unless otherwise indicated.
[†]Rifampin is not recommended for pregnant women, because the drug is teratogenic in laboratory animals. Because the reliability of oral contraceptives may be affected by rifampin therapy, consideration should be given to using alternative contraceptive measures while rifampin is being administered.
[‡]Ciprofloxacin is not generally recommended for persons younger than 18 years or for pregnant or lactating women, because the drug causes cartilage damage in immature laboratory animals. However, ciprofloxacin can be used for chemoprophylaxis in children if no acceptable alternative therapy is available.
Source: Rosenstein NE, Perkins BA, Stephens DS, et al: Meningococcal disease. N Engl J Med 344:1378–1388, 2001. By permission of the Massachusetts Medical Society.

due to totally different pathogens is unknown, but it appears most effective in *S. pneumoniae.*[30] A recently completed small, prospective controlled trial found significantly fewer neurologic complications and hearing loss in adults using dexamethasone 0.6 mg/kg per day in 4 divided doses for the first 4 days of antibiotic therapy.[29] Another study found improved outcome but no effect on hearing loss.[18] It may be effective in tuberculous meningitis[17,49] but only in selected patients with more severe disease, evidence of increased intracranial pressure, or deterioration despite antituberculosis therapy.[17] A major concern is that vancomycin penetration into the CSF is markedly reduced by dexamethasone. Some studies claimed reductions in concentration of vancomycin up to 77%.[10,46] Addition of rifampin could enhance absorption, or a larger dose of vancomycin could be used. Our practice is to give dexamethasone (0.6 mg/kg per day in four divided doses) for 4 days before the first dose of an antibiotic[52] to patients with fulminant bacterial meningitis if they are seen within hours of presentation, to patients with cerebral edema, and to patients with a high likelihood of tuberculous meningitis.[61] We add rifampin to vancomycin until susceptibility is known.

Recommendations for the duration of antibiotic therapy vary, but we attend to recent guidelines: *H. influenzae* and *N. meningitidis,* 7 days; *S. pneumoniae,* 10 to 14 days; *L. monocytogenes* and group B streptococci, 14 to 21 days; and other gram-negative bacilli, 21 days.[50]

DETERIORATION: CAUSES AND MANAGEMENT

Many patients do well after antibiotic therapy, but in a few, further deterioration is marked by progression to persistent coma. The course of this progression is rapid, usually beginning soon after admission. In the advanced stage of cerebral edema, pupils become sluggish and dilated and papilledema appears. Computed tomography scanning may show signs of cortical effacement, but this may be very difficult to appreciate in young patients with less prominent sulci. Progressive effacement of the sylvian fissure and compression of ventricles and the basal cisterns are more diagnostic for cerebral edema on CT scans. Patients with acute brain edema require intubation and mechanical ventilation to a respiratory alkalosis with

PaCO₂ in the low 30s. Cerebral blood flow autoregulation is impaired in acute bacterial meningitis because of acidosis-induced arteriolar dilatation. Hyperventilation seemed to improve autoregulation in a recent study.[43] Administration of a bolus of mannitol (1 g/kg) guided by standard criteria and goals may follow (Chapter 8). A parenchymal intracranial pressure monitor is placed to determine the effect of treatment. The development of brain edema is an ominous sign and may indicate progression to brain death.

In a rapidly worsening patient, subdural empyema should be considered for what at first seems to be acute bacterial meningitis. The clinical presentation of headache and worsening coma can be analogous to acute bacterial meningitis. Important clues are prior paranasal

sinusitis and recent sinus surgery, both of which are associated with subdural empyema in a considerable number of patients. To complicate matters further, CT scanning can yield normal results or may not have been performed initially. Magnetic resonance imaging may demonstrate multilocular collections that cannot be seen with CT scanning, particularly those localized at the convexity[63] (Fig. 19–3). In most patients, however, CT scanning with contrast demonstrates the subdural pus pocket (Fig. 19–4). A large craniotomy is needed to salvage the patient.[4] Outcome is poor if patients are comatose.

Another important cause for clinical deterioration is therapeutic failure. In recent years, penicillin-resistant *S. pneumoniae* strains have increased in frequency.[1,11,24] Any

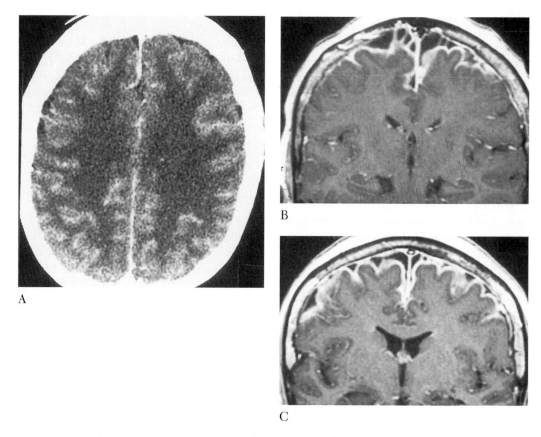

Figure 19–3. Neuroimaging in a patient with rapidly developing coma after sinus surgery. (*A*) Computed tomography scan with contrast shows normal findings. (*B* and *C*) Magnetic resonance images show significant multilocular subdural collections suspicious for subdural empyema.

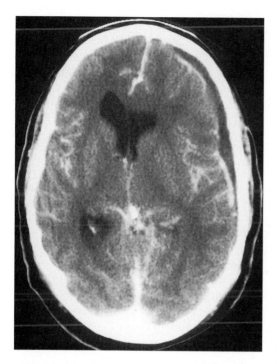

Figure 19–4. Contrast computed tomography scan showing subdural empyema with mass effect.

patient with bacterial meningitis, rapid clinical deterioration, persistent high fever despite antibiotic treatment, and diplococci in a repeated CSF culture after several days of treatment may have a penicillin-resistant strain of *S. pneumoniae*. As mentioned earlier, the addition of vancomycin to the initial empirical antibiotic treatment should reduce therapeutic failures. Rarely, intrathecal vancomycin with monitoring of CSF levels is needed in addition to systemic therapy.

The patient's condition may deteriorate from seizures, but the low incidence of 10% does not justify prophylactic treatment. Nonconvulsive status epilepticus is a rare cause of deterioration in patients with meningitis, but we monitor patients with electroencephalograms and video when seizures have occurred, if they fail to awaken promptly or their level of consciousness waxes and wanes.

Systemic causes of neurologic deterioration are infrequent. Some patients treated with high doses of cephalosporins may become disoriented, and their condition may deteriorate from toxic levels with generalized myoclonus, predominantly when renal failure is present.

OUTCOME

Prognostic factors in acute bacterial meningitis depend on the organism.[8] Other well-recognized risk factors are age and duration of illness before effective antibiotic therapy begins, hypotension, and seizures.[3,15] The case fatality rate is 19% for *S. pneumoniae* and 13% for *N. meningitidis*, and even in the current era, one in five adults with bacterial meningitis dies.[55] Mortality is higher in *N. meningitidis* meningitis when septicemia is present.[26] *Klebsiella*, a rare cause of acute bacterial meningitis, has a much higher reported mortality of 43%.[57]

Long-term neurologic deficits remain uncommon and are less than 10%.[3] Outcome in meningitis-associated traumatic CSF leak is good when the cause is *S. pneumoniae* and treatment with a third-generation cephalosporin is begun early. Nonetheless, the major disabling sequelae of acute bacterial meningitis are hearing loss and a seizure disorder. The risk of significant hearing impairment is approximately 15% in patients with *N. meningitidis* meningitis. Gadolinium-enhanced, high-resolution magnetic resonance imaging documented abnormalities in the cochlear nerve, but because many patients in the study received brief courses of gentamycin besides standard therapy, the relationship between meningitis and cochlear damage was clouded.[19]

The effects of empirical administration of vancomycin on outcome are unclear. One survey found that vancomycin-treated patients were less likely to be transferred to long-term care facilities but still had neurologic deficits. It is possible that vancomycin was used preferentially in patients with greater illness and deteriorating condition.[22]

An outcome algorithm for acute bacterial meningitis is shown in Figure 19–5.

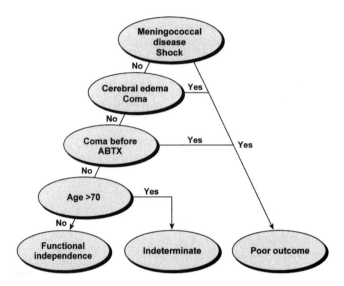

Figure 19–5. Outcome algorithm for bacterial meningitis. ABTX, antibiotic therapy. Functional independence: no assistance needed, minor handicap may remain. Indeterminate: any statement would be a premature conclusion. Poor outcome: severe disability or death, vegetative state.

CONCLUSIONS

- *S. pneumoniae* is the cause of most cases of adult bacterial meningitis. *S. aureus* can be implicated in penetrating trauma and intravenous drug abuse. In immunosuppressed patients, alcoholics, and debilitated patients with diabetes, *L. monocytogenes* or *P. aeruginosa* should be considered.
- Empirical therapy for adult bacterial meningitis consists of cefotaxime or ceftriaxone. Ampicillin is added in immunosuppressed patients and in patients older than 50 years.
- Vancomycin is currently recommended in the empirical regimen to treat penicillin-resistant pneumococci.
- Rapid deterioration in patients with presumed acute bacterial meningitis has three major causes: (*1*) fulminant meningitis or penicillin-resistant *S. pneumoniae* not properly covered with vancomycin, (*2*) cerebral edema, and (*3*) failure to diagnose empyema.

REFERENCES

1. Allen KD: Penicillin-resistant pneumococci. *J Hosp Infect* 17:3–13, 1991.
2. American Academy of Pediatrics Committee on Infectious Diseases: Dexamethasone therapy for bacterial meningitis in infants and children. *Pediatrics* 86: 130–133, 1990.
3. Aronin SI, Peduzzi P, Quagliarello VJ: Community-acquired bacterial meningitis: risk stratification for adverse clinical outcome and effect of antibiotic timing. *Ann Intern Med* 129:862–869, 1998.
4. Bannister G, Williams B, Smith S: Treatment of subdural empyema. *J Neurosurg* 55:82–88, 1981.

5. Barry B, Delattre J, Vie F, et al: Otogenic intracranial infections in adults. *Laryngoscope* 109:483–487, 1999.
6. Behrman RE, Meyers BR, Mendelson MH, et al: Central nervous system infections in the elderly. *Arch Intern Med* 149:1596–1599, 1989.
7. Beninger PR, Savoia MC, Davis CE: *Listeria monocytogenes* meningitis in a patient with AIDS-related complex (letter to the editor). *J Infect Dis* 158:1396–1397, 1988.
8. Bohr V, Rasmussen N, Hansen B, et al: Pneumococcal meningitis: an evaluation of prognostic factors in 164 cases based on mortality and on a study of lasting sequelae. *J Infect* 10:143–157, 1985.
9. Brown EM, de Louvois J, Bayston R, et al: Distin-

guishing between chemical and bacterial meningitis in patients who have undergone neurosurgery (letter to the editor). *Clin Infect Dis* 34:556–557, 2002.

10. Cabellos C, Martinez-Lacasa J, Martos A, et al: Influence of dexamethasone on efficacy of ceftriaxone and vancomycin therapy in experimental pneumococcal meningitis. *Antimicrob Agents Chemother* 39:2158–2160, 1995.

11. Catalán MJ, Fernández JM, Vazquez A, et al: Failure of cefotaxime in the treatment of meningitis due to relatively resistant *Streptococcus pneumoniae*. *Clin Infect Dis* 18:766–769, 1994.

12. Cherubin CE, Eng RH, Norrby R, et al: Penetration of newer cephalosporins into cerebrospinal fluid. *Rev Infect Dis* 11:526–548, 1989.

13. Clark WC, Metcalf JC Jr, Muhlbauer MS, et al: *Mycobacterium tuberculosis* meningitis: a report of twelve cases and a literature review. *Neurosurgery* 18:604–610, 1986.

14. Connolly KJ, Hammer SM: The acute aseptic meningitis syndrome. *Infect Dis Clin North Am* 4:599–622, 1990.

15. Conte HA, Chen YT, Mehal W, et al: A prognostic rule for elderly patients admitted with community-acquired pneumonia. *Am J Med* 106:20–28, 1999.

16. Corless CE, Guiver M, Borrow R, et al: Simultaneous detection of *Neisseria meningitidis*, *Haemophilus influenzae*, and *Streptococcus pneumoniae* in suspected cases of meningitis and septicemia using real-time PCR. *J Clin Microbiol* 39:1553–1558, 2001.

17. Coyle PK: Glucocorticoids in central nervous system bacterial infection. *Arch Neurol* 56:796–801, 1999.

18. de Gans J, van de Beek D, for the European Dexamethasone in Adulthood Bacterial Meningitis Study Investigators. *N Engl J Med* 347:1549–1556, 2002.

19. Dichgans M, Jager L, Mayer T, et al: Bacterial meningitis in adults: demonstration of inner ear involvement using high-resolution MRI. *Neurology* 52:1003–1009, 1999.

20. Durand ML, Calderwood SB, Weber DJ, et al: Acute bacterial meningitis in adults. A review of 493 episodes. *N Engl J Med* 328:21–28, 1993.

21. Dwelle TL, Dunkle LM, Blair L: Correlation of cerebrospinal fluid endotoxinlike activity with clinical and laboratory variables in gram-negative bacterial meningitis in children. *J Clin Microbiol* 25:856–858, 1987.

22. Fiore AE, Moroney JF, Farley MM, et al: Clinical outcomes of meningitis caused by *Streptococcus pneumoniae* in the era of antibiotic resistance. *Clin Infect Dis* 30:71–77, 2000.

23. Forgacs P, Geyer CA, Freidberg SR: Characterization of chemical meningitis after neurological surgery. *Clin Infect Dis* 32:179–185, 2001.

24. Friedland IR, Klugman KP: Failure of chloramphenicol therapy in penicillin-resistant pneumococcal meningitis. *Lancet* 339:405–408, 1992.

25. Fukui MB, Williams RL, Mudigonda S: CT and MR imaging features of pyogenic ventriculitis. *AJNR Am J Neuroradiol* 22:1510–1516, 2001.

26. Gedde-Dahl TW, Bjark P, Hoiby EA, et al: Severity of meningococcal disease: assessment by factors and scores and implications for patient management. *Rev Infect Dis* 12:973–992, 1990.

27. Geiman BJ, Smith AL: Dexamethasone and bacterial meningitis. A meta-analysis of randomized controlled trials. *West J Med* 157:27–31, 1992.

28. Geiseler PJ, Nelson KE, Levin S, et al: Community-acquired purulent meningitis: a review of 1,316 cases during the antibiotic era, 1954–1976. *Rev Infect Dis* 2:725–745, 1980.

29. Gijwani D, Kumhar MR, Singh VB, et al: Dexamethasone therapy for bacterial meningitis in adults: a double blind placebo control study. *Neurol India* 50:63–67, 2002.

30. Girgis NI, Farid Z, Mikhail IA, et al: Dexamethasone treatment for bacterial meningitis in children and adults. *Pediatr Infect Dis J* 8:848–851, 1989.

31. Gould IA, Belok LC, Handwerger S: *Listeria monocytogenes*: a rare cause of opportunistic infection in the acquired immunodeficiency syndrome (AIDS) and a new cause of meningitis in AIDS. A case report. *AIDS Res* 2:231–234, 1986.

32. Gray LD, Fedorko DP: Laboratory diagnosis of bacterial meningitis. *Clin Microbiol Rev* 5:130–145, 1992.

33. Hart CA, Cuevas LE, Marzouk O, et al: Management of bacterial meningitis. *J Antimicrob Chemother* 32 Suppl A:49–59, 1993.

34. Hasbun R, Abrahams J, Jekel J, et al: Computed tomography of the head before lumbar puncture in adults with suspected meningitis. *N Engl J Med* 345:1727–1733, 2001.

35. Havens PL, Wendelberger KJ, Hoffman GM, et al: Corticosteroids as adjunctive therapy in bacterial meningitis. A meta-analysis of clinical trials. *Am J Dis Child* 143:1051–1055, 1989.

36. Hussein AS, Shafran SD: Acute bacterial meningitis in adults. A 12-year review. *Medicine* (Baltimore) 79:360–368, 2000.

37. Jensen AJ, Espersen F, Skinhoj P, et al: *Staphylococcus aureus* meningitis. A review of 104 nationwide, consecutive cases. *Arch Intern Med* 153:1902–1908, 1993.

38. Jurado RL, Farley MM, Pereira E, et al: Increased risk of meningitis and bacteremia due to *Listeria monocytogenes* in patients with human immunodeficiency virus infection. *Clin Infect Dis* 17:224–227, 1993.

39. Kastenbauer S, Koedel U, Becker BF, et al: Oxidative stress in bacterial meningitis in humans. *Neurology* 58:186–191, 2002.

40. Koziol K, Rielly KS, Bonin RA, et al: *Listeria monocytogenes* meningitis in AIDS. *Can Med Assoc J* 135:43–44, 1986.

41. Lebel MH, Freij BJ, Syrogiannopoulos GA, et al: Dexamethasone therapy for bacterial meningitis. Results of two double-blind, placebo-controlled trials. *N Engl J Med* 319:964–971, 1988.

42. Lorber B: Listeriosis. *Clin Infect Dis* 24:1–9, 1997.

43. Moller K, Skinhoj P, Knudsen GM, et al: Effect of short-term hyperventilation on cerebral blood flow autoregulation in patients with acute bacterial meningitis. *Stroke* 31:1116–1122, 2000.

44. Moosa AA, Quortum HA, Ibrahim MD: Rapid diagnosis of bacterial meningitis with reagent strips. *Lancet* 345:1290–1291, 1995.

45. Ogawa SK, Smith MA, Brennessel DJ, et al: Tuberculous meningitis in an urban medical center. *Medicine (Baltimore)* 66:317–326, 1987.

46. Paris MM, Hickey SM, Uscher MI, et al: Effect of dexamethasone on therapy of experimental penicillin- and cephalosporin-resistant pneumococcal meningitis. *Antimicrob Agents Chemother* 38:1320–1324, 1994.

47. Paul R, Lorenzl S, Koedel U, et al: Matrix metalloproteinases contribute to the blood-brain barrier disruption during bacterial meningitis. *Ann Neurol* 44:592–600, 1998.

48. Porritt RJ, Mercer JL, Munro R: Detection and serogroup determination of *Neisseria meningitidis* in CSF by polymerase chain reaction (PCR). *Pathology* 32:42–45, 2000.

49. Prasad K, Volmink J, Menon GR: Steroids for treating tuberculous meningitis. *Cochrane Database Syst Rev* 3:2000.

50. Quagliarello VJ, Scheld WM: Treatment of bacterial meningitis. *N Engl J Med* 336:708–716, 1997.

51. Ragunathan L, Ramsay M, Borrow R, et al: Clinical features, laboratory findings and management of meningococcal meningitis in England and Wales: report of a 1997 survey. Meningococcal meningitis: 1997 survey report. *J Infect* 40:74–79, 2000.

52. Roos KL: Acute bacterial meningitis. *Semin Neurol* 20:293–306, 2000.

53. Rosenstein NE, Perkins BA, Stephens DS, et al: Meningococcal disease. *N Engl J Med* 344:1378–1388, 2001.

54. Schuchat A, Robinson K, Wenger JD, et al: Bacterial meningitis in the United States in 1995. Active Surveillance Team. *N Engl J Med* 337:970–976, 1997.

55. Sigurdardottir B, Bjornsson OM, Jonsdottir KE, et al: Acute bacterial meningitis in adults. A 20-year overview. *Arch Intern Med* 157:425–430, 1997.

56. Simon RP, Beckman JS: Why pus is bad for the brain (editorial). *Neurology* 58:167–168, 2002.

57. Tang LM, Chen ST: *Klebsiella pneumoniae* meningitis: prognostic factors. *Scand J Infect Dis* 26:95–102, 1994.

58. Tauber MG, Moser B: Cytokines and chemokines in meningeal inflammation: biology and clinical implications. *Clin Infect Dis* 28:1–11, 1999.

59. Thomas KE, Hasbun R, Jekel J, et al: The diagnostic accuracy of Kernig's sign, Brudzinski's sign, and nuchal rigidity in adults with suspected meningitis. *Clin Infect Dis* 35:46–52, 2002.

60. Tunkel AR: *Bacterial Meningitis*. Philadelphia: Lippincott Williams & Wilkins, 2001.

61. Tunkel AR, Scheld WM: Acute bacterial meningitis. *Lancet* 346:1675–1680, 1995.

62. Villalobos T, Arango C, Kubilis P, et al: Antibiotic prophylaxis after basilar skull fractures: a meta-analysis. *Clin Infect Dis* 27:364–369, 1998.

63. Weingarten K, Zimmerman RD, Becker RD, et al: Subdural and epidural empyemas: MR imaging. *AJR Am J Radiol* 152:615–621, 1989.

20

Brain Abscess

The number of patients with brain abscess in the NICU is not significant, and most of the time the diagnosis becomes apparent after elective biopsy for a solitary mass. Admission is mostly dictated by the complexity of management, such as fractionated drainage of the abscess, or by a complication, such as ventriculitis or cerebral edema. When a brain abscess is located in the brain stem,[14] it may cause impaired swallowing, difficulty with clearing of secretions, and respiratory problems. In some instances, merely the anticipation of clinical deterioration in a patient with a moderate-sized brain abscess qualifies admission to the NICU.

Several traditional causes of brain abscess, such as otitis media and sinusitis, have decreased in prevalence because of improved diagnosis and management and have been displaced by other causes, such as infections of molar teeth, staphylococcal endocarditis, and hematogenous dissemination from pulmonary infections.[25] The clinical spectrum of pathogens causing brain abscess has also most likely changed with the surge in human immunodeficiency virus infections and, to a lesser degree, with the increase in the number of immunocompromised transplant patients.

Definitive treatment of brain abscess is often neurosurgical, although several successful attempts have been reported with antibiotic therapy alone, particularly in patients with lesions that were not easily accessible. The management of brain abscess often requires expertise from specialists in infectious diseases, otolaryngologists, pulmonologists, and dental surgeons.

This chapter focuses on the diagnostic evaluation and options for medical treatment in brain abscess. It also proposes surgical indications.

CLINICAL RECOGNITION

A careful history and physical examination may provide additional clues in the evaluation of patients with a brain abscess. The potential source of infection may lie in dental abscess or periodontal disease, otitis media or suppurative sinusitis, congenital heart disease,[47] acquired valvular disease, pulmonary disease, skin infections, or recent travel or occupational exposure. Pulmonary arteriovenous malformations have been associated with brain abscesses, most frequently in patients with hereditary hemorrhagic telangiectasia (Osler's disease).[3,10,34]

Brain abscess is usually diagnosed on the basis of three important clinical signs: headache, focal neurologic deficit, and, perhaps less commonly, change in level of consciousness.[49,51] In a review from the University of California at San Francisco, 56% of the patients with a brain abscess were drowsy to stuporous at presentation.[29] In another report, full alertness was noted in approximately 70% of 140 patients, a discrepancy that may reflect recognition of cerebral abscess by early timing of neuroimaging studies.[51]

Pronounced neck stiffness is present in only 40% of patients with a brain abscess but may be more apparent in patients with a devastating ventriculitis. Fever and focal neurologic signs remain more distinctive signs, but both may also be absent.[49,51] Fever occurs in only 50% of patients in most series. Most patients have hemiparesis, which may be subtle; in others, a single cerebral abscess produces behavioral changes alone. Brain abscess frequently lodges in the frontal (or frontoparietal) lobe, and this location may explain the lack of obvious clinical signs. In patients with an abscess in the dominant hemisphere, symptoms may become more evident during reading, spelling out loud, or writing, although many patients have clearly recognizable Broca's aphasia. Seizures are common in patients with a solitary brain abscess, and the incidence in several studies approached 30%. Otogenic brain abscesses are most frequent in the temporal lobe or cerebellum.[41] An abscess in the brain stem can be associated with impaired consciousness if it abuts the reticular formation and involvement of major nuclei produces cranial nerve deficits. Depending on localization in the brain stem, patients have involvement of cranial nerves VI and VII and, less commonly, III, and these findings are almost always associated with marked horizontal nystagmus, ataxia, or hemiparesis. Localization in the medulla may produce primary abnormalities in breathing patterns but more often results in impaired swallowing and aspiration.

The clinical characteristics in patients with multiple brain abscesses are fairly similar, and most have headache, impaired consciousness, and focal neurologic deficits.[28] Symptoms depend on size and tissue shift, and one lesion may be responsible for the clinical presentation.

NEUROIMAGING AND LABORATORY TESTS

Advances in neuroimaging leading to early recognition may have improved the outcome in brain abscess. Currently, MRI is the preferred neuroimaging technique, but CT scanning remains important in the initial diagnosis, during stereotactic biopsy, and in serial monitoring after antibiotic therapy and surgical drainage.[31]

Typically, an abscess is manifested as a round, thick capsule with a central low density, representing pus. Surrounding edema in the white matter usually is found and often is the only clearly visible determinant of the lesion in a non-contrast CT scan. In cerebritis, these CT features are less developed. Contrast enhancement is seen in most cases but can be insignificant in patients treated with corticosteroids. The inner wall layer becomes smooth when the abscess is firm, which occurs almost invariably 2 weeks after the first symptoms. Multiloculation within the abscess is also an important CT feature, because it indicates that surgical intervention is a less favorable option. Features that require attention are shift of midline structures and release of pus into the ventricular system. Contrast enhancement in the ventricular wall is seen in ventriculitis or ependymitis. Bone windows on CT scans are necessary to carefully evaluate the sinuses and mastoids for loss of air pockets and presence of fluid collection, which may be a source of the infection.[32]

The differential diagnosis of a single mass on CT scan is shown in Table 20–1. Biopsy is preferred not only to confirm the diagnosis but also to obtain pus, if present, for cultures.

The advantage of MRI is a greater sensitivity in detection of cerebritis and abscesses that are either not detected or uncertain by CT.[6] Diffusion-weighted MRI may also be helpful in differentiating cerebral abscess from necrotic tumor and ventricular extension of pus.[37] Increased signal on echo-planar imaging and marked reduction of apparent diffusion coefficient were documented in two recent cases, findings not noted in gliomas or metastasis.[8]

Table 20–1. Differential Diagnosis of a Single Mass Suspicious for Bacterial Abscess

Noncompromised Host	Compromised Host
Cysticercosis	Cryptococcus neoformans
Glioma	Kaposi's sarcoma
Herpes simplex	Listeria monocytogenes
Metastasis	Lymphoma
Multiple sclerosis	Mycobacterium
Sarcoid	Nocardia
	Progressive multifocal leukoencephalopathy
	Toxoplasma

Table 20–2. Laboratory Studies in the Initial Evaluation of Brain Abscess

Cultures	Blood, urine, sputum, cerebrospinal fluid
	Selected cases: gastric washings, bronchial brushing, pleural or ascitic fluid, aspirate or biopsy
Serologic studies	Viral, fungal, *Toxoplasma gondii*
Imaging studies	Chest radiograph, sinus and dental radiographs, electrocardiogram, echocardiography, computed tomography images of chest or abdomen (optional)

Lumbar puncture may not be helpful, and rapid deterioration after the procedure has been demonstrated, not necessarily only in patients with massive shift on CT scans. However, one study reported no complications after lumbar puncture in 17 patients, including 3 with papilledema.[42] The yield of cerebrospinal fluid cultures in patients with brain abscess is low. The frequency varies from 0% to 7%,[5] although the number of reported patients who have had cerebrospinal fluid examination is small. As expected, identification of the organism is more common in surgical specimens. One series claimed that only 4% of the patients had sterile cultures.[29]

Findings on peripheral blood examination can be supportive, with increased sedimentation rate and increased leukocyte count in most patients. Blood cultures should be part of the evaluation in any patient with brain abscess. Three consecutive blood samples should be taken; they may demonstrate, for example, *Staphylococcus aureus* or *Aspergillus* in highly susceptible patients, such as intravenous drug abusers and transplant recipients. The bacteriologic cause of pyogenic brain abscess depends on its source, but cultures may yield a polymicrobial flora. *Streptococcus milleri* is most common in abscesses associated with paranasal sinusitis.[11] Otogenic abscesses are commonly caused by *Proteus* anaerobes, *Streptococcus* species, Enterobacteriaceae, or *Pseudomonas aeruginosa*.[41] Unusual species are *Klebsiella* bacteria,[27] *Streptococcus pneumoniae*,[18] and *Streptococcus bovis*.[30] Diagnostic criteria for neurocysticercosis have been published and should be considered in individuals from an endemic area.[7] In brief, they include cystic lesions showing the scolex on neuroimaging and funduscopic demonstration of subretinal parasites, positive serum enzyme-linked immunoelectrotransfer blot assay, and response to albendazole and praziquantel.[7] The essential laboratory tests in evaluation of brain abscess are summarized in Table 20–2.

FIRST STEPS IN MANAGEMENT

The argument in favor of medical management of cerebral abscess is compelling. Early antibiotic therapy alone in patients with an abscess is indicated for a small solitary abscess (< 3 cm), an abscess in a surgically inaccessible area, multilocular or multiple localizations, brain stem localization,[4,15,16] early abscess formation without clear capsule formation (cerebritis stage), and a paucity of clinical signs. In other patients, surgical aspiration, not necessarily with reduction of the mass itself, should be considered to obtain pus for cytologic examination and cultures. Obviously, antibiotic coverage is of utmost importance, but if surgery is performed within hours and the diagnosis of cerebral abscess is very uncertain, administration probably should be postponed to reduce the risk of sterile cultures.

Location and multiplicity of brain abscesses are important factors in surgical decision-making. When surgical aspiration is considered, the stereotactic approach is preferred. The risk of further morbidity from the stereotactic procedure remains low. A study from the University of Lille, France, comparing medical management, surgical aspiration, and excision in brain abscess found no differences in survival, but seizures and focal deficits occurred more often in the surgically approached group.[26] In general, for lesions that are very superficially located and are not over the motor strip of the cortex, catheter drainage can be tried by placing a bur hole and puncturing the parenchyma with a small soft catheter. Catheter drainage is continued for at least 1 week, with alternative aspiration and saline irrigation.

In deep-seated lesions, stereotactic aspiration can be considered, but most argue that antibiotic therapy is the first therapeutic choice.[44,45] Excision of the abscess by open craniotomy with additional damage to the surrounding white matter is not an attractive first option, even in large encapsulated abscesses. On the other hand, cerebellar abscesses are preferably healed surgically, and the outcome is much better than that with supratentorial abscess.

Multiple abscesses occur in 1% to 15% of the patients.[1,24] Surgical treatment is controversial,[2,38,39] and antimicrobial therapy seems more appropriate in patients with superficially located abscesses and in immunosuppressed patients with a chance of toxoplasmosis or aspergillosis.[9] Stereotactic aspiration by CT-guided techniques should be considered in patients with deep lesions larger than 3 cm.

It is difficult to marshal all the different options for the management of cerebral abscess (Fig. 20–1). The surgical technique usually consists of stereotactic aspiration, aspiration after craniotomy, or excision.[19,21,25,33] Surgical management is clearly indicated for superficial abscesses, lesions with a well-defined wall on imaging studies, and abscesses abutting the ventricles

at risk of rupture, causing ventriculitis. Abscesses located in the parieto-occipital region are more commonly associated with ventricular rupture than are those in other locations.[48] Abscesses originating from the sinus or middle ear may rupture into the subarachnoid space.[35] Abscesses in the posterior fossa should be surgically removed if the fourth ventricle is effaced and, as in cerebellar infarcts and hematomas, if features of a crowded tight posterior fossa are evident. Aspiration is clearly indicated if the lesion causes significant mass effect or produces coma or rapid clinical deterioration.[22] Conversely, medical management is more reasonable in patients with deep-seated lesions that are surgically inaccessible, multiple small abscesses, or multilocular abscesses. A primary lesion in the brain stem probably should be managed medically and may not need stereotactic aspiration. However, in a survey of 71 patients with brain stem masses who had stereotactic surgery, there was no procedure-related mortality and only one patient had permanent morbidity.[36]

Surgical intervention by stereotactic aspiration must be strongly considered in immunosuppressed patients with acquired immunodeficiency syndrome or human immuno-

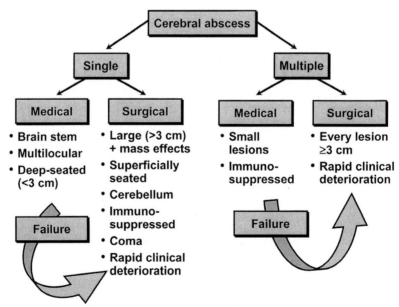

Medical: Empirical or specific antimicrobial therapy IV for 8 weeks using central venous access
Surgical: Stereotactic or open aspiration; excision

Figure 20–1. Guideline for management of brain abscess.

Table 20–3. Initial Management in Patients with Brain Abscess

Airway management	Intubation in patients with motor response less than localization to pain, progressive infiltrates from aspiration, or swallowing difficulties from brain stem localization
Fluid management	Insertion of Hickman-Broviac catheter 2 L of 0.9% sodium chloride (adjust with fever)
Medical management	Nafcillin or third-generation cephalosporin and metronidazole (vancomycin with penicillin allergy)
Surgical management	Rapid deterioration, coma, mass effect, and > 3 cm
Prophylactic measures	(Fos)phenytoin, 300 mg daily

deficiency virus infection. A 2-week trial with therapy directed against *Toxoplasma gondii* is recommended, but tissue must be obtained for culture and histologic examination if failure to improve is apparent clinically or by CT scan. On the other hand, an abscess caused by *Nocardia* is difficult to cure with aspiration and antibiotics and probably must be excised.[13] Local instillation of amphotericin B, next to systemic treatment, was entertained in a patient with cerebellar aspergillosis.[9]

Another approach favors surgically aggressive treatment of multiple cerebral abscesses, albeit based on a review of 16 patients.[28] In this protocol, every abscess greater than 2.5 cm in diameter was treated surgically (excision or drainage). Antibiotic therapy followed, CT scans or MRI was repeated in 2 weeks, and stereotactic drainage or craniotomy was re-

peated if new large lesions emerged. Abscesses with more than two aspirations were surgically excised. This management protocol reflects a very low threshold for drainage in large lesions (≥ 2.5 cm) and the investigators' willingness to repeat drainage if a good response was not observed by clinical and neuroimaging criteria. Very low mortality resulted.

The initial medical management in patients with a brain abscess is summarized in Table 20–3. Brain abscess is treated empirically by cephalosporins in combination with metronidazole.[17,43,50] Vancomycin should be administered in patients with penicillin allergy. Parenteral treatment should be continued for 3 to 4 weeks after excision and 4 to 6 weeks after aspiration.[20] Empirical treatment in immunocompromised patients or in patients who most likely have an unusual infection is complex (Table 20–4).

Table 20–4. Initial Empirical Antibiotic Treatment for Patients with Brain Abscess

Nonimmunocompromised Patients

Cefotaxime	8–12 g/day IV in divided doses q4h
Metronidazole	15 mg/kg IV load: 7.5 mg/kg IV q6h/day
Vancomycin (with penicillin allergy)	2 g/day IV in divided doses q12h

Immunocompromised Patients or Those with Possible Unusual Bacterial Infection, Atypical Bacteria, or Nonbacterial Infection

Antituberculous therapy	Isoniazid, 5 mg/kg per day p.o. Rifampin, 10 mg/kg per day p.o. Ethambutol, 15 mg/kg per day p.o. Pyrazinamide, 15–30 mg/kg per day p.o.
Antifungal therapy	Amphotericin B, 0.25–1.0 mg/kg per day IV to total dose of 1.5 mg/kg per day infused over 2–6 hours
Antiparasitic therapy	
Toxoplasma gondii	Pyrimethamine, initially 200 mg p.o. and then 50–100 mg per day p.o. Sulfadiazine, 1–1.5 g q6h/day (leucovorin [folinic acid], 10 mg p.o.)
Taenia solium°	Praziquantel, 60 mg/kg per day (in divided doses t.i.d.) or albendazole, 15 mg/kg per day (in divided doses t.i.d.)
Atypical bacteria	
Nocardia asteroides	Trimethoprim (160 mg)-sulfamethoxazole (800 mg), IV or p.o. q.i.d. per day or sulfisoxazole, 4–8 g per day

°Neurocysticercosis.

Central access should be obtained in expectation of several weeks of antibiotic administration. Preferably, a Hickman-Broviac catheter is inserted. This catheter is tunneled under the skin and brought out several inches from the site of insertion. (The silver-impregnated antibiotic cuff proximal to the Dacron cuff may reduce bacterial growth.) The catheter should be placed in the superior vena cava or the proximal right atrium, because malpositioning in smaller veins may produce phlebitis and thrombosis (Fig. 20–2). The complications of long-term placement of a central venous catheter are few, and most are related to insertion. Nonetheless, we observed pulmonary emboli in one patient at the end of an 8-week course of intravenously administered antibiotics.[16] Daily flushing with heparin is advised.

Fluid intake should not exceed maintenance amounts but must be adjusted if fever occurs. (Fos)phenytoin, 300 mg, is given when surgical treatment is planned but can be deferred in patients receiving medical management alone. Antiepileptic coverage is reasonable, however, when considerable edema and shift are seen on CT scans. Furthermore, the risk of late seizures is considerable in patients with abscess. Phenytoin or fosphenytoin is indicated if a single seizure has occurred. If level of consciousness waxes and wanes, one should also consider cephalosporin toxicity causing nonconvulsive status epilepticus.[23]

There is no rationale to use corticosteroids in patients without increased intracranial pressure from edema.

DETERIORATION: CAUSES AND MANAGEMENT

Most patients with a solitary abscess remain neurologically stable and begin to improve soon after antibiotic treatment. Deterioration in level of consciousness with rapid subsequent tentorial herniation is common in patients with multiple abscesses and in patients with multilocular abscesses; as expected, mortality is very high. In two series of patients who died before surgical procedures could be performed, multiple abscesses and rupture of abscesses into the ventricular system were prevalent.[40,51]

Enlargement of the abscess with gradual clinical deterioration is an absolute indication for stereotactic aspiration or extirpation. Brain edema surrounding the abscess may be the cause

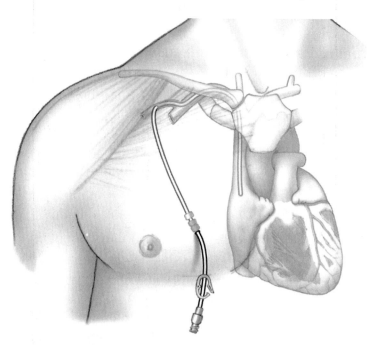

Figure 20–2. Placement of Hickman-Broviac catheter.

of significant displacement and can be determined only by comparison of recent and previous CT images. The size of the abscess may have increased as well, but cerebral edema adjacent to the abscess can be overwhelming and add to the mass effect. Corticosteroids to reduce edema may not have the disadvantage of spreading the infection, as commonly thought, and should be administered promptly in deteriorating patients (dexamethasone: loading dose of 0.2 mg/kg followed by 0.75 mg/kg in four divided doses). Waiting for the effect of dexamethasone, which may take hours, is ill-advised, and one should proceed with surgery. Patients should be intubated, and a bolus of mannitol (1 g/kg intravenously) should be used additionally to reduce intracranial pressure in anticipation of surgery. Surgical intervention is the only lifesaving measure if deterioration is rapid. Brain edema may also occur in patients with multiple abscesses, and patients may gradually dwindle to a vegetative state associated with more diffuse edema despite aspiration and intensive antibiotic treatment (Fig. 20–3).

In unfortunate circumstances, the abscess ruptures into the ventricular system and the outcome is often fatal.[12,48] Magnetic resonance imaging often shows enhancement of the ventricular wall adjacent to the abscess (Fig. 20–4), which may precede frank rupture.

Deterioration from hydrocephalus associated with abscess located in the posterior fossa has been reported. Extirpation of the compressing abscess alone with antibiotic therapy is sufficient. Ventriculostomy alone probably should be avoided to reduce the risk of upward herniation.

OUTCOME

Intravenous antibiotic therapy may cure a solitary brain abscess with or without aspiration. Use of a Hickman-Broviac catheter allows administration of antibiotics on an outpatient basis, greatly reducing hospital costs. Outcome in patients with medically treated brain stem abscesses is quite good; most neurologic function returns, and ataxia and diplopia diminish significantly (Fig. 20–5). Outcome seems correlated with location of lesion (deep-seated), progression to coma before intervention, and,

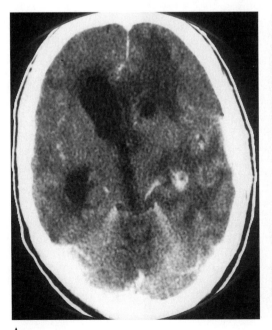
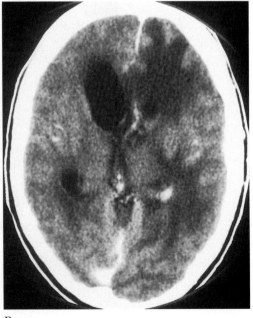

A   B

Figure 20–3. Computed tomography images of enlarging multiple abscesses and the effect of edema showed their evolution (A through D) within 2 weeks.

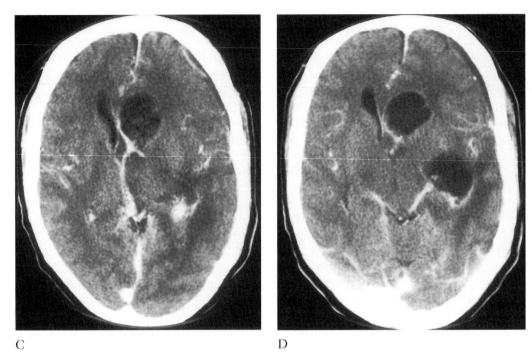

C D

Figure 20–3. (*Continued*)

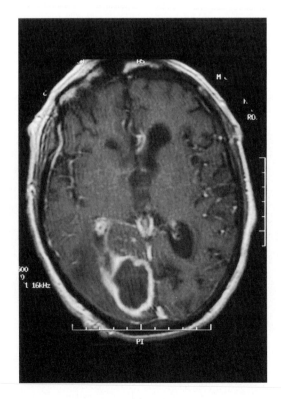

Figure 20–4. Brain abscess suspicious for early rupture to the ventricles. Note dumbbell shape and enhancement, suggesting ventriculitis.

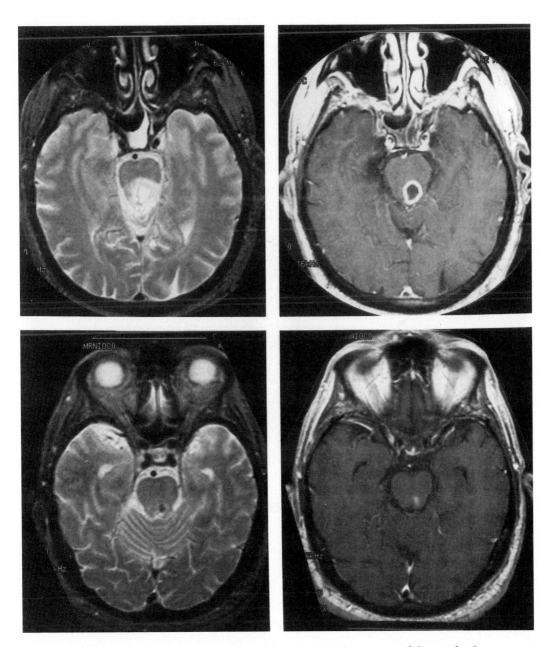

Figure 20–5. Magnetic resonance images of brain stem abscess cured by medical treatment alone. (From Fulgham et al.[16] By permission of the American Academy of Neurology.)

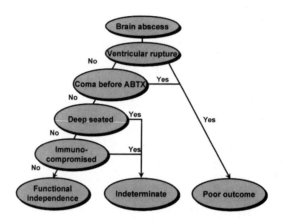

Figure 20–6. Outcome algorithm for brain abscess. ABTX, antibiotic therapy. Functional independence: no assistance needed, minor handicap may remain. Indeterminate: any statement would be a premature conclusion. Poor outcome: severe disability or death, vegetative state.

particularly, ventricular rupture.[46] However, outcome in patients with brain abscess also depends on the clinical features on admission, the type of infectious agent, or whether abscess is single or multiple. Multiple staphylococcal abscesses associated with endocarditis are often fatal. Cerebral abscesses in immunocompromised patients have a less favorable outcome because of fungal origin in most patients. In contrast, brain abscesses caused by *Toxoplasma* may virtually disappear after appropriate therapy, although the underlying illness may shorten the long-term outcome.

Mortality varies considerably in most series and currently probably approaches 20%. One study found that a shorter duration of symptoms before admission predicted death or severe sequelae, reflecting a fulminant course and its consequences.[42] Outcome prediction is shown in an algorithm (Fig. 20–6).

CONCLUSIONS

- Medical treatment is indicated for brain stem abscess, multilocular abscesses, and surgically inaccessible deep-seated lesions.
- Surgical treatment is indicated (craniotomy or stereotactic aspiration) if abscesses are causing mass effect and clinical deterioration is rapid. The threshold for a surgical approach should also be low if the abscess is superficially placed or in the cerebellum.
- Empirical therapy in nonimmunocompromised patients is cefotaxime with metronidazole.
- Empirical therapy in immunocompromised patients (particularly those infected with human immunodeficiency virus) is indicated if multiple abscesses suggestive of toxoplasmosis are found. Therapy is guided by repeat CT scan or MRI.

REFERENCES

1. Basit AS, Ravi B, Banerji AK, et al: Multiple pyogenic brain abscesses: an analysis of 21 patients. *J Neurol Neurosurg Psychiatry* 52:591–594, 1989.
2. Boom WH, Tuazon CU: Successful treatment of multiple brain abscesses with antibiotics alone. *Rev Infect Dis* 7:189–199, 1985.
3. Brydon HL, Akinwunmi J, Selway R, et al: Brain abscesses associated with pulmonary arteriovenous malformations. *Br J Neurosurg* 13:265–269, 1999.
4. Carpenter JL: Brain stem abscesses: cure with medical

therapy, case report, and review. *Clin Infect Dis* 18: 219–226, 1994.

5. Chun CH, Johnson JD, Hofstetter M, et al: Brain abscess. A study of 45 consecutive cases. *Medicine (Baltimore)* 65:415–431, 1986.

6. Davidson HD, Steiner RE: Magnetic resonance imaging in infections of the central nervous system. *AJNR Am J Neuroradiol* 6:499–504, 1985.

7. Del Brutto OH, Rajshekhar V, White AC Jr, et al: Proposed diagnostic criteria for neurocysticercosis. *Neurology* 57:177–183, 2001.

8. Desprechins B, Stadnik T, Koerts G, et al: Use of diffusion-weighted MR imaging in differential diagnosis between intracerebral necrotic tumors and cerebral abscesses. *AJNR Am J Neuroradiol* 20:1252–1257, 1999.

9. Erdogan E, Beyzadeoglu M, Arpaci F, et al: Cerebellar aspergillosis: case report and literature review. *Neurosurgery* 50:874–876, 2002.

10. Faughnan ME, Lui YW, Wirth JA, et al: Diffuse pulmonary arteriovenous malformations: characteristics and prognosis. *Chest* 117:31–38, 2000.

11. Fenton JE, Smyth DA, Viani LG, et al: Sinogenic brain abscess. *Am J Rhinol* 13:299–302, 1999.

12. Ferre C, Ariza J, Viladrich PF, et al: Brain abscess rupturing into the ventricles or subarachnoid space. *Am J Med* 106:254–257, 1999.

13. Fried J, Hinthorn D, Ralstin J, et al: Cure of brain abscess caused by *Nocardia asteroides* resistant to multiple antibiotics. *South Med J* 81:412–413, 1988.

14. Fuentes S, Bouillot P, Regis J, et al: Management of brain stem abscess. *Br J Neurosurg* 15:57–62, 2001.

15. Fujino H, Kobayashi T, Goto I, et al: Cure of a man with solitary abscess of the brain-stem. *J Neurol* 237: 265–266, 1990.

16. Fulgham JR, Wijdicks EFM, Wright AJ: Cure of a solitary brainstem abscess with antibiotic therapy: case report. *Neurology* 46:1451–1454, 1996.

17. Green HT, O'Donoghue MA, Shaw MD, et al: Penetration of ceftazidime into intracranial abscess. *J Antimicrob Chemother* 24:431–436, 1989.

18. Grigoriadis E, Gold WL: Pyogenic brain abscess caused by *Streptococcus pneumoniae*: case report and review. *Clin Infect Dis* 25:1108–1112, 1997.

19. Hasdemir MG, Ebeling U: CT-guided stereotactic aspiration and treatment of brain abscesses. An experience with 24 cases. *Acta Neurochir (Wien)* 125:58–63, 1993.

20. Infection in Neurosurgery Working Party of the British Society for Antimicrobial Chemotherapy: The rational use of antibiotics in the treatment of brain abscess. *Br J Neurosurg* 14:525–530, 2000.

21. Itakura T, Yokote H, Ozaki F, et al: Stereotactic operation for brain abscess. *Surg Neurol* 28:196–200, 1987.

22. Kala M: Aspiration or extirpation in cerebral abscess surgery? *Neurosurg Rev* 16:121–124, 1993.

23. Klion AD, Kallsen J, Cowl CT, et al: Ceftazidime-related nonconvulsive status epilepticus. *Arch Intern Med* 154:586–589, 1994.

24. Kratimenos G, Crockard HA: Multiple brain abscess: a review of fourteen cases. *Br J Neurosurg* 5:153–161, 1991.

25. Kulai A, Ozatik N, Topcu I: Otogenic intracranial abscesses. *Acta Neurochir (Wien)* 107:140–146, 1990.

26. Leys D, Christiaens JL, Derambure P, et al: Management of focal intracranial infections: Is medical treatment better than surgery? *J Neurol Neurosurg Psychiatry* 53:472–475, 1990.

27. Liliang PC, Lin YC, Su TM, et al: *Klebsiella* brain abscess in adults. *Infection* 29:81–86, 2001.

28. Mamelak AN, Mampalam TJ, Obana WG, et al: Improved management of multiple brain abscesses: a combined surgical and medical approach. *Neurosurgery* 36:76–85, 1995.

29. Mampalam TJ, Rosenblum ML: Trends in the management of bacterial brain abscesses: a review of 102 cases over 17 years. *Neurosurgery* 23:451–458, 1988.

30. Maniglia RJ, Roth T, Blumberg EA: Polymicrobial brain abscess in a patient infected with human immunodeficiency virus. *Clin Infect Dis* 24:449–451, 1997.

31. Miller ES, Dias PS, Uttley D: CT scanning in the management of intracranial abscess: a review of 100 cases. *Br J Neurosurg* 2:439–446, 1988.

32. Nalbone VP, Kuruvilla A, Gacek RR: Otogenic brain abscess: the Syracuse experience. *Ear Nose Throat J* 71:238–242, 1992.

33. Nauta HJ, Contreras FL, Weiner RL, et al: Brain stem abscess managed with computed tomography-guided stereotactic aspiration. *Neurosurgery* 20:476–480, 1987.

34. Preston DC, Shapiro BE: Pulmonary arteriovenous fistula and brain abscess. *Neurology* 56:418, 2001.

35. Quijano M, Schuknecht HF, Otte J: Temporal bone pathology associated with intracranial abscess. *ORL J Otorhinolaryngol Relat Spec* 50:2–31, 1988.

36. Rajshekhar V, Chandy MJ: Computerized tomography-guided stereotactic surgery for brainstem masses: a risk-benefit analysis in 71 patients. *J Neurosurg* 82: 976–981, 1995.

37. Rana S, Albayram S, Lin DD, et al: Diffusion-weighted imaging and apparent diffusion coefficient maps in a case of intracerebral abscess with ventricular extension. *AJNR Am J Neuroradiol* 23:109–112, 2002.

38. Rousseaux M, Lesoin F, Destee A, et al: Developments in the treatment and prognosis of multiple cerebral abscesses. *Neurosurgery* 16:304–308, 1985.

39. Ruelle A, Zerbi D, Zuccarello M, et al: Brain stem abscess treated successfully by medical therapy. *Neurosurgery* 28:742–745, 1991.

40. Schliamser SE, Backman K, Norrby SR: Intracranial abscesses in adults: an analysis of 54 consecutive cases. *Scand J Infect Dis* 20:1–9, 1988.

41. Sennaroglu L, Sozeri B: Otogenic brain abscess: review of 41 cases. *Otolaryngol Head Neck Surg* 123:751–755, 2000.

42. Seydoux C, Francioli P: Bacterial brain abscesses: factors influencing mortality and sequelae. *Clin Infect Dis* 15:394–401, 1992.

43. Sjolin J, Lilja A, Eriksson N, et al: Treatment of brain abscess with cefotaxime and metronidazole: prospective study on 15 consecutive patients. *Clin Infect Dis* 17:857–863, 1993.

44. Stapleton SR, Bell BA, Uttley D: Stereotactic aspiration of brain abscesses: Is this the treatment of choice? *Acta Neurochir (Wien)* 121:15–19, 1993.

45. Stroobandt G, Zech F, Thauvoy C, et al: Treatment by aspiration of brain abscesses. *Acta Neurochir (Wien)* 85:138–147, 1987.

46. Takeshita M, Kagawa M, Izawa M, et al: Current treatment strategies and factors influencing outcome in patients with bacterial brain abscess. *Acta Neurochir* 140:1263–1270, 1998.

47. Takeshita M, Kagawa M, Yato S, et al: Current treatment of brain abscess in patients with congenital cyanotic heart disease. *Neurosurgery* 41:1270–1278, 1997.

48. Takeshita M, Kawamata T, Izawa M, et al: Prodromal signs and clinical factors influencing outcome in patients with intraventricular rupture of purulent brain abscess. *Neurosurgery* 48:310–316, 2001.

49. Wispelwey B, Scheld WM: Brain abscess. *Semin Neurol* 12:273–278, 1992.

50. Yamamoto M, Jimbo M, Ide M, et al: Penetration of intravenous antibiotics into brain abscesses. *Neurosurgery* 33:44–49, 1993.

51. Yang SY, Zhao CS: Review of 140 patients with brain abscess. *Surg Neurol* 39:290–296, 1993.

21

Acute Viral Encephalitis

One of the most challenging admissions to the NICU is the patient with clinical characteristics of rapidly progressive encephalitis but no inkling of its source. Neurologists are adept at recognizing the emerging clinical picture, but a critically important part in the care of these patients is to identify pathogens that may radically change specific therapy. For example, the availability of polymerase chain reaction (PCR) for the diagnosis of herpes simplex encephalitis and cytomegalovirus (CMV) encephalitis has simplified evaluation in these patients and, most importantly, often obviated stereotactic brain biopsy.

Encephalitis is not an uncommon neurologic critical illness. For example, on average, New York City reports 10 cases of encephalitis each year.[6] When acute viral encephalitis is seen sporadically, herpes simplex encephalitis is statistically most common. On the other hand, the ability to recognize the beginning of an outbreak of arboviral encephalitis is difficult, and it may take time for the disease to become fully established. The season is important in epidemic forms of encephalitis, with peak occurrence often from June to September. In addition, an immunosuppressed state (including human immunodeficiency virus [HIV] infection) requires specific attention, because it places the patient in a much different category of differential diagnosis and outcome.

Patients with acute viral encephalitis are admitted to the NICU when they are in an altered state of awareness, have an urgent need for airway protection and mechanical ventilation, or re-

quire control of increased intracranial pressure (ICP). Admission to the NICU is also justified if seizures have developed and in some situations progressed to status epilepticus. Many other patients in earlier stages are agitated and combative, difficult to restrain effectively, and in need of sedation and respiratory monitoring.

This chapter discusses the most pertinent therapeutic targets in the management of acute viral encephalitis. The treatment of herpes simplex encephalitis is a major focus.

CLINICAL RECOGNITION

Typical clinical characteristics of acute viral encephalitis are the rapid development of fever (which may begin cyclically and reach 40°C), headache, acute confusional state, and localizing neurologic signs.[8,68] No clinical feature is characteristic of a certain viral encephalitis, but clues in the history may help in sorting out possible causes. Essential inquiries in the evaluation of any encephalitis are recent vaccination, travel, animal contact (pets, bats, or wild animals), deaths in horse populations, or tick exposure; long-term immunosuppression or possible exposure to HIV; and recent diagnosis of acquired immunodeficiency syndrome (AIDS).[8,68] Prodromal cervical lymphadenopathy, splenomegaly, or exudative pharyngitis may suggest CMV or Epstein-Barr virus (EBV) as a potential pathogen.

Cytomegalovirus encephalitis may develop in patients with AIDS. This type of encephalitis is often associated with hyponatremia from CMV adrenalitis, and half the patients have previously been treated for CMV retinitis.[32] Immunosuppressed patients are also at risk for herpes zoster encephalitis when disseminated cutaneous zoster is present.

Numerous clinical neurologic conditions can closely mimic viral encephalitis. The most commonly proposed alternative diagnoses for viral encephalitis are cerebral venous thrombosis, isolated granulomatous angiitis, central nervous system intravascular lymphoma, acute hemorrhagic leukoencephalitis,[26,52] acute disseminated encephalomyelitis, progressive multifocal leukoencephalopathy, subdural empyema, fulminant bacterial meningitis, brain abscess, and neurosyphilis.[10,62] More remote causes and mimicking disorders are *Listeria monocytogenes*,[3] tuberculosis, *Cryptococcus*, mucormycosis, Q fever encephalitis,[16] *Rickettsia rickettsii*, malignant glioma and metastasis, limbic encephalitis,[21] connective tissue disease with central nervous system manifestations, such as systemic lupus erythematosus, and any toxic encephalitis (cytostatic drugs, exposure to toxins, cocaine, or toluene). Obviously, each of these alternative explanations—albeit rare—in a rapidly progressive disorder may lead to a totally different therapeutic approach and thus should be considered early for treatment to affect outcome.

In herpes simplex encephalitis, the clinical features are altered consciousness, fever ($> 39°C$), and malaise. The predictive value of herpes labialis or vaginalis for herpes simplex encephalitis is poor. Focal neurologic signs, such as seizures, visual field defects, aphasia, and bizarre behavior, including hypomania,[24] have been reported. Memory impairment with abnormal recall alone and complete absence of fever and other accompanying signs has been reported as a presentation of herpes simplex encephalitis.[73] In other patients, marked abulia or signs of an anterior operculum syndrome (anarthria and marked dysphagia from faciopharyngoglossomasticatory diplegia)[45,71] seem more prominent. A proclivity for brain stem involvement exists in immunosuppressed patients with herpes simplex encephalitis.

The progression of the disorder is rapid in some patients, but in most patients neurologic symptoms reach their maximum within days. Coma with bilateral extensor posturing may be seen in patients with relentless progression in a matter of hours. Approximately 40% of patients have seizures, which can be focal and may evolve into complex partial seizures, generalized tonic-clonic seizures, or status epilepticus.

Herpes zoster encephalitis occurs more often in the elderly, in immunosuppressed patients, and in patients with malignant disease.[34] Cutaneous localization of herpes zoster is invariably present. Herpes zoster encephalitis is not common in patients with herpes zoster infection involving several dermatomes alone but is more often present in patients with a disseminated form. Reduced state of arousal may be accompanied by borderline fever, acute hemiparesis, language abnormalities, or apraxia, which can be due to ischemic stroke from vasculitis. Seizures are less common. Cranial nerve involvement in herpes zoster encephalitis may be more prevalent than in other types of encephalitis.

Cytomegalovirus encephalitis occurs predominantly in patients with a severely impaired cellular immune system. It occurs often in patients with therapy for another manifestation of CMV infection (e.g., CMV retinitis). Patients with CMV encephalitis may manifest confusion, apathy, and social withdrawal that closely mimic AIDS dementia.

Epstein-Barr virus-related encephalitis is very rare, but the outcome is quite good, even in patients with coma.[57] Epstein-Barr virus encephalitis usually occurs in systemic infections, and the classic findings are lymphadenopathy, pharyngitis, and splenomegaly.

Encephalitis may occur during the yearly influenza season, and both influenza A and influenza B have been implicated. The damage may be quite impressive, including akinetic mutism.

The clinical manifestations of other viral encephalitides can be very similar. However, several features are noticeable, such as involvement of facial, glossopharyngeal, and oculomotor nerves (St. Louis encephalitis); marked abulia (Colorado tick fever); high incidence of focal and generalized seizures with propensity toward development of status epilepticus (La Crosse encephalitis); and fear of water, vigorous muscle spasms in swallowing muscles, and violent behavior (rabies encephalitis).

Arboviral encephalitis is caused by a mosquito or tick vector. Outbreaks are seasonal, usually occurring in the summer. In encephalitides transmitted by ticks, outbreaks occur in high-risk areas during the tick feeding season (late spring and early summer).

One of the most dramatic types of encephalitis in the United States, occurring in freshwater and swampy areas, along the eastern seaboard, and on the Gulf coast, is the mosquito-borne eastern equine encephalomyelitis (EEE), in which mortality is 40%. The agent is a single-stranded RNA alpha virus. The onset is rather sudden, with a high incidence of seizures and dysautonomia, manifested by sympathetic storm. A short prodrome of several days is common, with headache and abdominal distress. Focal weakness occurs in half the patients. Cranial nerve palsies (III, VII, XII) have been noted in one-third of the patients. Virtually all patients have progression to coma and become markedly hypertonic. In contrast, western equine encephalomyelitis (WEE) is less often characterized by a devastating clinical course.

Japanese encephalitis, caused by a flavivirus transmitted through mosquitoes and amplified in young pigs during the wet season, is endemic in Asia and Australia.[28] Tick-borne encephalitides due to Flavivirus have been prevalent in eastern and central Europe.[22] Headache and fever may be the only signs, and the disorder may remain limited as an aseptic meningitis. The most severe form is a meningoencephalomyelitis occurring up to 2 weeks after resolution of the febrile prodrome. Flaccid paralysis and involvement of the cranial nerve nuclei, particularly the bulbar nuclei, lead to very poor outcome and often death.

More recently, U.S. states on the Atlantic seaboard and in the Midwest, particularly Illinois, experienced outbreaks of West Nile encephalitis due to a mosquito-borne fla-

vivirus, preceded by unexpected deaths in birds and horses. The patients were older than 50 years and had fever, severe muscle pain, conjunctivitis, and roseola. A flaccid asymmetric motor paralysis mimicking poliomyelitis with ventilator dependency, prominent pleocytosis, and cranial nerve deficits has been noted.[42] Pathologically, the medulla oblongata was significantly involved, but the virus also had a proclivity for the cranial nerve roots and possibly anterior horn cells. The virus genome can be detected by PCR but is insensitive.[6,30,49,56,65] An update on this emerging new cause of encephalitis has been published recently for review.[50]

A newly emerging pathogen in immunosuppressed transplant recipients is human herpesvirus 6. Its presentation may be acute, usually 2 to 4 weeks after transplantation, and its predilection for the limbic system produces amnesia.[43]

The epidemic encephalitides vary not only in presentation but also considerably in severity and mortality. The most common epidemic forms of encephalitis and their outcomes are shown in Table 21–1.

NEUROIMAGING AND LABORATORY TESTS

Cerebrospinal fluid examination is the preferred diagnostic test after the initial CT scan with contrast has excluded some of the most obvious mimicking disorders. Cerebrospinal fluid examination probably should be deferred in patients with mass effect, particularly those with swollen temporal lobes from herpes simplex encephalitis. When CSF is analyzed, pleocytosis with predominant lymphocytes is common at the first presentation, but exceptions exist. A fivefold to tenfold increase in protein concentration can be expected,[39] although protein values may be normal. Lactate in CSF is increased, particularly in patients with a viral encephalitis that carries a poor prognosis.[13] Red blood cells may be present, but this finding is not specific for any type of encephalitis. Cerebrospinal fluid glucose concentration

Table 21–1. Adult Epidemic Viral Encephalitis

Type	Virus	Severity	Mortality (%)
Eastern equine encephalomyelitis	Alphavirus	+++	50–70
Western equine encephalomyelitis	Alphavirus	++	5–10
Venezuelan equine encephalomyelitis	Alphavirus	+	< 1
Japanese encephalitis	Flavivirus	+++	25–50
St. Louis encephalitis	Flavivirus	++	~70°
Murray Valley encephalitis	Flavivirus	++	10–20
Colorado tick fever	Orbivirus	+	< 1
La Crosse encephalitis	Bunyavirus	++	< 5
Lymphocytic choriomeningitis	Arenavirus	++	< 1
Argentine hemorrhagic fever	Arenavirus	++	~10
Lassa fever	Arenavirus	++	~15
Rabies	Rabies virus	+++	~100[†]
West Nile	Flavivirus	++	~70[‡]

+++, often progressing to coma; ++, variable presentations; +, often mild.
°In elderly patients only.
[†]Occasional survivors in a severely disabled state have been reported.
[‡]Experience too limited for findings to be entirely accurate.

tends to be in the normal range but may be decreased in herpes simplex encephalitis and EEE.[39] In patients with EEE, the CSF formula may strongly suggest acute bacterial meningitis.[53]

Serologic testing may identify the cause of encephalitis, and acute and convalescent serum samples separated by 6 weeks should be obtained. Cerebrospinal fluid samples must be obtained for identification of the most common epidemic encephalitides, such as EEE, WEE, La Crosse, and St. Louis, which may demonstrate at least a fourfold increase in immunoglobulin M antibody responses.[14,15,47] A guideline for serologic testing of CSF is presented in Table 21–2. Other samples for virus identification may include throat swab (influenza, enterovirus), rectal swab (enterovirus), urine (adenovirus, CMV), saliva (rabies), and skin exudate (herpes).

The detection of virus by PCR may markedly facilitate the diagnosis of viral encephalitis from herpes simplex, CMV, EBV, enteroviruses, and, recently, influenza B.[44] The laboratory procedure can be completed within 10 hours. The sensitivity and specificity of PCR in the CSF in herpes simplex are very high, but false-negative samples very occasionally exist when collection is early.[1,25,36,40,51,55] Possible reasons for a negative PCR finding are the absence of DNA in the CSF sample from early

clearing of the viral genome (as early as 5 days after symptoms), variation in the amplification of HSV strains, and, less likely, institution of antiviral therapy.[4,5] Nested PCR includes a second amplification and increases detection.[67] In a study of 28 patients, 30% still had a positive herpes simplex virus PCR up to 1½ months after acyclovir treatment.[38] The PCR result can be positive as early as the first day into the illness, and only very rarely is herpes simplex virus DNA genome detected in patients without encephalitis, including those with active herpes labialis infection.

Table 21–2. Mandatory Serologic Tests of Cerebrospinal Fluid in Encephalitis of Unknown Cause

Herpes simplex
Cytomegalovirus
Human immunodeficiency virus (HIV-1 and HIV-2)
Varicella-zoster virus
Epstein-Barr virus
Toxoplasma gondii
Borrelia burgdorferi
Mycoplasma pneumoniae
Leptospira species
Legionella pneumophila
Brucella species
Chlamydia species
Syphilis
Aspergillus

Reexamination of CSF samples by the National Institute of Allergy and Infectious Diseases Collaborative Antiviral Study Group found a sensitivity of 98% and a specificity of 94% when CSF PCR was compared with brain biopsy. Of 54 patients with biopsy-proven herpes simplex encephalitis, 53 had a positive PCR result. Of 47 patients with a negative biopsy result, 44 had a negative PCR finding. The three positive PCR test results in biopsy-negative patients were considered to represent herpes simplex encephalitis and a "missed" biopsy. In virtually all patients, PCR could detect herpes simplex encephalitis DNA within 1 week of therapy. One study suggested that chemiluminescence assay (detecting viral fragments with antigenicity) can supplement a negative PCR finding, but most laboratories have reached excellent predictive value.[36]

The CT scan findings are abnormal in 60% of patients with biopsy-proven herpes simplex encephalitis but are often normal in other encephalitides. The yield of contrast-enhanced CT scanning increases significantly in comatose patients. Brain swelling may involve one or both temporal lobes (Fig. 21–1).

Magnetic resonance imaging is much more sensitive than CT scan in patients with herpes simplex encephalitis but, because of fulminant characteristics leading to death, has been performed less often in other types of encephalitis.[58] Magnetic resonance imaging demonstrates lesions that are hypointense on T1-weighted and hyperintense on T2-weighted images, with occasional mass effect and additional petechial hemorrhages in at least 50 percent of the patients. A very suggestive finding for herpes simplex encephalitis on MRI is a density change in the inferomedial temporal lobe, including the limbic system and extending into the insular cortex, with typical sparing of the putamen (Fig. 21–2). The internal cap-

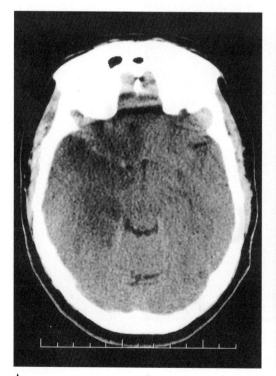 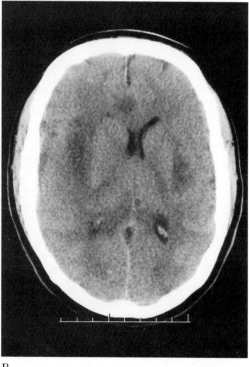

A   B

Figure 21–1. (*A, B*) Computed tomography scan images in a patient with herpes simplex encephalitis (confirmed by polymerase chain reaction) and unilateral swelling of the temporal lobe.

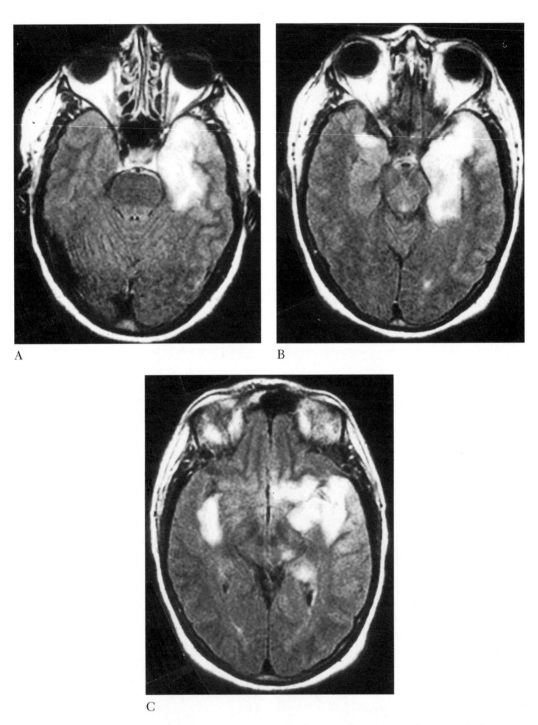

Figure 21–2. (*A–C*) Magnetic resonance imaging findings in herpes simplex encephalitis (see text for description).

sule, cingulate gyrus, and frontal lobe can be involved.[19] However, involvement of the medial and temporal lobes has also been described in a patient with limbic encephalitis associated with carcinoma of the lung[21] and in a patient with Q fever[16,60] and neurosyphilis,[62] again emphasizing the need for proper diagnosis with PCR or brain biopsy. Strictly unilateral lesions are uncommon in herpes simplex encephalitis and should raise suspicion of other causes (e.g., brain abscess, multiple sclerosis, malignant glioma, central nervous system lymphoma, brain metastasis). Diffusion-weighted imaging in patients with herpes simplex encephalitis may be more sensitive than conventional MRI and point to the development of cytotoxic edema.[64]

In patients with CMV encephalitis, MRI findings may be normal or later show nonspecific atrophy, diffuse white matter or periventricular hyperintensity, and meningeal enhancement.[32] Magnetic resonance imaging findings in EEE and rabies are predominantly in the basal ganglia and thalamus and nearly always abnormal in comatose patients.[7] Magnetic resonance imaging findings in a review of St. Louis encephalitis were mostly nonspecific, but edema in the substantia nigra was noted in two patients.[66] The MRI findings in different types of viral encephalitis are summarized in Table 21–3.[20,32,67]

Electroencephalography is an important test in patients with herpes simplex encephalitis in whom neuroimaging findings are normal. Electroencephalography demonstrates diffuse arrhythmic-rhythmic delta activity or diffuse polymorphic slowing of the background arrhythmic delta activity but more typically shows periodic lateralized epileptiform discharges in the temporal lobe as early as the second day, although it lacks specificity[33] (for further details, see Chapter 10).

Single-photon emission computed tomography found abnormalities in herpes simplex encephalitis but not in other encephalitides.[41] However, a study of eight patients with Japanese encephalitis showed fairly typical thalamic hypoperfusion and, less commonly, frontal lobe hypoperfusion.[35]

Although many authoritative reviews include apodictic truths emphasizing brain biopsy, open brain biopsy is currently indicated only in patients with atypical clinical presentation and unusual MRI findings, in patients with clinical deterioration despite antiviral treatment, and in patients with nondiagnostic PCR test findings.[17] In addition, the threshold for brain biopsy in immunosuppressed patients should be lower, particularly because opportunistic infection (CMV, *Toxoplasma*, fungi) may mimic herpes simplex encephalitis and result in a different therapeutic approach. Brain biopsy in patients with acute encephalitis without any CT or MRI abnormalities most likely has a very low yield if performed blindly.

Brain biopsy has a low complication rate in patients with encephalitis, with approximately 1% morbidity in the National Institute of Allergy and Infectious Diseases collaborative study, and virtually no mortality.[69,70] Higher complication rates from intracranial hemorrhage and edema have been reported. How-

Table 21–3. Magnetic Resonance Imaging Findings in Viral Encephalitis

Site	HSE	EEE	CMV	La Crosse	St. Louis	Rabies
Frontal	+			+		
Temporal	+			+		
Basal ganglia		+				+
Thalamus		+				+
White matter			+			
Substantia nigra					+	
Meningeal enhancement			+			

CMV, cytomegalovirus; EEE, eastern equine encephalomyelitis; HSE, herpes simplex encephalitis.
+, Abnormal signal.

ever, brain biopsies may have been performed in moribund patients, and further progressive temporal lobe edema in these cases may simply have represented the natural history of herpes simplex encephalitis. On the other hand, perioperative use of corticosteroids before the biopsy may reduce the risk of postbiopsy cerebral edema. Intracranial hematoma at the biopsy site may be devastating, and this risk may indeed be increased in patients with herpes simplex encephalitis and a hemorrhagic necrotic lesion. (For comparison, in a series of 300 patients with stereotactic biopsies for other types of intra-axial brain lesions, major morbidity or mortality occurred in 3%;[12] see Chapter 28.)

Brain tissue should be targeted at the lesion; and if no lesion can be identified or if neurosurgeons are reluctant to biopsy the temporal lobe of the dominant hemisphere, tissue in the form of a large sample of white matter should be obtained from the right frontal cortex. Handling of specimens from patients with HIV-associated encephalitis requires efficiency and care. However, the risk of HIV infection to the neurosurgeon is low.

Tissue should be processed unfixed in a special medium for subsequent viral culture and routine bacterial, fungal, and mycobacterial studies. (Usually, brain tissue is fixed in formaldehyde not only for routine hematoxylin-eosin examination but also for studies of lymphoma surface markers.) In patients with undiagnosed encephalitis, a major portion of the tissue should remain unfixed for cultures, and a portion should be fixed in glutaraldehyde for electron microscopic examination, which may identify certain viral particles. The specimen should be kept cool, but freezing destroys many viruses. The time to isolation of herpes simplex virus from brain tissue is 1 to 7 days. Immunohistochemical staining can diagnose the virus after microscopic examination.

Rabies encephalitis requires pathologic confirmation of hemorrhages and necrosis in the basal ganglia and brain stem, which can be documented on MRI if time allows. Intraneuronal, round eosinophilic intracytoplasmic bodies (Negri bodies) emerge in the hippocampal cortex and Purkinje cells. Corneal impression smears and biopsy of oral mucosa or skin can be diagnostic. However, antemortem diagnosis can be achieved in only a few cases, because the centrifugal spread of the virus takes time.

FIRST STEPS IN MANAGEMENT

Treatment of patients with viral encephalitis is largely by supportive measures (Table 21–4).

Airway management has the highest priority, especially in patients who are becoming progressively more drowsy and in patients who have had a flurry of seizures. The adequacy of ventilation must be immediately assessed. Endotracheal intubation must be performed in patients with hypoxemia. Most patients have normal respiratory drive and mechanics and breathe spontaneously on a T-piece only, but continuous positive airway pressure (5 to 10 cm H_2O) can be added. In addition, patients may become progressively agitated (restraints may intensify agitation), and aspiration becomes a

Table 21–4. Initial Management in Acute Viral Encephalitis

Airway management	Intubate early if deterioration rapid	
	T-piece (+ CPAP, 5–10 cm H_2O)	
Fluid management	Maintenance, 3 L of 0.9% NaCl (500 mL increase/°C); in patients with hyponatremia, consider dilution (treat with free-water restriction) or Addison's disease (treat with corticosteroids)	
Nutrition	Preferably enteral feeding	
Specific treatment	Antiviral	CMV: ganciclovir, 10 mg/kg q12 h
		HSE: acyclovir, 10 mg/kg q8h
	Seizures	Fosphenytoin, 20 mg/kg followed by 300 mg orally or IV
	Prophylaxis	Subcutaneous heparin or intermittent pneumatic devices
	Agitation	Midazolam or propofol infusion

CMV, cytomegalovirus; CPAP, continuous positive airway pressure; HSE, herpes simplex encephalitis.

great risk in patients who are thrashing around. Particularly vexing are patients who are floridly delirious. In these patients, the combination of sedation (e.g., with propofol or midazolam) and ventilatory support is more appropriate than trying to combat these episodes with haloperidol alone or a variety of benzodiazepines.

Normal maintenance fluids consist of 2 L of isotonic saline and incremental increases in intake in patients with fever (500 mL for every 1°C increase). Daily fluid balance must be estimated by measuring fluid intake and output, with sensible losses of 500 to 1000 mL per day. Renal function should be evaluated daily. Certain viral encephalitides may coincide with acute renal involvement (St. Louis encephalitis, rabies); renal failure may be caused by direct nephrotoxicity associated with acyclovir but more commonly by dehydration associated with fever.

It is important to supply proper nutrition, because protein catabolism begins early and continues throughout the period of relative starvation that follows. Protein wasting cannot be allowed, and adequate calories must be provided to counteract the effects of infection (Chapter 7).

The use of corticosteroids is very uncertain. A reported trial of dexamethasone in Japanese encephalitis did not show any effect on outcome, a result that may discourage its use in other types of encephalitis.[31] However, corticosteroids are advised in patients scheduled for diagnostic brain biopsy.

In patients with a strong likelihood of viral encephalitis, treatment is begun with acyclovir. Specific antiviral therapy is limited in viral encephalitides other than herpes simplex encephalitis, but acyclovir therapy is typically started while awaiting PCR results. Randomized clinical studies in patients treated with acyclovir have found that mortality is reduced to 25% (predominantly in patients with Glasgow coma scale scores of 10 or less) and that almost 40% of the treated patients have good recovery or only minimal deficits.[69] Acyclovir is administered at a dose of 10 mg/kg every 8 hours and is continued for 10 to 14 days. If recognized, the side effects of acyclovir are reversible; they include renal failure with increases in creatinine and blood urea nitrogen in 10% of patients. An adjusting schedule based on calculated creatinine clearance is shown in Table 21–5. Other side effects are thrombocytopenia (6%), aspartate transaminase elevation (3%), fever, and, less commonly (< 1%), leukopenia and tremors.

In patients with CMV encephalitis, ganciclovir is the preferred drug (10 mg/kg every 12 hours). Ganciclovir is much more toxic and is associated with bone marrow depression, nausea, and vomiting. Not infrequently, patients

Table 21–5. Acyclovir Doses in Renal Impairment

CRCL, mL/minute*	ACYCLOVIR	
	mg/kg	Frequency
>50	10	q8h
30–50	10	q12h
10–30	10	q24h
<10	5	q24h

*Calculation of creatinine clearance (CRCL).

Male: CRCL (mL/minute) = $\dfrac{(140 - age) \times (\text{ideal body weight [kg]})}{\text{serum creatine (mg/dL)} \times 72}$

Female: 0.85 × CRCL for men

Ideal body weight: males, 50 kg + 2.3 kg for each inch over 5 feet; females, 45.5 kg + 2.3 kg for each inch over 5 feet.

with CMV encephalitis have already been treated for CMV retinitis with a maintenance dose of ganciclovir. In these patients, foscarnet is indicated as additional therapy (40 mg/kg infused over 1 hour, every 8 hours) along with restarting of the intravenous dose of ganciclovir.[11,59] Toxicity, including electrolyte abnormalities and renal failure, is common with foscarnet.

DETERIORATION: CAUSES AND MANAGEMENT

Deterioration in a patient with viral encephalitis is most often the result of an overwhelming infection and may be associated with the development of cerebral edema. Deterioration can be expected in patients with a more virulent encephalitis. In the collaborative antiviral study, two-thirds of the patients had progression after the diagnosis was confirmed by brain biopsy, and one-third of the patients lapsed into coma.[70] Occasionally, sudden deterioration occurs in a patient who has recently had a diagnostic brain biopsy and may be caused by hemorrhage into a necrotic biopsy site.

In any patient with acute viral encephalitis who has rapid deterioration in level of consciousness and a marked febrile response, the possibility of early sepsis must be considered. Patients with acute viral encephalitis are at considerable risk of urosepsis and aspiration pneumonia that may evolve into bilateral pneumonia and adult respiratory distress syndrome (Chapter 33).

Hyponatremia is another potential problem in patients with encephalitis, because in some cases it becomes severe (plasma sodium concentration less than 120 mmol/L) (Chapter 31). Fluid restriction corrects dilutional hyponatremia and possibly its incumbent risks of cerebral edema and seizures. In many patients, fluid restriction with replacement of insensible loss and urine output alone corrects hyponatremia. Hyponatremia in CMV encephalitis may be due to adrenalitis. Adrenalitis may cause a characteristic addisonian syndrome with hyponatremia, hyperkalemia,

and shock, and corticosteroids are urgently indicated.

Seizures occur more often in certain viral encephalitides, and repeated electroencephalography is important at least to exclude the possibility that deterioration or fluctuation in consciousness is associated with nonconvulsive status epilepticus.

Intracranial monitoring should be considered if the level of consciousness deteriorates to coma. Placement of a ventricular catheter is very difficult, because slitlike ventricles may have appeared on CT scans. Whether aggressive management of increased ICP changes outcome is not known. The most extensive experience (albeit observations in only eight comatose patients), predominantly in patients with herpes simplex encephalitis, was reported from Massachusetts General Hospital.[9] Placement of an extradural catheter in comatose patients with encephalitis revealed that ICP was initially abnormal in only one of the eight; continuous ICP monitoring showed a progressive increase in ICP approximately 2 weeks after onset. Patients in whom increased ICP was controlled had a better outcome than those in whom no change in ICP was observed. The latter patients often had progression to brain death or died from sepsis while remaining in a severely disabled or vegetative state.[9] Elevation of the head position and mannitol may control ICP. There is virtually no clinical experience with the use of barbiturates or propofol infusion in this situation, but they may be the last resort.

Patients whose condition deteriorates despite optimal treatment of increased ICP and who have unilateral swelling of a nondominant temporal lobe can be salvaged with craniotomy and decompression by careful removal of the necrotic tissue of the anterior temporal lobe.[23,63,72] The options in patients with bilateral swelling or brain stem compression from a swollen dominant temporal lobe are very limited. Decompressive craniotomy increases the probability of survival in patients with bilateral involvement, but unlike patients with unilateral swelling, they are virtually certain to have a devastating handicap.

OUTCOME

Outcome varies and depends on the type of viral encephalitis. In the United States, rabies, EEE, and more recently West Nile are the most severe forms of encephalitis, and the probability of a poor outcome is high. Outcome in any type of viral encephalitis is determined by a multiplicity of factors. These include the virulence of the virus, age greater than 30 years, absent or late initiation (later than 4 days) of antiviral treatment, altered consciousness or status epilepticus at presentation, and whether secondary complications, such as brain edema, have occurred. Coma from brain edema in herpes simplex encephalitis implies a poor prognosis and increases the likelihood of fatal outcome. Early electroencephalographic findings, such as diffuse slowing, spikes, and sharp waves, do not predict poor outcome or future seizure disorder. However, later diffuse slowing of the background pattern on electroencephalograms correlates with poor outcome.[61]

In patients with treated herpes simplex encephalitis, mortality is 20%, and only 40% of the patients truly survive without any appreciable functional deficit.[54] Marked cognitive deficits as well as seizures[2] (up to 20%) are well-recognized sequelae. The cognitive deficits can be devastating, with loss of memory, significant intellectual decline, and behavioral and personality changes.[37] Young age and early administration of acyclovir increase the probability of a successful outcome.[18] Early treatment with acyclovir may not prevent cognitive sequelae; patients treated as early as 5 days into

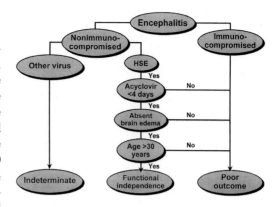

Figure 21–3. Outcome algorithm in viral encephalitis. HSE, herpes simplex encephalitis. Indeterminate: any statement would be a premature conclusion. Functional independence: no assistance needed, minor handicap may remain. Poor outcome: severe disability or death, vegetative state.

the illness have shown marked neurologic deficits and the inability to function at a similar intellectual level.[27] Average survival with CMV encephalitis in AIDS is 2 months after diagnosis despite therapy, and successful outcome is exceptional. La Crosse encephalitis, mostly reported in children, may result in profound defects in neurobehavior and IQ score.[46]

Brain death is a possible outcome in many patients with viral encephalitis. Patients with rabies encephalitis[29] obviously cannot become organ donors[48] because of the potential risk of cross-contamination (Chapter 34). An outcome algorithm for viral encephalitis is shown in Figure 21–3.

CONCLUSIONS

- PCR can reliably detect herpes simplex DNA in CSF and probably will replace the need for brain biopsy. (PCR is also available for CMV, EBV, and enteroviruses.)
- Treatment is largely supportive, with airway management, seizure control, prevention of aspiration and deep venous thrombosis, and management of agitation with midazolam or propofol.
- Acyclovir administration is started at a dose of 10 mg/kg every 8 hours, continued for up to 14 days, and adjusted to creatinine clearance.
- Brain edema in acute viral encephalitis warrants ICP monitoring, and aggressive management may increase the chance of survival.

REFERENCES

1. Anderson NE, Powell KF, Croxson MC: A polymerase chain reaction assay of cerebrospinal fluid in patients with suspected herpes simplex encephalitis. *J Neurol Neurosurg Psychiatry* 56:520–525, 1993.
2. Annegers JF, Hauser WA, Beghi E, et al: The risk of unprovoked seizures after encephalitis and meningitis. *Neurology* 38:1407–1410, 1988.
3. Armstrong RW, Fung PC: Brainstem encephalitis (rhombencephalitis) due to *Listeria monocytogenes*: case report and review. *Clin Infect Dis* 16:689–702, 1993.
4. Aslanzadeh J, Garner JG, Feder HM, et al: Use of polymerase chain reaction for laboratory diagnosis of herpes simplex virus encephalitis. *Ann Clin Lab Sci* 23: 196–202, 1993.
5. Aslanzadeh J, Skiest DJ: Polymerase chain reaction for detection of herpes simplex virus encephalitis. *J Clin Pathol* 47:554–555, 1994.
6. Asnis DS, Conetta R, Waldman G, et al: The West Nile virus encephalitis outbreak in the United States (1999–2000): from Flushing, New York, to beyond its borders. *Ann N Y Acad Sci* 951:161–171, 2001.
7. Awasthi M, Parmar H, Patankar T, et al: Imaging findings in rabies encephalitis. *AJNR Am J Neuroradiol* 22:677–680, 2001.
8. Bale JF Jr: Viral encephalitis. *Med Clin North Am* 77:25–42, 1993.
9. Barnett GH, Ropper AH, Romeo J: Intracranial pressure and outcome in adult encephalitis. *J Neurosurg* 68:585–588, 1988.
10. Bash S, Hathout GM, Cohen S: Mesiotemporal T2-weighted hyperintensity: neurosyphilis mimicking herpes encephalitis. *AJNR Am J Neuroradiol* 22:314–316, 2001.
11. Berman SM, Kim RC: The development of cytomegalovirus encephalitis in AIDS patients receiving ganciclovir. *Am J Med* 96:415–419, 1994.
12. Bernstein M, Parrent AG: Complications of CT-guided stereotactic biopsy of intra-axial brain lesions. *J Neurosurg* 81:165–168, 1994.
13. Büttner T, Dorndorf W: Prognostic value of computed tomography and cerebrospinal fluid analysis in viral encephalitis. *J Neuroimmunol* 20:163–164, 1988.
14. Calisher CH, Berardi VP, Muth DJ, et al: Specificity of immunoglobulin M and G antibody responses in humans infected with eastern and western equine encephalitis viruses: application to rapid serodiagnosis. *J Clin Microbiol* 23:369–372, 1986.
15. Calisher CH, Pretzman CI, Muth DJ, et al: Serodiagnosis of La Crosse virus infections in humans by detection of immunoglobulin M class antibodies. *J Clin Microbiol* 23:667–671, 1986.
16. Cameron DA, Freedman AR, Wansbrough-Jones MH: Q fever encephalitis. *J Infect* 20:159–162, 1990.
17. Coren ME, Buchdahl RM, Cowan FM, et al: Imaging and laboratory investigation in herpes simplex encephalitis. *J Neurol Neurosurg Psychiatry* 67:243–245, 1999.
18. Counsell CE, Taylor R, Whittle IR: Focal necrotising herpes simplex encephalitis: a report of two cases with good clinical and neuropsychological outcomes. *J Neurol Neurosurg Psychiatry* 57:1115–1117, 1994.
19. Demaerel P, Wilms G, Robberecht W, et al: MRI of herpes simplex encephalitis. *Neuroradiology* 34:490–493, 1992.
20. Deresiewicz RL, Thaler SJ, Hsu L, et al: Clinical and neuroradiographic manifestations of eastern equine encephalitis. *N Engl J Med* 336:1867–1874, 1997.
21. Dirr LY, Elster AD, Donofrio PD, et al: Evolution of brain MRI abnormalities in limbic encephalitis. *Neurology* 40:1304–1306, 1990.
22. Dumpis U, Crook D, Oksi J: Tick-borne encephalitis. *Clin Infect Dis* 28:882–890, 1999.
23. Ebel H, Kuchta J, Balogh A, et al: Operative treatment of tentorial herniation in herpes encephalitis. *Childs Nerv Syst* 15:84–86, 1999.
24. Fisher CM: Hypomanic symptoms caused by herpes simplex encephalitis. *Neurology* 47:1374–1378, 1996.
25. Gasecki AP, Steg RE: Correlation of early MRI with CT scan, EEG, and CSF: analyses in a case of biopsy-proven herpes simplex encephalitis. *Eur Neurol* 31: 372–375, 1991.
26. Gillies CG, Grunnet M, Hamilton CW: Tubular inclusions in macrophages in the brain of a patient with acute hemorrhagic leukoencephalitis (Weston-Hurst syndrome). *Ultrastruct Pathol* 18:19–22, 1994.
27. Gordon B, Selnes OA, Hart J Jr, et al: Long-term cognitive sequelae of acyclovir-treated herpes simplex encephalitis. *Arch Neurol* 47:646–647, 1990.
28. Hanna JN, Ritchie SA, Phillips DA, et al: Japanese encephalitis in north Queensland, Australia, 1998. *Med J Aust* 170:533–536, 1999.
29. Hantson P, Guérit JM, de Tourtchaninoff M, et al: Rabies encephalitis mimicking the electrophysiological pattern of brain death. A case report. *Eur Neurol* 33:212–217, 1993.
30. Hochberg LR, Sims JR, Davis BT: West Nile encephalitis in Massachusetts. *N Engl J Med* 346:1030–1031, 2002.
31. Hoke CH Jr, Vaughn DW, Nisalak A, et al: Effect of high-dose dexamethasone on the outcome of acute encephalitis due to Japanese encephalitis virus. *J Infect Dis* 165:631–637, 1992.
32. Holland NR, Power C, Mathews VP, et al: Cytomegalovirus encephalitis in acquired immunodeficiency syndrome (AIDS). *Neurology* 44:507–514, 1994.
33. Illis LS, Taylor FM: The electroencephalogram in herpes-simplex encephalitis. *Lancet* 1:718–721, 1972.
34. Jemsek J, Greenberg SB, Taber L, et al: Herpes zoster-associated encephalitis: clinicopathologic report of 12 cases and review of the literature. *Medicine (Baltimore)* 62:81–97, 1983.
35. Kalita J, Das BK, Misra UK: SPECT studies of regional cerebral blood flow in 8 patients with Japanese en-

cephalitis in subacute and chronic stage. *Acta Neurol Scand* 99:213–218, 1999.

36. Kamei S, Takasu T, Morishima T, et al: Comparative study between chemiluminescence assay and two different sensitive polymerase chain reactions on the diagnosis of serial herpes simplex virus encephalitis. *J Neurol Neurosurg Psychiatry* 67:596–601, 1999.

37. Kennedy PG, Adams JH, Graham DI, et al: A clinico-pathological study of herpes simplex encephalitis. *Neuropathol Appl Neurobiol* 14:395–415, 1988.

38. Koskiniemi M, Piiparinen H, Mannonen L, et al: Herpes encephalitis is a disease of middle aged and elderly people: polymerase chain reaction for detection of herpes simplex virus in the CSF of 516 patients with encephalitis. *J Neurol Neurosurg Psychiatry* 60:174–178, 1996.

39. Koskiniemi M, Vaheri A, Taskinen E: Cerebrospinal fluid alterations in herpes simplex virus encephalitis. *Rev Infect Dis* 6:608–618, 1984.

40. Lakeman FD, Whitley RJ, and the National Institute of Allergy and Infectious Diseases Collaborative Antiviral Study Group: Diagnosis of herpes simplex encephalitis: application of polymerase chain reaction to cerebrospinal fluid from brain-biopsied patients and correlation with disease. *J Infect Dis* 171:857–863, 1995.

41. Launes J, Nikkinen P, Lindroth L, et al: Diagnosis of acute herpes simplex encephalitis by brain perfusion single photon emission computed tomography. *Lancet* 1:1188–1191, 1988.

42. Leis AA, Stokic DS, Polk JL: A poliomyelitis-like syndrome from West Nile virus infection (letter). *N Engl J Med* 347:1279–1280, 2002.

43. MacLean HJ, Douen AG: Severe amnesia associated with human herpesvirus 6 encephalitis after bone marrow transplantation. *Transplantation* 73:1086–1089, 2002.

44. McCullers JA, Facchini S, Chesney PJ, et al: Influenza B virus encephalitis. *Clin Infect Dis* 28:898–900, 1999.

45. McGrath NM, Anderson NE, Hope JK, et al: Anterior opercular syndrome, caused by herpes simplex encephalitis. *Neurology* 49:494–497, 1997.

46. McJunkin JE, de los Reyes EC, Irazuzta JE, et al: La Crosse encephalitis in children. *N Engl J Med* 344:801–807, 2001.

47. Monath TP, Nystrom RR, Bailey RE, et al: Immunoglobulin M antibody capture enzyme-linked immunosorbent assay for diagnosis of St. Louis encephalitis. *J Clin Microbiol* 20:784–790, 1984.

48. Mrak RE, Young L: Rabies encephalitis in a patient with no history of exposure. *Hum Pathol* 24:109–110, 1993.

49. Nash D, Mostashari F, Fine A, et al: The outbreak of West Nile virus infection in the New York City area in 1999. *N Engl J Med* 344:1807–1814, 2001.

50. Petersen LR, Marfin AA: West Nile virus. A primer for the clinician. *Ann Intern Med* 137:173–179, 2002.

51. Pohl-Koppe A, Dahm C, Elgas M, et al: The diagnostic significance of the polymerase chain reaction and isoelectric focusing in herpes simplex virus encephalitis. *J Med Virol* 36:147–154, 1992.

52. Posey K, Alpert JN, Langford LA, et al: Acute hemorrhagic leukoencephalitis: a cause of acute brainstem dysfunction. *South Med J* 87:851–854, 1994.

53. Przelomski MM, O'Rourke E, Grady GF, et al: Eastern equine encephalitis in Massachusetts: a report of 16 cases, 1970–1984. *Neurology* 38:736–739, 1988.

54. Rao N, Costa JL: Rehabilitation of three patients after treatment for herpes encephalitis. *Am J Phys Med Rehabil* 70:73–75, 1991.

55. Rowley AH, Whitley RJ, Lakeman FD, et al: Rapid detection of herpes-simplex-virus DNA in cerebrospinal fluid of patients with herpes simplex encephalitis. *Lancet* 335:440–441, 1990.

56. Sampson BA, Armbrustmacher V: West Nile encephalitis: the neuropathology of four fatalities. *Ann NY Acad Sci* 951:172–178, 2001.

57. Schnell RG, Dyck PJ, Bowie EJ, et al: Infectious mononucleosis: neurologic and EEG findings. *Medicine (Baltimore)* 45:51–63, 1966.

58. Schroth G, Gawehn J, Thron A, et al: Early diagnosis of herpes simplex encephalitis by MRI. *Neurology* 37:179–183, 1987.

59. Schwarz TF, Loeschke K, Hanus I, et al: CMV encephalitis during ganciclovir therapy of CMV retinitis. *Infection* 18:289–290, 1990.

60. Sempere AP, Elizaga J, Duarte J, et al: Q fever mimicking herpetic encephalitis. *Neurology* 43:2713–2714, 1993.

61. Siren J, Seppalainen AM, Launes J: Is EEG useful in assessing patients with acute encephalitis treated with acyclovir? *Electroencephalogr Clin Neurophysiol* 107:296–301, 1998.

62. Szilak I, Marty F, Helft J, et al: Neurosyphilis presenting as herpes simplex encephalitis. *Clin Infect Dis* 32:1108–1109, 2001.

63. Taferner E, Pfausler B, Kofler A, et al: Craniectomy in severe, life-threatening encephalitis: a report on outcome and long-term prognosis of four cases. *Intensive Care Med* 27:1426–1428, 2001.

64. Tsuchiya K, Katase S, Yoshino A, et al: Diffusion-weighted MR imaging of encephalitis. *AJR Am J Roentgenol* 173:1097–1099, 1999.

65. Tyler KL: West Nile virus encephalitis in America. *N Engl J Med* 344:1858–1859, 2001.

66. Wasay M, Diaz-Arrastia R, Suss RA, et al: St Louis encephalitis: a review of 11 cases in a 1995 Dallas, Tex, epidemic. *Arch Neurol* 57:114–118, 2000.

67. Weil AA, Glaser CA, Amad Z, et al: Patients with suspected herpes simplex encephalitis: rethinking an initial negative polymerase chain reaction result. *Clin Infect Dis* 34:1154–1157, 2002.

68. Whitley RJ: Viral encephalitis. *N Engl J Med* 323:242–250, 1990.

69. Whitley RJ, Alford CA, Hirsch MS, et al: Vidarabine

versus acyclovir therapy in herpes simplex encephalitis. *N Engl J Med* 314:144–149, 1986.

70. Whitley RJ, Soong SJ, Dolin R, et al: Adenine arabinoside therapy of biopsy-proved herpes simplex encephalitis. National Institute of Allergy and Infectious Diseases collaborative antiviral study. *N Engl J Med* 297:289–294, 1977.

71. Wolf RW, Schultze D, Fretz C, et al: Atypical herpes simplex encephalitis presenting as operculum syndrome. *Pediatr Radiol* 29:191–193, 1999.

72. Yan HJ: Herpes simplex encephalitis: the role of surgical decompression. *Surg Neurol* 57:20–24, 2002.

73. Young CA, Humphrey PR, Ghadiali EJ, et al: Short-term memory impairment in an alert patient as a presentation of herpes simplex encephalitis. *Neurology* 42:260–261, 1992.

22

Acute Spinal Cord Disorders

The management of patients with a rapid development of quadriplegia or paraplegia is frustratingly complicated because the handicap may be permanent. The spectrum of causes is wide, and there are glaring regional differences in the cause of spinal cord injury in recently published series. In a study from France of 79 patients with acute myelopathy, the most common causes were multiple sclerosis, systemic disease such as cancer, and spinal cord infarction.[11] In contrast, tuberculosis of the spine, acute transverse myelitis, and primary cord tumor were common in a series of patients with paraplegia from India.[33]

The immediate priorities in the NICU are stabilization of respiration, cardiac rhythm, and blood pressure and management of neurogenic bladder and bowel dysfunction.[1] Moreover, decubitus prophylaxis is important because skin lesions may appear rapidly. Uncertainty about the etiology of an acute myelopathy also justifies a brief admission to the NICU not only to observe the clinical course but also to continue the search for a cause.

This chapter provides a template for rapid clinical localization and interpretation of neuroimaging studies. These two pieces of information are key to clinical diagnosis. The overarching theme of this chapter is management of acute spinal cord injury, with less attention to fractures and cancerous destruction of the bony structures. Damage to the bony structures from trauma or cancer as a source of acute myelopathy is discussed in other monographs,[7,35] and management should be appropriately relegated to neurosurgeons or spine surgeons.

CLINICAL RECOGNITION

The course of development of symptoms (insidious, rapid, saltatory, or maximal at onset) could indicate a certain cause but without much specificity. Tumors in the spinal cord may have different and unpredictable courses of development. Even a remitting, relapsing course can occur, and some benign tumors can cause rapid progression to quadriplegia (in days).

Sensory symptoms are the most frequent presenting symptoms in patients with multiple sclerosis, whereas motor and sphincter dysfunction appear to be more frequent in other causes.[11]

The manifestations of acute transverse myelitis at onset may be paresthesias (mimicking Guillain-Barré syndrome), interscapular pain followed by paraparesis, and urinary retention. Acute catastrophic onset has been reported.[2,9,29] The clinical course in necrotic myelopathy may be vacillating: Rapid decline is common, but gradual worsening alternating with sudden progression and followed by slow progression may be observed.[19,36] An ascending sensory level, pain, and urinary incontinence are common presenting symptoms of acute transverse myelitis, together with lower motor neuron signs (areflexia, atrophy, and flaccidity) on examination.

Spinal cord ischemia due to occlusion of the anterior spinal artery and tributaries results in acute maximal motor paralysis and sensory level. Causes are invariably dissecting aneurysm, shock, ruptured abdominal aneurysm, trauma, and, in young patients, fibrocartilaginous embolization. Neuromyelitis optica (Devic's disease) is possibly linked to multiple sclerosis, but its pathologic substrate of severe necrosis and axonal degeneration indicates that it could be a separate disorder. Absence of demyelinating lesions outside the optic nerve and spinal cord is required for the diagnosis. Respiratory failure due to cervical cord involvement in Devic's disease is common in relapsing forms. The optic neuritis and myelitis may not coincide with each other and may occur several years apart.

Pain is an important clinical feature that may point to a certain cause, but it may also result in a mistaken referral to a cardiologist (pain involving the T1–T5 roots), gastroenterologist (pain referred to the upper abdomen; T6–T10 roots), or urologist (pain involving the lower back and radiation to genitalia; T12–S4). The pain associated with spinal cord disease is sharp and stabbing and therefore can be differentiated from the more dull, nagging pain associated with visceral disease. Percussion pain may be elicited over the spine, but this symptom is generally considered unreliable. Patients with extensive metastatic disease and collapsed vertebrae may not feel any pain with percussion. Pain that feels as if something were "ripped open" is fairly typical in a patient with an acute epidural hematoma. It commonly mimics a ruptured abdominal aorta or ureter obstruction due to a kidney stone. Failure to support one's weight and urinary retention within the first few hours after onset of an excruciating stab of back pain are fairly diagnostic.

Neurologic examination specifically embodies determination of the level and the extent of spinal cord involvement in the horizontal axis. The function of the spinal cord is graded to determine whether the lesion is complete or incomplete. It is complete when absence of both motor and sensory function below the lesion level is documented.

Table 22–1. Medical Research Council Scale of Muscle Strength

0	No muscular contraction
1	A flicker of contraction either seen or palpated but insufficient to move a joint
2	Muscular contractions sufficient to move a joint but not against the force of gravity
3	Muscular contractions sufficient to maintain a position against the force of gravity
4	Muscular contractions sufficient to resist the force of gravity plus additional force
5	Normal motor power

Modified from *Aids to the Examination of the Peripheral Nervous System*. 4th ed. Edinburgh: WB Saunders, 2000. By permission of *The Guarantors of Brain*.

The degree of weakness can be assessed by grading muscle strength on the grading scale of the British Medical Research Council (Table 22–1). Although one may grade the weakness of all muscles for documentation and comparison over time, some muscles are localizing: arm abduction (C5), forearm extension (C5), forearm flexion (C5 and C6), knee extension (L3 and L4), foot and great toe dorsiflexion (L5), and plantar flexion (S1). Assessing muscle tone is also important, although many patients have a flaccid paralysis due to so-called spinal shock—a poorly understood pathophysiologic phenomenon. Muscle tone, or the resistance a muscle has against passive movement of the joint, may distinguish between upper motor neuron disease and lower motor neuron disease. Upper motor neuron disease typically causes spasticity in which the flexors in the upper extremities and extensors to the lower extremities are more commonly involved. It is worthwhile to inspect the muscles for atrophy, which may indicate a long-standing process that has evolved into cord compression. Acute radiculopathy does not produce atrophy, but long-standing compression root lesions produce fasciculations and significant atrophy of the muscle bulk. Myoclonic twitching may occur and can be widespread in the early hours of acute spinal cord injury.

The sensory level can be assessed by dermatomes (Fig. 22–1). Again, important pointers are nipple at level T4, umbilicus at level T10, and thumb, middle finger, and fifth digit

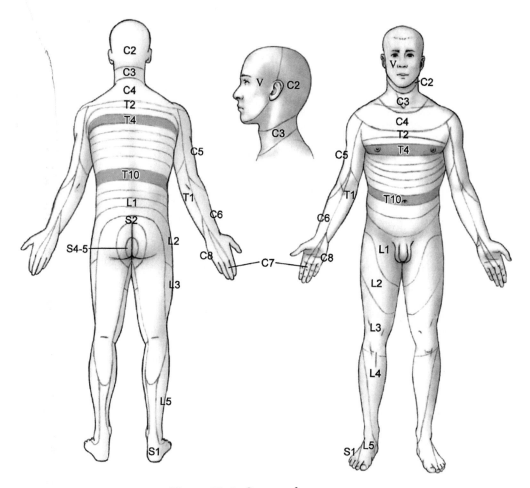

Figure 22–1. Sensory dermatomes.

innervated by C6, C7, and C8. The C4 and T2 dermatomes are continuous. A notable finding, when present, is preservation of sacral sensation, implying an intra-axial lesion due to ventrolateral localization of sacral spinothalamic tracts. Other patterns are Brown-Séquard's syndrome, with contralateral loss of pain and temperature (involvement of the crossed spinothalamic tract), ipsilateral loss of position and vibration sense (involvement of the ascending posterior column tracts), and paralysis (corticospinal tract).

It is important to assess anal sphincter tone (S3–S4). The examining finger should be held firmly against the anal verge to allow gradual passive relaxation. The strength of the external anal sphincter can be assessed by having the patient tighten the pelvic floor as if to prevent stool from escaping. The puborectalis should also be palpated a few inches inside the anal canal. Gentle pressure is applied toward the sacrum to assess the puborectalis for tone, strength, and spasticity. In addition, the bulbocavernous reflexes are elicited by pinching the dorsal glans penis or by pressing the clitoris and palpating for bulbocavernosus and external anal sphincter contraction. If these reflexes are intact, conus medullaris function probably is normal.

The spinal cord injury can be classified by the American Spinal Injury Association impairment scale specifically designed for traumatic injury (Table 22–2).

Clinical differentiation of an extramedullary tumor from an intramedullary tumor of the

Table 22–2. American Spinal Injury Association Impairment Scale

Grade *Description*	
A	Complete; no sensory or motor function preserved in the sacral segments S4–S5
B	Incomplete; sensory but not motor function preserved below the neurologic level and extending through the sacral segment S4–S5
C	Incomplete; motor function preserved below the neurologic level; most key muscles have a MRC grade < 3
D	Incomplete; motor function preserved below the neurologic level; most key muscles have a MRC grade > 3
E	Normal motor and sensory function

MRC, Medical Research Council.
Source: From McDonald JW, Sadowsky C: Spinal-cord-injury. *Lancet* 359:417–425, 2002. By permission of Elsevier Science.

spinal cord can be extremely difficult and unreliable. Nonetheless, an extramedullary tumor may appear as a Brown-Séquard type of lesion and then become more widespread. Extramedullary tumors often produce radicular and regional pain rather than the poorly localized burning pain of intramedullary tumors. Sphincter disturbances are also considered very unusual in patients with extramedullary and intramedullary tumors. (Magnetic resonance imaging may eventually resolve this clinical uncertainty.)

Two specific problems need to be addressed. First, respiration can be very seriously affected when the lesion involves the cervical cord C3 and C4 segments. Patients often have shortness of breath and heavy breathing with an increased work of breathing but also may have a sensation of air hunger and chest tightness. When lesions reach C3, diaphragmatic expansion and abdominal muscle function are absent, so that rapid intubation and full mechanical ventilation are needed. Tracheostomy is indicated with use of cannulas that allow for speech. Noninvasive assisted ventilation could be tried, but the criteria have not been well outlined in this condition. In spinal cord injury, weakness of the respiratory muscles, as in any type of impaired neuromuscular respiratory function, is determined by weakness of the diaphragm and the

intercostal and abdominal muscles. Innervation of these muscles is organized as follows: diaphragm (phrenic nerve, C3–C5), intercostal muscles (T1–T12), and abdominal muscles (T7–L1).[26] Therefore, effective coughing is determined by the level of injury. Lower levels of injury may spare intercostal muscles, resulting in better volume of expiratory reserve.[30] When myelitis or myelopathy involves levels in the lower cervical segments, breathing depends on posture. Vital capacity increases in the supine position (unlike diaphragmatic failure in Guillain-Barré syndrome and myasthenia gravis, which worsens breathing in this position). The abdominal contents produce a pressure effect, and this is the principle underlying use of abdominal binders.

Second, the delicate autonomic balance of sympathetic and parasympathetic output is skewed toward vagal output in lesions involving the low cervical midthoracic cord (C1–T6). This leads to hypotension (absent sympathetic arteriolar tone) and bradycardia (vagal innervation unopposed). Tonic and reflex control of sympathetic and sacral parasympathetic function in cord lesions above T5 leads to hypotension with head-up tilt but also to frequent bradycardia. Bradycardia (up to 20 beats a minute) can remain asymptomatic (Fig. 22–2), but cardiac pauses are common reasons for "calling a code." Bradycardia usually resolves within 6 weeks,[21] but the patient may need a temporary pacemaker. Injury to the cervical cord completely disrupts sympathetic traffic, which explains the much higher frequency of bradycardia with a lesion in this location. Tracheal suctioning is perhaps the most noticeable trigger. These vagal discharges clearly respond to 1 mg of atropine or revert spontaneously.

Many patients are poikilothermic (temperature fluctuations due to ambient temperature up to 2°C). Hypothermia may occur from lack of shivering and profound vasodilatation, and some patients may not notice decreases in bladder temperature to 33°C. It may also lead to a prolonged QT interval on the electrocardiogram. Lack of sweating from loss of sympathetic control of the apocrine glands may pro-

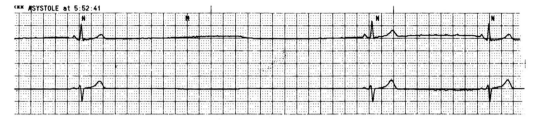

Figure 22–2. Bradycardia spell with brief pause in a patient with cervical necrotic myopathy.

duce hyperthermia. However, sweating above the lesion often prevents hyperthermia.

Gastric atony may be evident on a routine chest radiograph that reveals large air pockets. Atony also affects the bladder.[17] Catheterization and placement of an indwelling catheter are required to assess possible retention. Bladder retention of more than 1 L may not be noted by the patient. Retention may continue even when the patient is catheterized, particularly if urinary flow is minimal or obstructed. Bowel dysfunction significantly affects management, and most reflex activity below the level of spinal cord injury is lost.

NEUROIMAGING AND LABORATORY TESTS

Magnetic resonance imaging of the spine has become an essential test in acute spinal cord disorder and should be performed promptly. Imaging clearly identifies the location of the abnormality, compartment affected, degree of compression, destruction of surrounding structures, and intraspinal lesions not visualized by other neuroimaging tests. Spinal cord MRI should include routine 1.5 tesla T1-weighted sequences, supplemented by gadolinium, and T2-weighted sequences. Contrast enhancement with gadolinium is frequently present in multiple sclerosis and less common in other causes. Spinal cord swelling can also accompany multiple sclerosis and initially suggests a tumor. In multiple sclerosis, the lesions are frequently small and localized in the lateral or posterior regions.[32] In addition, MRI of the brain

detects areas of demyelination, typically in the corpus callosum. An isolated increased centromedullary signal on MRI is diagnostic for a spinal cord infarct. Magnetic resonance imaging of the spine is also more sensitive in visualizing vertebral metastasis, because a metastasis located in the medullary cavity could skip the cortex of the vertebral body and thus may not be detected by bone scintigraphy.[34] An acute spinal epidural hematoma may be isointense on T1-weighted images for 5 days, but the lesion is hyperintense with focal heterogeneous hypointensity on T2-weighted images.[15,16] The patterns of abnormality on MRI commonly encountered in acute spinal cord disorders are shown in Figure 22–3.

Visual evoked potentials are possibly helpful in documenting previous or simultaneous involvement of the optic nerves, pointing to Devic's (optic neuromyelitis) disease.[37] Somatosensory evoked potentials or corticomotor evoked potentials are not helpful in diagnosis but may hold promise as an indicator of prognosis. Tibial and pudendal somatosensory evoked potentials seem to indicate recovery of ambulatory capacity,[10] but one study suggested that this finding applied only to ischemic spinal cord lesions.[18]

Cerebrospinal fluid analysis can be helpful because oligoclonal bands and a cell count higher than 30 cells are common in multiple sclerosis. Pleocytosis (> 30 cells without oligoclonal bands) suggests an infectious cause and may indicate a postinfectious myelopathy. In spinal cord infarction, the cerebrospinal fluid should be normal, although a mild pleocytosis has been reported. The diagnostic tests are summarized in Table 22–3.

FIRST STEPS IN MANAGEMENT

The first crucial decision in any patient with acute spinal cord symptoms is whether immediate neurosurgical intervention is needed. Many neurosurgical conditions of the spinal cord, particularly acute epidural hematoma and penetrating injury, are successfully treated only when decompression has been achieved early in the course.

Acute epidural hematoma due to rupture of the epidural venous plexus is commonly associated with use of warfarin. Immediate administration of fresh frozen plasma and evacuation within 12 hours result in good ambulatory function and bladder control.[13] A nonsurgical approach should be considered only in patients with stable or improving minimal neurologic deficits and a lesion not compressing the cord. It is not commonly an option. Above all, these conservatively managed patients belong in the NICU with a neurosurgeon in attendance.[12]

Other emergency neurosurgical indications are removal of foreign objects (e.g., bullet), obtaining tissue samples of an unknown tumor, and spinal instability from any cause in a patient whose condition is rapidly worsening. Patients with significant traumatic displacement, perching, and burst fracture need stabilization with instrumentation.[4] However, an uncertain neurosurgical indication is pro-

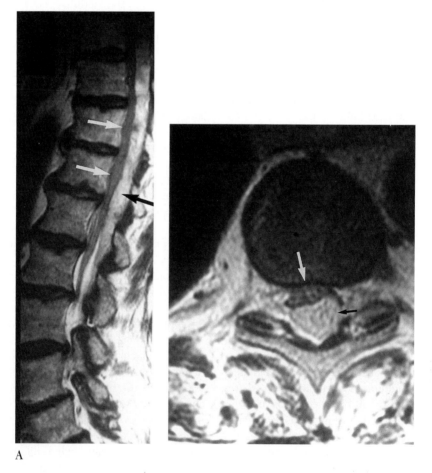

A

Figure 22–3. Magnetic resonance imaging examples of acute spinal cord injury (*arrows* denote lesions). (A) Epidural hematoma (*black arrows*); *white arrows* show compressed cord.

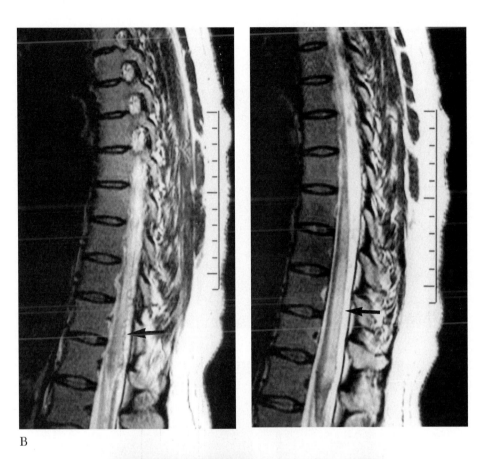

B

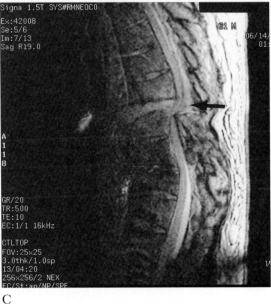

C

Figure 22–3. (*Continued*) (*B*) Dural arteriovenous fistula with a typical dilated vein and T2 hyperintensity in patient with progressive paraplegia. (*C*) Central cord lesion due to trauma.

361

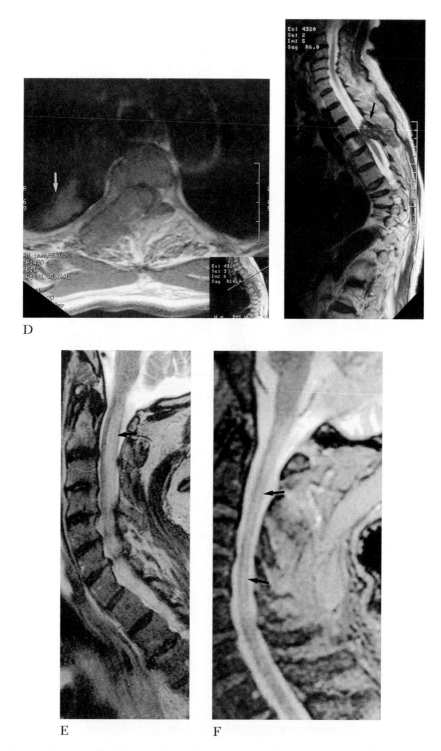

D

E   F

Figure 22–3. (*Continued*) (*D*) Spinal cord compression due to a paraspinal mass. Also shown (*left image*) is lung cancer (*arrow*). (*E*) Acute necrotic myelopathy with swollen cord. (*F*) De-myelinating lesion in cervical cord associated with respiratory failure.

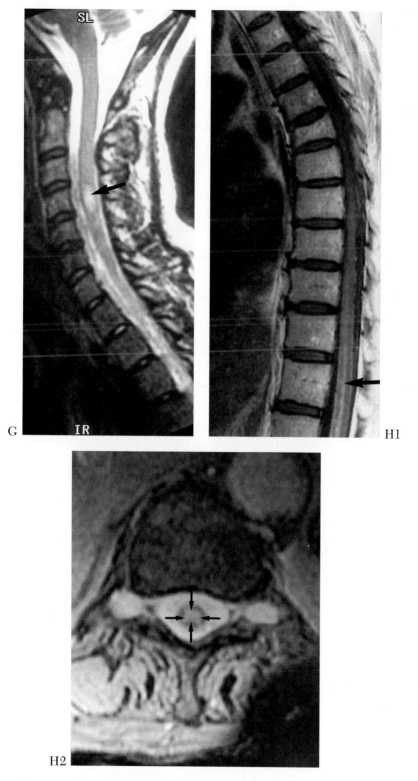

Figure 22–3. (*Continued*)(*G*) Transverse myelitis. (*H1* and *H2*) Spinal cord infarction (*arrows*). (*A* from Henderson et al.[16] By permission of the American Medical Association. *F* from Pittock et al.[28] By permission of the International Anesthesia Research Society.)

Table 22–3. Common Diagnostic Considerations in Acute Spinal Cord Disease

Disorder	Diagnostic Test
Myelopathy	
Compressive myelopathy	MRI of spine
Acute necrotic myelopathy	MRI of spine, biopsy
Vacuolar myelopathy	CSF (PMN), HIV-1
Anterior spinal artery occlusion	MRI of spine, RF, SLE, ANA
Foix-Alajouanine syndrome	MRI of spine, spinal angiogram
Radiation myelopathy	Radiation field, irradiation dose
Paraneoplastic myelopathy	CT scan of chest-abdomen, bone marrow, thyroid scan
Myelitis	
Acute disseminated encephalomyelitis	CSF (MN), MRI of brain
Postinfectious myelitis	Echovirus, coxsackievirus
Demyelinating myelitis	CSF (protein, IgG, oligoclonal bands)
Neuromyelitis optica	VEP, MRI of spine, CSF (protein)
Viral myelitis	Herpes zoster, CSF (PCR)
Bacterial myelitis	VDRL, FTA-ABS, CSF (cells, protein)
Human T-cell lymphotropic virus type I (HTLV-I) myelitis	HTLV-I
Tropical myelitis	Circulating antigen, stools, ELISA (schistosomiasis, trichinosis)

ANA, antinuclear antibody; CSF, cerebrospinal fluid; CT, computed tomography; ELISA, enzyme-linked immunosorbent assay; FTA-ABS, fluorescent treponemal antibody absorption test; HIV, human immunodeficiency virus; MN, mononuclear leukocytes; MRI, magnetic resonance imaging; PCR, polymerase chain reaction; PMN, polymorphonuclear leukocytes; RF, rheumatoid factor; SLE, systemic lupus erythematosus; VEP, visual evoked potential.
Source: Berman M, Feldman S, Alter M, et al: Acute transverse myelitis: incidence and etiologic considerations. *Neurology* 31:966–971, 1981, and Campi A, Filippi M, Comi G, et al: Acute transverse myelopathy: spinal and cranial MR study with clinical follow-up. *AJNR Am J Neuroradiol* 16:115–123, 1995.

gression of paraplegia after or during radiotherapy.

The initial measures for patients with acute spinal cord injury are fairly standard for each of the disorders (Table 22–4). After admission to the NICU, the patient should be placed in a special rotating or air-fluidized bed to decrease decubitus ulcers. These turning beds and specialty care beds may also reduce the complication of pulmonary embolization, although no hard data are available. Every patient should receive heparin subcutaneously

Table 22–4. Initial Management in Acute Spinal Cord Disorder

Airway management	Incentive spirometry
	AC or IMV mode in high cervical lesions (C3–C5)
Hemodynamic management	2 L of 0.9% NaCl
	Consider crystalloid infusions with shock
	Consider temporary pacemaker
	Consider atropine, 0.5 mg, or isoproterenol infusion, 2–10 μg per minute
	Avoid vasopressors
	Abdominal binders with upright position
Specific management	Surgical stabilization and instrumentation in spinal cord compression from cancer
	Immediate evacuation in epidural spinal hematoma
	In spinal cord compression and acute myelitis: dexamethasone, 100 mg IV, followed by 24 mg/day q.i.d.
	In traumatic spine injury: methylprednisolone ≤3 hr (30 mg/kg bolus, followed by infusion of 5.4 mg/kg for 23 hours); 3–8 hr (30 mg/kg bolus, followed by infusion of 5.4 mg/kg for 48 hours)
	Aggressive postural drainage, rotating beds
Prophylactic management	Heparin, 5000 U subcutaneously b.i.d.
	Pantoprazole 40 mg IV

AC, asissted control; IMV, intermittent mandatory ventilation.

(5000 U twice a day) or intermittent pneumonic devices. Subcutaneous heparin is not contraindicated in patients after surgery for an acute epidural hematoma, and the claim that heparin increases the risk of recurrence after the operation is somewhat baseless. Aggressive pulmonary techniques and prevention are important to reduce the development of pulmonary complications, which substantially increase length of hospital stay and costs.[38] In many patients, pulmonary complications are due to mechanical ventilation; therefore, endotracheal intubation and mechanical ventilation should be considered only with clear evidence of diaphragmatic dysfunction. Abdominal binders and leg wraps are needed when patients are placed in an upright position (Fig. 22–4). Bradycardia associated with hypotension can

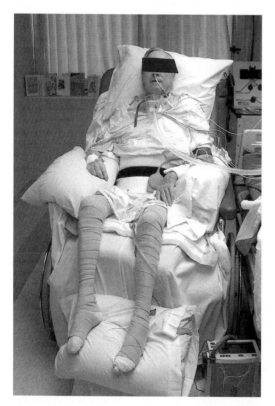

Figure 22–4. Patient with cervical lesion is in sitting position. Note abdominal binders and leg wraps.

be treated with 0.5 mg of atropine intravenously, a low-dose infusion of isoproterenol, titrating to response (2–10 μg per minute), or a temporary pacemaker.[21] Neurogenic bladder is prone to become associated with asymptomatic bacteriuria. Antimicrobial therapy reduces its frequency but not symptomatic infections and therefore is not recommended for prophylaxis.[25]

Corticosteroids are indicated if an acute spinal cord lesion is due to a tumor, trauma, or demyelination. In patients with acute cord compression, 100 mg of dexamethasone intravenously is given immediately and is followed by 4 to 25 mg four times a day. A tapering of the high doses of corticosteroid is started after 3 days. We routinely administer proton pump inhibitors (pantoprazole, 40 mg IV) to patients receiving corticosteroids. Corticosteroids or plasma exchange has also been useful in patients with acute spinal cord injury due to exacerbation of multiple sclerosis. We reversed ventilatory dependence in one patient after use of high-dose corticosteroid treatment.[28]

In patients with traumatic spinal cord injury seen within 3 hours of injury, an intravenous bolus of methylprednisolone, 30 mg/kg, is followed by infusion of 5.4 mg/kg per hour for 23 hours.[3,6] For patients seen between 3 and 8 hours, similar doses are given by intravenous bolus and infusion, but treatment is maintained for 48 hours. (Patients with cauda equina syndromes have been excluded from study protocols.) The design and results of the National Acute Spinal Cord Injury Study 2 and 3 trials have been criticized, and claims of success are not generally accepted.[5,27] One study found that gastrointestinal and pulmonary complications were higher with methylprednisolone (17% and 35%, respectively) compared with placebo (0% and 4%).[22]

DETERIORATION: CAUSES AND MANAGEMENT

Deterioration in the intensive care unit because of earlier surgical intervention is not very common. A fixed deficit or improvement in function is more commonly observed. In some specific disorders, further deterioration is possible despite early stabilization that prompted a conservative wait-and-see approach. Progressive deterioration in acute myelopathy is typically due to acute necrotic myelopathy or acute enlarging epidural hematoma in patients initially treated conservatively. In epidural hematoma, outcome is clearly linked to prompt intervention, and any delay reduces chances of later ambulation, adequate pain control, and bladder and bowel control. Postoperative deterioration due to recurrence is rarely observed, and usually an epidurally placed drain prevents further accumulation of a sizable hematoma.

Necrotic myelopathy may be rapidly ascending without response to corticosteroids. Immunomodulating therapy, such as plasma exchange or intravenous immune gamma globulin, may not be helpful but is used in these patients without much optimism. In some of these patients, it may be difficult to clearly distinguish between multiple sclerosis and necrotic myelopathy (considered a separate entity), and these aggressive modes of therapy are considered.

Spinal epidural abscess may worsen insidiously despite aggressive antibiotic therapy and surgical drainage, all of which hinder recovery. Delay in early recognition—understandable because of the mimicking of infectious disease—possibly is partly to blame. Rapid progression of signs in patients with spinal metastasis may be due to vertebral collapse, and some patients continue to worsen after radiotherapy, but indications for surgical decompression remain uncertain.

OUTCOME

Acute complete loss of spinal cord function rarely results in significant improvement.[8,24] Impaired respiratory function in high cervical lesions is permanent, and long-term mechanical ventilation is needed. Ventilatory support may be needed in many patients with cervical or high-thoracic lesions, but improvement and weaning from the ventilator can be expected in lesions lower than C4 (estimated 50% to 80% of patients). Pulmonary function test results improve gradually and may increase to 60% of predicted values at 5 months.[20] Stiffening of the chest wall associated with spasticity of the abdominal and intercostal muscles reduces collapse with breathing, but also the diaphragm may condition itself to larger workloads of breathing.

Mortality in spinal cord infarction remains high (22%).[31] Some spinal cord disorders, such as epidural hematoma and acute vertebral collapse due to cancer, have surprisingly good outcomes if surgical intervention is prompt. Relapse is uncommon after one bout of transverse myelitis, but one study found that 80% of patients with acute partial transverse myelitis had acquired definite multiple sclerosis within a 3-year follow-up period.[14]

Outcome in acute spinal cord injury[23] is difficult to judge, but sparing of pinprick sensation in the sacral area could predict improvement. It has been claimed that more than 50% of patients with sacral sensory sparing may have conversion from American Spinal Injury Association grade B to grade C–D.[23] An outcome algorithm is shown in Figure 22–5.

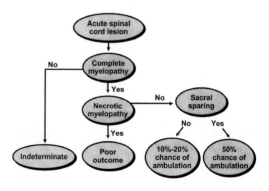

Figure 22–5. Algorithm of outcome in acute spinal cord disorder. Poor outcome: severe disability or death; vegetative state. Indeterminate: any statement would be a premature conclusion.

CONCLUSIONS

- MRI complements clinical localization and should be performed urgently.
- Respiratory compromise and severe bradycardia should be expected in patients with complete cervical lesions.
- Methylprednisolone may be effective in traumatic spinal cord injury if administration begins within 3 hours. An intravenous bolus of 30 mg/kg is followed by infusion of 5.4 mg/kg per hour for 23 hours.
- Plasma exchange should be considered in acute demyelinating disorders not responding to corticosteroids.
- Prompt neurosurgical intervention is generally indicated for acute epidural hematoma, spinal instability from trauma or cancer destruction, and removal of a foreign object.

REFERENCES

1. Ball PA: Critical care of spinal cord injury. *Spine* 26:S27–S30, 2001.
2. Berman M, Feldman S, Alter M, et al: Acute transverse myelitis: incidence and etiologic considerations. *Neurology* 31:966–971, 1981.
3. Blight AR, Zimber MP: Acute spinal cord injury: pharmacotherapy and drug development perspectives. *Curr Opin Investig Drugs* 2:801–808, 2001.
4. Botel U, Glaser E, Niedeggen A: The surgical treatment of acute spinal paralysed patients. *Spinal Cord* 35:420–428, 1997.
5. Bracken MB: Methylprednisolone and spinal cord injury. *J Neurosurg* 93:175–179, 2000.
6. Bracken MB, Shepard MJ, Holford TR, et al: Administration of methylprednisolone for 24 or 48 hours or tirilazad mesylate for 48 hours in the treatment of acute spinal cord injury. Results of the Third National Acute Spinal Cord Injury Randomized Controlled Trial. National Acute Spinal Cord Injury Study. *JAMA* 277:1597–1604, 1997.
7. Byrne TN, Benzel EC, Waxman SG: *Diseases of the Spine and Spinal Cord.* Oxford: Oxford University Press, 2000.
8. Cheshire WP, Santos CC, Massey EW, et al: Spinal cord infarction: etiology and outcome. *Neurology* 47:321–330, 1996.
9. Christensen PB, Wermuth L, Hinge HH, et al: Clinical course and long-term prognosis of acute transverse myelopathy. *Acta Neurol Scand* 81:431–435, 1990.
10. Curt A, Dietz V: Ambulatory capacity in spinal cord injury: significance of somatosensory evoked potentials and ASIA protocol in predicting outcome. *Arch Phys Med Rehabil* 78:39–43, 1997.
11. de Seze J, Stojkovic T, Breteau G, et al: Acute myelopathies: clinical, laboratory and outcome profiles in 79 cases. *Brain* 124:1509–1521, 2001.
12. Duffill J, Sparrow OC, Millar J, et al: Can spontaneous spinal epidural haematoma be managed safely without operation? A report of four cases. *J Neurol Neurosurg Psychiatry* 69:816–819, 2000.
13. Foo D: Operative treatment of spontaneous spinal epidural hematomas: a study of the factors determining postoperative outcome. *Neurosurgery* 41:1218–1220, 1997.
14. Ford B, Tampieri D, Francis G: Long-term follow-up of acute partial transverse myelopathy. *Neurology* 42:250–252, 1992.
15. Fukui MB, Swarnkar AS, Williams RL: Acute spontaneous spinal epidural hematomas. *AJNR Am J Neuroradiol* 20:1365–1372, 1999.
16. Henderson RD, Pittock SJ, Piepgras DG, et al: Acute spontaneous spinal epidural hematoma. *Arch Neurol* 58:1145–1146, 2001.
17. Inatomi Y, Itoh Y, Fujii N, et al: The spinal cord descending pathway for micturition: analysis in patients with spinal cord infarction. *J Neurol Sci* 157:154–157, 1998.
18. Iseli E, Cavigelli A, Dietz V, et al: Prognosis and recovery in ischaemic and traumatic spinal cord injury: clinical and electrophysiological evaluation. *J Neurol Neurosurg Psychiatry* 67:567–571, 1999.
19. Katz JD, Ropper AH: Progressive necrotic myelopathy: clinical course in 9 patients. *Arch Neurol* 57:355–361, 2000.
20. Ledsome JR, Sharp JM: Pulmonary function in acute cervical cord injury. *Am Rev Respir Dis* 124:41–44, 1981.
21. Lehmann KG, Lane JG, Piepmeier JM, et al: Cardiovascular abnormalities accompanying acute spinal cord injury in humans: incidence, time course and severity. *J Am Coll Cardiol* 10:46–52, 1987.
22. Matsumoto T, Tamaki T, Kawakami M, et al: Early complications of high-dose methylprednisolone sodium succinate treatment in the follow-up of acute cervical spinal cord injury. *Spine* 26:426–430, 2001.
23. McDonald JW, Sadowsky C: Spinal-cord injury. *Lancet* 359:417–425, 2002.
24. McKinley WO, Seel RT, Gadi RK, et al: Nontraumatic vs. traumatic spinal cord injury: a rehabilitation outcome comparison. *Am J Phys Med Rehabil* 80:693–699, 2001.
25. Morton SC, Shekelle PG, Adams JL, et al: Antimicrobial prophylaxis for urinary tract infection in persons

with spinal cord dysfunction. *Arch Phys Med Rehabil* 83:129–138, 2002.

26. Murray JF, Nadel JA (eds): *Textbook of Respiratory Medicine*. 3rd ed. Philadelphia: WB Saunders, 2000.

27. Nesathurai S: Multiple sclerosis presenting as transverse myelopathy: clinical and MRI features. *Neurology* 48:65–73, 1998.

28. Pittock SJ, Rodriguez M, Wijdicks EFM: Rapid weaning from mechanical ventilator in acute cervical cord multiple sclerosis lesion after steroids. *Anesth Analg* 93:1550–1551, 2001.

29. Ropper AH, Poskanzer DC: The prognosis of acute and subacute transverse myelopathy based on early signs and symptoms. *Ann Neurol* 4:51–59, 1978.

30. Roth EJ, Lu A, Primack S, et al: Ventilatory function in cervical and high thoracic spinal cord injury: relationship to level of injury and tone. *Am J Phys Med Rehabil* 76:262–267, 1997.

31. Salvador de la Barrera S, Barca-Buyo A, Montoto-Marques A, et al: Spinal cord infarction: prognosis and recovery in a series of 36 patients. *Spinal Cord* 39:520–525, 2001.

32. Simnad VI, Pisani DE, Rose JW: Multiple sclerosis presenting as transverse myelopathy: clinical and MRI features. *Neurology* 48:65–73, 1997.

33. Srivastava S, Sanghavi NG: Nontraumatic paraparesis: aetiological, clinical and radiological profile. *J Assoc Physicians India* 48:988–990, 2000.

34. Taoka T, Mayr NA, Lee HJ, et al: Factors influencing visualization of vertebral metastases on MR imaging versus bone scintigraphy. *AJR Am J Roentgenol* 176:1525–1530, 2001.

35. Wijdicks EFM: *Neurologic Complications of Critical Illness*. 2nd ed. Oxford: Oxford University Press, 2002, pp 302–336.

36. Wiley CA, VanPatten PD, Carpenter PM, et al: Acute ascending necrotizing myelopathy caused by herpes simplex virus type 2. *Neurology* 37:1791–1794, 1987.

37. Wingerchuk DM, Hogancamp WF, O'Brien PC, et al: The clinical course of neuromyelitis optica (Devic's syndrome). *Neurology* 53:1107–1114, 1999.

38. Winslow C, Bode RK, Felton D, et al: Impact of respiratory complications on length of stay and hospital costs in acute cervical spine injury. *Chest* 121:1548–1554, 2002.

23

Traumatic Brain Injury

Assault or accidental trauma to the brain merits stabilization in the emergency department and, as a matter of course, admission to a NICU or trauma unit for expeditious management. Traumatic brain injury is a major cause of disability in young persons and leads to the expenditure of billions of dollars. Epidemiologic surveys have estimated that the number of new disabled survivors of traumatic brain injury in the United States each year is nearly 80,000,[27] labeled a "silent epidemic." One of the most tragic, and often entirely avoidable, events is admission to the NICU of an inebriated teenager extracted from a rolled-over motor vehicle, resulting in an empty and unfulfilled life.

The management of patients with traumatic brain injury requires a multidisciplinary approach. There are also some indications that outcome in severe head injury is better if patients are managed in recognized trauma centers with extensive experience in managing deterioration.[27] In large hospitals, trauma to the central nervous system is primarily managed by neurosurgical services. Patients with multiple trauma are often cared for in surgical trauma units with a neurologic or neurosurgical consultative service. However, most pioneering clinical and basic research has originated from investigations in neurosurgical departments.

A large proportion of patients with traumatic brain injury are not considered candidates for neurosurgical intervention to remove contusional brain or extra-axial hematomas. Management is largely directed to reducing increased ICP and maintaining cerebral perfusion pressure, closely observing patients at high risk of deterioration, and preventing systemic complications associated with coma. This chapter discusses the management of severe head injury and the neurosurgical options in a patient whose condition is deteriorating. Every adept neurologist or neurosurgeon involved in management of head injury, whether seeing patients in the emergency department or in the NICU, recognizes that outcome after head injury could depend greatly on whether or not the injury is accompanied by hypoxemia, hypercapnia, and hypovolemia.[28,47] In reality, outcome may already have been determined by failure to correct these factors early. Moreover, these factors may obscure the neurologic examination.[2]

Admission to the NICU is warranted in patients who have impaired consciousness or are at risk for further deterioration. The threshold for observation in the intensive care unit should be very low in older patients and in patients with skull fracture, trauma by fall, blunt head trauma from fists, or a temporal or frontal lobe intracranial hematoma on CT scan even though the Glasgow coma scale score is normal.[1,83]

CLINICAL RECOGNITION

The vast majority of patients with severe traumatic brain injury have clinical symptoms of diffuse axonal brain injury. Depending on the impact and the damage to brain parenchyma, patients may be alert and able to follow commands, combative, agitated, or comatose with abnormal motor responses. The Glasgow coma scale score is the most important measure of the severity of the head injury and is related to prognosis. Grading of this scale, however, can be greatly confounded if recent alcohol or illicit drug use led to head trauma. Other patients may have received intravenous benzodiazepines to control agitation and these substances continue to be disseminated in large quantities. The responses measured by the Glasgow coma scale may significantly improve after successful fluid replacement in patients in shock. Thus, the Glasgow coma score after any type of resuscitation may have changed greatly from that at first evaluation. In an analysis of 746 patients from the Traumatic Coma Data Bank, approximately 40% had a Glasgow coma sum score of 3 at presentation, whereas 20% had this score after resuscitation.[63]

Of all available brain stem reflexes, pupillary size and light reflex have been tested most often, and they are still considered the most important indicators of brain damage. The diagnostic value of all other brain stem reflexes or certain combinations has not been tested. Although intuitively obvious, it is not known whether absence of pontomesencephalic reflexes portends poor outcome as it does in expanding lobar hematomas (Chapter 13). In the Traumatic Coma Data Bank analysis, 74% of patients with initial bilateral fixed pupils from all causes became vegetative.[63] In addition, 50% of patients with developing abnormal pupils after admission died or became vegetative. However, good outcome is particularly possible in patients with an extradural hematoma and fixed pupils.[69] Bilateral miotic pupils may be seen in the early stages of central diencephalic herniation (e.g., in patients with bilateral subdural hematomas), but in many patients the use of opioids can be implicated. In the absence of direct trauma to the globe, dilatation of one pupil and absent or sluggish light response usually suggest an intracranial contusional mass that produces compartmental shifts. Often, the ipsilateral pupil di-

lates and becomes fixed, and this reaction soon follows in the opposite pupil. The presenting signs of epidural and subdural hematomas are similar, with a decline in consciousness, focal signs, and unilateral pupil enlargement. The course in epidural hematoma is very rapid because of the arterial source.

Trauma to the cervical spine should be clinically very unlikely before eye movements are investigated with use of oculocephalic responses, and determination of oculovestibular responses by cold caloric testing is safer in comatose patients. Abnormal responses with failure to adduct or abduct may suggest a third or sixth cranial nerve palsy.

Post-traumatic injury may involve cranial nerves I, II, VI, and VII. Post-traumatic anosmia due to shearing of olfactory fibers at the cribriform plate is permanent, with some return and regeneration, although rarely noticeable, in one-third of the patients.[36] Traumatic optic neuropathy may result in no light perception, and if it is associated with orbital fracture, visual loss is not likely to improve. Visual acuities of at least 20/400 may improve with corticosteroids alone (10 mg of dexamethasone every 6 hours for 2 days). In any patient with less visual acuity, optic decompression needs to be considered.[86]

Sixth nerve palsy may be seen and in extreme cases is bilateral. Inability to abduct past the midline, bilateral involvement at presentation, and female sex predict poor outcome, and incisional strabismus surgery is needed.[33] Traumatic facial palsy is predominantly in the geniculate ganglion area. Surgical decompression is indicated if facial palsy is total and noted immediately after trauma.[16] Many patients recover well within 6 months.

In the initial assessment, it is important to examine the patient for facial fractures. Midface fractures are more frequently associated with traumatic brain injuries than mandibular fractures. Facial fractures increase the chance of severe intracranial injury and are more often present in patients with lower Glasgow coma sum scores.[31] As part of a routine trauma examination, one should specifically note if the patient has Battle's sign (clearly visible bruising at the level of the mastoid, which indicates

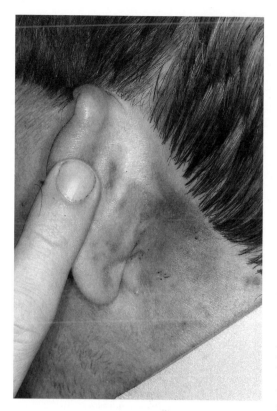

Figure 23–1. Retroauricular hematoma (Battle's sign, after William Henry Battle, English surgeon).

fracture of the basal skull and mastoid) (Fig. 23–1) or "raccoon eyes" (periorbital ecchymosis, indicating facial fractures or a frontobasal skull fracture).

The motor response of the Glasgow coma score is the most important clinical guide in patients with severe head injury, particularly those with facial trauma or the need for endotracheal intubation for airway protection in whom eye opening and verbal response cannot be adequately assessed. Absence of motor response should always prompt further imaging of the spinal column.

Seizures are comparatively uncommon in patients with traumatic brain injury (5% to 10%). The incidence of seizures in patients with mild head injury is probably very low (< 1%). In patients with severe head injury, alcohol-related seizures should be considered, especially if there is a history of heavy drinking. The most significant risk factors associated with developing late post-traumatic seizures are a Glasgow coma score of less than 10, cortical contusion, depressed skull fracture and dural tear, penetrating head wound, and a seizure within 24 hours of injury. The additional presence of an intracranial hematoma may markedly increase the risk of seizures, with incidences up to 35%.[17]

Patients with severe head injury and coma on admission may be affected by a significant and often dramatic sympathetic outburst. Besides agitation, clenching of fists, and grinding of teeth, profuse sweating, sustained tachycardia, and marked hypertension occur. These episodes are typically associated with hyperthermia (to 40°C) and increased respiratory rate, often with inadequate gas exchange, and ICP often increases during these episodes (Fig. 23–2). These sympathetic storms are inappropriately termed "diencephalic seizures"[4,11] (electroencephalographic recordings during these episodes have not shown epileptiform activity).

After an initial neurologic examination, the physical examination should be repeated to recognize possible additional systemic injuries, such as lung and heart contusion, splenic rupture, and any type of bony fracture. Hypotension usually signals hypovolemia from bleeding somewhere and should not be considered a manifestation of severe head injury. Hypotension occurs only in patients who fulfill the clinical criteria for brain death, patients with marked spinal cord injury, and children with large epidural hematomas. Hypotension indicates significant blood loss. The head should be carefully examined for lacerations of the scalp. Blood loss from facial fractures or scalp lacerations can be profound and is never completely appreciated in the initial assessment. Hypotension is commonly associated with fractures of the pelvis or femur, and blood loss (> 1 to 2 L) can be life-threatening. However, even when long bone fractures are found in a patient with hypotension, other sites need to be considered, including the chest, peritoneal cavity, and retroperitoneal space. Chest radio-

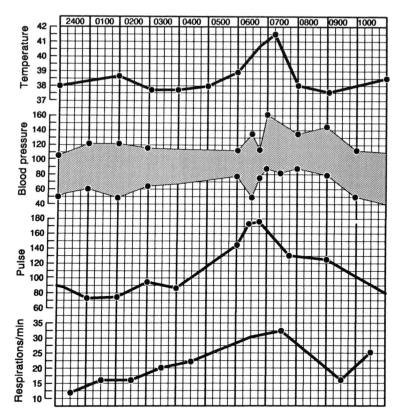

Figure 23–2. Alterations in core body temperature (in °C), blood pressure (in mm Hg), pulse (in beats per minute), and respiratory rate (in respirations per minute) during a sympathetic storm. Note the increase in systolic pressure and decrease in diastolic pressure (with widening of pulse pressure) time-locked with the tachycardia. Hyperthermia occurred later and was not precisely time-locked with the hemodynamic changes. Hyperhidrosis and posturing were maximal during the periods of intense hyperthermia.

graphs, thoracocentesis, and diagnostic peritoneal lavage are fairly reliable tests to demonstrate internal bleeding. (For guidance in evaluation, see Chapter 32.)

In a patient with multitrauma, one must consider fat embolism syndrome from bone marrow of fractured long bones. Generally 12 to 72 hours after the traumatic impact, the patient's condition suddenly deteriorates in parallel with laboratory changes. The common manifestations are acute confusional state, focal neurologic signs, and generalized tonic-clonic seizures. A pathognomonic sign, present in 50% of patients, is a petechial rash appearing suddenly on the chest, axillary folds, and, occasionally, conjunctiva.[10,42] A typical fat em-

bolization syndrome, however, appears in only 3% to 4% of the patients, and clinical signs may resolve within 24 hours.[42]

To summarize, assessing the severity of traumatic brain injury is important for several reasons. First, systemic manifestations of a hypermetabolic response and trauma to other organs are more common and require careful management. Second, neurologic or medical worsening is expected. Third, outcome can be projected, and this may strongly influence the degree of aggressive management, including neurosurgical intervention. The most important clinical components in the determination of outcome are motor response, pupillary responses to light, and oculocephalic responses, but therapy-refractory increased intracranial pressure, shock or prolonged cardiovascular resuscitation, and spinal cord injury are nearly as important.

NEUROIMAGING AND LABORATORY TESTS

Computed tomography scan of the brain has become the rule in any head injury. The current use for alert and stable patients with trauma is not very selective, but it is very difficult to identify a set of criteria that may result in a firm recommendation of CT scan deferral. Moreover, normal findings on CT do not preclude delayed traumatic hemorrhage. Five high-risk factors have been identified (100% sensitive for neurosurgical intervention). They are failure to reach the maximal Glasgow coma score within 2 hours, suspected open skull fracture, signs of basal skull fracture, vomiting more than twice, and age over 65 years.[81] In contrast, in a large series of consecutive patients with maximal Glasgow coma scores, only 9% had CT scan abnormalities, and only two of these patients required neurosurgical intervention.[43] Although these recommendations are pragmatic, it is doubtful that most emergency departments and trauma units in the United States will adopt this policy. Because of possible medicolegal consequences, many patients, if not all, irrespective of any type of head injury, are likely to have a CT scan in the emergency department.

The types of abnormalities that can be seen on CT scans in traumatic brain injury are summarized in Table 23–1.[41,46] Many patients have small hemorrhages in both hemispheres, with only minimal shift of the midline structures. Figure 23–3A illustrates diffuse axonal injury with multiple parenchymal contusions. Tissue tear hemorrhages (Fig. 23–3B) can also be seen in traumatic brain injury, usually in the frontal cortex, white and gray matter interface, basal ganglia, thalamus, internal capsule,[92] and brain stem (Fig. 23–4). In 50% of these patients, there is additional traumatic subarachnoid or intraventricular blood. When tissue tear hem-

Table 23–1. Types of Computed Tomography Scan Abnormalities in Traumatic Brain Injury

Intraparenchymal
    Diffuse axonal injury
    Hemorrhagic contusion
    Tissue tear (shear) hemorrhage
    Brain stem hemorrhage
Extra-axial compartment
    Subarachnoid hemorrhage (sulci, vertex)
    Intraventricular
    Subdural hematoma
    Epidural hematoma
Secondary lesions
    Diffuse brain swelling
    Watershed, thalamus infarcts, multiple localizations
      (anoxic-ischemic)
    Posterior cerebral artery territory infarct
      (transtentorial herniation)
    Middle cerebral artery territory infarct (traumatic
      carotid lesion)

orrhages are found in both the corpus callosum and the interpeduncular midbrain, the outcome is poor, but the predictive value of these shear lesions in other locations is much less clear.

It is important to note the visibility of the basal cistern, an indicator of cerebral swelling, on CT scans. If a CT scan shows compressed or absent cisterns without a large intracranial mass lesion or if absence of cisterns is accompanied by marked midline shift, the outcome is poor. In the Traumatic Coma Data Bank study, however, these ominous CT scans were seen in only 32 of 746 patients.[46]

A traumatic intracerebral hematoma may not appear on the first CT scan.[20] Identification of an intracerebral hematoma on CT scan may be delayed for 8 hours, even 13 days after the impact, although in most patients, the hematoma can be identified within 2 days of admission.[29] Specifically, frontal hemorrhagic contusions should alert the physician to the potential for further deterioration from edema and brain stem compression.[80] CT scanning should also be repeated if the initial scan was performed within hours of the impact or if the patient has documented coagulopathy.[54] Less common localizations of intracranial hematomas are hemorrhages in the posterior fossa, basal ganglia, or intraventricular compartment. However, in these pa-

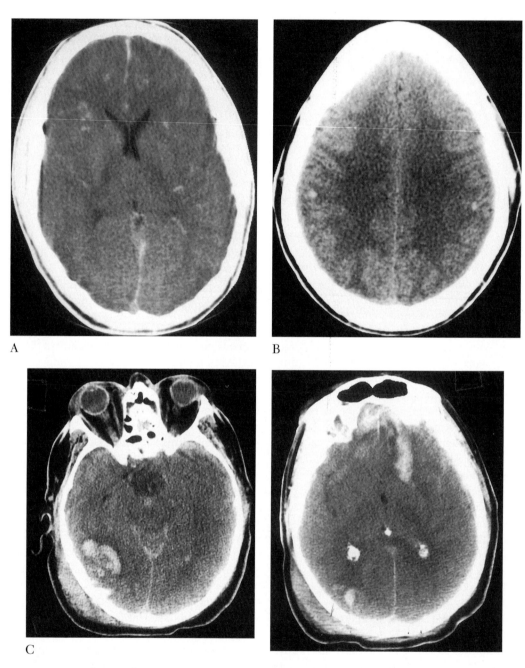

Figure 23–3. Abnormalities in traumatic brain injury. (*A*) Multiple small parenchymal hemorrhages with significant cerebral edema. (*B*) Multiple typical shear ("tissue tear") lesions. (*C*) Diffuse axonal injury with multiple lobar (contrecoup) hemorrhagic contusions.

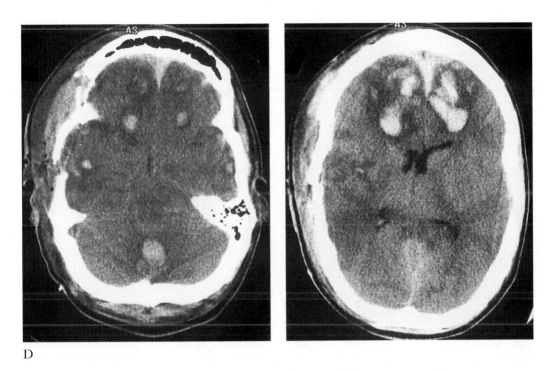

D

Figure 23–3. (*Continued*) (*D*) Multiple hemorrhagic lesions with frontal contusion.

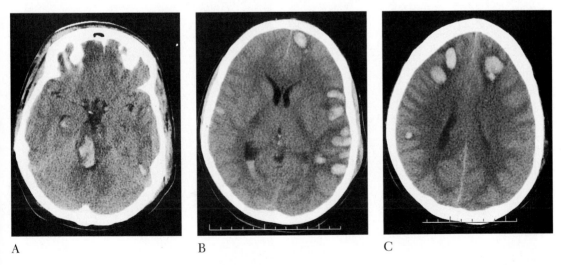

A   B   C

Figure 23–4. (*A–C*) Multiple large contusional lesions with primary brain stem hemorrhage.

tients, hemorrhagic contusions are found in other locations, all indicating a very significant traumatic impact.[5]

Computed tomography scans may show traumatic subarachnoid hemorrhage, usually located at the superficial cortical sulci. In patients with blood specifically localized in the sylvian fissure, trauma cannot be distinguished from aneurysmal rupture, and cerebral angiography is warranted (see Chapter 12).

Epidural hematomas appearing on CT scans are a neurosurgical emergency (Fig. 23–5A).[76] If the hematomas are small, they probably are associated with tear of a dural vessel rather

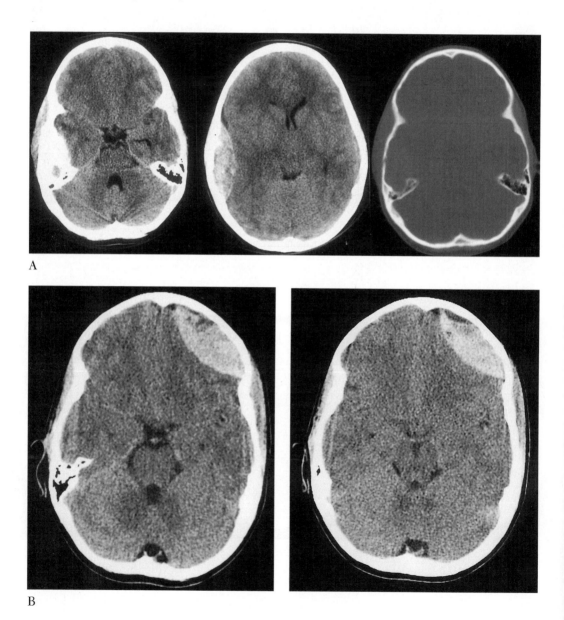

Figure 23–5. Epidural hematomas. (*A*) Typical convex configuration. (Note associated skull fracture on bone window setting.) (*B*) Hyperlucent area.

than with rupture of a meningeal artery from a skull fracture. One study suggested that a radiolucent region (Fig. 23–5B) within a denser clot may be a sign of active bleeding and may prompt early evacuation.[38] Epidural hematomas in the posterior fossa are generally neurosurgical emergencies, and postponement of evacuation in clinically alert patients may be inappropriate (Fig. 23–6).

A subdural hematoma and its mass effect can usually be easily recognized on CT scans. However, when isodense and in patients with marked anemia, the size may be difficult to estimate (Fig. 23–7). Bilateral subdural hematomas are common, but when they are isodense, the classic appearance of "hypernormal CT scan" may be apparent (Fig. 23–7). (This descriptive term is derived from the fact that sulci are not visible and, together with the slit-like ventricular system, suggests a much younger patient.)

Any patient with significant head trauma (Glasgow coma scale score of less than 8) needs radiographs of the cervical spine.[34] Patients with cervical fractures may have double fractures in the cervical region or an additional lumbar body fracture and may need a full radiographic series of the spine. Cervical spine films should be carefully scrutinized for soft tissue abnormalities, abnormalities in alignment, abnormalities in disk space and height, and fractures. Questionable plain film radiologic findings should prompt additional imaging with CT scan. However, important cervical spine fractures may be overlooked with 4- to 10-mm slices, because occasionally a segment is not displayed on CT scan. An overview with graphic display of the most common spine fractures is found in a recent monograph.[89]

Magnetic resonance imaging has a much higher sensitivity than conventional CT but in the hectic emergency department setting should be deferred to a later stage. The clinical usefulness of MRI in acute brain injury remains unclear. Its contribution is mostly in the demonstration of diffuse injury and secondary abnormalities from anoxia or brain swelling.[26,79,90] The first prospective studies of

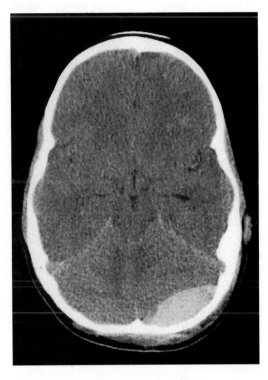

Figure 23–6. Posterior fossa epidural hematoma.

MRI documented a higher frequency of abnormalities than that with CT, and corpus callosum and brain stem lesions particularly seemed to predict poor outcome. Cognitive tasks were much worse in patients with MRI-documented lesions in the corpus callosum.[60] Follow-up MRI has also documented compression of the cerebral peduncle as a sign of prior major trauma and shift.[39] Magnetic resonance imaging could also be useful in confirming fat emboli to the brain. A case report suggested that a specific pattern of white spots on a dark background appears on diffusion-weighted imaging ("starfield" pattern).[58]

Laboratory tests in patients with severe head injury should include electrolytes, glucose, activated partial thromboplastin time, liver function tests, and urinalysis for hematuria. A blood sample must be sent to the blood bank for typing. An electrocardiogram should be obtained in all patients; in a young patient, it may detect additional cardiac contusion, although myocar-

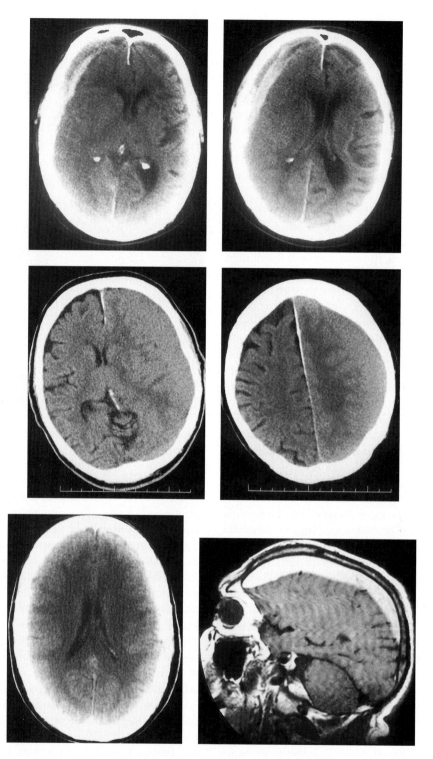

Figure 23–7. Subdural hematomas. (*Top row*) Acute traumatic subdural hematoma. (*Middle row*) Unilateral isodense subdural hematoma. Note loss of sulcal definition and shift of septum pellucidum and pineal gland. (*Bottom row*) Computed tomography scan (*left*) in an 85-year-old man with bilateral isodense subdural hematoma. Demonstration by magnetic resonance imaging (*right*).

dial damage may be associated with increased circulating catecholamines. Severe head injury progressing to brain death may be associated with cardiac stunning and significant wall motion abnormalities that can be diagnosed on echocardiograms; this condition currently precludes cardiac transplantation if the patient becomes an eligible donor (see Chapter 34). Chest radiography should be repeated regularly for signs of possible aspiration or secondary bacterial infection after aspiration. There is a considerable risk of nosocomial pneumonia, usually within days of the impact, and significant lung contusions, and they may become more evident days after the impact.

FIRST STEPS IN MANAGEMENT

The management of traumatic brain injury has been reviewed by the Brain Trauma Foundation. This review should be readily available in the NICU.[61]

Many patients are stabilized in the emergency department, and often the decision is made there whether to transfer the patient to an NICU, a trauma unit, or an operating room. Transfer of a patient with severe head injury is fraught with potential danger. A study that audited transfer of conscious patients with head injury to a neurosurgical unit found that hypoxemia, hypotension, and failure to diagnose major extracranial injuries before transfer were prevalent.[25] In 25% of comatose patients, no endotracheal tube was inserted, and many patients were transported supine. This landmark study in Glasgow pertained to patients admitted to the neurosurgical intensive care unit from outside hospitals, but intrahospital transfer may pose the same threats.

The airway should be assessed immediately after the patient enters the NICU. The patient should be intubated if there is evidence of inadequate gas exchange on pulse oximetry or arterial blood gas determinations. Massive aspiration may already have occurred in patients with severe head injury, and adult respiratory distress syndrome may have developed. Neuromuscular blockade and sedation should be reserved only for this situation, because they make any type of monitoring impossible. Moreover, patients with severe head injury who are given neuromuscular blockade prophylactically have a higher incidence of pneumonia, more frequent sepsis, and longer intensive care stay. Neuromuscular blockade has no place in the treatment of increased ICP and in general should be used sparingly. When neuromuscular blockade is used, ICP monitoring with an intraparenchymal fiberoptic device becomes essential to observe the patient's clinical status.

Securing adequate oxygenation throughout the clinical course is important. Episodes of hypoxemia, with PaO_2 less than 60 mm Hg, are frequently seen and must be immediately corrected. Mechanical ventilation in most patients is in the intermittent mandatory mode with pressure support. Breaths per minute vary from 8 to 10, and pressure support is usually set at 10 cm H_2O.

The ideal management of fluids in patients with severe traumatic brain injury is not exactly known. Currently, most investigators believe that adequate volume status with a maintenance dose of at least 3 L of isotonic saline a day is warranted. There is no reason to believe that fluid restriction in traumatic brain injury is beneficial. In addition, many patients receive mannitol for control of ICP, and this in combination with marginal fluid intake may lead to rapid hypovolemia if urinary losses are not replaced by maintenance fluids.[22] Moreover, a recent analysis of fluid balance associated with poor outcome found a strong and independent correlation with a negative cumulative fluid balance of more than 500 mL over 4 days.[14]

Blood pressure should be titrated, if possible, to acceptable cerebral perfusion pressure (> 70 mm Hg) and ICP (< 20 mm Hg). Experimental data have also shown that the compensatory cardiovascular response to hypotension is, for some reason, significantly muted in patients with high ICP. Blood loss may more easily cause a shock syndrome in patients with increased ICP. The true mechanism is unclear.[37] A general guideline is avoidance of both hypotension, defined as systolic blood pressure of less than 100 mm Hg, and persistent hypertension, defined as mean arterial pressure greater than 130 mm Hg, particularly because the upper breakpoint of the autoregulation curve is situated at that level and edema may occur.[15] Persistent hypertension may be particularly deleterious in patients with diffuse brain swelling on CT scans. Most patients with severe head injury are young, and brief episodes of hypertension are well tolerated, but surges of hypertension may trigger plateau waves. However, treatment of hypertension may have the detrimental effect of decreasing cerebral perfusion pressure, particularly in areas with lost autoregulation. Blood pressure management should be titrated to a cerebral perfusion pressure of 70 mm Hg or higher. Patients with persistent hypertension are best treated with esmolol or labetalol because the duration of action is brief. Patients in a sympathetic overdrive with hypertension should receive morphine (10 mg) and bromocriptine (10 mg three times a day) to mute these responses. Thorazine (10 mg orally every 6 hours) could also reduce fever and autonomic manifestations.

A randomized trial in 82 patients with a Glasgow coma scale score of 3 to 7 showed that initial 24-hour management with hypothermia (32°C to 33°C) and vecuronium and fentanyl to prevent shivering improved outcome.[44] The benefit could be demonstrated only in patients with coma scores of 5 to 7, with an approximately 50% reduction in death and poor outcome. Moreover, hypothermia reduced ventricular glutamate, an effect suggesting an additional benefit through reduction of central ischemia.[44] (Glutamate, an excitatory neurotransmitter released by ischemic neurons, results in calcium and sodium influx, leading to cell death.)

A recent trial found that hypothermia (cooling to a core temperature of 33°C within 8 hours after injury and for 2 days) did not result in improvement of outcome. However, active rewarming of moderately hypothermic patients should be discouraged[13,50] (see also Chapter 9).

Insertion of an ICP monitor should be strongly considered.[51,55,56] Intracranial pressure monitoring has not been subjected to a prospective study to evaluate its effect on outcome but may help detect delayed hematomas, limit indiscriminate use of measures to lower ICP, and indicate lack of response and thus poor outcome. Use of the monitoring device may be limited to patients with a Glasgow coma sum score of less than 8 after correction of confounding factors and patients with a CT scan showing an intracranial hematoma[56] (especially in the temporal or frontal lobe) or brain edema. Patients in need of neuromuscular blockade for adequate ventilation (e.g., because of severe lung contusion or flail chest) almost certainly need ICP monitoring, because clinical neurologic signs, except for sudden pupillary changes, are lost.

The goals of management of increased ICP have not been well established, but 20 mm Hg should be considered the threshold above which treatment to lower ICP is initiated. Cerebral perfusion pressure should be maintained at more than 70 mm Hg.[68] The ICP monitoring devices have been discussed in Chapter 10. There is considerable controversy about whether a ventricular catheter connected to an external strain gauge transducer is as accurate and reliable as a parenchymal fiber-optic transducer device. The ventricular catheter has a comparatively low risk of infection, may not necessarily increase morbidity, and has the major advantage of withdrawal of cerebrospinal fluid (Chapter 10). The infection rate increases to 20% when these fluid-coupled ICP devices are irrigated, but bacterial colonization is low (5%).[48,78] The most compelling drawback of fluid-coupled ventricular catheters is malfunction from obstruction, particularly in patients with cerebral edema that compresses the lateral horns. Parenchymal fiber-optic probes are most often used, and clinical experience is very satisfactory[73,93] (Chapter 10).

The treatment of increased ICP in the initial management of patients with severe head injury is guided toward changes in ICP and cerebral perfusion pressure. The management of increased ICP includes control of hyperthermia, elevation of the head of the bed to 30° in neutral position while avoiding obstruction of jugular venous outflow (generally, head elevation enhances jugular venous outflow and decreases ICP),[67] sedation in markedly combative patients, normal volume status, and adequate arterial oxygenation. Rigid collars may distort or compress neck veins and increase ICP.[35] Patients with increased ICP, a large mass, and no initial response to osmotic agents may need immediate neurosurgical evacuation of the contused brain.

Prophylactic hyperventilation should be avoided. A prospective, randomized clinical study found that patients with an initial Glasgow coma sum score of 4 or 5 who received prophylactic hyperventilation had significantly worse outcomes than patients with normocapnia.[49] Cerebral blood flow measurements in patients with severe traumatic brain injury have shown that blood flow is decreased and may reach values consistent with ischemia.[6] The use of aggressive hyperventilation (defined as $PaCO_2 < 30$ mm Hg) may further reduce cerebral blood flow, and it is not certain whether this reduction is matched by increased cerebral oxygen extraction. In addition, the response to hyperventilation is muted in patients who have severe head injury, typically those with diffuse multiple hemorrhagic contusions and those with extra-axial hematomas[70] (Chapter 9).

Although the use of hyperventilation as first-line treatment of increased ICP can be questioned, many patients have spontaneous hyperventilation causing $PaCO_2$ to be in the lower 30s. Hyperventilation in patients with a primary lung injury or aspiration is simply a compensatory response to hypoxemia.

Patients with increased ICP probably should be treated first with osmotic agents.

Administration of mannitol remains the preferred treatment. Mannitol has an osmotic effect after 15 to 30 minutes of infusion. Mannitol is excreted entirely in the urine and may cause acute tubular necrosis if serum osmolarity exceeds 320 mOsm/L. Mannitol should be administered in repeat boluses rather than by continuous infusion, because it may accumulate in the brain if infused for long periods. Serum osmolarity of 310 to 320 mOsm/L is

considered the therapeutic goal. Reduction of ICP can be expected 20 minutes after a bolus, and the first-pass effect may last up to 6 hours.

Another method of osmotic diuresis is the use of hypertonic saline (3% NaCl; 50 mL in 10 minutes), probably equal to mannitol in effect[18] (see Chapter 9). Alternatively, tromethamine (THAM) can be considered. Tromethamine at a rate of 1 mL/kg per hour was effective in reduction of ICP in a pilot study (see Chapter 9 for further details).

If patients with severe head injury cannot be managed with mannitol,[77] tromethamine,[94] hypertonic saline,[24,95] or propofol,[32] barbiturate treatment can be considered.[19,65,75,87] Barbiturate therapy lowers ICP and reduces mortality in patients with increased intracranial hypertension.[62] However, the side effects are considerable and include marked hypotension, hypocalcemia, hepatic and renal dysfunction, and sepsis.[71] Barbiturates may also depress lung mucociliary clearance, thereby accounting for an increased risk of pulmonary infections[23] (Chapter 22). Corticosteroids are strongly discouraged,[7,72] except in patients with severe additional spinal cord injury seen within 8 hours.[8]

The incidence of seizures after traumatic brain injury can be significantly reduced in the first week by administration of phenytoin.[84] A 7-day course of antiepileptic agents is considered in patients with marked cerebral swelling on CT scan. Seizures may greatly increase ICP and trigger plateau waves. (Even in pharmacologically paralyzed patients, seizures may increase ICP.)[74] Intravenous loading with (fos)phenytoin, 20 mg/kg, is preferred to achieve high blood concentration rapidly.

A subgroup analysis of a head injury study on the efficacy of nimodipine suggested that nimodipine may have a beneficial effect in patients with head injury and subarachnoid blood. A study of 130 patients with traumatic subarachnoid hemorrhage claimed to find delayed cerebral ischemia in 7%,[82] but the clinical relevance remains uncertain. Nimodipine, 60 mg every 6 hours for 10 days,[21] can be considered in patients with massive subarachnoid hemorrhage unless blood pressure is unstable from visceral trauma.

Table 23–2. Initial Management of Traumatic Brain Injury

Airway management	Intubation if gas exchange is inadequate or motor response is to localization or less; evidence of aspiration or lung contusion
	Mechanical ventilation with IMV/PS mode; consider PEEP if gas exchange is inadequate
Fluid management	0.9% NaCl, 3 L/day
Blood pressure management	Esmolol or labetalol if MAP > 130 mm/kg
ICP management	Placement of ICP monitoring device (fiber-optic parenchymal catheter or ventriculostomy) if GCS < 8, ICH or brain swelling on CT, use of neuromuscular blockade
	CPP, ≥ 70 mm Hg; ICP, < 20 mm Hg
	Head elevation, 30°
	Mannitol, 0.25–1 g/kg, or THAM, 1 mg/kg per hour infusion
	Consider brief periods of hyperventilation, propofol or barbiturate coma
Nutrition	Early enteral feeding when stable
	Start parenteral feeding when signs of underlying malnutrition appear
Additional measures	No corticosteroids (unless additional spinal cord lesion)
	(Fos)phenytoin, 300 mg for 7 days, in ICH, dural leak, or edema on CT
	Consider nimodipine, 60 mg q6h, for traumatic SAH with stable blood pressures
	Normothermia

CPP, cerebral perfusion pressure; CT, computed tomography; GCS, Glasgow coma scale score; ICH, intracranial hemorrhage; ICP, intracranial pressure; IMV, intermittent mandatory ventilation; MAP, mean arterial blood pressure; PEEP, positive end-expiratory pressure; PS, pressure support; SAH, subarachnoid hemorrhage; THAM, tromethamine.

Early enteral nutrition is preferred but complicated.[53,57] The early use of parenteral nutrition in patients with marked catabolic response is controversial[30] (see Chapter 7 for details).

The initial management of patients with severe traumatic brain injury[23] is summarized in Table 23–2.

DETERIORATION: CAUSES AND MANAGEMENT

The condition of patients with severe head injury may deteriorate from enlargement of hemorrhagic contusions, massive malignant cerebral edema, or further extension of an extra-axial hematoma. Diffuse brain swelling has a poor outcome. The initial CT scan in patients susceptible to malignant diffuse brain swelling is more often abnormal, revealing diffuse shear injury and subarachnoid hemorrhage. In one study, approximately half the patients with severe head injury had an episode of hypoxemia and hypotension preceding diffuse cerebral edema; this finding emphasized the possible relationship between extracranial insults and development of diffuse brain swelling. In another study, prominent leukocytosis that could not be explained by nosocomial infection was thought to be associated with a secondary increase in ICP from generalized brain swelling,[85] but the mechanism remains unexplained.

Malignant brain swelling often leads to brain death, and virtually no therapeutic option is available other than aggressive ICP management with the previously mentioned pharmacologic agents.[40] Whether barbiturate treatment improves outcome in this situation is not known, and, as mentioned earlier, it is associated with complications of its own[71] (Chapter 9). Craniotomy with removal of frontoparietal bone flaps (often bilateral) and use of an expansile duraplasty is a last resort. This measure, however, can be successful in post-traumatic cerebral infarction from a traumatic carotid lesion (often middle cerebral artery territory), most likely only when infarction involves the nondominant hemisphere.

Many patients have deterioration from enlargement of a hemorrhagic contusion[3] (Fig. 23–8). A bifrontal hematoma or temporal lobe hematoma increases the chance of herniation and marked deterioration. These patients, who typically "talk and deteriorate," need to be rushed to the operating room at the first signs of deterioration.[66,92] If the temporal lobe is damaged, a lobectomy is done in the inferior

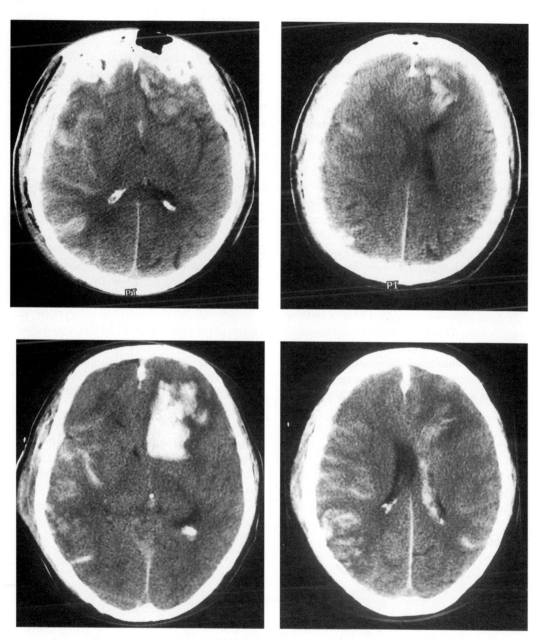

Figure 23–8. Worsening parenchymal traumatic hemorrhage. (*Top row*) Frontal lobe contusion, significant traumatic subarachnoid blood, and contusional parietal lobe. (*Bottom row*) Repeat computed tomography scan images at the time of worsening in level of consciousness show extension of the hematoma and ventricular dissection.

segment of the damaged temporal lobe, and any other severely damaged brain tissue is resected.

Extra-axial hematomas can be watched closely, but the hematomas in most patients are evacuated before they are admitted to the NICU.[52,66] Initial management of acute subdural hematoma may remain conservative if the thickness of the hematoma is similar to the thickness of the skull bone and no midline shift is noted. However, if enlargement is associated with clinical deterioration, craniotomy must be timely for a potentially successful outcome. Delayed epidural hematoma has been noted in patients with hypotension whose condition deteriorated after correction of hypotension, which most likely increased perfusion pressure and thus caused recurrent bleeding.[9]

Patients with severe traumatic brain injury may have clinical deterioration from a systemic complication. The risk of nosocomial pneumonia and adult respiratory distress syndrome is high. Rarely, disseminated coagulopathy or pulmonary embolus develops. The management of respiratory complications is described in Chapter 29.

OUTCOME

The most important factors with high predictive power are postresuscitation Glasgow coma score of 3, age of 65 years, abnormal pupils or abnormal pupils for at least one observation, shock on admission, persistently increased ICP, hypoxemia on admission, and CT scan abnormalities representing multiple contusions.[88,96] The overall percentage of patients left in a permanent vegetative state is low (3% to 5%). Patients who become severely disabled after a severe head injury may be able to return to work in sheltered workplaces, usually with responsibilities far less challenging than those before injury. Only a minority are cared for in nursing homes. In many trauma data banks, prediction of good or poor outcome was more powerful than prediction of moderate disability (independent but with a significant handicap). A useful prediction tree in diffuse brain injury[12] is shown in Figure 23–9.

In general, elderly patients do very poorly. In a series of patients older than 65 years, comatose patients had only a 10% chance of survival and a 4% chance of independent functional outcome.[45] Most likely, elderly patients more often have extradural hematomas, associated vascular disease, or multitrauma that jeopardizes recovery.[64] Nonetheless, acute traumatic subdural hematoma per se remains associated with poor outcome in the elderly.[59,91]

Two-thirds of patients with an epidural hematoma and Glasgow coma score of 3 or less die or remain in a vegetative state.[69] Outcome

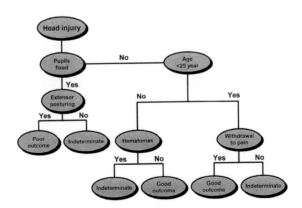

Figure 23–9. Outcome algorithm for head injury. Poor outcome: severe disability or death. Indeterminate: any statement would be a premature conclusion. Good outcome: no assistance needed, minor handicap may remain. (Data from Choi et al.[12])

is excellent with posterior fossa epidural hematomas after immediate surgical evacuation.

Permanent vegetative state is a much-feared outcome for family members confronted with a patient who is unresponsive after trauma. Patients can remain in a permanent vegetative state for 15 to 20 years, a situation extremely disruptive for families. However, in most patients, mortality for permanent vegetative state (defined as beginning 1 month after trauma) is 82% at 3 years and 95% at 5 years. Mortality in permanent vegetative state is highly dependent on whether the family requests resuscitative efforts and antibiotic therapy for infections. Recovery from a vegetative state associated with trauma is very rare (only a few well-documented instances have been reported), but most patients remain severely disabled despite the ability to communicate.

CONCLUSIONS

- ICP monitoring is strongly indicated in patients with traumatic brain injury and Glasgow coma scale score of 8 or less, in patients with brain swelling or multiple contusions on CT scan, and in patients who need sedation or neuromuscular blockade.
- Mannitol remains the preferred therapeutic agent. Prophylactic hyperventilation is strongly discouraged. Brief hyperventilation may be useful if ICP is not controlled. Alternatively, propofol or barbiturate treatment or decompressive craniotomy are measures of last resort with unproven efficacy.
- Bilateral fixed, dilated pupils in patients with traumatic hematomas are a sign of poor prognosis, but 25% of patients may recover with independent function.
- Poor outcome is expected in patients with a postresuscitation Glasgow coma scale score of 3, age of 65 years, abnormal pupils, hypoxemia or shock on admission, or multiple contusions on CT scans.

REFERENCES

1. Alcantara AL, Roszler MH, Guyot AM, et al: Blunt head trauma: comparison of various weapons with intracranial injury and neurologic outcome. *J Trauma* 37:521–524, 1994.
2. Andrews BT (ed): *Neurosurgical Intensive Care.* New York: McGraw-Hill, 1993.
3. Andrews BT, Chiles BW III, Olsen WL, et al: The effect of intracerebral hematoma location on the risk of brain-stem compression and on clinical outcome. *J Neurosurg* 69:518–522, 1988.
4. Boeve BF, Wijdicks EFM, Benarroch EE, et al: Paroxysmal sympathetic storms ("diencephalic seizures") after severe diffuse axonal head injury. *Mayo Clin Proc* 73:148–152, 1998.
5. Boto GR, Lobato RD, Rivas JJ, et al: Basal ganglia hematomas in severely head injured patients: clinicoradiological analysis of 37 cases. *J Neurosurg* 94:224–232, 2001.
6. Bouma GJ, Muizelaar JP: Cerebral blood flow, cerebral blood volume, and cerebrovascular reactivity after severe head injury. *J Neurotrauma* 9 Suppl 1:S333–S348, 1992.
7. Braakman R, Schouten HJ, Blaauw-van Dishoeck M, et al: Megadose steroids in severe head injury. Results of a prospective double-blind clinical trial. *J Neurosurg* 58:326–330, 1983.
8. Bracken MB, Shepard MJ, Collins WF, et al: A randomized, controlled trial of methylprednisolone or naloxone in the treatment of acute spinal-cord injury. Results of the Second National Acute Spinal Cord Injury Study. *N Engl J Med* 322:1405–1411, 1990.
9. Bucci MN, Phillips TW, McGillicuddy JE: Delayed epidural hemorrhage in hypotensive multiple trauma patients. *Neurosurgery* 19:65–68, 1986.
10. Bulger EM, Smith DG, Maier RV, et al: Fat embolism syndrome. A 10-year review. *Arch Surg* 132:435–439, 1997.
11. Bullard DE: Diencephalic seizures: responsiveness to bromocriptine and morphine. *Ann Neurol* 21:609–611, 1987.
12. Choi SC, Muizelaar JP, Barnes TY, et al: Prediction tree for severely head-injured patients. *J Neurosurg* 75:251–255, 1991.
13. Clifton GL, Miller ER, Choi SC, et al: Lack of effect of induction of hypothermia after acute brain injury. *N Engl J Med* 344:556–563, 2001.
14. Clifton GL, Miller ER, Choi SC, et al: Fluid thresholds and outcome from severe brain injury. *Crit Care Med* 30:935–945, 2002.
15. Czosnyka M, Smielewski P, Piechnik S, et al: Cerebral

autoregulation following head injury. *J Neurosurg* 95:756–763, 2001.

16. Darrouzet V, Duclos JY, Liguoro D, et al: Management of facial paralysis resulting from temporal bone fractures: our experience in 115 cases. *Otolaryngol Head Neck Surg* 125:77–84, 2001.

17. De Santis A, Cappricci E, Granata G: Early posttraumatic seizures in adults. Study of 84 cases. *J Neurosurg Sci* 23:207–210, 1979.

18. Doyle JA, Davis DP, Hoyt DB: The use of hypertonic saline in the treatment of traumatic brain injury. *J Trauma* 50:367–383, 2001.

19. Eisenberg HM, Frankowski RF, Contant CF, et al: High-dose barbiturate control of elevated intracranial pressure in patients with severe head injury. *J Neurosurg* 69:15–23, 1988.

20. Elsner H, Rigamonti D, Corradino G, et al: Delayed traumatic intracerebral hematomas: "Spat-Apoplexie." Report of two cases. *J Neurosurg* 72:813–815, 1990.

21. The European Study Group on Nimodipine in Severe Head Injury: A multicenter trial of the efficacy of nimodipine on outcome after severe head injury. *J Neurosurg* 80:797–804, 1994.

22. Feldman JA, Fish S: Resuscitation fluid for a patient with head injury and hypovolemic shock. *J Emerg Med* 9:465–468, 1991.

23. Forbes AR, Gamsu G: Depression of lung mucociliary clearance by thiopental and halothane. *Anesth Analg* 58:387–389, 1979.

24. Freshman SP, Battistella FD, Matteucci M, et al: Hypertonic saline (7.5%) versus mannitol: a comparison for treatment of acute head injuries. *J Trauma* 35:344–348, 1993.

25. Gentleman D, Jennett B: Audit of transfer of unconscious head-injured patients to a neurosurgical unit. *Lancet* 335:330–334, 1990.

26. Gentry LR, Godersky JC, Thompson B: MR imaging of head trauma: review of the distribution and radiopathologic features of traumatic lesions. *AJR Am J Roentgenol* 150:663–672, 1988.

27. Ghajar J: Traumatic brain injury. *Lancet* 356:923–929, 2000.

28. Golding EM, Robertson CS, Bryan RM Jr: The consequences of traumatic brain injury on cerebral blood flow and autoregulation: a review. *Clin Exp Hypertens* 21:299–332, 1999.

29. Gudeman SK, Kishore PR, Miller JD, et al: The genesis and significance of delayed traumatic intracerebral hematoma. *Neurosurgery* 5:309–313, 1979.

30. Hadley MN, Grahm TW, Harrington T, et al: Nutritional support and neurotrauma: a critical review of early nutrition in forty-five acute head injury patients. *Neurosurgery* 19:367–373, 1986.

31. Haug RH, Savage JD, Likavec MJ, et al: A review of 100 closed head injuries associated with facial fractures. *J Oral Maxillofac Surg* 50:218–222, 1992.

32. Herregods L, Verbeke J, Rolly G, et al: Effect of propofol on elevated intracranial pressure. Preliminary results. *Anaesthesia* 43 Suppl:107–109, 1988.

33. Holmes JM, Beck RW, Kip KE, et al: Predictors of nonrecovery in acute traumatic sixth nerve palsy and paresis. *Ophthalmology* 108:1457–1460, 2001.

34. Holly LT, Kelly DF, Counelis GJ, et al: Cervical spine trauma associated with moderate and severe head injury: incidence, risk factors, and injury characteristics. *J Neurosurg* 96 Suppl: 285–291.

35. Hunt K, Hallworth S, Smith M: The effects of rigid collar placement on intracranial and cerebral perfusion pressures. *Anaesthesia* 56:511–513, 2001.

36. Kern RC, Quinn B, Rosseau G, et al: Post-traumatic olfactory dysfunction. *Laryngoscope* 110:2106–2109, 2000.

37. Kirkeby OJ, Rise IR, Nordsletten L, et al: Cardiovascular response to blood loss during high intracranial pressure. *J Neurosurg* 83:1067–1071, 1995.

38. Knuckey NW, Gelbard S, Epstein MH: The management of "asymptomatic" epidural hematomas: a prospective study. *J Neurosurg* 70:392–396, 1989.

39. Kole MK, Hysell SE: MRI correlate of Kernohan's notch. *Neurology* 55:1751, 2000.

40. Lang DA, Teasdale GM, Macpherson P, et al: Diffuse brain swelling after head injury: More often malignant in adults than children? *J Neurosurg* 80:675–680, 1994.

41. Levi L, Guilburd JN, Lemberger A, et al: Diffuse axonal injury: analysis of 100 patients with radiological signs. *Neurosurgery* 27:429–432, 1990.

42. Levy D: The fat embolism syndrome. A review. *Clin Orthop* 261:281–286, 1990.

43. Lobato RD, Sarabia R, Rivas JJ, et al: Normal computerized tomography scans in severe head injury. Prognostic and clinical management implications. *J Neurosurg* 65:784–789, 1986.

44. Marion DW, Penrod LE, Kelsey SF, et al: Treatment of traumatic brain injury with moderate hypothermia. *N Engl J Med* 336:540–546, 1997.

45. Marshall LF, Gautille T, Klauber MR, et al: The outcome of severe closed head injury. *J Neurosurg* 75 Suppl:S28–S36, 1991.

46. Marshall LF, Marshall SB, Klauber MR, et al: A new classification of head injury based on computerized tomography. *J Neurosurg* 75 Suppl:S14–S20, 1991.

47. Matsushita Y, Bramlett HM, Kuluz JW, et al: Delayed hemorrhagic hypotension exacerbates the hemodynamic and histopathologic consequences of traumatic brain injury in rats. *J Cereb Blood Flow Metab* 21:847–856, 2001.

48. Mayhall CG, Archer NH, Lamb VA, et al: Ventriculostomy-related infections. A prospective epidemiologic study. *N Engl J Med* 310:553–559, 1984.

49. Muizelaar JP, Marmarou A, Ward JD, et al: Adverse effects of prolonged hyperventilation in patients with severe head injury: a randomized clinical trial. *J Neurosurg* 75:731–739, 1991.

50. Narayan RK: Hypothermia for traumatic brain injury—a good idea proved ineffective. *N Engl J Med* 344: 602–603, 2001.

51. Narayan RK, Kishore PR, Becker DP, et al: Intracranial pressure: To monitor or not to monitor? A review of our experience with severe head injury. *J Neurosurg* 56:650–659, 1982.

52. Nelson AT, Kishore PR, Lee SH: Development of delayed epidural hematoma. *AJNR Am J Neuroradiol* 3:583–585, 1982.

53. Norton JA, Ott LG, McClain C, et al: Intolerance to enteral feeding in the brain-injured patient. *J Neurosurg* 68:62–66, 1988.

54. Oertel M, Kelly DF, McArthur D, et al: Progressive hemorrhage after head trauma: predictors and consequences of the evolving injury. *J Neurosurg* 96:109–116, 2002.

55. Ostrup RC, Luerssen TG, Marshall LF, et al: Continuous monitoring of intracranial pressure with a miniaturized fiberoptic device. *J Neurosurg* 67:206–209, 1987.

56. O'Sullivan MG, Statham PF, Jones PA, et al: Role of intracranial pressure monitoring in severely head-injured patients without signs of intracranial hypertension on initial computerized tomography. *J Neurosurg* 80:46–50, 1994.

57. Ott L, Young B, Phillips R, et al: Altered gastric emptying in the head-injured patient: relationship to feeding intolerance. *J Neurosurg* 74:738–742, 1991.

58. Parizel PM, Demey HE, Veeckmans G, et al: Early diagnosis of cerebral fat embolism syndrome by diffusion-weighted MRI (starfield pattern). *Stroke* 32:2942–2944, 2001.

59. Phonprasert C, Suwanwela C, Hongsaprabhas C, et al: Extradural hematoma: analysis of 138 cases. *J Trauma* 20:679–683, 1980.

60. Pierallini A, Pantano P, Fantozzi LM, et al: Correlation between MRI findings and long-term outcome in patients with severe brain trauma. *Neuroradiology* 42:860–867, 2000.

61. Povlishock JT (ed): Management and prognosis of severe traumatic brain injury. *J Neurotrauma* 17:449–628, 2000.

62. Rea GL, Rockswold GL: Barbiturate therapy in uncontrolled intracranial hypertension. *Neurosurgery* 12:401–404, 1983.

63. Report on the Traumatic Coma Data Bank. *J Neurosurg* 75 Suppl:S1–S66, 1991.

64. Rivas JJ, Lobato RD, Sarabia R, et al: Extradural hematoma: analysis of factors influencing the courses of 161 patients. *Neurosurgery* 23:44–51, 1988.

65. Rockoff MA, Marshall LF, Shapiro HM: High-dose barbiturate therapy in humans: a clinical review of 60 patients. *Ann Neurol* 6:194–199, 1979.

66. Rockswold GL, Leonard PR, Nagib MG: Analysis of management in thirty-three closed head injury patients who "talked and deteriorated." *Neurosurgery* 21:51–55, 1987.

67. Ropper AH, O'Rourke D, Kennedy SK: Head position, intracranial pressure, and compliance. *Neurology* 32:1288–1291, 1982.

68. Rosner MJ, Rosner SD, Johnson AH: Cerebral perfusion pressure: management protocol and clinical results. *J Neurosurg* 83:949–962, 1995.

69. Sakas DE, Bullock MR, Teasdale GM: One-year outcome following craniotomy for traumatic hematoma in patients with fixed dilated pupils. *J Neurosurg* 82:961–965, 1995.

70. Salvant JB Jr, Muizelaar JP: Changes in cerebral blood flow and metabolism related to the presence of subdural hematoma. *Neurosurgery* 33:387–393, 1993.

71. Sato M, Tanaka S, Suzuki K, et al: Complications associated with barbiturate therapy. *Resuscitation* 17:233–241, 1989.

72. Saul TG, Ducker TB, Salcman M, et al: Steroids in severe head injury: a prospective randomized clinical trial. *J Neurosurg* 54:596–600, 1981.

73. Schickner DJ, Young RF: Intracranial pressure monitoring: fiberoptic monitor compared with the ventricular catheter. *Surg Neurol* 37:251–254, 1992.

74. Schierhout G, Roberts I: Anti-epileptic drugs for preventing seizures folowing acute traumatic brain injury (Cochrane Review). *Cochrane Database Syst Rev* 4:2001.

75. Schwartz ML, Tator CH, Rowed DW, et al: The University of Toronto Head Injury Treatment Study: a prospective, randomized comparison of pentobarbital and mannitol. *Can J Neurol Sci* 11:434–440, 1984.

76. Smith HK, Miller JD: The danger of an ultra-early computed tomographic scan in a patient with an evolving acute epidural hematoma. *Neurosurgery* 29:258–260, 1991.

77. Smith HP, Kelly DL Jr, McWhorter JM, et al: Comparison of mannitol regimens in patients with severe head injury undergoing intracranial monitoring. *J Neurosurg* 65:820–824, 1986.

78. Smith RW, Alksne JF: Infections complicating the use of external ventriculostomy. *J Neurosurg* 44:567–570, 1976.

79. Snow RB, Zimmerman RD, Gandy SE, et al: Comparison of magnetic resonance imaging and computed tomography in the evaluation of head injury. *Neurosurgery* 18:45–52, 1986.

80. Statham PF, Johnston RA, Macpherson P: Delayed deterioration in patients with traumatic frontal contusions. *J Neurol Neurosurg Psychiatry* 52:351–354, 1989.

81. Stiell IG, Wells GA, Vandemheen K, et al: The Canadian CT Head Rule for patients with minor head injury. *Lancet* 357:1391–1396, 2001.

82. Taneda M, Kataoka K, Akai F, et al: Traumatic subarachnoid hemorrhage as a predictable indicator of delayed ischemic symptoms. *J Neurosurg* 84:762–768, 1996.

83. Teasdale GM, Murray G, Anderson E, et al: Risks of acute traumatic intracranial haematoma in children and adults: implications for managing head injuries. *BMJ* 300:363–367, 1990.

84. Temkin NR, Dikmen SS, Wilensky AJ, et al: A randomized, double-blind study of phenytoin for the prevention of post-traumatic seizures. *N Engl J Med* 323:497–502, 1990.

85. Unterberg A, Kiening K, Schmiedek P, et al: Long-term observations of intracranial pressure after severe head injury. The phenomenon of secondary rise of intracranial pressure. *Neurosurgery* 32:17–23, 1993.

86. Wang BH, Robertson BC, Girotto JA, et al: Traumatic optic neuropathy: a review of 61 patients. *Plast Reconstr Surg* 107:1655–1664, 2001.

87. Ward JD, Becker DP, Miller JD, et al: Failure of prophylactic barbiturate coma in the treatment of severe head injury. *J Neurosurg* 62:383–388, 1985.

88. Wardlaw JM, Easton VJ, Statham P: Which CT features help predict outcome after head injury? *J Neurol Neurosurg Psychiatry* 72:188–192, 2002.

89. Wijdicks EFM: *Neurologic Complications of Critical Illness.* 2nd ed. Oxford: Oxford University Press, 2002.

90. Wilberger JE Jr, Deeb Z, Rothfus W: Magnetic resonance imaging in cases of severe head injury. *Neurosurgery* 20:571–576, 1987.

91. Wilberger JE Jr, Harris M, Diamond DL: Acute subdural hematoma: morbidity, mortality, and operative timing. *J Neurosurg* 74:212–218, 1991.

92. Wilberger JE Jr, Rothfus WE, Tabas J, et al: Acute tissue tear hemorrhages of the brain: computed tomography and clinicopathological correlations. *Neurosurgery* 27:208–213, 1990.

93. Winfield JA, Rosenthal P, Kanter RK, et al: Duration of intracranial pressure monitoring does not predict daily risk of infectious complications. *Neurosurgery* 33:424–430, 1993.

94. Wolf AL, Levi L, Marmarou A, et al: Effect of THAM upon outcome in severe head injury: a randomized prospective clinical trial. *J Neurosurg* 78:54–59, 1993.

95. Worthley LI, Cooper DJ, Jones N: Treatment of resistant intracranial hypertension with hypertonic saline. Report of two cases. *J Neurosurg* 68:478–481, 1988.

96. Zink BJ: Traumatic brain injury outcome: concepts for emergency care. *Ann Emerg Med* 37:318–332, 2001.

24

Status Epilepticus

Status epilepticus is a neurologic emergency that not only needs rapid pharmacologic intervention but also is more properly treated when its cause is identified. Fortunately, 70% to 80% of patients with status epilepticus become seizure-free in the emergency department from treatment with repeated boluses of benzodiazepines and intravenous loading with a sufficient amount of phenytoin. Thus, persistent and therapy-refractory generalized tonic-clonic seizures after admission to the NICU indicate a more severe form of status epilepticus with undoubtedly higher probability of permanent neurologic damage. A critical juncture is time of successful administration of antiepileptic agents. Delay in treatment (more than 30 minutes to 1 hour) could lead to persistent neurologic damage, mostly from memory deficits.

The cause of tonic-clonic status epilepticus is diverse. Withdrawal of antiepileptic medication or poor compliance has traditionally been implicated. One study noted that the vast majority of patients with status epilepticus and a seizure disorder had therapeutic or subtherapeutic antiepileptic drug levels at the time of presentation.[5] Clearly identified causes of status epilepticus in adults are alcohol withdrawal, primary brain tumors, head injury, ischemic and hemorrhagic stroke, encephalitis, meningitis, poisoning, illicit drug abuse, and, occasionally, metabolic derangements, such as marked shifts in plasma sodium and serum glucose.[52] In older adults without a history of epilepsy, half of all instances could be attributed to acute stroke.[22] Worldwide, neurocysticercosis is a common cause of seizures and status epilepticus.

Some drugs used in the NICU can lower the seizure threshold and trigger a single seizure, particularly in patients with a proclivity to seizures (Table 24–1).

Nonconvulsive status epilepticus is infrequent in patients without a previously diagnosed seizure disorder. Nonconvulsive status epilepticus most often follows seizures, which may occur with a new structural brain lesion, but other possible causes are withdrawal of antiepileptic agents or benzodiazepines, psychotropic drugs (neuroleptics, tricyclic antidepressants), and, rarely, diagnostic procedures in the hospital, such as cerebral angiography and electroconvulsive therapy.

Status epilepticus in adults can be classified broadly into tonic-clonic status epilepticus, nonconvulsive status epilepticus, and complex partial status epilepticus. This chapter mainly concentrates on tonic-clonic status epilepticus.

CLINICAL RECOGNITION

Tonic-clonic status epilepticus is difficult to define, and spontaneous resolution, albeit uncommon, may occur. The definition "continuous seizures of more than 5-minute duration or two or more discrete seizures without full recovery of consciousness" is currently considered the most reasonable operational definition, and the time limit of several minutes allows rapid intervention.[47]

Table 24–1. Pharmaceutical Agents Used in the Neurologic Intensive Care Unit That Can Reduce Seizure Threshold

Antibiotics	Imipenem
	Norfloxacin
	Ciprofloxacin
	Cefepime
	Penicillin derivatives
Antidepressants	Amitriptyline
	Doxepin
	Nortriptyline
	Fluoxetine, sertraline
Antipsychotics	Chlorpromazine
	Haloperidol
	Thioridazine
	Perphenazine
	Trifluoperazine

Tonic-clonic status epilepticus may begin as a single seizure with initial full recovery of consciousness. In typical tonic-clonic status epilepticus, the fits begin to overlap one another. In the extreme case, some body parts may be in a resolving clonic stage and others in a new tonic spell as status epilepticus progresses.[3,7,14,63] The tonic phase seems to become progressively shorter or may even disappear. Additionally, the clonic phase may lose its characteristics and become brief and less intense, even dispersing into multiple twitches.

Most of the time, a tonic-clonic seizure starts with a tonic contraction lasting 15 to 30 seconds and continues with several minutes of repeated muscle contractions, loss of pupillary light response and corneal reflexes, and emergence of bilateral Babinski's signs. Very notable at this stage in some patients, as the result of a sympathetic outpouring, is profuse sweating, tachycardia, increased bronchial secretion, and marked hypertension. Before the next seizure begins, patients cannot be roused, and this interval is often marked by labored breathing with frothing at the mouth. The lack of full recovery between spells is characteristic, but use of benzodiazepines to counter an initial series of seizures may cause drowsiness; conversely, patients may shiver from the use of sedative medication, and this reaction should not be immediately interpreted as imminent status epilepticus.

The prerogatives in the recognition and management of myoclonus status epilepticus are different.[42] This subset of status epilepticus, seen immediately after cardiopulmonary resuscitation and defibrillation, is linked to extensive cortical, thalamic, brain stem, and even spinal cord infarction and twitches could perpetuate for 1 or 2 days before subsiding. Brief but continuous widespread multifocal myoclonus is seen and may look like "shivering." It is a phenomenon in extremis rather than a different type of status epilepticus that has to be treated aggressively. (We could mute the myoclonus using propofol.[78])

Nonconvulsive status epilepticus is less characteristic in presentation. Clinical hallmarks are decrease in the level of consciousness and, more important, daily fluctuation in responsiveness. Patients may have facial grimacing as a clinical feature or a puzzled, expressionless, trance-like demeanor. Patients in nonconvulsive status epilepticus may continue to follow very simple commands when prodded repeatedly. The manifestations can be as subtle as acute reluctance to follow commands and eyelid twitching, with eye deviation noted only when eyelids are lifted, and thus cannot be discovered by video alone. Nonconvulsive status epilepticus with waxing and waning of level of consciousness may last for days without being noticed.

Complex partial status epilepticus may have a strong clinical resemblance to generalized nonconvulsive status epilepticus with its characteristic fluctuating level of responsiveness, but often automatism or some type of bizarre ritual is seen[4] (e.g., face rubbing, lip smacking, pinching on blankets, or episodic loquacious speech). Isolated aphasia is on record.[33] Agitated paranoid behavior may occur, suggesting a psychiatric emergency. As expected, complex partial status epilepticus is most common in patients with a previously documented partial seizure disorder, but it may appear first in acute neurologic disorders such as herpes simplex encephalitis.

Convulsive status epilepticus is usually recognized by astute clinicians, but psychogenic status epilepticus may at times mimic its manifestations and even lead to intubation and use of barbiturates. The typical features are absent dysautonomia, lateral tongue bite (biting of the tip is often psychogenic), and flailing and rocking movements rather than tonic-clonic periodicity. Prolonged EEG-videomonitoring may also document lack of stereotypical movements. Measurement of arterial blood gas commonly reveals absent lactic acidosis.

Tonic-clonic status epilepticus can lead to remote effects involving vital organs;[19,26,31,64,76] the most pertinent consequences are illustrated in Figure 24–1. These manifestations of status epilepticus can be brief and transient but also are potentially life-threatening (e.g., pulmonary edema or aspiration).

NEUROIMAGING AND LABORATORY TESTS

Computed tomography scan may document a structural lesion and is mandatory in patients with tonic-clonic status epilepticus. It may not be sensitive enough to rule out an underlying new structural lesion and therefore at some point must be supplemented by MRI. Computed tomography scan changes—effacement of sulci from edema or infarction in watershed territories—can be seen in patients who have had a major additional hypoxic-ischemic insult to the brain. Traumatic subarachnoid blood or small hemorrhagic contusions may be noted that could be a consequence of trauma from a fall rather than a trigger for status epilepticus.

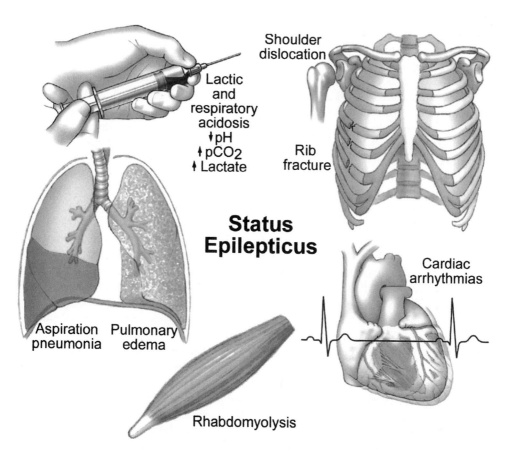

Figure 24–1. Systemic effects of status epilepticus.

Magnetic resonance imaging may document evidence of encephalitis, evolution of an ischemic stroke, a low-grade astrocytoma, or cavernous malformations. Magnetic resonance imaging scanning may also show small areas of hyperintensity on T2-weighted images in the gray and white matter, often in the posterior vascular watershed areas, abnormalities that resolve after seizures are under control. Cerebral edema is the most likely cause for these reversible MRI abnormalities.[84] Diffusion-weighted MRI may document transient increased diffusion in the subcortical white matter and decrease in the cortex, possibly from water flux toward the seizing cortical neurons.[77] Damage to the hippocampus with subsequent hippocampal sclerosis and amygdala kindling may occur as a direct result of status epilepticus and appear as hyperintensity on T2-weighted images with fluid-attenuated inversion recovery.[39,67] Single-photon emission CT in the interictal phase may show global reduced perfusion after sampling of both hemispheres but has less value in localizing an epileptic focus. Single-photon emission CT coregistered with MRI may be a helpful test in documentation of seizure focus after recovery from status epilepticus, particularly when epilepsy surgery is under consideration.[66]

Examination of the cerebrospinal fluid is obligatory in patients with fever and increased white blood cell counts to exclude bacterial meningitis. Status epilepticus may transiently increase the cell count up to 65 total nucleated cells. Obviously, an increased cell count in the cerebrospinal fluid in any patient with status epilepticus should prompt further cultures and empirical antibiotic or antiviral therapy.[14,62] Polymerase chain reaction should be performed for certain types of encephalitis (e.g., herpes simplex). Herpes simplex encephalitis should be considered if family members mention that acute confusion, aphasia, and abruptly high temperatures occurred before seizures began. *Aspergillus* and *Cryptococcus* antigens need to be determined in immunosuppressed patients (Chapter 21). Neuron-specific enolase may be found in increased titers in the cerebrospinal fluid (a less robust association in serum) and indicate brain injury, but usefulness of this finding in determining outcome is not known.[17]

Results of arterial blood gas examination are often abnormal after status epilepticus. Respiratory acidosis (due to reduced respiratory drive) is common, occurring alone or in combination with metabolic acidosis (due to lactate from muscle injury). Most acid–base abnormalities disappear spontaneously within hours. There is no consistent relation of any of the acid–base abnormalities to cardiac arrhythmias occurring after status epilepticus.[79]

Chest radiography may give an early indication of gastric aspiration. Seldom are typical features of neurogenic pulmonary edema shown[19] (see Chapter 29 for details). Fractures of the long bones and vertebral bodies may occur, more often, as expected, in elderly patients. Bilateral posterior fracture-dislocation of the humeral head is a characteristic fracture, but rib fractures and vertebral body compression fractures should be considered when pain suggests those regions.[26] Radiographs are indicated in patients with localized pain, and sometimes MRI of the shoulder is needed to document a major tear. Pain in the shoulder should not be attributed simply to muscle soreness following seizures.

Conventional EEG documents status epilepticus, and it becomes even more important in patients who need second-line drugs for treatment (Chapter 11). Many EEG patterns are seen, and a five-phase evolution has been proposed.[70] The initial stage shows single epileptic activity followed by high-voltage slow activity. The EEG characteristically shows an episode of silence in the postictal phase. The next stages are characterized by merging of electrographic seizures accompanied by fluctuating amplitude and frequency of EEG rhythms, continuous ictal activity, or continuous ictal activity punctuated by low-voltage flat periods that finally evolve into a burst-suppression pattern of periodic epileptiform discharges on a flat background. This classification has been criticized because the progressive temporal evolution observed in animal experiments does not appear in clinically encountered cases. A major controversy exists about whether the periodic epileptic discharges in the final stage represent continuing seizure activity requiring more aggressive treatment or merely reflect very severe brain damage. The claim that the response to treatment declines proportionally with each stage, with a response of almost 20% remaining in patients with periodic epileptic discharges, requires confirmation.[70]

Electroencephalography infrequently captures all elements of status epilepticus because of aggressive early treatment. An EEG should be obtained in a patient with prolonged (exceeding 30 minutes) postictal unresponsiveness, to differentiate coma due to continuing seizures from postictal sleep; in a patient who has received neuromuscular blocking agents and sedative agents with a prolonged anesthetic effect; and in a patient with atypical features suggesting the possibility of pseudoseizures.[42] However, we strongly believe EEG-videomonitoring is required in any patient with status epilepticus. Electroencephalographic recordings characteristically show a discrete seizure with intermittent flattening that may evolve into periodic lateralized epileptiform discharges (PLEDs). During the course of status epilepticus, EEG may continue to demonstrate outbursts of epileptic activity without any clinically observed motor accompaniment. Whether PLEDs represent potentially reversible continuing epileptic activity or severe cerebral damage is uncertain,[28] but many experts consider PLEDs (bilaterally independent or bilaterally synchronous-generalized) an interictal phenomenon if no motor manifestations occur.

Burst suppression may be seen as a consequence of status epilepticus, its treatment, or its cause. Generalized slowing and attenuation are clearly not ictal and should not be treated as such, even in a comatose patient. If the seizures are controlled clinically and there is no EEG evidence of continuing seizure activity, any EEG pattern is acceptable. Titration of an anesthetic agent to an isoelectric or burst-

suppression pattern is not known to be beneficial, and the high dose of antiepileptic agent needed to produce this EEG pattern may cause profound hypotension.

FIRST STEPS IN MANAGEMENT

Management of status epilepticus should begin during transportation and in the emergency department. The first measure at arrival in the NICU is airway control. Many patients have been aspirating, may have copious secretions, and, in fact, may already have an obstructed bronchial branch. Often, endotracheal intubation is necessary because large doses of benzodiazepines have caused drowsiness and upper airway collapse. Invariably, all benzodiazepines greatly depress respiratory drive, causing hypoventilation, transient apneic episodes, and, occasionally, tongue obstruction. However, not all patients in status epilepticus need endotracheal intubation, and "manual bagging" may be considered if a therapeutic response seems likely. Endotracheal intubation is definitely needed when a second-line agent (midazolam or propofol) is administered.

Endotracheal intubation should follow the oral route, facilitated by succinylcholine (1.5 mg/kg) and thiopental sodium (3 mg/kg). If status epilepticus is due to increased intracranial pressure, lidocaine (1.5 mg/kg) or fentanyl (3 μg/kg) can mute the increase in pressure during the procedure.[75]

Mechanical ventilation may not be strictly necessary after endotracheal intubation, although oxygen delivery is substantially improved by, for example, an initial intermittent mandatory ventilation of 8, FIO_2 of 60, and pressure support of 5 cm H_2O. A pulse oximeter is needed to monitor episodes of oxygen desaturation. If oxygenation does not noticeably improve, fiber-optic bronchoscopy may be indicated to investigate possible bronchial obstruction from a foreign body (e.g., tooth fragment) or mucus plug. In the rare situation of neurogenic pulmonary edema, mechanical ventilation with high settings of positive end-expiratory pressure is necessary, but pulmonary edema is short-lived. Aspiration occurred much more often than pulmonary edema in one series of patients with status epilepticus.[79] In none of a consecutive series of 35 patients with treatment-refractory status epilepticus could neurogenic pulmonary edema be implicated as a potential cause for hypoxemia and respiratory acidosis,[79] but others have reported well-documented instances.[19]

After the airway has been secured, two intravenous peripheral catheters must be placed in large arm veins for administration of antiepileptic and possibly inotropic agents. Antiepileptic drugs, predominantly diazepam, 0.5 to 1 mg/kg, have been administered rectally in patients with no intravenous access (e.g., drug addicts).[57] However, in patients with very difficult venous access, it is better to proceed with femoral vein catheterization than to try to counter status epilepticus with rectal medication. Femoral vein catheterization is much easier than subclavian catheterization (the femoral vein lies medial to the femoral artery, and the searching needle is pointed cephalad) and does not require much technical experience. In addition, femoral vein catheterization does not have the potential complication of pneumothorax accompanying placement of a subclavian catheter.

In patients with multiple seizures, hydration with 0.9% saline (200 mL/hour) is started immediately to reduce the risk of renal failure from rhabdomyolysis, particularly if the admission serum creatine kinase is considerably increased.

Excessive muscle activity depletes glycogen, promotes anaerobic glycolysis, and results in lactate production; thus, metabolic acidosis is frequently found but should not be corrected until the pH has declined to 7.0. The use of bicarbonate in patients with overt lactic acidosis is potentially dangerous because it may increase the likelihood of an overcorrection to alkalosis, which reduces the seizure threshold.

The effect of status epilepticus on heart muscle has been poorly studied in humans, but recent animal experiments suggest that myocardial hemorrhage, contraction bands, and cardiac pump failure occur within minutes after seizure induction.[37] Cardiac arrhythmias are present in 50% of the patients.[63,64,79] Sinus tachycardia is most prevalent. In other patients, multifocal atrial tachycardia, ventricular tachycardia, or a brief asystole after bradycardia has been found. Although ST depressions can be transient in patients with electrocardiographic abnormalities suggesting ventricular strain or myocardial ischemia, selective protective beta-blockade (e.g., with metoprolol) should be considered.[68]

Benzodiazepines are the first line of treatment and are virtually immediately followed by intravenous phenytoin loading.[21] The choice of benzodiazepine is arbitrary. Diazepam has traditionally been one of the most successful agents, but it is associated with severe respiratory depression when used repeatedly and may lead to unnecessary intubation. Lorazepam is the preferred benzodiazepine and has the advantage of terminating seizures in almost 80% of patients.[43,44] It is active for approximately 1 to 3 hours and is administered in a dose of 4 mg at 1 to 2 mg/minute to a maximum of 10 mg. Lorazepam is not more effective than phenobarbital or a combination of diazepam and phenytoin for initial treatment, but a randomized trial found the highest response rate and fewest side effects in lorazepam-treated patients.[71] Lorazepam appeared to be more effective than diazepam in a trial investigating its safety when administered by paramedics.[2] Lorazepam should, therefore, be considered the most appropriate first-line agent to terminate status epilepticus.

The use of midazolam in status epilepticus for initial treatment has not been carefully investigated. Because its effectiveness is brief, continuous infusion is necessary (the recommended dose is a 0.2 mg/kg bolus followed by infusion of 0.1 to 0.6 mg/kg per hour). With continuous administration of midazolam, full mechanical ventilation becomes necessary, whereas this is not yet a concern in patients with phenytoin loading. Moreover, it is not known whether intravenous midazolam or clonazepam (more commonly used outside the United States) in a single bolus is as effective as lorazepam.

In general, intravenous loading with phenytoin is standard after patients have been treated with benzodiazepines.[60] Oral administration of 300 mg of phenytoin after intravenous loading should begin 6 hours after infusion and produces steady serum levels of phenytoin after 4 days of treatment.[18] Phenytoin is infused in isotonic saline, the infusion rate must not exceed 50 mg/minute, and the rate must be halved in elderly patients. Infusion in a typical patient of 80 kg takes 30 minutes, but seizures should stop after approximately 10 minutes. A more rapid infusion has the disadvantage of increasing the risk of hypotension and cardiac arrhythmias. These side effects are more common in elderly patients and, in addition to a direct cardiotoxic effect, may be more common in poorly hydrated patients. Other, much less common, side effects are vomiting, choreoathetosis, nystagmus, thrombophlebitis, purple hand syndrome, and hypersensitivity.[25]

Some of the major side effects have been overcome with the introduction of fosphenytoin. Fosphenytoin (Cerebyx), a water-soluble disodium phosphate ester of phenytoin, does not require the propylene glycol vehicle that is often responsible for hypotension and cardiac arrhythmias.[59] We have been using fosphenytoin intravenously for status epilepticus; the dose is similar to that of phenytoin and is expressed in phenytoin equivalents. The drug, however, is not widely available outside the United States. The recommended rate for status epilepticus is 100 to 150 mg of phenytoin equivalents per minute two to three times, considerably faster than that for intravenous phenytoin. Careful checking of labels is required, because rapid infusion of phenytoin, mistaken for fosphenytoin, may cause life-threatening cardiac arrhythmias.[80] The initial management of convulsive status epilepticus is summarized in Table 24–2.

Nonconvulsive status epilepticus usually is managed by intravenous administration of benzodiazepines alone.[15,32] Identification of the trigger is important (e.g., recent withdrawal of large doses of benzodiazepines or severe metabolic derangements).

The most commonly used drugs in nonconvulsive status epilepticus are diazepam, 0.2 to 0.3 mg/kg, and lorazepam, 0.1 mg/kg. Benzodiazepines are very effective in most patients, but doses may need to be repeated regularly. Long-term treatment with valproate or phenytoin must begin almost immediately, orally or through the nasogastric tube, in patients with recurrent events.

Partial complex seizures are treated in a similar manner, but the relative resistance to benzodiazepines often dictates a higher dose (diazepam, 0.4 to 0.6 mg/kg) or initial intravenous loading with phenytoin. In many patients, oral therapy with carbamazepine (200 mg three times a day) or divalproex sodium (Depakote) (20 mg/kg loading as a starting dose and infusion of 5 mg/kg per hour until seizure free) is instituted. Valproate should not be used if focal status epilepticus is due to an intracerebral hematoma. The negative effect of valproate— a decrease in platelet aggregation and an increase in bleeding time—has been well established and can be expected in the high doses used to treat focal status epilepticus.[29]

Table 24–2. Initial Management of Status Epilepticus

Airway management	Intubation if evidence of aspiration, hypoxemia, or pulmonary edema
	Elective endotracheal intubation if second-line treatment (propofol or midazolam) is anticipated
	IMV mode may have to change to AC if barbiturates needed for seizure control
Fluid management	Two large-bore intravenous catheters
	2–3 L of 0.9% NaCl; increase with fever or evidence of rhabdomyolysis
Anticonvulsants	Lorazepam, 4 mg (total dose, 10 mg)
	Phenytoin loading, 20 mg/kg (rate, 50 mg/minute or, in elderly, 25 mg/minute), or fosphenytoin, 20 mg PE/kg (100–150 mg PE/minute)
Prophylactic measures	Intermittent pneumatic devices
	Consider beta-blockade if electrocardiogram changes

AC, assist-control; IMV, intermittent mandatory ventilation; PE, phenytoin equivalents.

Treatment of epilepsia partialis continua is one of the most frustrating experiences. Patients may potentially go through the whole gamut of antiepileptic medications. Intravenous administration of high doses of phenobarbital, nimodipine, or valproate may be a last resort.[11]

DETERIORATION: CAUSES AND MANAGEMENT

Two major forms of clinical deterioration occur in status epilepticus: first, recurrence of seizures almost immediately after completion of phenytoin (or fosphenytoin) infusion, and second, breakthrough seizures every time the anesthetic agent is tapered. Both forms are considered therapy-refractory status epilepticus.

Failure to control seizures has several causes, and each should be explored. The most common cause is an inadequate dose of phenytoin. Most often, a typical but highly insufficient "1000 mg" infusion of phenytoin has been ordered. (This dose, originally from the landmark paper by Wallis et al.,[74] is most likely used because a dose of 1 g is easily remembered.) Other causes of failure to control seizures, besides an acute structural brain lesion, are persistence of a metabolic derangement (e.g., hyponatremia, recurrent hypoglycemia, or hyperglycemia), drug toxicity, and central nervous system infection. In some patients, the cause of the poor initial response remains unknown and treatment with lorazepam and phenytoin is simply not sufficient to control seizures.

Treatment of status epilepticus in this second phase of management is difficult and regrettably guided by personal opinion and trends. Therapy algorithms may suddenly change after premature enthusiasm for a new drug.[7,14,36,63] However, it remains important to have a predetermined idea of which agent to use rather than to frequently switch agents. A reasonable guideline is shown in Figure 24–2. Before a new antiepileptic agent is considered, an additional infusion of phenytoin at one-third or half of the original infusion dose (usually 5–10 mg/kg) is useful to maximize phenytoin loading. This probably should be given after an additional intravenous dose of 4 mg of lorazepam.

The next antiepileptic agent in a patient with status epilepticus has traditionally been phenobarbital. Its use in status epilepticus can be questioned, and many neurointensivists now directly proceed with midazolam, propofol, or pentobarbital anesthesia. In our experience, phenobarbital remains a useful drug in patients with significant underlying cardiac disease and epilepsia partialis continua and should by no means be considered a relic of the past. The recommended starting dose is 10 to 20 mg/kg infused at a rate of less than 100 mg/minute, and this is followed by a maintenance infusion of 1 to 4 mg/kg per hour. Onset of action is rapid, relapse is uncommon, and the risk of marked hypotension and significant sedation with respiratory hypoventilation is comparably low with this starting dose. If seizures continue, the dose of phenobarbital can be gradually increased to 30 to 40 mL/kg but at the expense of marked sedation and hypoventilation, and many patients then need full mechanical ventilation. The major drawback of barbiturates is long elimination time and significant accumulation, and weaning from the mechanical ventilator is significantly prolonged.[54]

Midazolam has emerged as a second-line antiepileptic drug for status epilepticus (Fig. 24–2).[8,41,55] The recommended loading dose is 0.2 mg/kg intravenously in a bolus, and this is followed by an infusion of 0.1 to 0.6 mg/kg per hour until the EEG is free of seizure activity.[8,27,41,55] However, midazolam is severalfold more expensive than barbiturates when used in an intravenous infusion. In addition, with increasing doses, blood pressure may decrease significantly, with a need for dopamine support as well. A comparative study with pentobarbital is not available.

An alternative approach is to use high doses of propofol.[1,48,82] Propofol is administered in a bolus of 2 mg/kg followed by an infusion of 5 mg/kg per hour, later tapered to 1 to 5 mg/kg per hour. Propofol acts through enhancement of γ-aminobutyric acid-mediated transmission, possibly at the chloride ion channel, different from that with benzodiazepines and barbiturates.[12] The preconvulsive effect, largely discounted, has been estimated to affect 1 in 47,000 patients.[6] The enthusiasm for propofol

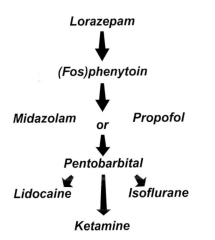

Figure 24–2. Algorithm for treatment-refractory status epilepticus.

may diminish if an early report of fourfold higher mortality in patients with APACHE scores of more than 20 is confirmed and explained.[55] For now, midazolam and propofol remain the leading pharmaceutical agents for treatment of refractory status epilepticus.

As a last resort, pentobarbital is administered if prior drugs fail. Pentobarbital is administered intravenously in 1 to 2 minutes as an initial bolus of 10 to 15 mg/kg followed by infusion of 1 to 3 mg/kg per hour until seizures stop clinically and on EEG.[46,56,85] A burst-suppression pattern, up to 30 seconds, is preferable, but one may argue that an EEG without superimposed epileptic discharges is equally effective. In fact, burst suppression on EEG recording does not mean intermittent brief seizures cannot occur. Pushing the pentobarbital dosage to a burst-suppression or flat EEG pattern may markedly increase the need for more dopamine support. Thus, aiming for an EEG without seizure activity may considerably reduce the side effects of pentobarbital. However, in daily practice, the EEG may fluctuate from burst suppression to bilateral PLEDs without appreciable bursts of seizures. This EEG recording may be a satisfactory end point.

Pentobarbital has a marked cardiodepressant effect, and many patients need dopamine for blood pressure support. Dopamine in a dose of 5 to 10 μg/kg per minute increases cardiac output and reverses hypotension in the vast majority of patients treated with pentobarbital. Phenylephrine may be needed in addition to dopamine in resistant cases when pentobarbital levels must necessarily be high to control status epilepticus.

Pentobarbital infusion is administered for at least 24 hours. Adjusting the dose of pentobarbital to a lower infusion rate is not always successful and may lead to breakthrough seizures.

The dose of pentobarbital is reduced when initial blood levels of phenytoin are therapeutic. The patient is closely observed clinically, and continuous EEG recordings are used to monitor for possible recurrence.[9] The infusion should be halved after 24 hours to limit the toxic exposure of barbiturates. For example, the risk of pulmonary edema and *Pseudomonas* and *Staphylococcus* pneumonia is increased from a direct effect on ciliary function.[54] There is no good pharmacologic rationale to discontinue pentobarbital infusion gradually over days. Time to recovery is very difficult to estimate, may take days, and often depends on total body fat and underlying liver function.

A major management problem arises when generalized tonic-clonic seizures are not controlled or continue to recur after discontinuation of barbiturate therapy. Failure to control seizures with barbiturate anesthesia seems very uncommon, but if it happens, the chance of effectively controlling seizures is low and mortality is high in these patients. Secondary brain damage may perpetuate status epilepticus,[14,63] or the initial trigger can be implicated.

The third line of therapy in status epilepticus is entirely anecdotal. Lidocaine has shown efficacy in therapy-refractory status epilepticus.[14,63,73] Lidocaine is injected in a bolus of 2 to 3 mg/kg in several minutes, followed by an infusion of 3 mg/kg per hour. The infusion should not be continued for more than 12 hours. Its use is limited in patients with a history of cardiac arrhythmias or electrocardiographic evidence of any type of heart block and poor ejection fraction on echocardiography. Use in patients with liver failure is also contraindicated due to decreased hepatic clearance, and a high level of lidocaine, which itself can lead to seizures, may result.

Table 24–3. Antiepileptic Agents Used to Treat Convulsive Status Epilepticus

Drug	Initial Dose (Bolus)	Rate	Infusion (Maintenance)	Precautions
Diazepam	10–20 mg	≤ 5 mg/minute	8 mg/hour	Endotracheal intubation and mechanical ventilation with repeated doses
Midazolam	0.2 mg/kg	≤ 4 mg/minute	0.1–0.6 mg/kg per hour	Mechanical ventilation invariably needed; dopamine for occasional hypotension
Lorazepam	4 mg	1–2 mg/minute	NA	Cardiac monitoring for cardiac arrhythmias (bradycardia)
Phenytoin	18–20 mg/kg	50 mg/minute	NA	Cardiac and blood pressure monitoring
Fosphenytoin	18–20 mg PE/kg	100–150 mg PE/minute	NA	Cardiac and blood pressure monitoring
Phenobarbital	10–20 mg/kg	≤ 100 mg/minute	1–4 mg/kg per hour	Mechanical ventilation with high dose (≥ 20 mg/kg) may be preferred
Pentobarbital	10–15 mg/kg	1–2 mg/kg over 5 minutes	1–3 mg/kg per hour	Dopamine, 5–10 µg/kg per minute; chest radiograph for pneumonia
Lidocaine	2–3 mg/kg	≤ 50 mg/minute	3 mg/kg per hour	Cardiac monitoring (bradycardia, heart block)
Isoflurane	Inhalation to end-tidal volume concentration of 0.8%–3%	NA	NA	Anesthetic system with scavenging
Propofol	2 mg/kg initially	Slow push	1–5 mg/kg per hour	Blood pressure monitoring (blood gas for metabolic acidosis)
Ketamine	2 mg/kg	NA	10–50 mg/kg per minute	Tachyphylaxis (increasing dose needed)
Valproate	20–30 mg/kg	NA	20–50 mg/minute	Monitoring of albumin

Max, maximum; NA, not applicable; PE, phenytoin equivalents.

Isoflurane, suggested as another last-resort treatment, is cumbersome to use in the NICU because of the complexity of inhalational anesthetic systems.[40,49,58] In a series of 11 patients with treatment-refractory status epilepticus, mortality remained high despite seizure control. However, isoflurane anesthesia should be strongly considered in patients with recurrent status epilepticus. In one personally observed patient, control of seizures was achieved almost immediately. Isoflurane is used in concentrations of 0.8% to 3%, and progressively higher concentrations are often needed to control seizures.

The doses of antiepileptic drugs are summarized in Table 24–3 (see also Appendix for drug interactions).

New alternative agents for treatment of refractory status epilepticus include ketamine and valproate. Experience is very limited, and undoubtedly only successful cases have been published. One should not run away with the notion that these agents have an established role in the treatment of status epilepticus. Ketamine, an N-methyl-D-aspartate receptor antagonist, may become the next choice after propofol or midazolam. A short-acting anticonvulsant, ketamine surprisingly controlled status epilepticus in one patient refractory to phenytoin, phenobarbital, midazolam, propofol, valproate, and lidocaine infusion. This unconfirmed experience is valuable. Ketamine was used in a bolus of 2 mg/kg followed by an infusion of 10 to 50 mg/kg per minute, a dose that does not cause respiratory depression.[2,10,61] Intravenous valproate was recently introduced, but its efficacy is unknown and control of seizures was only 30% in one study. Its major advantage may be that it does not reduce blood pressure and thus may be a good alternative in patients who have become cardiovascularly unstable with midazolam and propofol.[35,65] It also has virtually no respiratory depression. Intravenous loading doses of valproate can be 25 to 30 mg/kg, with infusion rates of 20 to 50 mg/minute to attain a steady-state serum concentration of 75 mg/L. It is highly bound to albumin, and toxicity may rapidly arise in patients with poor nutritional intake (e.g., alcoholics).[23,38]

In patients with recurrent seizures after discontinuation of pentobarbital or midazolam, readministering the drug seems reasonable but with infusion for several more days and perhaps more gradual reduction of dose. A difficult situation arises with patients in coma who have continuous epileptic activity, no clinical accompaniment, and no response to a series of different antiepileptic medications. Control cannot be expected, awakening from coma is uncommon, and mortality is very high. An aggressive approach with prolonged use of anesthetic drugs for several weeks may be justified only in young patients with traumatic brain injury, in encephalitis, and in patients with MRI findings that do not suggest widespread cortical damage.

OUTCOME

The prognosis of status epilepticus depends on several factors.[34] The most important clinically relevant finding has been the association of the actual time that patients remain in tonic-clonic status epilepticus and later morbidity. This finding, however, probably does not hold for patients in nonconvulsive status epilepticus. Nonconvulsive status epilepticus lasting many days may result in a favorable outcome,[81] but data are sparse in this category of patients.

Patients with tonic-clonic status epilepticus have a considerable risk of permanent morbidity. Neuropathologic studies in humans have unequivocally shown that status epilepticus can damage the brain.[50,51] The most striking abnormalities have been found in the hippocampus and reflect the clinically observed memory deficits in some patients. The hippocampus may swell and have complete cell loss in the CA1 region.[20] As noted earlier, the major confounding factor in clinicopathologic correlation of hippocampal damage is hypoxemia, which may be particularly severe in patients with prolonged status epilepticus. Nonetheless, carefully controlled experimental studies have shown that despite adequate oxygenation, 2 hours of status epilepticus can produce neuronal changes not only in the Sommer sector but also in thalamic nuclei and pyramidal cortical layers.[50] The duration of status epilepticus, therefore, is a decisive factor.

However, complete neurologic improvement can be expected. A neuropsychologic study in nine patients with previous epilepsy who were tested before and after status epilepticus found no substantial changes in cognitive ability.[24]

Mortality in status epilepticus is based on hospital series alone; therefore, considerable referral bias exists. A review of deaths related to status epilepticus found a mortality of 2% in adult status epilepticus.[62] In a study of 282 consecutive admissions, mortality from status epilepticus could be linked to an underlying disorder in all but 2 patients.[30] Mortality was higher in patients with stroke if status epilepticus occurred within 7 days of stroke.[72] Anoxic-ischemic insult to the brain and older age predicted mortality in status epilepticus and could be related to cardiac resuscitation in the first place.[16,44,83]

The risk of subsequent epilepsy in adult patients with de novo status epilepticus is 12% and includes a small risk of recurrent status epilepticus.[62] Risks are higher in patients with known structural lesions, onset of seizure disorder during adolescence, and neurologic abnormalities.[13] In general, predictive factors for poor outcome include the lack of response to first treatment and the underlying cause of sta-

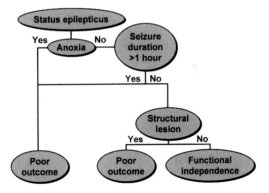

Figure 24–3. Outcome algorithm for status epilepticus. Poor outcome: severe disability or death, vegetative state. Functional independence: no assistance needed, minor handicap may remain.

tus epilepticus, particularly when they are associated with anoxic-ischemic encephalopathy, acute stroke, encephalitis, diffuse axonal head injury, or a primary malignant tumor.[45] Status epilepticus lasting more than 1 hour and status epilepticus associated with anoxic ischemic injury and age significantly increase the odds of a higher incidence of mortality and severe, persistent disability.[69] An outcome algorithm is shown in Figure 24–3.

CONCLUSIONS

- One can expect that a large proportion of patients with status epilepticus can be controlled with benzodiazepines (lorazepam, 4 to 8 mg) and an adequate loading dose of phenytoin (20 mg/kg, 50 mg/minute).
- Fosphenytoin should be preferred over phenytoin and can be given at a rate of 100 to 150 mg of phenytoin equivalents per minute.
- Recurrence of seizures after adequate phenytoin loading could be treated with midazolam or propofol infusion.
- If all fail, intravenous administration of ketamine, valproate, pentobarbital, or lidocaine should be considered.
- Outcome of status epilepticus is strongly related to the response to the first dose of antiepileptic agent and to the underlying trigger.

REFERENCES

1. Alia G, Natale E, Mattaliano A, et al: On two cases of status epilepticus treated with propofol (abstract). *Epilepsia* 32 Suppl 1:77, 1991.

2. Alldredge BK, Gelb AM, Isaacs SM, et al: A comparison of lorazepam, diazepam, and placebo for the treatment of out-of-hospital status epilepticus. *N Engl J Med* 345:631–637, 2001.

3. Aminoff MJ, Simon RP: Status epilepticus. Causes,

clinical features and consequences in 98 patients. *Am J Med* 69:657–666, 1980.

4. Ballenger CE III, King DW, Gallagher BB: Partial complex status epilepticus. *Neurology* 33:1545–1552, 1983.

5. Barry E, Hauser WA: Status epilepticus and antiepileptic medication levels. *Neurology* 44:47–50, 1994.

6. Bevan JC: Propofol-related convulsions. *Can J Anaesth* 40:805–809, 1993.

7. Bleck TP: Convulsive disorders: status epilepticus. *Clin Neuropharmacol* 14:191–198, 1991.

8. Bleck TP: Advances in the management of refractory status epilepticus (editorial). *Crit Care Med* 21:955–957, 1993.

9. Bleck TP: Management approaches to prolonged seizures and status epilepticus. *Epilepsia* 40 Suppl 1:S59–S63, 1999.

10. Borris DJ, Bertram EH, Kapur J: Ketamine controls prolonged status epilepticus. *Epilepsy Res* 42:117–122, 2000.

11. Brandt L, Saveland H, Ljunggren B, et al: Control of epilepsy partialis continuans with intravenous nimodipine. Report of two cases. *J Neurosurg* 69:949–950, 1988.

12. Brown LA, Levin GM: Role of propofol in refractory status epilepticus. *Ann Pharmacother* 32:1053–1059, 1998.

13. Browne TR, Holmes GL: Epilepsy. *N Engl J Med* 344:1145–1151, 2001.

14. Browne TR, Mikati M: Status epilepticus. In Ropper AH, Kennedy SF (eds): *Neurological and Neurosurgical Intensive Care*. 2nd ed. Rockville, MD: Aspen Publishers, 1988, pp 269–288.

15. Cascino GD: Nonconvulsive status epilepticus in adults and children. *Epilepsia* 34 Suppl 1:S21–S28, 1993.

16. Claassen J, Lokin JK, Fitzsimmons BF, et al: Predictors of functional disability and mortality after status epilepticus. *Neurology* 58:139–142, 2002.

17. Correale J, Rabinowicz AL, Heck CN, et al: Status epilepticus increases CSF levels of neuron-specific enolase and alters the blood-brain barrier. *Neurology* 50:1388–1391, 1998.

18. Cranford RE, Leppik IE, Patrick B, et al: Intravenous phenytoin: clinical and pharmacokinetic aspects. *Neurology* 28:874–880, 1978.

19. Darnell JC, Jay SJ: Recurrent postictal pulmonary edema: a case report and review of the literature. *Epilepsia* 23:71–83, 1982.

20. DeGiorgio CM, Tomiyasu U, Gott PS, et al: Hippocampal pyramidal cell loss in human status epilepticus. *Epilepsia* 33:23–27, 1992.

21. Delgado-Escueta AV, Enrile-Bacsal F: Combination therapy for status epilepticus: intravenous diazepam and phenytoin. *Adv Neurol* 34:477–485, 1983.

22. DeLorenzo RJ, Hauser WA, Towne AR, et al: A prospective, population-based epidemiologic study of status epilepticus in Richmond, Virginia. *Neurology* 46:1029–1035, 1996.

23. Devinsky O, Leppik I, Willmore LJ, et al: Safety of intravenous valproate. *Ann Neurol* 38:670–674, 1995.

24. Dodrill CB, Wilensky AJ: Intellectual impairment as an outcome of status epilepticus. *Neurology* 40 Suppl 2:23–27, 1990.

25. Earnest MP, Marx JA, Drury LR: Complications of intravenous phenytoin for acute treatment of seizures. Recommendations for usage. *JAMA* 249:762–765, 1983.

26. Finelli PF, Cardi JK: Seizure as a cause of fracture. *Neurology* 39:858–860, 1989.

27. Fountain NB, Adams RE: Midazolam treatment of acute and refractory status epilepticus. *Clin Neuropharmacol* 22:261–267, 1999.

28. Garzon E, Fernandes RM, Sakamoto AC: Serial EEG during human status epilepticus: evidence for PLED as an ictal pattern. *Neurology* 57:1175–1183, 2001.

29. Gidal B, Spencer N, Maly M, et al: Valproate-mediated disturbances of hemostasis: relationship to dose and plasma concentration. *Neurology* 44:1418–1422, 1994.

30. Goulon M, Lévy-Alcover MA, Nouailhat F: Etat de mal epileptique de l'adulte. Etude epidemiologique et clinique en réanimation. *Rev Electroencephalogr Neurophysiol Clin* 14:277–285, 1985.

31. Gravenstein JS, Anton AH, Wiener SM, et al: Catecholamine and cardiovascular response to electro-convulsion therapy in man. *Br J Anaesth* 37:833–839, 1965.

32. Guberman A, Cantu-Reyna G, Stuss D, et al: Nonconvulsive generalized status epilepticus: clinical features, neuropsychological testing, and long-term follow-up. *Neurology* 36:1284–1291, 1986.

33. Hamilton NG, Matthews T: Aphasia: the sole manifestation of focal status epilepticus. *Neurology* 29:745–748, 1979.

34. Hauser WA: Status epilepticus: epidemiologic considerations. *Neurology* 40 Suppl 2:9–13, 1990.

35. Hodges BM, Mazur JE: Intravenous valproate in status epilepticus. *Ann Pharmacother* 35:1465–1470, 2001.

36. Jagoda A, Riggio S: Refractory status epilepticus in adults. *Ann Emerg Med* 22:1337–1348, 1993.

37. Johnston SC, Siedenberg R, Min JK, et al: Central apnea and acute cardiac ischemia in a sheep model of epileptic sudden death. *Ann Neurol* 42:588–594, 1997.

38. Kaplan PW: Intravenous valproate treatment of generalized nonconvulsive status epilepticus. *Clin Electroencephalogr* 30:1–4, 1999.

39. Kim JA, Chung JI, Yoon PH, et al: Transient MR signal changes in patients with generalized tonicoclonic seizure or status epilepticus: periictal diffusion-weighted imaging. *AJNR Am J Neuroradiol* 22:1149–1160, 2001.

40. Kofke WA, Young RS, Davis P, et al: Isoflurane for refractory status epilepticus: a clinical series. *Anesthesiology* 71:653–659, 1989.

41. Kumar A, Bleck TP: Intravenous midazolam for the treatment of refractory status epilepticus. *Crit Care Med* 20:483–488, 1992.

42. Lawn ND, Wijdicks EFM: Status epilepticus: a critical review of management options. *Can J Neurol Sci* 29:206–215, 2002.

43. Leppik IE, Derivan AT, Homan RW, et al: Double-blind study of lorazepam and diazepam in status epilepticus. *JAMA* 249:1452–1454, 1983.

44. Logroscino G, Hesdorffer DC, Cascino GD, et al: Long-term mortality after a first episode of status epilepticus. *Neurology* 58:537–541, 2002.

45. Lowenstein DH, Alldredge BK: Status epilepticus at an urban public hospital in the 1980s. *Neurology* 43:483–488, 1993.

46. Lowenstein DH, Aminoff MJ, Simon RP: Barbiturate anesthesia in the treatment of status epilepticus: clinical experience with 14 patients. *Neurology* 38:395–400, 1988.

47. Lowenstein DH, Bleck T, Macdonald RL: It's time to revise the definition of status epilepticus. *Epilepsia* 40:120–122, 1999.

48. Mackenzie SJ, Kapadia F, Grant IS: Propofol infusion for control of status epilepticus. *Anaesthesia* 45:1043–1045, 1990.

49. Meeke RI, Soifer BE, Gelb AW: Isoflurane for the management of status epilepticus. *DICP* 23:579–581, 1989.

50. Meldrum BS, Brierley JB: Prolonged epileptic seizures in primates. Ischemic cell change and its relation to ictal physiological events. *Arch Neurol* 28:10–17, 1973.

51. Nevander G, Ingvar M, Auer R, et al: Status epilepticus in well-oxygenated rats causes neuronal necrosis. *Ann Neurol* 18:281–290, 1985.

52. Oxbury JM, Whitty CW: Causes and consequences of status epilepticus in adults. A study of 86 cases. *Brain* 94:733–744, 1971.

53. Parent JM, Lowenstein DH: Treatment of refractory generalized status epilepticus with continuous infusion of midazolam. *Neurology* 44:1837–1840, 1994.

54. Parviainen I, Uusaro A, Kälviäinen R, et al.: High-dose thiopental in the treatment of refractory status epilepticus in intensive care unit. *Neurology* 59:1249–1251, 2002.

55. Prasad A, Worrall BB, Bertram EH, et al: Propofol and midazolam in the treatment of refractory status epilepticus. *Epilepsia* 42:380–386, 2001.

56. Rashkin MC, Youngs C, Penovich P: Pentobarbital treatment of refractory status epilepticus. *Neurology* 37:500–503, 1987.

57. Remy C, Jourdil N, Villemain D, et al: Intrarectal diazepam in epileptic adults. *Epilepsia* 33:353–358, 1992.

58. Ropper AH, Kofke WA, Bromfield EB, et al: Comparison of isoflurane, halothane, and nitrous oxide in status epilepticus (letter to the editor). *Ann Neurol* 19:98–99, 1986.

59. Runge JW, Allen FH: Emergency treatment of status epilepticus. *Neurology* 46 Suppl 1:S20–S23, 1996.

60. Shaner DM, McCurdy SA, Herring MO, et al: Treatment of status epilepticus: a prospective comparison of diazepam and phenytoin versus phenobarbital and optional phenytoin. *Neurology* 38:202–207, 1988.

61. Sheth RD, Gidal BE: Refractory status epilepticus: response to ketamine. *Neurology* 51:1765–1766, 1998.

62. Shorvon S: Tonic clonic status epilepticus. *J Neurol Neurosurg Psychiatry* 56:125–134, 1993.

63. Shorvon SD: *Status Epilepticus: Its Clinical Features and Treatment in Children and Adults*. Cambridge, NY: Cambridge University Press, 1994.

64. Simon RP: Physiologic consequences of status epilepticus. *Epilepsia* 26 Suppl 1:58–66, 1985.

65. Sinha S, Naritoku DK: Intravenous valproate is well tolerated in unstable patients with status epilepticus. *Neurology* 55:722–724, 2000.

66. So EL: Integration of EEG, MRI, and SPECT in localizing the seizure focus for epilepsy surgery. *Epilepsia* 41 Suppl 3:S48–S54, 2000.

67. Tien RD, Felsberg GJ: The hippocampus in status epilepticus: demonstration of signal intensity and morphologic changes with sequential fast spin-echo MR imaging. *Radiology* 194:249–256, 1995.

68. Tigaran S, Rasmussen V, Dam M, et al: ECG changes in epilepsy patients. *Acta Neurol Scand* 96:72–75, 1997.

69. Towne AR, Pellock JM, Ko D, et al: Determinants of mortality in status epilepticus. *Epilepsia* 35:27–34, 1994.

70. Treiman DM: Generalized convulsive status epilepticus in the adult. *Epilepsia* 34 Suppl 1:S2–S11, 1993.

71. Treiman DM, Meyers PD, Walton NY, et al: A comparison of four treatments for generalized convulsive status epilepticus. Veterans Affairs Status Epilepticus Cooperative Study Group. *N Engl J Med* 339:792–798, 1998.

72. Velioglu SK, Ozmenoglu M, Boz C, et al: Status epilepticus after stroke. *Stroke* 32:1169–1172, 2001.

73. Walker IA, Slovis CM: Lidocaine in the treatment of status epilepticus. *Acad Emerg Med* 4:918–922, 1997.

74. Wallis W, Kutt H, McDowell F: Intravenous diphenylhydantoin in treatment of acute repetitive seizures. *Neurology* 18:513–525, 1968.

75. Walls RM, Sagarin MJ: Status epilepticus. *N Engl J Med* 339:409, 1998.

76. Walton NY: Systemic effects of generalized convulsive status epilepticus. *Epilepsia* 34 Suppl 1:S54–S58, 1993.

77. Wieshmann UC, Symms MR, Shorvon SD: Diffusion changes in status epilepticus. *Lancet* 350:493–494, 1997.

78. Wijdicks EF: Propofol in myoclonus status epilepticus in comatose patients following cardiac resuscitation. *J Neurol Neurosurg Psychiatry* 73:94–95, 2002.

79. Wijdicks EFM, Hubmayr RD: Acute acid-base disorders associated with status epilepticus. *Mayo Clin Proc* 69:1044–1046, 1994.

80. Wilder BJ (ed): The use of parenteral antiepileptic drugs and the role for fosphenytoin. *Neurology* 46 Suppl 1:S1–S28, 1996.

81. Williamson PD, Spencer DD, Spencer SS, et al: Complex partial status epilepticus: a depth-electrode study. *Ann Neurol* 18:647–654, 1985.

82. Wood PR, Browne GP, Pugh S: Propofol infusion for the treatment of status epilepticus (letter to the editor). *Lancet* 1:480–481, 1988.

83. Wu YW, Shek DW, Garcia PA, et al: Incidence and mortality of generalized convulsive status epilepticus in California. *Neurology* 58:1070–1076, 2002.

84. Yaffe K, Ferriero D, Barkovich AJ, et al: Reversible MRI abnormalities following seizures. *Neurology* 45:104–108, 1995.

85. Young GB, Blume WT, Bolton CF, et al: Anesthetic barbiturates in refractory status epilepticus. *Can J Neurol Sci* 7:291–292, 1980.

25

Guillain-Barré Syndrome

Guillain-Barré syndrome (GBS) is an acute, self-limiting, inflammatory, demyelinating polyneuropathy. The incidence has remained fairly constant at 1 per 100,000, but outbreaks, often of unknown cause, continue to occur.

Guillain-Barré syndrome is commonly precipitated by an infection, often a trivial viral respiratory infection. Certain pathogens predominate as triggers in GBS, mainly *Campylobacter jejuni*, cytomegalovirus, Epstein-Barr virus, and *Mycoplasma pneumoniae*.[32,42] Other, less robust, associations are vaccinations, surgery, and cancer.[43,64] A puzzling finding is that no preceding illness can be identified in one-third of the patients.

The immunopathogenesis of GBS has remained elusive since its original description in 1916.[29,37,88] Recent studies have suggested that complement activation triggers myelin destruction. Complement cascade activation is mediated by the binding of antibodies to the Schwann cells and results in vesicular myelin degeneration.[33] The axon may be a target as well, often after *Campylobacter jejuni* infection, or may be involved in more severe manifestations of GBS ("the innocent bystander theory"). The proclivity of motor axonal involvement has led to the designation "acute motor axonal neuropathy (AMAN)." Lack of demyelinization but presence of macrophages within the periaxonal spaces of myelinated fibers in these patients is highly suggestive of direct macrophage invasion.[28] A competing explanation involves antibodies to ganglioside

epitopes or myelin proteins.[37] *Campylobacter* infection from undercooked poultry has been confirmed as a prominent trigger for severe forms of GBS, and the putative immunologic pathways have been characterized better than those of any other possible infection. The lipopolysaccharide of *Campylobacter* shows a homology with epitopes in gangliosides of the peripheral nerves, a suggestion of molecular mimicry. The risk of GBS developing after *Campylobacter* infection is very low, probably 1 in every 1000 cases of *Campylobacter* infection.[50,51,58]

First and foremost, patients with GBS usually are managed on wards, but if their clinical condition is deteriorating, admission to the NICU or at least to a room with a monitored bed is justified. Unchallenged admission criteria are respiratory muscle failure, accumulating secretions from oropharyngeal weakness and poor coughing, and evolving aspiration pneumonia. Dysautonomia—usually onset of a cardiac arrhythmia or fluctuations in blood pressure—clearly should prompt admission to the NICU. Similarly, chest tightness or marked hypotension during the first course of plasma exchange necessitates transfer to the unit. Medical reasons for admission to a neurologic or medical intensive care unit are sepsis syndrome, suspected pulmonary embolism, and gastrointestinal complications. Uncertainty about progression of respiratory muscle weakness warrants brief admission to the neurologic unit for overnight monitoring of respiratory mechanics. This concern is particularly legitimate in a bed-bound patient with rapid onset of upper limb weakness and oropharyngeal involvement, bilateral facial palsy, and worsening pulmonary function.[44]

CLINICAL RECOGNITION

To some extent, GBS is easy to diagnose. The diagnosis becomes more difficult in circumstances in which the clinical presentation is more protean.

Limb paresthesias, germane to typical GBS, are presenting signs. They often begin in the wrists and ankles and are experienced as a "tight band" or "nagging prickling sensation" but also as a "feeling of rocks in the shoes." The paresthesias gradually become scattered over the limbs and include the more proximal parts. Weakness is notable 1 to 2 days after the onset of pares-

thesias and begins in the more proximal muscles, causing difficulty with climbing stairs, getting out of a chair, and, if the disease progresses rapidly, lifting the arms. The tendon reflexes become absent or depressed in weak limbs but may be initially spared in limbs that are not affected or are mildly weak and still can overcome the pull of gravity. Complete areflexia occurs in virtually all bed-bound patients. Thus, retained tendon reflexes in an otherwise seemingly clear-cut case of GBS may point to other causes such as thallium or arsenic poisoning or to botulism.

Cramping, deep aching pain, and limb dysesthesias are accompanying symptoms in most patients, specifically in the proximal muscles, back, and buttocks (often referred to as "charley horse").[57] Shooting pain may occur when sudden movements are made and can be excruciating for several seconds[68] (Chapter 4).

Facial weakness, very common in early GBS, does not necessarily imply further progression

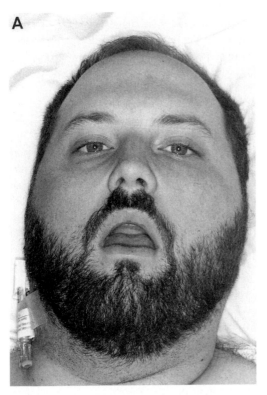
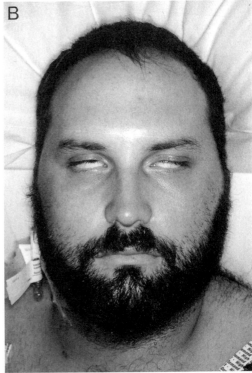

Figure 25–1. Guillain-Barré syndrome with prominent bifacial palsy. Patient is asked to (*A*) smile and (*B*) attempts to close both eyes with force.

to bulbar involvement or ophthalmoplegia but is more commonly associated with respiratory failure and may precede it[44] (Fig. 25–1).

The emergence of ptosis, ophthalmoplegia, or oropharyngeal weakness during progression of limb weakness clearly suggests an overwhelming inflammatory reaction and a possibility of axonal damage with longer recuperation. Oropharyngeal weakness is manifested by difficulty in swallowing solid foods and clearing secretions, loss of vocal clarity, and some degree of dysarthria. Oropharyngeal weakness may occur in approximately one-third of hospitalized patients. With each breath, aspiration of unswallowed saliva may occur, and patients

seem to consciously plan their breathing efforts. Intubation for airway protection alone is imperative at this stage.

Ptosis is often severe, up to a point that effort is needed to briefly open the eyelids (Fig. 25–2).

Respiratory failure occurs on average within 1 week after the onset of paresthesias. It is unusual for diaphragmatic failure to develop more than 2 weeks into the illness. The clinical signs and symptoms of neuromuscular failure have been detailed in Chapter 5. Again, respiratory failure in GBS is evident by interrupted speech; patients tend to speak with only a few syllables to each breath. Besides in-

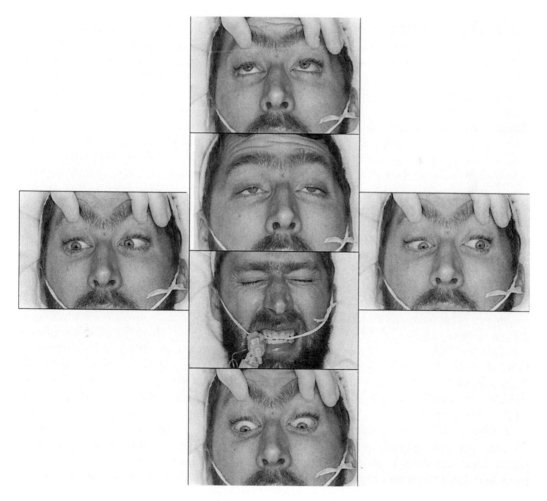

Figure 25–2. Patient with Guillain-Barré syndrome who has bilateral ptosis and partial ophthalmoplegia. There is no facial muscle weakness.

creased respiratory rate and small tidal volumes, many patients have mild tachycardia and sweating on the forehead. Rapid decline within the day of admission, including "crash" (sudden respiratory distress), may occur quite unexpectedly. In our study, intubation between 6 P.M. and 8 A.M. was common, a suggestion that the early signs of acute neuromuscular failure during the day were not recognized.[44] Nocturnal decompensation could also be due to impairment of central respiratory drive along with poor pulmonary mechanics.[44] A gradual decline (e.g., 30% reduction in vital capacity over more than 1 day) is much less common.

Regional variants introduced by Ropper[65] include pharyngeal-cervical-brachial weakness, paraparetic weakness, bilateral facial weakness and paresthesias, sixth-nerve paresis with paresthesias, and lumbar plexopathy. Other well-established, but no more frequent, clinical presentations are Fisher's variant (recently also described with pharyngeal-cervical-brachial weakness), pure motor GBS without the classic presenting paresthesias, pure sensory GBS, and pure dysautonomia. The typical clinical findings in the Fisher variant are characterized by various degrees of ophthalmoplegia, ptosis, gait ataxia, and areflexia and virtually no limb, facial, or oropharyngeal weakness. Half the patients may have progression to a more generalized weakness, often within a week of presentation.[71] Patients with these variants of GBS are admitted to the intensive care unit, because many of the disorders produce considerable difficulty in the clearing of secretions, and endotracheal intubation is often imminent. Whether any of these subtypes are defined by a certain infection trigger is not clear. Early data, however, suggest links between severe (axonal) GBS and *Campylobacter* and cytomegalovirus with a fulminant form.[82]

In patients with predominant ptosis, ophthalmoplegia, and oropharyngeal weakness at presentation, one should consider myasthenia gravis and other myasthenic syndromes, polymyositis, and botulism. Often the evaluation needs to be completed during their stay in the intensive care unit. Careful clinical and electrodiagnostic examinations should suffice to differentiate the disorders. Although most likely uncommon in any patient with acute flaccid paralysis, fulminant vasculitis, botulism, organophosphate poisoning, ingestion of the fruit of the buckthorn shrub, glue sniffing, and snake and spider bites should be considered. A remarkable presentation is tick paralysis, a disorder in children but also in young adults.[19,73,80] Within hours to days after neurotoxin from the female tick interferes with voltage-gated sodium channels of axons, ascending paralysis occurs. It is common in spring and summer and in southeastern and northwestern parts of the United States. The ticks may settle in the scalp (young girls with long hair may be predisposed), axilla, or perineum. Recovery occurs within 24 hours after removal of the tick, baffling all description.[19,73,80]

Porphyria may be manifested by an acute flaccid paralysis and should certainly be suspected when barbiturates have recently been administered. In certain areas (e.g., Caribbean islands), ciguatera (puffer fish) poisoning is endemic and a more common cause for paresthesias and rapid weakness than GBS.

The most frequent diseases mimicking GBS and their distinguishing features are summarized in Table 25–1.[71]

NEUROIMAGING AND LABORATORY TESTS

Exclusion of acute spinal cord disease or brain stem involvement may require neuroimaging studies, but they generally have a low priority in the evaluation of GBS. Magnetic resonance imaging of the spine is often performed in patients with atypical presentations, such as predominant paraparesis. Pronounced gadolinium enhancement (indicating breakdown of the blood–nerve barrier) of the anterior spinal nerve roots, conus medullaris, and cauda equina has been reported in GBS,[10,14,26,60] most often in the most severe cases.

Magnetic resonance imaging findings in the brain are normal, but cranial nerve enhancement has been noted.[23] In Fisher's variant, a

Table 25–1. Disorders Frequently Mimicking Guillain-Barré Syndrome

Disease	Relevant Clinical Features	Helpful Laboratory Tests
Transverse myelitis	Sensory level	MRI of spine with gadolinium
	Urinary incontinence	CSF: pleocytosis (> 200 cells)
	No facial or bulbar involvement	
Myasthenia gravis	Marked fatiguing ptosis and ophthalmoplegia	EMG, NCV, repetitive stimulation
	Intact tendon reflexes	CSF: normal
	Masseter weakness	Neostigmine test
	No dysautonomia	
Vasculitic neuropathy	History of PAN, SLE, WG, RA	Chest and sinus radiographs or CT scan of thorax
	Pain without paresthesias	
	Marked asymmetry of weakness	Nerve and muscle biopsies
Carcinomatous or lymphomatous meningitis	Mental changes	CSF cytology
	Radicular pain	MRI with gadolinium
	Asymmetrical cranial nerve involvement	MRI of spine or brain with gadolinium

CSF, cerebrospinal fluid; CT, computed tomography; EMG, electromyography; MRI, magnetic resonance imaging; NCV, nerve conduction velocity; PAN, polyarteritis nodosa; RA, rheumatoid arthritis; SLE, systemic lupus erythematosus; WG, Wegener's granulomatosis.

double dose of gadolinium enhanced the third, sixth, and seventh nerves.[25] Occasionally, a chronic inflammatory demyelinating polyneuropathy is manifested as acute GBS. Abnormal magnetic resonance imaging findings of multifocal white matter lesions in periventricular and brain stem locations have been reported in patients with chronic inflammatory demyelinating polyneuropathy, but neither their diagnostic value nor their significance is known.[54]

Electrodiagnostic studies remain the most sensitive tests in the evaluation of GBS. The most common patterns are motor nerve conduction block (Fig. 25–3), prolonged distal latency, temporal dispersion, slowing of nerve conduction, and increased F-wave latency. Sural nerve conduction can be normal in combination with abnormal median sensory conduction.[1] Detection of these abnormalities is contingent on a competent and comprehensive electrophysiologic study. This could be arbitrarily defined as stimulation of at least two motor and sensory nerves each in the arms or legs, assessment of conduction block, recording of F waves with attention to impersistence, determination of H reflex and blink reflexes, testing of the trigeminal and facial nerves, and needle examination in at least one distal and one proximal muscle, with confirmation in contralateral muscles when findings are abnormal.

This protocol invariably produces abnormal study results in patients with GBS who are several days into the illness. When study results appear normal, the electromyographer typically should refocus attention on early abnormalities, such as prolongation, dispersion, or

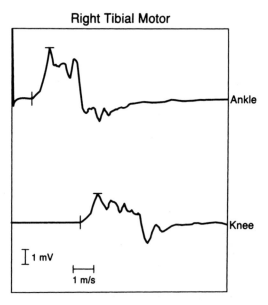

Figure 25–3. Conduction block (decline in compound motor action potential amplitude) in Guillain-Barré syndrome.

absence of F waves.[70,83] The results of a comprehensive study in 113 consecutive patients at the Massachusetts General Hospital are summarized in Table 25–2.[70]

Prolonged phrenic nerve latency was common in one study (78%) but occurred in both ventilated and nonventilated patients with GBS. This study also emphasized that normal phrenic nerve conduction (the minority of the patients) was associated with normal respiratory mechanics.[92] Phrenic nerve conduction studies may help in establishing the diagnosis,[12] but whether a documented abnormality predicts pending respiratory failure more reliably than abnormal clinical findings or respiratory function variables is uncertain.

Table 25–2. Electrodiagnostic Findings in 113 Consecutive Patients with Guillain-Barré Syndrome*

	PATIENTS	
Finding	No.	%
PCB and DL	30	27
Isolated PCB	31	27
Generalized slowing	25	22
PCB and DCB	11	10
Isolated DL	6	5
PCB and ICB	4	4
Absent response	2	2
PCB, ICB, and DL	1	1
DL and ICB	1	1
Isolated ICB	1	1
Normal†	1	1
Total	113‡	

*The major motor nerve abnormalities were categorized as follows:

1. *Distal lesion* (DL): > 15% increase in duration of compound muscle action potential (CMAP) or increased distal motor latency on distal stimulation, with motor nerve conduction velocity > 80% of the lower limit of normal.

2. *Distal conduction block* (DCB): decreased CMAP amplitude (median or ulnar CMAP, < 4000 μV; peroneal or tibial CMAP, < 2000 μV) in at least two nerves, with normal motor nerve conduction velocity, duration of CMAP, and distal motor latency.

3. *Proximal conduction block* (PCB): absent F waves or decreased F-wave persistence in the presence of motor nerve conduction velocity > 80% of the lower limit of normal, and no distal or intermediate block in the same nerve.

4. *Intermediate conduction block* (ICB): > 40% reduction between distal (D) and proximal (P) stimulation sites, specifically in the following ratio: [CMAP (D) − CMAP (P)] / [CMAP (D)] × 100 with < 10% difference in duration between sites without distal conduction block, increased duration, or distal motor latency in the same nerve.

5. *Generalized slowing*: maximum motor conduction velocity < 80% of the lower limit of normal in at least two of the median, ulnar, peroneal, or tibial nerves.

6. *Absent response*: no evoked motor response with distal stimulation sites in at least three nerves.

7. *Multiple abnormalities*: a combination of two or more of abnormalities 1 through 4, above; the same combination was found in at least two nerves.

8. *Denervation*: at least two muscles in the arms and two in the legs were examined for spontaneous activity in the form of fibrillation potentials or positive sharp deflections.

†Prolonged F-wave latencies were found on repeated testing 2 days later.

‡Electromyography demonstrated extensive fibrillation in 10 patients.

Source: Ropper AH, Wijdicks EFM, Shahani BT: Electrodiagnostic abnormalities in 113 consecutive patients with Guillain-Barré syndrome. Arch Neurol 47:881–887, 1990. By permission of the American Medical Association.

Nerve biopsy in typical GBS is rarely performed and, as mentioned, the sural nerve may be spared in acute motor axonal variants.[49] Biopsy could be considered if the clinical suspicion of a rapidly progressive polyneuropathy from vasculitis is very strong, but usually other laboratory abnormalities point to the diagnosis.

Examination of the CSF typically shows normal cell counts and increased protein in the early days of the illness, and abnormal findings level off after 1 month (Fig. 25–4). Marked pleocytosis (> 20 cells) is associated with human immunodeficiency virus and Lyme disease, and if this abnormality is found, serology and polymerase chain reaction testing should be done. Greatly increased protein values may be associated with papilledema. Papilledema may be due to decreased CSF absorption from high protein concentration, but this mechanism has been questioned.[4] In patients with variants of GBS, cerebrospinal fluid protein values tend to be normal, causing additional diagnostic confusion, but often electrophysiologic studies clinch the diagnosis.

Many other laboratory test results can be abnormal. These include liver function abnormalities that can be associated with coexisting hepatitis (A, B, or C), cytomegalovirus, or Epstein-Barr virus. Liver function abnormalities are more often observed (up to severalfold more than the upper limits of normal) in patients treated with intravenous immune gamma globulin (IVIG)[59] but may occur in 10% to 20% of untreated patients.[71] Currently, pretreatment (including treatment with a solvent and detergent) of IVIG preparations to inactivate hepatitis C and other membrane-enveloped viruses excludes this possible explanation. The

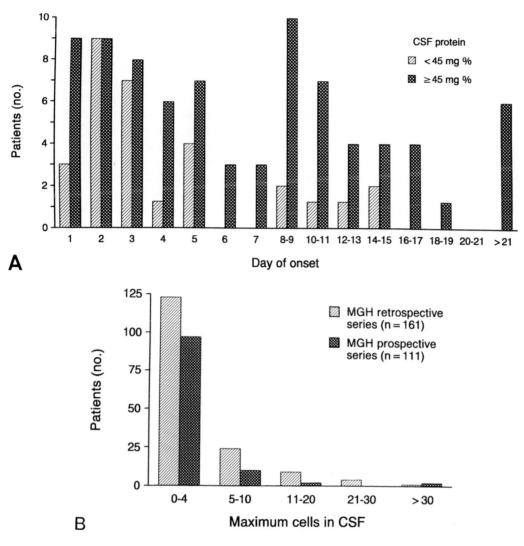

Figure 25–4. (A) Cerebrospinal fluid (CSF) protein and (B) cell counts. MGH, Massachusetts General Hospital. (Modified from Ropper et al.[71] By permission of FA Davis Company.)

mechanism of liver function abnormalities in GBS is unknown.

Patients with GBS may have a transient increase in sedimentation rate and increased white blood cell counts without concomitant infections. Because the creatine kinase level may become markedly elevated in patients with severe pain, some degree of muscle necrosis is suggested as a mechanism rather than a neurogenic cause for the increase.

Autoantibodies targeting gangliosides have been characterized and can be fairly easily obtained by serologic tests. GM_1 is a major ganglioside that is diffusely located in either the myelin or the axon. Both clinically and in an animal model, antibody reactivity to GM_1 has been linked to a severe and pure motor variant of GBS. Anti-GM_{1b} antibodies were found more commonly in *Campylobacter*-associated GBS, and progression was more severe.[90,91] Antibodies to another ganglioside, GQ_{1b}, are highly specific for the Fisher variant and are found in high titers.[37] Measurement of these antibodies is not common practice but may have implications for prognosis and therapy. A recent unconfirmed study suggested that a subgroup with anti-GM_{1b}-positive antibodies had a better response with IVIG.[90]

Respiratory variables remain important, and serial measurements are very helpful in anticipating mechanical ventilation. Vital capacity of less than 20 mL, maximum inspiratory pressure (PImax) of less than 30 cm H_2O, and maximum expiratory pressure (PEmax) of less than 40 cm H_2O ("20–30–40 rule") or any reduction of more than 30% from baseline in any of these values highly predicts the need for endotracheal and mechanical ventilation.[44]

FIRST STEPS IN MANAGEMENT

The initial steps in management of a patient with GBS depend on several clinical features. Pivotal factors that direct the way at the bedside are severity of weakness or rapidity of progression, involvement of neuromuscular respiratory weakness, dysautonomia, an early systemic complication, and comorbid disease. The initial management in GBS is summarized in Table 25–3.

Management in GBS, more than in any other neurologic critical illness, is guided by the physiologic changes during prolonged bed rest. These changes do not always pertain to dysautonomia. In any patient confined to bed, plasma volume tends to decrease by 10% in the first week and by 20% in the second week because of venous pooling in the lower extremities. Other cardiovascular alterations in bed rest are

sinus tachycardia, an exaggerated increase in pulse rate, and decreased cardiac output with any type of exercise. The mechanism of orthostasis associated with bed rest may be related to decreased venous return and certainly also to decreased gain of the baroreceptor reflexes.

Fluid intake in patients with GBS includes a 2-L infusion of isotonic saline, which should be adjusted when enteric feeding is started. Larger volumes are needed in patients receiving mechanical ventilation and in those with fever to compensate for imperceptible fluid loss. Hypotension commonly occurs in patients who are transferred to the NICU for mechanical ventilation. The sudden introduction of positive pressure lung inflation diminishes venous return, and in patients who are relatively dehydrated, blood pressure may significantly decrease.

Bed rest alters gastrointestinal function, and the most salient changes are an almost two-thirds reduction in transit time through the stomach, reduced gastric bicarbonate secretion, and slowing of small bowel activity, rapidly leading to constipation. Enteral nutrition is started almost immediately after admission. In patients with diminished swallowing mechanics, a nasogastric tube is placed and daily residuals (less than 50% of infused volume) are carefully monitored. At later stages, high caloric feeding is contraindicated, because energy-rich formulas may seriously hamper weaning from the mechanical ventilator (see Chapter 7). Most patients need a stool softener such as bisacodyl (two tablets a day). Enteral feeding is contraindicated in patients with adynamic ileus.

Table 25–3. Initial Management in Guillain-Barré Syndrome

Airway management	Incentive spirometry, assisted coughing
	Intubation if vital capacity $\leq$ 20 mL/kg and maximum inspiratory pressure $\leq$ -30 mm Hg
Fluid management	2 L of isotonic saline
Nutrition	Full strength enteral nutrition
Specific treatment	IVIG, 0.4 g/kg for 5 days
	Plasma exchange on 5 alternate days for a total of 250 mL/kg if IVIG is not tolerated
	Pantoprazole, 40 mg daily, in mechanically ventilated patients and in patients with previous use of aspirin or other nonsteroidal anti-inflammatory drugs
	Heparin, 5000 U subcutaneously b.i.d.
	Oxycodone or corticosteroids intramuscularly for pain; consider tramadol or epidural morphine

IVIG, intravenous immune globulin.

The possible development of ileus must be monitored daily, but it occurs in only a minority of patients. Adynamic ileus may occur early in the course of GBS and during a bout of dysautonomia, but more commonly it occurs from secondary causes, including opiates given for pain.[9] One must be familiar with the early signs and symptoms of abdominal discomfort, thirst, and increase in pulse rate pari passu with the degree of distention. Auscultation of the abdomen yields typical findings of silence interrupted by transmitted heart sounds and tinkles and occasional successive splashes when the patient moves. Ileus should be treated conservatively with continuous suctioning, liberal intravenous administration of fluids, and placement of a flatus tube. Neostigmine (2 mg intravenously), a parasympathomimetic agent that stimulates colonic contraction, has been considered in patients without response to conservative management.[62] Because of associated bradycardia (despite prophylactic use of atropine or glycopyrrolate), neostigmine is less attractive in GBS and in fact contraindicated in patients with GBS and dysautonomia. Colonic perforation from adynamic ileus is a potential threat but very uncommon (Chapter 32). Parenteral nutrition may be needed if the signs do not subside within days.

Bladder paralysis is not uncommon. Intermittent catheterization, although favored over an indwelling catheter, is impractical and time-consuming; careful attention to sterile handling of a closed system may be preferable. Voiding in patients with detrusor areflexia usually cannot be enhanced by pharmacologic agents.

The management of respiration is a major component of care in severe GBS. Any patient with GBS, and certainly one on the verge of diaphragmatic akinesis, is at considerable risk of atelectasis. The supine position relocates a large proportion of lung tissue into the most dependent third zone, resulting in a tendency toward accumulation of interstitial fluid and closing of alveoli. Bed rest, therefore, produces ventilation and perfusion mismatch, culminating in oxygen desaturation. It is prudent to monitor desaturation with a pulse oximeter.

Lung expansion techniques are important, and in patients with near-marginal tidal volume capacities, a rigorous protocol may prevent deterioration from progressive atelectasis, leading to intubation. Patients with GBS should be helped to perform incentive spirometry hourly (Chapter 3). In addition, patients could be instructed to perform sustained maximal inspiration with cough maneuvers every 30 minutes, a method that has proved effective in reducing postsurgical pulmonary complications and that can also be useful in patients with GBS.[3] Aerosols are useless in nonintubated patients because most of the spray does not reach the most peripheral and lower parts of the respiratory tract. No benefit has been demonstrated with expectorants or aminophylline.

The indications for intubation in patients with neuromuscular failure, including GBS, are summarized in Chapter 5. It is important to emphasize that the use of succinylcholine in paralyzed patients to facilitate endotracheal intubation is contraindicated. Massive potassium release may occur, leading to cardiac arrest. (The risk is most likely increased in patients with long-standing paralysis.)

Most patients are well served with an intermittent mandatory ventilation mode and low settings of positive end-expiratory pressure. Tracheostomy must be postponed for at least 3 weeks in many patients to await the effect of specific therapy,[46,47,86] as described in Chapter 5. We have used a sum score of the pulmonary function tests (vital capacity [mL/kg] + PImax [cm H_2O] + PEmax [cm H_2O]) and compared this score with the score at intubation. Persistent improvement of this sum score may suggest a possibility of weaning within 3 weeks, so that deferral of tracheostomy is indicated. Worsening of the score at the end of the second week of intubation highly predicts prolonged mechanical ventilation, and tracheostomy should be pursued[47] (Chapter 5). Early tracheostomy can also be considered when a prolonged course seems inevitable, such as in axonal motor variants. In these patients, quadriplegia has developed rapidly over several days, with electrodiagnostic findings of widespread fibrillations, low amplitudes or absent responses, and no response after a course of IVIG or plasma exchange. In this circumstance, early tracheostomy allows significantly more comfort and much more effective respiratory care. Tracheostomy may also be considered for comfort in patients with marked bulbar weakness and pooling of secretions but normal respiratory function.[36] Percutaneous dilatory tracheostomy has clear advantages over traditional surgical tracheostomy. Cosmetic disfiguration, which can be substantial and may require later plastic surgery for correction,[86] is not expected in dilatory tracheostomy, which requires an incision of only 1 to 2 inches (Chapter 5).

Skin, eye, and mouth care is crucial to the comfort of quadriplegic patients. The skin must be kept dry, and after washing, lanolin cream should be applied. Special beds may be required, but whether they prevent decubitus is not certain. Eyedrops are necessary in patients who cannot close their eyes completely. Patients with marked ptosis should be asked whether they want their eyes taped open for brief periods. Mouth care includes toothbrushing and careful inspection for oral candidiasis (Chapter 3).

The patient is positioned in the lateral decubitus or frog-like resting position (Chapter 3). The limbs should be maintained in a good anatomical position. Splints, foot boards, or sneakers are needed to prevent contractures. Patients with complete quadriplegia should be asked whether they are in a comfortable position, and a small change in alignment of the limbs and shoulders is often greatly appreciated.

Hot packs relieve pain in many patients, and they are certainly of use before initiation of passive range of movements. Severe pain can be relieved by narcotics, nonsteroidal antiinflammatory drugs, and, in resistant cases, epidural morphine. In patients with excruciating pain and marginal diaphragmatic function, it is probably better to intubate and to treat pain aggressively. Brief, but significant, relief is possible by a single intramuscular injection of 60 mg of methylprednisolone. Burning pain (at the recovery stage) may be treated with amitriptyline or mexiletine (mexiletine is contraindicated in patients with dysautonomia). Carbamazepine, 100 mg three times a day, reduces the opiate requirement (Chapter 4).[77]

Prophylaxis of deep venous thrombosis is important, although the true risk of deep venous thrombosis and pulmonary embolus is low. It is not certain whether intermittent pneumatic compression devices on the calf are sufficient in bed-bound patients. (We have noticed deep venous thrombosis within a week despite intermittent pneumatic devices.) In addition, many patients with GBS cannot tolerate these high-frequency devices. We continue to use heparin administered subcutaneously. However, in a recent series with prophylaxis in the majority of patients, 60% still developed deep venous thrombosis.[24] Prophylaxis for stress ulcers with proton pump inhibitors should be limited to patients who have previously used aspirin or other nonsteroidal anti-inflammatory agents or who are receiving mechanical ventilation and thus seem to be at increased risk for gastrointestinal bleeding (Chapter 32).

Psychologic support must be provided. Some patients are calm and try to obtain adequate rest, but others are anxious, depressed, and dysphoric. High-strung persons may not accept complete immobility and complete dependence on others, and in the end they may put an almost unacceptable burden on family members. Discussions with the patient are necessary daily in the plateau phase, and patients with severe GBS should be told unequivocally that they have been hit hard but that improvement is expected. The future course should be projected as clearly as possible. Many patients need to master patience, and every time a gain in strength is made, even if subtle, one should show enthusiasm in a realistic manner. Depression must be recognized, but the incidence is low in the earlier stages of GBS.

Intravenous immune gamma globulin or plasma exchange is the preferred treatment in typical GBS and in any other type of GBS that produces a bed-bound state or severe ataxia, such as Fisher's variant of GBS.[21,31,34,61] The mode of action of plasma exchange or IVIG has remained speculative. Plasma exchange may remove any of the mediators in the immune response, and IVIG could, by means of anti-idiotypic antibodies, block autoantibodies and neutralize their action on epitopes for nerve conduction.[8] Intravenous immune gamma globulin typically costs less and is definitely much easier to use, but the therapy had been under serious scrutiny after several earlier reports of relapse and continued worsening after treatment. Corticosteroids alone in any dose are of no benefit,[30,38] but outcome is not negatively influenced when continued use is mandated (e.g., in asthma or immunosuppressed patients).[39]

Evidence for a beneficial effect of plasma exchange is based on randomized studies, none of which compared plasma exchange with sham exchange.[15,21,31] North American and French studies, using independent raters, both showed an increase in the number of patients with significant functional change and a reduction in the number of days ventilation was required.[21,31] In the North American study, the median time to walking unassisted was reduced from 85 to 53 days, and in the French study, from 111 to 70 days, both statistically and clinically significant reductions in time to recovery. In approximately one-third to one-half of the patients on a mechanical ventilator who were treated by plasma exchange, effective weaning could be achieved within 2 weeks, obviating tracheostomy.

The benefits of plasma exchange are more pronounced in patients treated within 2 weeks into the illness. The use of plasma exchange in patients who have not reached a bed-bound state has been investigated, because deferring plasma exchange in patients who have clear daily progression but who can still ambulate is too intimidating. Two plasma exchanges significantly reduced clinical deterioration or the later requirement of mechanical ventilation.[22] Plasma exchange is recommended in any patient with a variant syndrome, including Fisher's variant. In Fisher's variant of GBS, ataxia may resolve within weeks after a plasma exchange series (which makes the patient ambulant), but ophthalmoplegia may take considerably longer to abate.

Contraindications to plasma exchange are septic shock, recent myocardial infarction (6 months), marked dysautonomia, and active bleeding. Many surveys of large series of patients treated with plasma exchange have demonstrated that when plasma exchange is performed in hospitals with years of experience in exchange procedures, the incidence of serious complications is very low.[13] The side effects are vasovagal reactions, hypovolemia, allergic reactions, hemolysis from kinking in the tubing, and, uncommonly, air embolization and large hematomas.[6] Adverse reaction to fresh frozen plasma accounts for a comparatively high incidence of anaphylactoid reactions, recognized by fever, rigors, urticaria, wheezing, and hypotension. Currently, albumin 5% is used, with a much lower incidence of anaphylaxis. Plasma exchange using cubital veins is possible if they are spared daily venipuncture for routine laboratory tests, but in others, placement of a central venous catheter is necessary. A significant number of patients have a complication from placement of the venous catheter, and this may be related to operator experience. (In one trial, one patient died from aortic dissection during subclavian vein catheterization.[22]) Generally, it is possible that differences in complication rates in the plasma exchange trials may be related to a higher proportion of small contributing centers with much less experience than the organizing major contributing center. Management strategies to avoid complications of plasma exchange[56] are summarized in Table 25–4.

The actual amount of plasma removed varies from patient to patient but generally is 2 to 4 L, and the time ranges from 90 to 120 minutes. A total of five plasma exchanges on alternate days has remained standard.[22] Red blood cell loss must not be more than 25 mL after one series of five total plasma exchanges. The preferred replacement fluid is albumin 5% to provide the proper oncotic pressure.

A positive effect of plasma exchange can be expected in the week after the series has been completed. Occasionally, progression is halted

Table 25–4. Complications during and after Plasma Exchange

Complication	Potential Causes	Management
Hypocalcemia	Citrate	Prophylactic calcium administration (10 mL of 10% $CaCl_2$; rate, 30 minutes)
Hemorrhage	Depletion of coagulation factors by albumin	2 units of fresh frozen plasma (400–500 mL) at end of each exchange
Anaphylaxis or sensitivity	Anti-IgA antibodies Prekallikrein activator or bradykinin	Diagnostic evaluation after premedication with prednisone, 50 mg orally 13, 7, and 1 hour before treatment; diphenhydramine, 50 mg orally 1 hour before treatment; ephedrine, 25 mg orally 1 hour before treatment and before pheresis
Thrombocytopenia	Filter thrombosis Centrifugal methods	Plasma separation is substituted
Hypovolemia or hypotension	Inadequate or hypo-oncotic volume replacement Cardiac arrhythmia Dysautonomia	5% albumin, continuous flow separations with matched input and output
Postpheresis infection	Immunoglobulin or complement depletion	Intravenous immunoglobulin (100–400 mg/kg)
Hypothermia	Cold replacement fluids	Warming of fluids
Hypokalemia	Albumin devoid of potassium	Add 4 mmol of potassium to each liter of 5% albumin

IgA, immunoglobulin A.

after the first two exchanges. Plasma exchange in patients with rapid quadriplegia with mechanical ventilation almost never leads to rapid clinically appreciable improvement. Progression to neuromuscular respiratory failure resulting in the need for mechanical ventilation has not been prevented with any of the currently available specific therapies.[44]

More recently, IVIG was introduced, and on the basis of two trials that compared plasma exchange with high doses of gamma globulin, it can be concluded that gamma globulin is as effective as plasma exchange.[61,78] Gamma globulin treatment (IVIG, 0.4 g/kg per day for 5 days) should become the preferred treatment simply because of easy infusion through a peripheral catheter and lower costs. Additionally, some hospitals cannot provide timely plasma exchange services. A very small randomized trial of IVIG compared 3 days of therapy with 6 days. A significantly shorter time to walking without assistance was found in mechanically ventilated patients in the 6-day group.[63] However, the practical consequence is not certain, and we continue to give IVIG for 5 days. An infusion guideline is shown in Table 25–5.

Possible disadvantages of gamma globulin have accumulated over the years and have tempered enthusiasm. The adverse effects, all rare, are aseptic meningitis,[5,74,81] acute renal failure,[76] thromboembolic events (including ischemic stroke),[75] anaphylactic shock,[52] and pseudohyponatremia due to a laboratory arti-

Table 25–5. Infusion Guideline for Intravenous Immune Gamma Globulin*

Time (hour)	Rate of Infusion (mL/minute)	Total Dose (mL)
First 1/2	1	30
Second 1/2	3	90
Third 1/2	4	120
Fourth 1/2	5[†]	

*IVIG (intravenous immune gamma globulin) is contraindicated in patients with known anaphylaxis to blood products and in patients with immunoglobulin A deficiency. Usually, 10% IVIG is used; therefore, 0.4 g/kg becomes 4 mL/kg. For a 70 kg patient, the total volume infused would be 280 mL. The infusion dose is increased only if there is no headache (common) and no hypersensitivity reaction.

In case of anaphylaxis: (1) discontinue infusion; (2) epinephrine 1:1000, 0.5 mL intramuscularly; (3) if no improvement, epinephrine 1:10,000, 3 mL intravenously; (4) if refractory bronchospasm, aminophylline, 4 mg/kg intravenously at a rate of 10 mg/minute; maintenance: 0.5 mg/kg per minute intravenously.

[†]Maximum rate (300 mL/hour) until infusion is completed.

fact when an automated method does not correct for increased protein concentrations.[48] Small anecdotal series have suggested a high relapse rate in patients receiving IVIG.[11,41] A large comparative trial has not confirmed a higher relapse rate and again shows that anecdotal science can become biased science and lead to wrong conclusions.[7,61] The efficacy of IVIG is very comparable to that of plasma exchange, and results of a large British-North American trial suggest no difference in outcome at 48 weeks between IVIG and plasma exchange or between one alone and both together.[61] Intravenous immune gamma globulin and plasma exchange can probably both be used in GBS but not simultaneously; the choice is probably determined by availability (periodic shortages are common in the United States) and provider costs (less outside the United States). A trial comparing IVIG with short-term use of methylprednisolone seemed to indicate better outcome with the combination, but the results require confirmation to become generally applicable.[79]

If one accepts the flaws of previous studies (none had placebo or sham exchange), the position that plasma exchange should be used first is untenable because of its obviously greater potential for serious complications.[40] Patients very sensitive to IVIG should receive plasma exchange, but this is seldom seen.

A possible alternative to plasma exchange is CSF filtration. Up to six times, 30 to 50 mL of CSF was filtered and reinfused for several days. No difference in outcome was found compared with that of plasma exchange, but the study was underpowered, and the cost of this procedure has not been established. Its use should be considered highly experimental.[89]

DETERIORATION: CAUSES AND MANAGEMENT

The typical course in GBS is progression to a maximal deficit within 3 weeks after onset of the first paresthesias, a plateau phase ranging from 1 day to 6 months (median, 2 weeks), and gradual improvement in several months. Patients may have a halted progression, stuttering progression, virtually no identifiable plateau phase, recovery interrupted by a relapse that usually is less severe, or an intermittent course over weeks that suggests a chronic inflammatory demyelinating polyneuropathy. These clinical profiles were described before specific therapy, such as plasma exchange or IVIG, was introduced, but there is a possibility that plasma exchange or IVIG modifies the progression phase. Without a clear understanding of what plasma exchange and IVIG modify in the complex immunologic response, their effect on progression or relapse remains mysterious.

Gradual progression may occur during plasma exchange or IVIG, suggesting treatment failure. This situation becomes especially urgent if deterioration continues and intubation and mechanical ventilation are imminent. Typically, symptoms progress rapidly and there may be early electrophysiologic indicators of a severe form of GBS. Additional treatment with another series of IVIG or plasma exchange is unlikely to change this course and may only unnecessarily increase the costs. Supportive therapy is probably the only option.

If motor function unexpectedly worsens after completion of a plasma exchange or IVIG that seemed to have halted progression, another 5-day series of plasma exchange or IVIG should be considered. Data are sparse, and it is not known whether IVIG should follow plasma exchange or vice versa. The half-life of IVIG is 3 to 6 weeks, and there could be a concern that plasma exchange may wash out IVIG. Corticosteroids may be considered (and also other immunosuppressive agents, such as cyclosporine[2]) when it becomes clear that chronic inflammatory demyelinating polyneuropathy is a more likely explanation than a single bout of GBS. New criteria have recently been proposed.[72]

Another clinical course that should be clearly distinguished from the first one is relapse during improvement after the plateau phase.[66] Relapse fortunately is limited, occurs in 5% of patients treated with plasma exchange, and very seldom is as severe as the previous state. A second series of plasma exchange or IVIG in these patients is successful, reversal is more rapid in onset, and the patient's condition returns to the baseline state. The cause of this relapse during improvement is not known. Intercurrent infections have been suggested.[66]

When GBS is worsening, specific expertise is required for management of dysautonomia and the mechanical ventilator. Autonomic storms most commonly occur in patients with rapidly progressive GBS associated with ophthalmoplegia, but the autonomic nervous system may become involved in any degree of weakness. However, dysautonomia is very uncommon in Fisher's syndrome and in chronic inflammatory demyelinating polyneuropathy beginning as GBS.

The most common manifestations are spontaneous blood pressure changes and cardiac arrhythmias. In our series of 114 patients with severe GBS admitted to the NICU, 15% had cardiac arrhythmias, 23% had marked blood pressure fluctuation, and 6% had hypotension, particularly during intubation.[35] Blood pressure changes may be caused by sepsis, pulmonary embolus, or severe electrolyte disturbances, but the appearance of wide fluctuations over minutes is characteristic for dysautonomia (Fig. 25–5). These clinical manifestations are a result of impaired baroreceptor buffering.[69] (Baroreceptor function predominantly involves toning down acute changes in blood pressure. Baroreceptors in the carotid and aortic arch re-

lay to the nucleus solitarius, and vasoconstriction as well as increase in heart rate is seen after hypotensive episodes.) Spontaneous fluctuations in blood pressure are best left alone. Persistent hypotension could be treated by placement in Trendelenburg's position and administration of a bolus of albumin. The use of an alpha antagonist, such as phenylephrine, is problematic, because in some patients it may result in overcompensation to hypertension. Hypertension, which may lead to congestive heart failure in predisposed patients, can be treated with a morphine bolus of 5 to 30 mg and preferably not with beta-blockade (use of β-blockers has been linked to cardiac arrest).

Another dysautonomic feature is cardiac arrhythmia. Arrhythmias are usually insignificant, consisting of sinus bradycardia and sinus tachycardia. More easily than usual, pressure on the eyeball may bring on bradycardia. The procedure is dangerous. We have seen bradycardia with many sinus pauses and believe that the test should be discouraged for diagnosis. In approximately 35% of severely affected patients, vagal spells are recognized. These episodes of sinus bradycardia, sinus arrest, and atrioventricular block are potentially life-threatening. Tracheal suctioning commonly provokes these arrhythmias. Complete heart block may occur, necessitating a temporary pacemaker.[16,17,27] It is prudent to have atropine readily available. In our experience, cardiac arrhythmias are not a common cause of sudden death or significant hypotension, and a pacemaker has not been placed in the last

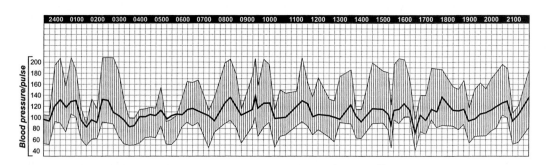

Figure 25–5. Labile blood pressures and pulse from dysautonomia.

100 patients with severe GBS admitted to the Mayo Clinic. Other dysautonomic features are profuse sweating, increased bronchial secretion, and impaired salivation; none of these observed transient phenomena have been carefully studied.

Long-term respiratory management in GBS is a complicated matter, and bronchopneumonia is a major cause of morbidity.[35] Most patients are well served with an intermittent mandatory mode of ventilation and tidal volume settings of 12 to 14 mL/kg to prevent atelectasis.[67] The intermittent mandatory ventilation rate is determined by $PaCO_2$ and pH and must secure normal alveolar ventilation. In many patients with GBS, 6 to 10 breaths per minute provide adequate support in conjunction with normal breathing at this stage of the disease. Only occasionally is a T-piece with pressure support alone sufficient, and in many patients, switching to intermittent mandatory ventilation is necessary, particularly at night.

Weaning from the ventilator in GBS can be expected within 20 to 30 days. The odds of prolonged ventilatory support are markedly increased if patients are not extubated 3 weeks after intubation.

It is very important not to link diaphragmatic weakness with limb weakness. Patients with GBS who have prolonged mechanical ventilation generally first begin to have improvement in diaphragmatic function, often at a time when no signs of motor improvement in the limbs have been noticed for weeks. Weaning should not be entertained when severe dysautonomia is still present, because the stress of weaning may trigger wide blood pressure fluctuations and cardiac arrhythmias.

Weaning trials in GBS have not been compared, but the preferred approach is to reduce intermittent mandatory ventilation and unload the ventilatory muscles with maximum pressure-support ventilation when vital capacity has reached 15 mL/kg and the patient can deliver tidal volumes of 10 to 12 mL/kg. Pressure support is gradually reduced to 5 cm H_2O, a critical value for the decision to extubate (for laboratory weaning criteria, see Chapter 5).

OUTCOME

Guillain-Barré syndrome is a one-time event in the overwhelming majority of patients. Recurrence is very unusual, and patients should be unequivocally told that the risk of recurrence, even with a similar trigger (e.g., vaccination, documented infection), remains low. Because recurrences have been reported in patients receiving vaccinations, it is prudent to refrain from vaccinations except when a premorbid condition (e.g., diabetes, emphysema) dictates vaccination or when the risk of infection is comparatively great (e.g., travel outside the United States). Avoidance of immunizations at least 1 year after the onset of GBS seems good advice, because most reported relapses have occurred within 1 year. Multiple influenza vaccinations have been tolerated in at least one patient after GBS.[84] When GBS has been associated with a specific vaccination, it is advised to avoid that type of vaccination.

Recurrence after a long asymptomatic interval (up to 36 years) has been reported but again with full recovery.[87]

Poor outcome is related to previous serologic documentation of *Campylobacter jejuni* infection, older age, comorbidity (particularly underlying lung disease), and inexcitable motor potentials. In ventilated patients with GBS, increasing age, upper limb paralysis, duration of ventilation (more than 4 months), and delayed transfer to a tertiary institution were significantly more likely to result in poor functional outcome and even mortality.[20] Although repeated claims have been made in the literature, we did not find increased pulmonary morbidity in patients intubated emergently.[85] Mortality is more common in older patients and patients with underlying pulmonary disease and may reach 20% in mechanically ventilated patients.[20,45] Chronic inflammatory demyelinating polyneuropathy may appear as GBS in fewer than 2% of patients, often with fluctuations, persistently elevated protein values, and, more important, very significant slowing of motor conduction velocity. The distinction between acute GBS and chronic inflammatory demyelinating polyneuropathy remains difficult. Most often, patients have a relapse within 2 months of initial treatment.

In at least one study, fatigue was a major component of disability, lasting for years.[55] Physical deconditioning and depression may have contributed, and these factors could be modified.

Patients with GBS recover completely, although examination will reveal that most have slight weakness and hyporeflexia that do not interfere with daily activities. In patients with persistent motor weakness (fewer than 5% of the total population with GBS), improvement may continue up to 2 years after the initial symptoms.[20] Some patients who remain wheelchair-bound recover to walking with splints and braces, often, but not always, with full use of the arms. Factors that have been associated with an increased likelihood of permanent disabling weakness that requires correction with orthopedic appliances are mechanical ventilation for more than 4 months and quadriplegia within a week of onset.[71]

A particularly severe course in GBS associated with rapid quadriplegia, cranial nerve involvement, dysautonomia, and anti-GM_1 antibodies has been linked to an axonal variant of GBS with very slow and often incomplete recovery.[18,28]

The findings on electrodiagnostic examination have marginal long-term prognostic value, but a reduced mean compound muscle action potential amplitude of less than 20% of the lower limit of normal has been identified in a post hoc analysis as predictive of persistent

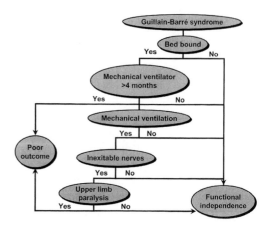

Figure 25–6. Outcome algorithm in Guillain-Barré syndrome. Poor outcome: severe disability and chance of fatal outcome from complications. Functional independence: no assistance needed, minor handicap may remain.

weakness with a need for braces, splints, and wheelchair. Early randomly distributed fibrillations, multifocal conduction block, or inexcitable motor responses in a quadriplegic patient in need of mechanical ventilation suggest a protracted course. Another study found that the combination of early fibrillations with compound muscle action potential amplitude of 10% (or less) often predicts permanent disabling weakness.[53] Factors that do not necessarily indicate poor outcome are the total protein value in CSF, presence of pleocytosis in CSF, profound pain at onset, and time in plateau.

The prediction of disability is summarized in Figure 25–6.

CONCLUSIONS

- Absolute indications for intensive care admission are recent 30% reduction in pulmonary function variables (vital capacity, PImax, PEmax), oropharyngeal weakness, evidence of aspiration on chest radiographs, and dysautonomia.
- IVIG (0.4 g/kg per day for 5 days) or plasma exchange (albumin 5% as replacement fluid) of 250 mL/kg in five sessions on alternate days can be instituted, and they seem equally effective.

- Intubation and mechanical ventilation are indicated in patients with vital capacity less than 20 mL, PImax less than 30 cm H_2O, and PEmax less than 40 cm H_2O ("20–30–40 rule"); hypoxemia; and rapid shallow breathing.
- Tracheostomy must be delayed at least 3 weeks unless there is evidence of the axonal form of GBS or significant bulbar weakness causing marked discomfort in handling secretions.
- Blood pressure changes could be a result of dysautonomia. Drugs used to treat blood pressure may cause exaggerated effects. Complete heart block is rare, and a temporary pacemaker may be necessary. Patients should be monitored for possible adynamic ileus.

REFERENCES

1. Bansal R, Kalita J, Misra UK: Pattern of sensory conduction in Guillain-Barré syndrome. *Electromyogr Clin Neurophysiol* 41:433–437, 2001.
2. Barnett MH, Pollard JD, Davies L, et al: Cyclosporin A in resistant chronic inflammatory demyelinating polyradiculoneuropathy. *Muscle Nerve* 21:454–460, 1998.
3. Bartlett RH: Postoperative pulmonary prophylaxis: breathe deeply and read carefully (letter to the editor). *Chest* 81:1–3, 1982.
4. Behan PO, Harrington H, Sekoni G: Papilloedema in the Landry-Guillain-Barré-Strohl syndrome. *Eur Neurol* 20:62–63, 1981.
5. Bertorini TE, Nance AM, Horner LH, et al: Complications of intravenous gammaglobulin in neuromuscular and other diseases. *Muscle Nerve* 19:388–391, 1996.
6. Bouget J, Chevret S, Chastang C, et al: Plasma exchange morbidity in Guillain-Barré syndrome: results from the French prospective, randomized, multicenter study. The French Cooperative Group. *Crit Care Med* 21:651–658, 1993.
7. Bril V, Ilse WK, Pearce R, et al: Pilot trial of immunoglobulin versus plasma exchange in patients with Guillain-Barré syndrome. *Neurology* 46:100–103, 1996.
8. Buchwald B, Ahangari R, Weishaupt A, et al: Intravenous immunoglobulins neutralize blocking antibodies in Guillain-Barré syndrome. *Ann Neurol* 51:673–680, 2002.
9. Burns TM, Lawn ND, Low PA, et al: Adynamic ileus in severe Guillain-Barré syndrome. *Muscle Nerve* 24:963–965, 2001.
10. Byun WM, Park WK, Park BH, et al: Guillain-Barré syndrome: MR imaging findings of the spine in eight patients. *Radiology* 208:137–141, 1998.
11. Castro LH, Ropper AH: Human immune globulin infusion in Guillain-Barré syndrome: worsening during and after treatment. *Neurology* 43:1034–1036, 1993.
12. Chen R, Collins S, Remtulla H, et al: Phrenic nerve conduction study in normal subjects. *Muscle Nerve* 18:330–335, 1995.
13. Couriel D, Weinstein R: Complications of therapeutic plasma exchange: a recent assessment. *J Clin Apheresis* 9:1–5, 1994.
14. Crino PB, Zimmerman R, Laskowitz D, et al: Magnetic resonance imaging of the cauda equina in Guillain-Barré syndrome. *Neurology* 44:1334–1336, 1994.
15. Dyck PJ, Kurtzke JF: Plasmapheresis in Guillain-Barré syndrome (editorial). *Neurology* 35:1105–1107, 1985.
16. Emmons PR, Blume WT, DuShane JW: Cardiac monitoring and demand pacemaker in Guillain-Barré syndrome. *Arch Neurol* 32:59–61, 1975.
17. Favre H, Foex P, Guggisberg M: Use of demand pacemaker in a case of Guillain-Barré syndrome. *Lancet* 1:1062–1063, 1970.
18. Feasby TE, Hahn AF, Brown WF, et al: Severe axonal degeneration in acute Guillain-Barré syndrome: Evidence of two different mechanisms? *J Neurol Sci* 116:185–192, 1993.
19. Felz MW, Smith CD, Swift TR: A six-year-old girl with tick paralysis. *N Engl J Med* 342:90–94, 2000.
20. Fletcher DD, Lawn ND, Wolter TD, et al: Long-term outcome in patients with Guillain-Barré syndrome requiring mechanical ventilation. *Neurology* 54:2311–2315, 2000.
21. French Cooperative Group on Plasma Exchange in Guillain-Barré Syndrome: Efficiency of plasma exchange in Guillain-Barré syndrome: role of replacement fluids. *Ann Neurol* 22:753–761, 1987.
22. French Cooperative Group on Plasma Exchange in Guillain-Barré Syndrome: Appropriate number of plasma exchanges in Guillain-Barré syndrome. *Ann Neurol* 41:298–306, 1997.
23. Fulbright RK, Erdum E, Sze G, et al: Cranial nerve enhancement in the Guillain-Barré syndrome. *AJNR Am J Neuroradiol* 16 Suppl:923–925, 1995.
24. Gaber TAK, Kirker SGB, Jenner JR: Current practice of prophylactic anticoagulation in Guillain-Barré syndrome. *Clin Rehabil* 16:190–193, 2002.
25. Garcia-Rivera CA, Zhou D, Allahyari P, et al: Miller Fisher syndrome: MRI findings. *Neurology* 57:1755, 2001.
26. Gorson KC, Ropper AH, Muriello MA, et al: Prospective evaluation of MRI lumbosacral nerve root enhancement in acute Guillain-Barré syndrome. *Neurology* 47:813–817, 1996.
27. Greenland P, Griggs RC: Arrhythmic complications in the Guillain-Barré syndrome. *Arch Intern Med* 140:1053–1055, 1980.
28. Griffin JW, Li CY, Ho TW, et al: Pathology of the motor-sensory axonal Guillain-Barré syndrome. *Ann Neurol* 39:17–28, 1996.
29. Guillain G, Barré J, Strohl A: Sur un syndrome de radiculo-neurite avec hyperalbuminose du liquide

cephalo-rachidien sans reaction cellulaire. Remarques sur les caracteres cliniques et graphiques des reflexes tendineux. *Rev Neurol* 40:1462–1470, 1916.

30. Guillain-Barré Syndrome Steroid Trial Group: Double-blind trial of intravenous methylprednisolone in Guillain-Barré syndrome. *Lancet* 341:586–590, 1993.

31. The Guillain-Barré Syndrome Study Group: Plasmapheresis and acute Guillain-Barré syndrome. *Neurology* 35:1096–1104, 1985.

32. Hadden RD, Karch H, Hartung HP, et al: Preceding infections, immune factors, and outcome in Guillain-Barré syndrome. *Neurology* 56:758–765, 2001.

33. Hafermacko CE, Sheikh KA, Li CY, et al: Immune attack on the Schwann cell surface in acute inflammatory demyelinating polyneuropathy. *Ann Neurol* 39:627–637, 1996.

34. Hammers A, Hardie RJ: Miller-Fisher syndrome with rapid recovery (letter to the editor). *Lancet* 343:1290, 1994.

35. Henderson RD, Lawn ND, Fletcher DD, et al: The morbidity of Guillain-Barré syndrome in patients admitted to the intensive care unit. *Neurology* 60:17–21, 2003.

36. Herschman Z: Tracheostomy in Guillain-Barré syndrome (letter to the editor). *Crit Care Med* 19:743, 1991.

37. Hughes RA, Hadden RD, Gregson NA, et al: Pathogenesis of Guillain-Barré syndrome. *J Neuroimmunol* 100:74–97, 1999.

38. Hughes RA, Newsom-Davis JM, Perkin GD, et al: Controlled trial prednisolone in acute polyneuropathy. *Lancet* 2:750–753, 1978.

39. Hughes RAC, van der Meché FGA: Corticosteroids for Guillain-Barré syndrome (Cochrane review). *The Cochrane Library* 4:2000.

40. Hughes RAC, Wijdicks EFM, Barohn R, et al: Immunotherapy in Guillain-Barré syndrome. American Academy of Neurology practice parameter (submitted for publication).

41. Irani DN, Cornblath DR, Chaudhry V, et al: Relapse in Guillain-Barré syndrome after treatment with human immune globulin. *Neurology* 43:872–875, 1993.

42. Jacobs BC, Rothbarth PH, van der Meché FG, et al: The spectrum of antecedent infections in Guillain-Barré syndrome: a case-control study. *Neurology* 51:1110–1115, 1998.

43. Lasky T, Terracciano GJ, Magder L, et al: The Guillain-Barré syndrome and the 1992–1993 and 1993–1994 influenza vaccines. *N Engl J Med* 339:1797–1802, 1998.

44. Lawn ND, Fletcher DD, Henderson RD, et al: Anticipating mechanical ventilation in Guillain-Barré syndrome. *Arch Neurol* 58:893–898, 2001.

45. Lawn ND, Wijdicks EFM: Fatal Guillain-Barré syndrome. *Neurology* 52:635–638, 1999.

46. Lawn ND, Wijdicks EFM: Tracheostomy in Guillain-Barré syndrome. *Muscle Nerve* 22:1058–1062, 1999.

47. Lawn ND, Wijdicks EFM: Post-intubation pulmonary function test in Guillain-Barré syndrome. *Muscle Nerve* 23:613–616, 2000.

48. Lawn N, Wijdicks EFM, Burritt MF: Intravenous immune globulin and pseudohyponatremia. *N Engl J Med* 339:632, 1998.

49. Lu JL, Sheikh KA, Wu HS, et al: Physiologic-pathologic correlation in Guillain-Barré syndrome in children. *Neurology* 54:33–39, 2000.

50. McCarthy N, Andersson Y, Jormanainen V, et al: The risk of Guillain-Barré syndrome following infection with *Campylobacter jejuni*. *Epidemiol Infect* 122:15–17, 1999.

51. McCarthy N, Giesecke J: Incidence of Guillain-Barré syndrome following infection with *Campylobacter jejuni*. *Am J Epidemiol* 153:610–614, 2001.

52. McCluskey DR, Boyd NA: Anaphylaxis with intravenous gammaglobulin (letter to the editor). *Lancet* 336:874, 1990.

53. McKhann GM, Griffin JW, Cornblath DR, et al: Plasmapheresis and Guillain-Barré syndrome: analysis of prognostic factors and the effect of plasmapheresis. *Ann Neurol* 23:347–353, 1988.

54. Mendell JR, Kolkin S, Kissel JT, et al: Evidence for central nervous system demyelination in chronic inflammatory demyelinating polyradiculoneuropathy. *Neurology* 37:1291–1294, 1987.

55. Merkies IS, Schmitz PI, Samijn JP, et al: Fatigue in immune-mediated polyneuropathies. European Inflammatory Neuropathy Cause and Treatment (INCAT) Group. *Neurology* 53:1648–1654, 1999.

56. Mokrzycki MH, Kaplan AA: Therapeutic plasma exchange: complications and management. *Am J Kidney Dis* 23:817–827, 1994.

57. Moulin DE, Hagen N, Feasby TE, et al: Pain in Guillain-Barré syndrome. *Neurology* 48:328–331, 1997.

58. Nachamkin I, Allos BM, Ho T: *Campylobacter* species and Guillain-Barré syndrome. *Clin Microbiol Rev* 11:555–567, 1998.

59. Oomes PG, van der Meché FGA, Kleyweg RP, et al: Liver function disturbances in Guillain-Barré syndrome: a prospective longitudinal study in 100 patients. *Neurology* 46:96–100, 1996.

60. Perry JR, Fung A, Poon P, et al: Magnetic resonance imaging of nerve root inflammation in the Guillain-Barré syndrome. *Neuroradiology* 36:139–140, 1994.

61. The Plasma Exchange/Sandoglobulin Guillain-Barré Syndrome Trial Group: Randomised trial of plasma exchange, intravenous immunoglobulin, and combined treatments in Guillain-Barré syndrome. *Lancet* 349:225–230, 1997.

62. Ponec RJ, Saunders MD, Kimmey MB: Neostigmine for the treatment of acute colonic pseudo-obstruction. *N Engl J Med* 341:137–141, 1999.

63. Raphael J-C, Chevret S, Harboun M, et al: Intravenous immune globulins in patients with Guillain-Barré syndrome and contraindications to plasma exchange: 3 days versus 6 days. *J Neurol Neurosurg Psychiatry* 71:235–238, 2001.

64. Re D, Schwenk A, Hegener P, et al: Guillain-Barré syndrome in a patient with non-Hodgkin's lymphoma. *Ann Oncol* 11:217–220, 2000.

65. Ropper AH: Further regional variants of acute immune polyneuropathy. Bifacial weakness or sixth nerve paresis with paresthesias, lumbar polyradiculopathy, and ataxia with pharyngeal-cervical-brachial weakness. *Arch Neurol* 51:671–675, 1994.

66. Ropper AH, Albert JW, Addison R: Limited relapse in Guillain-Barré syndrome after plasma exchange. *Arch Neurol* 45:314–315, 1988.

67. Ropper AH, Kehne SM: Guillain-Barré syndrome: management of respiratory failure. *Neurology* 35: 1662–1665, 1985.

68. Ropper AH, Shahani BT: Pain in Guillain-Barré syndrome. *Arch Neurol* 41:511–514, 1984.

69. Ropper AH, Wijdicks EFM: Blood pressure fluctuations in the dysautonomia of Guillain-Barré syndrome. *Arch Neurol* 47:706–708, 1990.

70. Ropper AH, Wijdicks EFM, Shahani BT: Electrodiagnostic abnormalities in 113 consecutive patients with Guillain-Barré syndrome. *Arch Neurol* 47:881–887, 1990.

71. Ropper AH, Wijdicks EFM, Truax BT: *Guillain-Barré Syndrome*. Philadelphia: FA Davis Company, 1991.

72. Saperstein DS, Katz JS, Amato AA, et al: Clinical spectrum of chronic acquired demyelinating polyneuropathies. *Muscle Nerve* 24:311–324, 2001.

73. Schaumburg HH, Herskovitz S: The weak child—a cautionary tale. *N Engl J Med* 342:127–129, 2000.

74. Sekul EA, Cupler EJ, Dalakas MC: Aseptic meningitis associated with high-dose intravenous immunoglobulin therapy: frequency and risk factors. *Ann Intern Med* 121:259–262, 1994.

75. Silbert PL, Knezevic WV, Bridge DT: Cerebral infarction complicating intravenous immunoglobulin therapy for polyneuritis cranialis. *Neurology* 42:257–258, 1992.

76. Tan E, Hajinazarian MO, Bay W, et al: Acute renal failure: serious complication of intravenous immunoglobulin G (IVIG) treatment (abstract). *Neurology* 42 Suppl 3:335, 1992.

77. Tripathi M, Kaushik S: Carbamazepine for pain management in Guillain-Barré syndrome patients in the intensive care unit. *Crit Care Med* 28:655–658, 2000.

78. van der Meché FG, Schmitz PI, and the Dutch Guillain-Barré Study Group: A randomized trial comparing intravenous immune globulin and plasma exchange in Guillain-Barré syndrome. *N Engl J Med* 326:1123–1129, 1992.

79. van der Meché FG, van Doorn PA: Guillain-Barré syndrome. *Curr Treat Options Neurol* 2:507–516, 2000.

80. Vedanarayanan VV, Evans OB, Subramony SH: Tick paralysis in children. *Neurology* 59:1088–1090, 2002.

81. Vera-Ramirez M, Charlet M, Parry GJ: Recurrent aseptic meningitis complicating intravenous immunoglobulin therapy for chronic inflammatory demyelinating polyradiculoneuropathy. *Neurology* 42:1636–1637, 1992.

82. Visser LH, van der Meché FG, Meulstee J, et al: Cytomegalovirus infection and Guillain-Barré syndrome: the clinical, electrophysiologic, and prognostic features. Dutch Guillain-Barré Study Group. *Neurology* 47:668–673, 1996.

83. Weinberg DH: AAEM case report 4: Guillain-Barré syndrome. American Association of Electrodiagnostic Medicine. *Muscle Nerve* 22:271–281, 1999.

84. Wijdicks EFM, Fletcher DD, Lawn ND: Influenza vaccine and the risk of relapse of Guillain-Barré syndrome. *Neurology* 55:452–453, 2000.

85. Wijdicks EFM, Henderson RR, McClelland R: Emergency intubation in Guillain-Barré syndrome. *Arch Neurol* 2003. In press.

86. Wijdicks EFM, Lawn ND, Fletcher DD: Tracheostomy scars in Guillain-Barré syndrome: A reason for concern? *J Neurol* 248:527–528, 2001.

87. Wijdicks EFM, Ropper AH: Acute relapsing Guillain-Barré syndrome after long asymptomatic intervals. *Arch Neurol* 47:82–84, 1990.

88. Wijdicks EFM, Ropper AH: Guillain-Barré syndrome. In Koehler PJ, Bruyn GW, Pearce JMS (eds): *Neurological Eponyms*. Oxford: Oxford University Press, 2000, pp 219–226.

89. Wollinsky KH, Hulser PJ, Brinkmeier H, et al: CSF filtration is an effective treatment of Guillain-Barré syndrome: a randomized clinical trial. *Neurology* 57: 774–780, 2001.

90. Yuki N, Ang CW, Koga M, et al: Clinical features and response to treatment in Guillain-Barré syndrome associated with antibodies to GM1b ganglioside. *Ann Neurol* 47:314–321, 2000.

91. Yuki N, Yamada M, Koga M, et al: Animal model of axonal Guillain-Barré syndrome induced by sensitization with GM1 ganglioside. *Ann Neurol* 49:712–720, 2001.

92. Zifko U, Chen R, Remtulla H, et al: Respiratory electrophysiological studies in Guillain-Barré syndrome. *J Neurol Neurosurg Psychiatry* 60:191–194, 1996.

26

Myasthenia Gravis

Among the disorders associated with neuro-muscular respiratory failure, myasthenia gravis is common. Many large institutions have specialized clinics dedicated to the care of patients with severe myasthenia gravis, and this concentration may also increase the annual number of hospital admissions in times of crisis. Serious exacerbation of myasthenia gravis can be encountered in two clinical situations. First, a myasthenic crisis can cause imminent respiratory failure or impairment of swallowing. Important triggers for myasthenic crisis are a viral upper respiratory infection and, less common, recent use of medication that exacerbates the disease. (Administration of certain pharmaceutical agents may be the first time that myasthenia gravis declares itself.) Second, patients with myasthenia gravis have worsened while admitted to a surgical intensive care unit after a surgical procedure, including thymectomy.

Myasthenia gravis is an autoimmune disease, and the pathologic and biochemical processes have been well elucidated. Its pathogenesis can be briefly summarized as an antibody reaction at the antigen epitopes of the acetylcholine receptor, eventually leading to destruction and simplification of the junctional fold and widening of the synaptic cleft.[23,38,58] Defective neurotransmission leads to fatigable muscle weakness. Myasthenia gravis has an incidence of 0.5 to 5 per 100,000 population, occurs at all ages, and may even be frequent in persons older than 60 years.[73] Many patients have lymphoid follicular hyperplasia or thymoma, cells of which

in culture secrete immunoglobulins and acetylcholine receptor antibodies.[38]

The most common reason for admission to the NICU is a need to intervene for acute exacerbation, but often patients are admitted for overnight monitoring of respiratory function as a precautionary measure because their condition may unexpectedly worsen suddenly. The clinical diagnosis of myasthenia gravis often is well established before deterioration, and diagnostic evaluation for generalized muscle weakness is seldom a major focus of attention in the NICU. In fact, many patients with myasthenia gravis have had previous experience with deterioration during intercurrent respiratory infection.

CLINICAL RECOGNITION

Patients admitted to the NICU who are worsening from myasthenia gravis often have abnormal eye movements, oropharyngeal weakness, and proximal limb weakness. Progressive failure of neuromuscular transmission in the diaphragmatic muscle may occur in 30% of patients with myasthenia gravis at the time of diagnosis.

The archetypal clinical finding in myasthenia is fatigability of several muscles.[58,61] Documentation of the severity of weakness at admission is important, but when done, one must take into account and document the time of the last dose of pyridostigmine or neostigmine. The maximal effect can be expected up to 4 hours after administration of either drug, and weakness may not be noticed.

Cranial nerve examination should include assessment of the degree of ptosis and ophthalmoplegia. Ptosis can be defined as a position of the eyelid just crossing the superior limbus.[74] Ptosis is one of the clinical hallmarks in patients with myasthenia gravis, and several tests have been proposed to aggravate it. Ptosis can be aggravated by upward gaze for 3 minutes (Fig. 26–1) and can be relieved by cooling. When ice packed in a surgical glove is placed over a closed eye for 2 minutes, ptosis can be significantly relieved.[74] The ice test is very specific and sensitive, with a positive result in 80% of patients with myasthenia gravis and not in patients without the disorder.[29] Resolution of ptosis may simply be due to resting the eyelid from closure, also known as the "mini-sleep test."[35,55] Interestingly, relief of ptosis on one side by elevation of the eyelid results in aggravation of ptosis on the contralateral side, explained by relaxation of the contracted frontalis muscle. Chronic blinking mimicking blepharospasm with prolonged ptosis, with a response to pyridostigmine, has been noted.[67]

Diplopia is difficult to assess. Fluctuating diplopia can be unmasked by sustained gaze to a fixed target but at a considerable distance to eliminate convergence weakness. Pseudointernuclear ophthalmoplegia has been reported (Fig. 26–2), but in most patients, ocular motility is limited in both vertical and horizontal directions, resulting in marked diplopia.

Bulbar function must be specifically assessed for fatigability and may determine the need for elective intubation. In patients with myasthenia gravis, muscle weakness occurs in the masseters, and jaw opening is typically stronger than jaw closure. The pterygoid muscles, which can be tested by resistance to lateral pressure against the jaw, can be normal. A few attempts at forceful biting on a tongue depressor for 20 seconds produce jaw weakness, and the examiner can easily slide the blade out between the teeth. Nasopharyngeal weakness can be examined by carefully listening for slurring of speech and the nasal tone after the patient is asked to

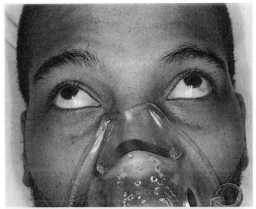

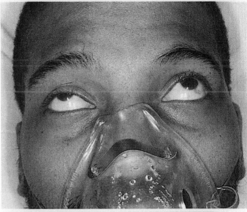

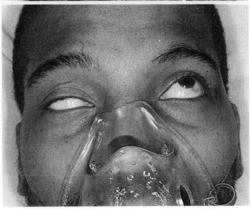

Figure 26–1. Typical "curtain" phenomenon with upgaze.

repeat brief sentences, or the weakness can be provoked by having the patient count to 100. After the patient is asked to puff out both cheeks and to attempt to resist pressure from the examiner's fingers, passage of air through

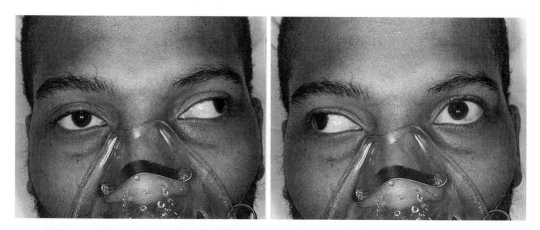

Figure 26–2. Bilateral pseudointernuclear ophthalmoplegia (failure of adduction with abduction nystagmus, often with only occasional brief jerks) in myasthenia gravis.

the nose is typical. Bifacial weakness may be present, shown as a depressed grin or snarl. It is frequently associated with a frown as the patient attempts to alleviate ptosis by lifting the eyebrows. Whistling is impossible (Fig. 26–3).

Dysphagia may be a presenting symptom and can be examined by having the patient take a few sips of water; nasal regurgitation or a flurry of weak and ineffective coughs may result. The gag reflex is often muted. However, careful history-taking may reveal a much longer period of choking on liquids or solid food.[40]

Isolated respiratory failure or exertional stridor[34] as the first manifestation of myasthenia gravis has been reported in a few patients, with bulbar or proximal muscle weakness found after a more careful history and detailed examination.[21,50,53] As in acute neuromuscular respiratory failure of any other cause, respiratory failure in the early stages of myasthenia gravis can be subtle; sweat at the frontal hairline, restless and anxious behavior, inability to count to 20 in one breath, and mild tachypnea are often present (see Chapter 5). In most patients with

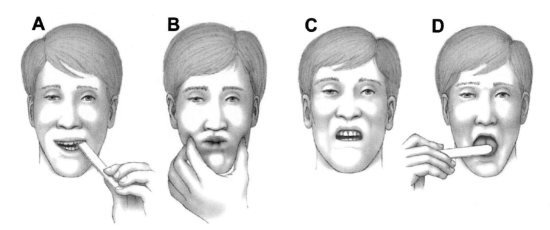

Figure 26–3. Clinical examination of pertinent features in myasthenia gravis. (*A*) Biting on tongue depressor for masseter weakness. (*B*) Puffing out cheeks and resisting pressure from examiner's fingers. (*C*) Ptosis and typical snarl of bifacial weakness. (*D*) Pushing away tongue depressor with tongue.

generalized myasthenia gravis, spontaneous breathing is characterized by short inspiratory and expiratory times with a smaller tidal volume.[76] Reflex tachypnea may result in normal to low PCO_2. An additional primary pulmonary process may cause a mixed clinical picture, often with early hypoxemia.

Weakness in proximal muscle groups should be examined and documented because the findings are valuable clinical guidelines to assess the effects of specific treatment. A useful test, suggested by Watson and Lisak, is the "pump handle" test.[46] (The examiner repeatedly depresses the patient's abducted arm to the side while the patient strongly resists.) Other methods of testing muscle weakness include sitting up from the supine position without the use of the arms and rising from a sitting position. In summary, it is useful to grade proximal muscle strength in patients with myasthenia gravis: the time in minutes a patient is able to hold the arms horizontally outstretched and to hold the legs above the plane of the bed while supine. The Myasthenia Gravis Foundation of America recently published a grading scale of severity[36] (Table 26–1).

Most patients are admitted because of myasthenic crisis,[78] but attention should also be focused on cholinergic signs. A mixed clinical picture is certainly possible if patients have been overmedicated. Excessive salivation, thick bronchial secretions, and diarrhea are important clinical symptoms. Fasciculations may be the only symptom and not immediately evident. (Cholinergic crisis is further described in the subsection on deterioration.)

NEUROIMAGING AND LABORATORY TESTS

The ocular or bulbar type of myasthenia gravis is usually confirmed by electrophysiologic studies. However, it may be mimicked by brain stem compression from a vertebrobasilar aneurysm,[24] intracranial metastasis in the midbrain,[37] or a midbrain glioma.[7] In some of these curious cases, results of edrophonium tests[19] have also been claimed to be positive. Magnetic resonance imaging of the brain therefore seems warranted in patients with the bulbar or ocular type of myasthenia gravis if there is serious concern about the validity of the diagnosis.

Table 26–1. Clinical Classification Proposed by the Myasthenia Gravis Foundation of America

Class I	Any ocular muscle weakness
	May have weakness of eye closure
	All other muscle strength is normal
Class II	Mild weakness affecting muscles other than ocular
	May also have ocular muscle weakness of any severity
IIa	Predominantly affecting limb or axial muscles, or both
	May also have lesser involvement of oropharyngeal muscles
IIb	Predominantly affecting oropharyngeal or respiratory muscles, or both
	May also have lesser or equal involvement of limb or axial muscles, or both
Class III	Moderate weakness affecting muscles other than ocular
	May also have ocular muscle weakness of any severity
IIIa	Predominantly affecting limb or axial muscles, or both
	May also have lesser involvement of oropharyngeal muscles
IIIb	Predominantly affecting oropharyngeal or respiratory muscles, or both
	May also have lesser or equal involvement of limb or axial muscles, or both
Class IV	Severe weakness affecting muscles other than ocular
	May also have ocular muscle weakness of any severity
IVa	Predominantly affecting limb or axial muscles, or both
	May also have lesser involvement of oropharyngeal muscles
IVb	Predominantly affecting oropharyngeal or respiratory muscles, or both
	May also have lesser or equal involvement of limb or axial muscles, or both
Class V	Defined by intubation, with or without mechanical ventilation, except when used during routine postoperative management. The use of a feeding tube without intubation places the patient in class IVb.

Myasthenia gravis is a clinical diagnosis, but the repetitive motor nerve stimulation test, single-fiber electromyography, intravenous administration of a short-acting anticholinesterase drug, such as edrophonium chloride, and measurement of serum acetylcholine receptor antibody titers are helpful tests with acceptable diagnostic accuracy.[5,28]

The edrophonium test is simple to perform when objective markers are available, such as considerable limb weakness, diplopia, and ptosis. Intravenous injection of edrophonium should not be done in patients with asthma and a history of cardiac arrhythmias. The test is less useful in patients with only minor symptoms when improvement cannot be reliably judged. Limb weakness can be quantified by a dynamometer. Diplopia and its response are ideally documented by Lancaster green tests in the office,[83] but only virtually complete disappearance of diplopia has sufficient diagnostic value. Pulmonary function tests can also be performed before and after the edrophonium test.

The edrophonium test can be performed in a blind manner if the cause of deterioration is sufficiently uncertain.[14] Two syringes of 1 mL each are used, one filled with edrophonium, 10 mg/mL, and one with isotonic saline. The best technique is gradual injection of the contents of each syringe in five small increments and subsequent recording of improvement, which should continue for at least 5 minutes. Many patients have a response within minutes after 2 mg has been injected. Atropine should be administered in a dose of 0.5 mg in an intravenous bolus if abdominal cramps, bronchospasm, vomiting, or bradycardia occurs. If bradycardia remains and is associated with a reduction in blood pressure, an additional dose of 1 mg of atropine should be administered.

Alternatively, neostigmine (1.5 mg intramuscularly), often in combination with atropine (0.4 mg subcutaneously), can be administered to test for myasthenia gravis. Its effect is present after 30 minutes and lasts for 1 hour, and although administration of neostigmine may allow more time for observation and additional testing, its delayed effect is not very useful for evaluation of a patient in a critical condition.

Electrodiagnostic studies are important for confirmation of the diagnosis, but the patient should ideally be without medication for 12 hours. Electrodiagnostic results are fairly reliable when testing is done on the day of plasma exchange (because significant improvement by plasmapheresis usually takes 2 or 3 days). The results are abnormal in all patients with severe generalized myasthenia gravis but in only half of them if the disorder is limited to ocular signs.[56]

Surface electrodes are used for repetitive stimulation at a stimulation rate of 2 to 5 Hz before and after maximal voluntary contraction of the tested muscle.[23,69] Recording is from the abductor digiti minimi in a limb warmed to 37°C (low temperatures can mute the decremental response). An abnormal result is usually defined as a 10% or greater decrement of the compound muscle action potential amplitude between the first and the fourth responses with supramaximal stimulation (Fig. 26–4). Response in testing of the proximal muscles is different, with better sensitivity in the deltoid than in the trapezius muscles.[72] Single-fiber electromyography requires special expertise, and the recording surface of the fine concentric needle measures single-fiber action potentials. Single-fiber electromyography has a sensitivity of 95% and typically demonstrates increased jitter and blocking.[28] Jitter, the variation in time intervals among the action potentials, increases with defective neuromuscular function; blocking occurs when nerve impulses fail to generate a muscle action potential.[69,71] Normal jitter in a weak muscle virtually excludes myasthenia gravis. A study suggested that the use of transeyelid techniques to insert a needle in the superior rectus muscle has a high yield in the diagnosis of ocular myasthenia gravis.[65] Needle examination may demonstrate fibrillation, which may indicate functional denervation of the muscle fibers and is generally a marker for more severe disease.

Radioimmunoassay with purified human acetylcholine receptor antigen may demonstrate an acetylcholine receptor binding anti-

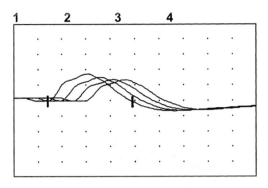

No.	Peak amp (mV)	Amp decr (%)	Area (mVms)	Area decr (%)	Stim level (mA)
1	1.75	0	7.01	0	73
2	1.54	12	6.11	13	73
3	1.40	20	5.50	22	73
4	1.37	22	5.39	23	73

Stimulus frequency 2 Hz, stimulus duration 0.1 ms

Figure 26–4. Repetitive stimulation of the ulnar nerve in a patient with myasthenia gravis and recording of decrement of the compound muscle action potential (CMAP).

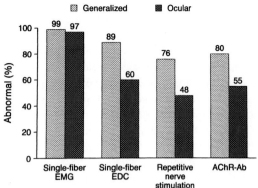

Figure 26–5. Comparison of several laboratory tests in myasthenia gravis. AChR-Ab, acetylcholine receptor antibody; EDC, extensor digitorum communis; EMG, electromyography. (From Howard JF Jr, Sanders DB, Massey JM: The electrodiagnosis of myasthenia gravis and the Lambert-Eaton myasthenic syndrome. *Neurol Clin* 12:305–330, May 1994. By permission of WB Saunders Company.)

body, which is positive in 86% of patients with generalized myasthenia.[70] In approximately 80% of patients with thymoma, striational antibodies against skeletal muscle proteins, such as titin, can be found. Titin antibodies have been associated with thymoma in patients younger than 60 years. Measurement of interferon and interleukin may be more useful to monitor thymoma recurrence.[8] In patients with seronegative myasthenia gravis, antibodies against thyroid or gastric parietal cells may support the diagnosis. The sensitivities of several diagnostic tests are shown in Figure 26–5.

Computed tomography scanning of the thorax must be performed in every patient to screen for thymoma. Thymomas vary in their malignancy potential, and CT scans may give a reasonable view of the invasive potential, a finding most often associated with well-differentiated thymic carcinoma. The essential laboratory tests in evaluation of myasthenia gravis are summarized in Table 26–2.

The diagnosis of myasthenia gravis should not pose insurmountable difficulties, but alternative diagnoses should be considered if any of these tests are nondiagnostic. Ocular myasthenia can be mimicked by mitochondrial cytopathy, oculopharyngeal muscular dystrophy, thyroid ophthalmopathy, and a brain stem lesion. Generalized myasthenia can be mimicked by Lambert-Eaton myasthenic syndrome, botulism, venoms, and many other inflammatory myopathies or acquired neuromyotonia.[80]

Imminent respiratory failure is the most common reason for admission to the NICU, and the early clinical signs of diaphragmatic

Table 26–2. Diagnostic Tests in Myasthenia Gravis

Electromyography, nerve conduction velocity, repetitive stimulation, single fiber study
Edrophonium or neostigmine test
Acetylcholine receptor blocking, titin antibodies
Thyroid, parietal cell antibodies
Thyroxine, triiodothyronine, thyrotropin
Computed tomography scan of the chest
Serial arterial blood gas determinations
Serial measurements of vital capacity and maximal inspiratory pressure
Preoperative pulmonary function test (with neostigmine provocation, optional)

failure should be well known (Chapter 5). Measurement of vital capacity remains an important bedside test, although it may not accurately reflect diaphragmatic function. A useful additional maneuver is to measure vital capacity in the supine position. Typically, patients with diaphragmatic failure but no apparent clinical signs have a significant decrease (up to 60% from the baseline value in the erect position) in vital capacity when supine. In patients without neuromuscular failure, the decrease in vital capacity with position change is seldom more than 20% from baseline. The development of paradoxical breathing in a patient lying down is often a prelude to the need for endotracheal intubation and mechanical ventilation. A study performed in patients with myasthenia gravis found that these maximal static pressures were more sensitive in the early detection of neuromuscular failure and that pressures clearly improved after administration of pyridostigmine.[51]

The frequency of measurements of vital capacity and inspiratory and expiratory pressures is often a matter of debate, but declining values must heighten the awareness of imminent respiratory failure. Risk factors for respiratory decline have not been studied prospectively, but it is prudent to measure vital capacity every 3 to 4 hours in a patient with myasthenic crisis. Unfortunately, the clinical course of myasthenia gravis is erratic, and repeated measurements of vital capacity with a documented decrease of 30% or more do not predict the need for intubation, as clearly shown in Guillain-Barré syndrome (Chapter 25).

However, patients with chest X-ray evidence of early atelectasis and right lower lobe infiltrates suggestive of aspiration are at considerable risk of worsening respiratory failure, as are patients with considerable bulbar dysfunction.

FIRST STEPS IN MANAGEMENT

Patients with myasthenia gravis can become critically ill rapidly. The severity of the exacerbation is commonly misjudged, and the timing of endotracheal intubation is particularly difficult.

Endotracheal intubation may be avoided with conservative measures, such as placing the patient in an erect position and using incentive spirometry and assisted coughing, and certainly can be avoided if plasma exchange or administration of IVIG is started promptly. However, conservative measures may fail, and one should probably electively intubate rather than procrastinate if the trend is a decline in respiratory function. We have tried to avoid intubation in patients with myasthenic crises using bilevel positive airway pressure ventilation (BiPAP) (see Chapter 5). In 11 episodes, a BiPAP trial prevented intubation in 7 (70%), but not in patients with $PaCO_2$ values greater than 50 mm Hg. In these patients, hypercapnea reflected a more profound degree of respiratory failure that could not be assisted with positive pressure and thus needed a volume-controlled mode.[63]

Elective intubation proceeds in an organized manner and is carefully explained to the patient. Patients should understand that mechanical ventilation is only a temporary supportive measure and that weaning is the rule. Obviously, neuromuscular blocking agents are discouraged during intubation, because patients with myasthenia gravis are very sensitive to these drugs, and in the case of succinylcholine, hyperkalemia may arise in paralyzed patients.

The cause of the myasthenic crisis must be identified. Several pharmaceutical agents have been reported to exacerbate myasthenia gravis (Table 26–3).[82] Patients with a bacterial respiratory infection can be empirically and safely treated with cephalosporins (see Chapter 33). The initial management is summarized in Table 26–4.

Specific treatment in myasthenic crisis is plasma exchange or IVIG.[1,11,15,16] A trial in 87 patients with worsening myasthenia gravis showed similar benefits but a better safety profile for IVIG.[26]

Intravenous immune gamma globulin treatment is reserved for patients with very difficult venous access, patients with possible sepsis as a trigger for myasthenic crisis, and, perhaps, children. Its effectiveness could be identical to that of plasma exchange. Similar outcome was

Table 26–3. Pharmaceutical Agents with the Potential to Aggravate Myasthenia Gravis

Antibiotics	Cardiovascular agents	Miscellaneous
Clindamycin	Quinidine	Penicillamine
Colistin	Propranolol	Chloroquine
Kanamycin	Procainamide	Succinylcholine
Neomycin	Practolol	chloride
Streptomycin	Lidocaine	Curare and other
Tobramycin	Verapamil	relaxants
Tetracyclines	Nifedipine	Decamethonium
Gentamicin	Diltiazem	Phenytoin
Polymyxin B	Psychotropic agents	Trimethadione
Bacitracin	Chlorpromazine	Carbamazepine
Trimethoprim-	Promazine	
sulfamethoxazole	Phenelzine	
Hormones	Lithium	
ACTH	Diazepam	
Corticosteroids		
Thyroid hormone		
Oral contraceptives		

ACTH, adrenocorticotrophic hormone.

demonstrated when plasma exchanges were compared with IVIG, 0.4 g/kg daily for 3 to 5 days, but very few patients required mechanical ventilation during the crisis.[26] A retrospective study, also limited by small patient numbers, suggested that intravenous IVIG was less effective in patients on a mechanical ventilator in a crisis episode.[62] Treatment failures in IVIG with subsequent response to plasma exchange have been reported.[77] Our limited experience agrees with these findings, and we could not liberate our patients from the mechanical ventilator with IVIG alone. We therefore prefer plasma exchange in mechanically ventilated patients with myasthenic crises.

Administration of pyridostigmine can be discontinued to facilitate mechanical ventilation and to improve bronchial suctioning.[4] Many patients have retained secretions from ineffective coughing and chest X-ray signs of early atelectasis.[78] Discontinuation of cholinesterase inhibitors leads to a considerable increase in

Table 26–4. Initial Management in Patients with Severe Myasthenic Crisis

Airway management	Incentive spirometry, assisted coughing
	BiPAP trial of $Paco_2 < 50$ mm Hg
	Endotracheal intubation and mechanical ventilation (IMV, PS) in patients with impaired swallowing mechanism leading to inability to clear secretions, ineffective cough and nasal voice, signs of aspiration pneumonitis on chest radiograph with marginal Po_2 or widening A-a gradient or any vital capacity near 15 mL/kg
	Tracheostomy is deferred
	A third-generation cephalosporin is added when pulmonary infiltrates appear
Fluid management	Maintenance with isotonic saline; amount increased during fever from infection
Nutrition	Nasogastric tube in severe bulbar dysfunction
	Proton inhibitors when corticosteroids are administered
Specific treatment	Administration of pyridostigmine is stopped during mechanical ventilation; pyridostigmine therapy is gradually reinstated intravenously or intramuscularly
	Plasma exchange: five plasma exchanges or 5 days of IVIG, 0.4 g/kg; 2 consecutive days of plasma exchange are followed by three exchanges on alternate days
	Corticosteroids (60 mg/day) are given if no improvement after 5 days of plasma exchange
	In refractory cases, cyclosporine (5 mg/kg per day in two divided doses) or mycophenolate mofetil (2 g in two divided doses) can be considered

A-a, alveolar-arterial; BiPAP, bilevel positive airway pressure ventilation; IMV, intermittent mandatory ventilation; IVIG, intravenous immune gamma globulin; PS, pressure support.

muscle weakness, but patients with severe myasthenic crisis, who are often exhausted, appreciate short-term mechanical ventilation and rest and often accept the consequences of discontinuation of cholinesterase inhibitors. Moreover, when plasma exchange is started immediately, improvement is quickly notable after a series of exchanges.

In some patients, plasma exchange is not effective, and only an increase in the intravenous dose of pyridostigmine with atropine or glycopyrrolate to counter hypersecretion is effective in weaning from the ventilator. One approach is to discontinue cholinesterase inhibitors and gradually increase the dose of pyridostigmine after completing a full series of plasma exchange. Intramuscular administration of pyridostigmine is more effective than intravenous, which has a very short effect. However, when multiple (often painful) intramuscular doses are needed, one could proceed with a continuous infusion. The risk of a cholinergic crisis from continuous infusion of pyridostigmine (initial infusion of 2 mg/hour, with a gradual increase in dose) is considerable, but administration seems safe in patients with normal renal function.[6,68]

In patients with considerable muscle weakness but no clinical or laboratory evidence of respiratory failure, it is reasonable to increase the dose of pyridostigmine in increments of 15 to 30 mg until a satisfactory response is apparent. In patients with difficulty swallowing, a syrup (60 mg/5 mL) should be administered or an intravenous dose can be tried (dose equivalents are shown in Table 26–5). High doses of pyridostigmine (up to 50 mg IV in divided doses) may be required.

Another complex management issue is preparation of the patient before thymectomy. The indications for thymectomy have been well outlined in several overviews.[33,41,42] A thymoma is an absolute indication for thoracotomy unless the tumor is malignant and significantly invades the mediastinum.[44,46] Thymoma, a slow-growing malignant lesion, has been staged by Masaoka[48] through modification of the Bergh[3] classification: stage I, tumor encapsulated, no invasion; stage II, macroscopic (IIa) or microscopic (IIb) invasion; stage III, invasion of the pericardium, great vessels, or lung; stage IV, pleural or pericardial dissemination (IVa) or metastasis (IVb).

Complete resection is associated with almost no recurrence but cannot be achieved with stage III thymoma. Relapse has been reported in 20% of patients, with distant metastasis developing in 5%. Postoperative radiation and chemotherapy with a cisplatin regimen are needed in these cases.

Absence of a thymoma on CT scan may guide the thoracic surgeon in deciding to proceed with transcervical thymectomy, which leaves a less deforming scar and reduces the risk of phrenic nerve damage. Many thoracic surgeons prefer the transsternal approach because this exposure almost certainly guarantees complete removal of the thymus. The thymus may have additional localizations within the mediastinum that are not in continuity with the bulk of its gland. A retrospective study of transcervical thymectomy in 53 patients with myasthenia gravis (but skewed toward milder disease) showed that 77% of the patients were in complete remission after 5 years of follow-up.[17] Only one patient (2%) had transsternal reexploration for relapse; residual thymus tissue was found.

It is not known whether less complete removal of thymus tissue, which is a possible consequence of limited surgical exposure, is

Table 26–5. Cholinesterase Inhibitor Doses in Myasthenia Gravis

	Oral (mg)	Intravenous (mg)
Pyridostigmine bromide (Mestinon)	60	2
Neostigmine bromide (Prostigmin)	15	NA
Neostigmine methylsulfate (Prostigmin)	NA	0.5

NA, not available.

as effective as complete removal. However, thymectomy has not been subjected to a rigorous controlled clinical trial. No randomized study comparing types of thymectomy or comparing thymectomy with the best medical treatment has been performed, and some remain doubtful about the benefit of the operation.[41,42] A recent systematic review using evidence-based criteria concluded that sufficient evidence of its benefit was lacking, and the need for thymectomy in myasthenia gravis was downgraded to "optional."[33,36] Others have argued persuasively that the course of myasthenia gravis is positively affected by surgery, and tentative evidence suggests that thymectomy improves the natural history in 50% of the patients, with the prospect of a complete remission. For now, thymectomy for myasthenia gravis without thymoma could be considered in patients with severe generalized myasthenia gravis, in relatively younger patients (less than 60 years), in patients who have a progressively decreasing response to medication, and in patients who have had several episodes of myasthenic crisis.[9,60]

Patients selected for thymectomy should have a preoperative pulmonary function test evaluation with neostigmine provocation (2 mg intramuscularly). Patients with normal lung function can be expected to have an uncomplicated postoperative course and early extubation. In patients with marginal pulmonary function that cannot be further improved with neostigmine preoperatively, plasma exchange for 5 consecutive days before planned surgery should be scheduled. Preoperative plasma exchange to reduce the risk of prolonged post-operative ventilation probably is not needed in patients with normal lung function, but any deviation of pulmonary function test values from normal probably should prompt a complete course of plasma exchange or, in resistant cases, corticosteroids.

Cholinesterase inhibitors are discontinued the morning of surgery. Atropine is recommended to reduce secretions, and in patients with corticosteroid maintenance, preoperative protection from surgical stress response is very important (125 mg of hydrocortisone intravenously every 8 hours beginning on the day before surgery and continuing for up to 3 days postoperatively).

DETERIORATION: CAUSES AND MANAGEMENT

Patients with myasthenia gravis are generally admitted because of a severe myasthenic crisis. A cholinergic crisis is less common, if not nonexistent, in its pure form. Differences traditionally highlighted are shown in Table 26–6. The causes of myasthenic crisis are intercurrent infection, recent tapering or first administration of large doses of corticosteroids, elective surgery, and delivery.

The condition of patients with myasthenic crisis may not improve or continues to deteriorate despite a series of plasma exchanges. It is reasonable practice to add prednisone (60 mg/day) if no hint of improvement appears after 5 days of plasma exchanges and an increase in the intravenous dose of pyridostigmine. The timing of

Table 26–6. Differentiation of Cholinergic and Myasthenic Crises

	Cholinergic Crises	Myasthenic Crises
Frequency[*]	Rare	Common
Trigger	Overdose, drug therapy for MG	Infection, certain drugs, corticosteroids
Pupils	Miosis	Mydriasis
Respiration	Bronchus plugging and spasm, marked salivation	Diaphragm failure
Fasciculations, cramps	Present	Absent
Diarrhea	Present	Absent

MG, myasthenia gravis.
[*]Combination of both crises is often clinically encountered.

administration of corticosteroids remains arbitrary, and others may wait for at least 2 weeks after plasma exchange to start corticosteroid treatment. An additional 3-day plasma exchange series can be considered to cover the delay in pharmaceutical effect of corticosteroids. The dose of corticosteroids is continued for 1 month, changed to alternate days, and then tapered to clinical response. At a later stage, azathioprine (2 mg/kg daily) can be added to reduce the side effects of corticosteroids[27] or to supplement prednisone if it is not adequately effective.[2] Some may even replace corticosteroids after several years of treatment.[59]

Some early experience suggests that high-dose intravenous methylprednisolone pulse therapy (2 g methylprednisolone administered in 250 mL of glucose, 50 mg/mL) for 2 consecutive days may reduce long-term side effects of prednisone. Its effect was sustained for a mean of 2 months.[45]

Before other immune-modulating therapies are considered, the effect of plasma exchange with corticosteroid supplementation must be observed for at least 2 weeks. Patients previously treated with IVIG who have deterioration should undergo a series of plasma exchanges, beginning with five exchanges. Alternative treatments have been studied in smaller populations, and their effects and side effects are less well known.

An alternative immunosuppressive therapy, administration of cyclosporine, has been evaluated in only two small controlled clinical trials.[30,79] Cyclosporine inhibits interleukin-2 production and helper T-cell release of cytokinesis but, most importantly, inhibits T-lymphocyte maturation. Its use (initially 5 mg/kg per day in two divided doses) is adjusted to maintain trough plasma levels of 100 to 150 ng/L. In the initial trial, administration of cyclosporine was discontinued in 25% of patients, mostly because of nephrotoxicity. In a more recent retrospective analysis from Duke University Medical Center,[13] nephrotoxicity was also a limiting factor and incidences of new-onset hypertension were similar, but control was good with antihypertensive agents. In an analysis of 57 patients treated with cyclosporine (mean use of 3.5

years), improvement began as early as 1 week but usually after 1 month and with maximal effect at approximately 6 months. Other side effects of cyclosporine were hirsutism, headache, tremor, gastrointestinal symptoms, and possibly increased risk of skin cancer.

Another immunosuppressive agent, mycophenolate mofetil (CellCept), has been widely used in organ transplantation and has found its way to autoimmune disorders. Mycophenolate mofetil has been tested in very few patients with myasthenia gravis, but improvement occurred in patients using an oral dose of 2 g (in two divided doses), again as early as 2 weeks, with sustained improvement for at least 6 months. The side effects may include and are similar to those of cyclosporine,[12,49,52] but the major advantage is that the incidence is low. The pros and cons of these newer drugs compared with those of corticosteroids have been debated recently. A major concern is high cost (300 times that of prednisone).[2,66]

If available, a less often used option, immunoadsorption therapy, should be considered in patients with a particularly severe myasthenic crisis.[32,75] Immunoadsorption therapy, a relatively new technique in this situation, uses a synthetic resin that adsorbs acetylcholine antibodies very effectively (e.g., tryptophan-linked polyvinyl alcohol gel). In a randomized study, this therapy had a striking effect on clinical response, and a 60% reduction in circulating acetylcholine antibodies was documented. Immunoadsorption therapy is accomplished with the exchange of one plasma volume during 5 consecutive days; the plasma separator consists of a cellulose diacetate membrane. Improvement can be expected in 48 hours, with a peak at 1 to 4 days after the last adsorption.[75]

Another cause of in-hospital deterioration in myasthenia gravis is significant worsening within the first days of corticosteroid administration. Often, this clinical worsening is observed in patients exposed to corticosteroids for the first time, but it also can occur when the initial doses are high. We usually continue giving corticosteroids (in a lower starting dose) and treat the exacerbation with plasma exchange and increasing doses of pyridostigmine.

Another cause of deterioration in myasthenia gravis is a cholinergic crisis. Whether a cholinergic crisis causes weakness is unresolved, and its full-fledged manifestation is rarely observed. In clinical practice, both conditions are more commonly present at the same time. Typically, in patients with a continuing downhill clinical course, the dose of pyridostigmine has been incrementally increased, and although the clinically observed muscle weakness may be a manifestation of the myasthenic crisis itself, the other symptoms are related to gradual overdosing of the inhibiting cholinesterase drug. The common observation that generalized weakness becomes more severe after discontinuation of drug therapy in patients with an alleged cholinergic crisis supports the contention that both conditions can exist at the same time.

The clinical signs of a cholinergic crisis are miosis (patients with a myasthenic crisis often tend to have some mydriasis); excessive, thick pulmonary secretions rapidly leading to atelectasis, shunting, and hypoxemia; muscle fasciculations; abdominal cramping and diarrhea; sweating; and extreme tearing (Table 26–6). The cause of respiratory dysfunction in a pure form of cholinergic crisis, therefore, may be bronchiolar spasm, aspiration, and difficulty clearing thick secretions rather than diaphragmatic failure.

Treatment of patients with cholinergic crisis consists of respiratory care, most likely intubation, and mechanical ventilation with discontinuation of medication until the symptoms above have subsided. Bronchoscopy through the endotracheal tube to clear the major parts of the tracheobronchial tree may be needed regularly. Antibiotic coverage becomes important if fever and pulmonary infiltrates develop, and reinstitution of pyridostigmine therapy must be postponed to facilitate bronchial drainage. When the chest radiograph shows sufficient clearing, pyridostigmine is administered intravenously in half the initial total daily dose, and then the dose is gradually increased until the optimal clinical effect is obtained.

When laboratory weaning criteria are fulfilled (see Chapter 5), weaning can begin and can often be expedited. Again we found BiPAP helpful in some patients.[64] After endotracheal extubation, swallowing must be assessed before soft food is allowed. Patients may still have considerable bulbar dysfunction despite recovery to fairly normal respiratory function, and premature feeding may lead to aspiration. When soft food is tolerated, the intravenous dose can be changed to an oral dose.

Postoperative deterioration following thymectomy in myasthenia gravis or failure to wean from the ventilator is less common with frequent use of preoperative plasma exchange[18,22] and meticulous preoperative pulmonary assessment. Several reports have highlighted risk factors for postoperative complications. Among these factors are duration of myasthenia gravis exceeding 6 years, preexisting respiratory illness, large doses of pyridostigmine before surgery, marginal pulmonary function measured by vital capacity, severity of bulbar dysfunction, and history of respiratory failure after any type of surgery with general anesthesia.[43,84]

Patients should not be extubated unless they can sustain a head lift for 5 seconds. Failure to wean from the ventilator may have several causes. The most significant complication is pneumothorax or hemothorax from transcervical thymectomy. With this operative approach, adherence of the thymus to the pleura and subsequent tearing after removal may cause right-sided pneumothorax. Immediate drainage is indicated.

In the transsternal approach, the phrenic nerve may become damaged, but this complication is rarely a reason for prolonged postoperative care. Seldom are parathyroid glands incidentally removed or is the recurrent laryngeal nerve severed. Stridor after thymectomy may be an early lead, and difficulty breathing should not be interpreted as worsening myasthenia.

Inadequate management of pain may be one of the reasons for failure to wean in the postoperative phase. Pain management with epidural catheterization has significantly improved postoperative pulmonary care,[10] which often is hampered by disruption of the thoracic cage. None of the currently used narcotics is contraindicated in myasthenia gravis, and most patients benefit from fentanyl by infusion at 10 mL/hour.

OUTCOME

In most patients, symptoms of myasthenia gravis become most severe within approximately 3 years of onset.[47] Large surveys of the natural history of myasthenia gravis have also reported spontaneous, mostly short, remissions.[31,39,57] Extreme examples of remissions lasting more than a decade have been reported as well.[39,57] The remission of myasthenia gravis after standard transsternal thymectomy can be impressive, and complete, persistent remission can be achieved in 25% to 40% of patients as early as 6 months.[25,54] In addition, studies of long-term outcome after thymectomy have shown continuing deterioration in only a very small proportion of patients.[20] The rate of remission may be lower with a transcervical approach.

Immunosuppressive therapy in patients who have not had a remission with thymectomy has improved life expectancy and remarkably improved quality of life. Permanent tracheostomy

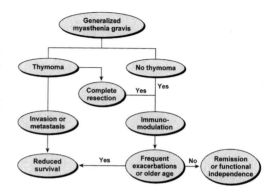

Figure 26–6. Outcome algorithm in myasthenia gravis. Functional independence: no assistance needed, minor handicap may remain.

and severe limb weakness leading to a wheelchair-bound state are currently unusual. Associated neoplasms, mostly colorectal cancers, develop in approximately one-third of the patients.[81]

An outcome algorithm is shown in Figure 26–6.

CONCLUSIONS

- Myasthenic crisis is possibly triggered by intercurrent infection, recent tapering of or first-time initiation of corticosteroids, and elective surgery. Initial steps in management of severe cases are endotracheal intubation, discontinuation of pyridostigmine therapy, mechanical ventilation, and plasma exchange. BiPAP may prevent intubation in some patients.
- If a myasthenic crisis has not abated after 5 days of plasma exchange, prednisone (1 mg/kg) should be continued or started. Cyclosporine (5 mg/kg) or mycophenolate mofetil (2 g) should be considered when treatment fails.
- Cholinergic crisis is characterized by miosis, thick bronchial secretions, muscle fasciculations, abdominal cramping, diarrhea, and tearing. Bronchospasm, aspiration, or difficulty in clearing very thick secretions may cause respiratory failure.
- Postoperative deterioration in myasthenia gravis can be largely eliminated by preoperative plasma exchange and postoperative pain control with fentanyl.

REFERENCES

1. Arsura EL, Bick A, Brunner NG, et al: High-dose intravenous immunoglobulin in the management of myasthenia gravis. *Arch Intern Med* 146:1365–1368, 1986.
2. Bedlack RS, Sanders DB: Steroid treatment for myasthenia gravis: steroids have an important role. *Muscle Nerve* 25:117–121, 2002.
3. Bergh NP, Gatzinsky P, Larsson S, et al: Tumors of the thymus and thymic region: I. Clinicopathological studies on thymomas. *Ann Thorac Surg* 25:91–98, 1978.
4. Berrouschot J, Baumann I, Kalischewski P, et al: Therapy of myasthenic crisis. *Crit Care Med* 25:1228–1235, 1997.
5. Besinger UA, Toyka KV, Homberg M, et al: Myasthenia gravis: long-term correlation of binding and bungarotoxin blocking antibodies against acetylcholine receptors with changes in disease severity. *Neurology* 33:1316–1321, 1983.
6. Borel CO: Management of myasthenic crisis: continuous anticholinesterase infusions (editorial). *Crit Care Med* 21:821–822, 1993.

7. Brodsky MC, Boop FA: Lid nystagmus as a sign of intrinsic midbrain disease. *J Neuroophthalmol* 15:236–240, 1995.

8. Buckley C, Newsom-Davis J, Willcox N, et al: Do titin and cytokine antibodies in MG patients predict thymoma or thymoma recurrence? *Neurology* 57:1579–1582, 2001.

9. Budde JM, Morris CD, Gal AA, et al: Predictors of outcome in thymectomy for myasthenia gravis. *Ann Thorac Surg* 72:197–202, 2001.

10. Burgess FW, Wilcosky B Jr: Thoracic epidural anesthesia for transsternal thymectomy in myasthenia gravis. *Anesth Analg* 69:529–531, 1989.

11. Chang I, Fink ME: Plasmapheresis in the treatment of myasthenic crisis (abstract). *Neurology* 42 Suppl 3:242, 1992.

12. Ciafaloni E, Massey JM, Tucker-Lipscomb B, et al: Mycophenolate mofetil for myasthenia gravis: an open-label pilot study. *Neurology* 56:97–99, 2001.

13. Ciafaloni E, Nikhar NK, Massey JM, et al: Retrospective analysis of the use of cyclosporine in myasthenia gravis. *Neurology* 55:448–450, 2000.

14. Daroff RB: The office Tensilon test for ocular myasthenia gravis. *Arch Neurol* 43:843–844, 1986.

15. Dau PC: Plasmapheresis therapy in myasthenia gravis. *Muscle Nerve* 3:468–482, 1980.

16. Dau PC, Lindstrom JM, Cassel CK, et al: Plasmapheresis and immunosuppressive drug therapy in myasthenia gravis. *N Engl J Med* 297:1134–1140, 1977.

17. DeFilippi VJ, Richman DP, Ferguson MK: Transcervical thymectomy for myasthenia gravis. *Ann Thorac Surg* 57:194–197, 1994.

18. d'Empaire G, Hoaglin DC, Perlo VP, et al: Effect of prethymectomy plasma exchange on postoperative respiratory function in myasthenia gravis. *J Thorac Cardiovasc Surg* 89:592–596, 1985.

19. Dirr LY, Donofrio PD, Patton JF, et al: A false-positive edrophonium test in a patient with a brainstem glioma. *Neurology* 39:865–867, 1989.

20. Durelli L, Maggi G, Casadio C, et al: Actuarial analysis of the occurrence of remissions following thymectomy for myasthenia gravis in 400 patients. *J Neurol Neurosurg Psychiatry* 54:406–411, 1991.

21. Dushay KM, Zibrak JD, Jensen WA: Myasthenia gravis presenting as isolated respiratory failure. *Chest* 97:232–234, 1990.

22. Eisenkraft JB, Papatestas AE, Kahn CH, et al: Predicting the need for postoperative mechanical ventilation in myasthenia gravis. *Anesthesiology* 65:79–82, 1986.

23. Engel AG: Myasthenia gravis and myasthenic syndromes. *Ann Neurol* 16:519–534, 1984.

24. Frisby J, Wills A, Jaspan T: Brain stem compression by a giant vertebrobasilar aneurysm mimicking seronegative myasthenia. *J Neurol Neurosurg Psychiatry* 71:125–126, 2001.

25. Frist WH, Thirumalai S, Doehring CB, et al: Thymectomy for the myasthenia gravis patient: factors influencing outcome. *Ann Thorac Surg* 57:334–338, 1994.

26. Gajdos P, Chevret S, Clair B, et al: Clinical trial of plasma exchange and high-dose intravenous immunoglobulin in myasthenia gravis. Myasthenia Gravis Clinical Study Group. *Ann Neurol* 41:789–796, 1997.

27. Gajdos P, Elkharrat D, Chevret S, et al: A randomised clinical trial comparing prednisone and azathioprine in myasthenia gravis. Results of the second interim analysis. *J Neurol Neurosurg Psychiatry* 56:1157–1163, 1993.

28. Gilchrist JM, Massey JM, Sanders DB: Single fiber EMG and repetitive stimulation of the same muscle in myasthenia gravis. *Muscle Nerve* 17:171–175, 1994.

29. Golnik KC, Pena R, Lee AG, et al: An ice test for the diagnosis of myasthenia gravis. *Ophthalmology* 106:1282–1286, 1999.

30. Goulon M, Elkharrat D, Lokiec F, et al: Results of a one-year open trial of cyclosporine in ten patients with severe myasthenia gravis. *Transplant Proc* 20 Suppl 4:211–217, 1988.

31. Grob D, Brunner NG, Namba T: The natural course of myasthenia gravis and effect of therapeutic measures. *Ann N Y Acad Sci* 377:652–669, 1981.

32. Grob D, Simpson D, Mitsumoto H, et al: Treatment of myasthenia gravis by immunoadsorption of plasma. *Neurology* 45:338–344, 1995.

33. Gronseth GS, Barohn RJ: Practice parameter: thymectomy for autoimmune myasthenia gravis (an evidence-based review): report of the Quality Standards Subcommittee of the American Academy of Neurology. *Neurology* 55:7–15, 2000.

34. Hanson JA, Lueck CJ, Thomas DJ: Myasthenia gravis presenting with stridor. *Thorax* 51:108–109, 1996.

35. Jacobson DM: The "ice pack test" for diagnosing myasthenia gravis. *Ophthalmology* 107:622–623, 2000.

36. Jaretzki A III, Barohn RJ, Ernstoff RM, et al: Myasthenia gravis: recommendations for clinical research standards. Task Force of the Medical Scientific Advisory Board of the Myasthenia Gravis Foundation of America. *Ann Thorac Surg* 70:327–334, 2000; *Neurology* 55:16–23, 2000.

37. Kao YF, Lan MY, Chou MS, et al: Intracranial fatigable ptosis. *J Neuroophthalmol* 19:257–259, 1999.

38. Katzberg HD, Aziz T, Oger J: In myasthenia gravis cells from atrophic thymus secrete acetylcholine receptor antibodies. *Neurology* 56:572–573, 2001.

39. Kennedy FS, Moersch FP: Myasthenia gravis: clinical review of 87 cases observed between 1915 and early part of 1932. *Can Med Assoc J* 37:216–223, 1937.

40. Khan OA, Campbell WW: Myasthenia gravis presenting as dysphagia: clinical considerations. *Am J Gastroenterol* 89:1083–1085, 1994.

41. Kissel JT, Franklin GM: Treatment of myasthenia gravis: a call to arms. *Neurology* 55:3–4, 2000.

42. Lanska DJ: Indications for thymectomy in myasthenia gravis. *Neurology* 40:1828–1829, 1990.

43. Leventhal SR, Orkin FK, Hirsh RA: Prediction of the need for postoperative mechanical ventilation in myasthenia gravis. *Anesthesiology* 53:26–30, 1980.

44. Lewis JE, Wick MR, Scheithauer BW, et al: Thymoma. A clinicopathologic review. *Cancer* 60:2727–2743, 1987.

45. Lindberg C, Andersen O, Lefvert AK: Treatment of

myasthenia gravis with methylprednisolone pulse: a double blind study. *Acta Neurol Scand* 97:370–373, 1998.

46. Lisak RP (ed): *Handbook of Myasthenia Gravis and Myasthenic Syndromes.* New York: Marcel Dekker, 1994.

47. Mantegazza R, Beghi E, Pareyson D, et al: A multicentre follow-up study of 1152 patients with myasthenia gravis in Italy. *J Neurol* 237:339–344, 1990.

48. Masaoka A, Monden Y, Nakahara K, et al: Follow-up study of thymomas with special reference to their clinical stages. *Cancer* 48:2485–2492, 1981.

49. Meriggioli MN, Rowin J: Treatment of myasthenia gravis with mycophenolate mofetil: a case report. *Muscle Nerve* 23:1287–1289, 2000.

50. Mier A, Laroche C, Green M: Unsuspected myasthenia gravis presenting as respiratory failure. *Thorax* 45:422–423, 1990.

51. Mier-Jedrzejowicz AK, Brophy C, Green M: Respiratory muscle function in myasthenia gravis. *Am Rev Respir Dis* 138:867–873, 1988.

52. Mowzoon N, Sussman A, Bradley WG: Mycophenolate (CellCept) treatment of myasthenia gravis, chronic inflammatory polyneuropathy and inclusion body myositis. *J Neurol Sci* 185:119–122, 2001.

53. Nagappan R, Kletchko S: Myasthenia gravis presenting as respiratory failure. *N Z Med J* 105:152, 1992.

54. Nieto IP, Robledo JP, Pajuelo MC, et al: Prognostic factors for myasthenia gravis treated by thymectomy: review of 61 cases. *Ann Thorac Surg* 67:1568–1571, 1999.

55. Odel JG, Winterkorn JM, Behrens MM: The sleep test for myasthenia gravis. A safe alternative to Tensilon. *J Clin Neuroophthalmol* 11:288–292, 1991.

56. Oh SJ, Kim DE, Kuruoglu R, et al: Diagnostic sensitivity of the laboratory tests in myasthenia gravis. *Muscle Nerve* 15:720–724, 1992.

57. Oosterhuis HJ: Observations of the natural history of myasthenia gravis and the effect of thymectomy. *Ann N Y Acad Sci* 377:678–690, 1981.

58. Oosterhuis HJ: *Myasthenia Gravis.* Edinburgh: Churchill Livingstone, 1984.

59. Palace J, Newsom-Davis J, Lecky B: A randomized double-blind trial of prednisolone alone or with azathioprine in myasthenia gravis. Myasthenia Gravis Study Group. *Neurology* 50:1778–1783, 1998.

60. Papatestas AE, Genkins G, Kornfeld P, et al: Effects of thymectomy in myasthenia gravis. *Ann Surg* 206:79–88, 1987.

61. Perlo VP, Poskanzer DC, Schwab RS, et al: Myasthenia gravis: evaluation of treatment in 1,355 patients. *Neurology* 16:431–439, 1966.

62. Qureshi AI, Choudhry MA, Akbar MS, et al: Plasma exchange versus intravenous immunoglobulin treatment in myasthenic crisis. *Neurology* 52:629–632, 1999.

63. Rabinstein AA, Wijdicks EFM: BiPAP in acute respiratory failure due to myasthenic crisis may prevent intubation. *Neurology* 59:1647–1649, 2002.

64. Rabinstein AA, Wijdicks EFM: Weaning from the ventilator using BiPAP in myasthenia gravis. *Muscle Nerve* 2003 (in press).

65. Rivero A, Crovetto L, Lopez L, et al: Single fiber electromyography of extraocular muscles: a sensitive method for the diagnosis of ocular myasthenia gravis. *Muscle Nerve* 18:943–947, 1995.

66. Rivner MH: Steroid treatment for myasthenia gravis: steroids are overutilized. *Muscle Nerve* 25:115–117, 2002.

67. Roberts ME, Steiger MJ, Hart IK: Presentation of myasthenia gravis mimicking blepharospasm. *Neurology* 58:150–151, 2002.

68. Saltis LM, Martin BR, Traeger SM, et al: Continuous infusion of pyridostigmine in the management of myasthenic crisis. *Crit Care Med* 21:938–940, 1993.

69. Sanders DB: The electrodiagnosis of myasthenia gravis. *Ann N Y Acad Sci* 505:539–556, 1987.

70. Sanders DB, Andrews PI, Howard JF Jr, et al: Seronegative myasthenia gravis. *Neurology* 48 (Suppl 5):S40–S45, 1997.

71. Sanders DB, Howard JF Jr: AAEE minimonograph 25: single-fiber electromyography in myasthenia gravis. *Muscle Nerve* 9:809–819, 1986.

72. Schady W, MacDermott N: On the choice of muscle in the electrophysiological assessment of myasthenia gravis. *Electromyogr Clin Neurophysiol* 32:99–102, 1992.

73. Schon F, Drayson M, Thompson RA: Myasthenia gravis and elderly people. *Age Ageing* 25:56–58, 1996.

74. Sethi KD, Rivner MH, Swift TR: Ice pack test for myasthenia gravis. *Neurology* 37:1383–1385, 1987.

75. Shibuya N, Sato T, Osame M, et al: Immunoabsorption therapy for myasthenia gravis. *J Neurol Neurosurg Psychiatry* 57:578–581, 1994.

76. Spinelli A, Marconi G, Gorini M, et al: Control of breathing in patients with myasthenia gravis. *Am Rev Respir Dis* 145:1359–1366, 1992.

77. Stricker RB, Kwiatkowska BJ, Habis JA, et al: Myasthenic crisis. Response to plasmapheresis following failure of intravenous gamma-globulin. *Arch Neurol* 50:837–840, 1993.

78. Thomas CE, Mayer SA, Gungor Y, et al: Myasthenic crisis: clinical features, mortality, complications, and risk factors for prolonged intubation. *Neurology* 48:1253–1260, 1997.

79. Tindall RS, Rollins JA, Phillips JT, et al: Preliminary results of a double-blind, randomized, placebo-controlled trial of cyclosporine in myasthenia gravis. *N Engl J Med* 316:719–724, 1987.

80. Vincent A, Drachman DB: Myasthenia gravis. *Adv Neurol* 88:159–188, 2002.

81. Wilkins KB, Sheikh E, Green R, et al: Clinical and pathologic predictors of survival in patients with thymoma. *Ann Surg* 230:562–572, 1999.

82. Wittbrodt ET: Drugs and myasthenia gravis: an update. *Arch Intern Med* 157:399–408, 1997.

83. Younge BR, Bartley GB: Lancaster test with Tensilon for myasthenia. *Arch Neurol* 44:472–473, 1987.

84. Younger DS, Braun NM, Jaretzki A III, et al: Myasthenia gravis: determinants for independent ventilation after transsternal thymectomy. *Neurology* 34:336–340, 1984.

PART IV

POSTOPERATIVE NEUROSURGICAL COMPLICATIONS

27

Carotid Endarterectomy

Carotid endarterectomy is an established procedure in patients with symptomatic carotid artery stenosis of more than 70%. Although it is considered the standard therapy, carotid endarterectomy will be compared with carotid stenting and angioplasty.[16,36,40] Stenting is currently limited to patients in whom carotid endarterectomy would be a high-risk procedure.[40] In keeping with many performance standards, patients who undergo carotid surgery for atherosclerotic carotid disease are briefly admitted to an intensive care unit (ICU). Depending on the surgeon, the patient is admitted to a neurologic intensive care unit (NICU) or a vascular intermediate unit. In-hospital mortality with carotid endarterectomy is 1% and may involve postoperative myocardial infarction.[43,48] The medical manifestations of carotid endarterectomy are equally important, and respiratory compromise may occur, with a need for endotracheal intubation. Whether these complications can be prevented or more effectively treated by having the patient in the NICU is uncertain. The criteria for admission to the NICU have not been well defined, and quite a few surgeons believe that routine admission leads to overutilization and excessive triage.[50] However, a survey of 91 carotid endarterectomies noted use of intravenous hypertensive medication in more than two-thirds of the patients and three reexplorations, most occurring within 12 hours of the procedure.[64] Other surgeons believe that NICU admission should be restricted to patients who awaken with a stroke; develop cardiac arrhythmias or

early electrocardiographic changes; have significant wound hemorrhage; are reintubated in the recovery room; or, particularly, require vasoactive medication more than 3 hours after surgery.[60] The implication is that for many other patients, the need for NICU admission is abrogated.

Unquestionably, neurosurgeons and vascular surgeons continue to shepherd their patients through the postoperative course. Personal interaction with the neurologist to address complications amounts to a few cases a year. Nonetheless, because a sizable number of patients with carotid endarterectomy are admitted to the NICU, the neurologist must be familiar with the surgical procedure and its potential neurologic complications.

SURGICAL PROCEDURE

Carotid endarterectomy is performed by vascular surgeons and neurosurgeons with additional expertise in vascular surgery.[9] Admission of these patients to our NICU is typically after surgery performed by neurosurgeons.

General anesthesia is in common use for carotid endarterectomy. Regional (cervical block) anesthesia could become a feasible alternative, and preliminary studies have claimed reduced complications and hospital stay.[13] Standard variables recommended for monitoring by the American Society of Anesthesiologists are end-tidal carbon dioxide, oxygen saturation (pulse oximetry), electrocardiographic changes, temperature, and blood pressure. Some institutions apply full-channel electroencephalographic monitoring or estimate cerebral blood flow by performing xenon Xe 133 cerebral blood flow studies. Continuous transcranial Doppler monitoring may identify hyperperfusion states, microemboli, or an increase in middle cerebral artery velocity during cross-clamping as signals of a developing postoperative stroke.[5,29] Somatosensory evoked potentials may show changes in scalp amplitudes with cross-clamping and could assist in determining the need for shunt insertion.[46] However, claims for these sophisticated monitoring tests remain premature. These tests may substantially increase the cost of the procedure and lack proof that complications are reduced.

Carotid endarterectomy requires approximately 2 to 3 hours, with average cross-clamping time between 30 and 40 minutes. A sketch of the anatomy is shown in Figure 27–1. The proximity of the cranial nerves predisposes them to injury during carotid exposure. Whether stretching from retraction or improper placement of the retractors can be implicated is uncertain. The common carotid artery is occluded with a vascular clamp, and smaller clamps or aneurysm clips are used to occlude the internal carotid artery and external carotid artery. The arteriotomy is made on the anterior surface of the internal carotid artery.

Intraoperative shunting is not a universal practice. Some surgeons systematically place a shunt in every patient and claim the benefits of improved cerebral protection. Other surgeons, however, believe that shunting may increase stroke rate because of embolization from placement of the shunt or distal intimal damage, an injury that eventually may lead to embolization and carotid artery dissection. Others use the shunt only if electroencephalographic changes are becoming apparent. In a few patients, shunt placement is technically not possible because of a high bifurcation, distal plaque, or diminutive internal carotid artery.

Another difference in technique is use of vein patching, and typically, saphenous veins are used.[19] Some surgeons justify patching and claim reduced late restenosis in follow-up. Postoperative complications do not differ significantly between vein and polyethylene fiber (Dacron) patching.[32]

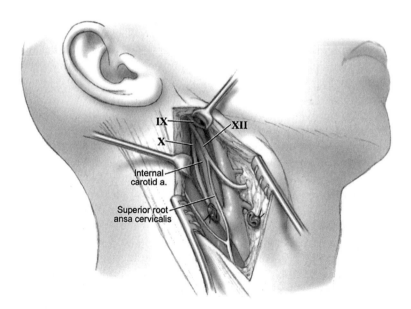

Figure 27–1. Proximity of cranial nerves to the carotid artery poses a risk of damage during carotid endarterectomy.

After removal of gross plaque, the artery is closed. A smooth arteriotomy bed is the best result but may be difficult to attain in patients with stone-hard plaque. One of the most important parts of the surgical procedure is to reduce stray adventitial tacks or suture ends sewn into the lumen, because they may eventually produce thrombosis or dissection.

NEUROLOGIC COMPLICATIONS

The American Heart Association guidelines imply that to maintain credibility, centers performing carotid endarterectomy have to limit postoperative complications to a minimum of 3%.[52] Many of the major neurologic complications are immediately evident after surgery. Stroke is the most prevalent. In some patients, ischemic stroke becomes apparent in the recovery room (Table 27–1). In others, a fatal intracranial hemorrhage occurs several days after surgery (Table 27–2). Lesions of the cranial nerves are of considerable postoperative concern, and the difficulty with swallowing and coughing should be appreciated. Recommendations for management follow in separate sections.

Hyperperfusion Syndrome

Notwithstanding major skepticism, hyperperfusion syndrome is very rare, estimated to occur in fewer than 0.5% of cases.[35,41,59,67,74] Risk factors include a large pressure gradient across the stenosis and contralateral carotid occlusion. Many patients have some increase in cerebral blood flow after a critically stenosed carotid artery is reopened,[74] but only a few symptoms occur. Irritability, frontotemporal or, more characteristically, periorbital headache, acute confusional state, and seizures have been described, most occurring within hours but often at the end of the first postoperative week and even at 3 weeks. Intracerebral hematoma and ischemic stroke should be excluded. Neuroimaging modalities, such as transcranial Doppler ultrasonography and single-photon emission computed tomography, document major asymmetries in flow distribution.[21]

An interesting, but unconfirmed, series reported brain edema on computed tomography scans, with fatal outcome in one patient due to massive edema. Symptoms developed in each patient 5 to 8 days after carotid endarterectomy and after an asymptomatic interval.[15] In another case example, the findings could represent edema associated with hemorrhagic infarction.[76] In the overwhelming number of remaining cases, brain edema cannot be documented on computed tomography or magnetic resonance imaging.

The syndrome always is accompanied by greatly increased blood pressure (> 250 mm Hg systolic).[59,67] Treatment is judicious reduction of blood pressure by esmolol or labetalol bolus.

Intracranial Hemorrhage

Intracranial hemorrhage following carotid endarterectomy is a very uncommon complication, but mortality and morbidity are high. It is estimated to occur in fewer than 1% of cases, but in the total of events after surgery, it may account for up to 25% of the complications. A recent study suggested the following predictive factors for intracerebral hemorrhage: young age, hypertension, and high degree of ipsilateral and contralateral carotid stenosis or high rate of contralateral carotid occlusion.[54] Mortality is very high, and many patients die within 72 hours of the hemorrhage.[17,30,33,39,54,56,57,70,71]

More than one mechanism appears to contribute to the development of intracranial hemorrhage. We found that doubling of the cerebral blood flow at surgery significantly increased the chance of an intracerebral hematoma.[33] This finding argues that a hyperperfusion syndrome is present to a greater degree in patients with intracranial hematomas. One of the mechanisms is that cerebral autoregulation is impaired in patients who have severe carotid artery stenosis. After endarterectomy, the increase in pressure in capillaries and vessels that are maximally dilated causes disruption of ep-

Table 27–1. Incidence of Postoperative Ischemic Stroke or Transient Ischemic Attack

	Year of Publication	Study Period	Number of Patients	NEUROLOGIC COMPLICATIONS	
				No.	%
Steed et al.[72]	1982	1967–1981	345	21°	
Sundt et al.[73]	1986	1972–1984	1935	58°	
Branchereau et al.[14]	1987	1980–1987	700	37	5°
L'AURC et al.[44]	1988	1987	927	52	6°
Riles et al.[61]	1994	1961–1991	3062	66	2†
Ouriel et al.[54]	1999	1992–1997	1471	31	2°
Radak et al.[58]	1999	1985–1997	2250	59	3†
Rockman et al.[63]	2000	1985–1997	2024	38	2°
Ayari et al.[8]	2001	1997–2000	364	19	5°

NA, not available.
° Postoperative transient ischemic attack and stroke.
† Postoperative stroke.
Source: Ayari R, Ede B, Bartoli M, et al: Neurologic complications of carotid surgery. In Branchereau A, Jacobs M (eds): *Complications in Vascular and Endovascular Surgery.* Part I. Armonk, NY: Futura Publishing Company, 2001, pp 119–131. By permission of Futura Publishing Company.

ithelial cells and breakdown of the blood-brain barrier. Loss of autoregulation hampers the countering vasoconstriction associated with reperfusion to limit a downstream effect of increased blood flow. This event is most pronounced in the first week after carotid endarterectomy. Systemic hypertension by itself is not the only primary event leading to intracranial hemorrhage after carotid endarterectomy, because anticoagulation may also contribute.[24,33] In addition, an intracranial hematoma may extend within a cerebral infarct. Our study suggests that estimating cerebral blood flow with ^{133}Xe may be a useful technique during surgery. Particularly in patients in whom doubling of flow is noted, postoperative anticoagulation should be deferred and aggressive blood pressure control is indicated (Table 27–2).

Massive hemorrhage commonly occurs with rapidly developing signs of cerebral herniation. Surgical evacuation of the hematoma thus can be seen as a salvaging procedure. Good recovery has been reported in patients in whom an intracerebral hematoma developed 7 weeks after the procedure and those in whom petechial hemorrhages were more common.[54] Examples are shown in Figures 27–2 through 27–4.

CRANIAL NERVE LESIONS

Cranial nerve lesions are uncommon, although frequency has varied significantly in prospective series.[20,47,79,80] Table 27–3 shows the incidence of cranial nerve lesions after carotid endarterectomy. The incidence of cranial or cervical nerve injuries is higher after repeat carotid endarterectomy. In a study by Abu-Rahma et al.,[1,2] 21% of 89 consecutive patients who had repeat carotid endarterectomy had lesions of the hypoglossal nerve, vagal nerve, and laryngeal nerves, but most neurologic deficits were reversible. Most frequently involved were the great auricular nerve, hypoglossal nerve (XII) (Fig. 27–5), mandibular branch of the facial nerve (VII), and vagus nerve (X). The recurrent laryngeal nerve was occasionally involved as well but much less frequently than the superior glossopharyngeal nerve (IX) and accessory nerve (XI). Clinical manifestations of

Table 27–2. Characteristics of 12 Patients with Intracerebral Hematoma after Carotid Endarterectomy

Case	Stroke or TIA	Time between IE and CEA (Days)	% Change in Xenon Flow	Time between CEA and Bleeding (Days)	Size of ICH (cm)	Mechanism of Bleeding
1	Stroke	17°	>100	<1	>4	PIE, HPS
2	TIA	30†	26	<1	>4	PIE, AC
3	TIA	25	>100	<1	>4	PIE, HPS, AC
4	TIA	48	18	1	>4	PIE, AC
5	Stroke	75	5	2	>4	Prior stroke
6	TIA	20	Not known	3	2–4	AC
7	Stroke	3	>100	3	>4	HPS, possible recent stroke
8	None	—	—	5	>4	HPS
9	Stroke	30†	>100	5	>4	HPS
10	Stroke	4	>100	5	>4	HPS, AC
11	Stroke	15	Not known	6	<2	Recent stroke
12	TIA	Not known	Not known	8	>4	HPS, AC

AC, anticoagulation; CEA, carotid endarterectomy; HPS, hyperperfusion syndrome; ICH, intracerebral hematoma; IE, preoperative ischemic event; PIE, perioperative cerebral ischemic event; TIA, transient ischemic attack.
°Similar transient event 7 days before surgery.
†Similar transient event 24 hours before surgery.
‡Stroke 4 years before CEA.
Source: Modified from Henderson RD, Phan TG, Piepgras DG, et al: Mechanisms of intracerebral hemorrhage after carotid endarterectomy. *J Neurosurg* 95:964–969, 2001. By permission of the American Association of Neurological Surgeons.

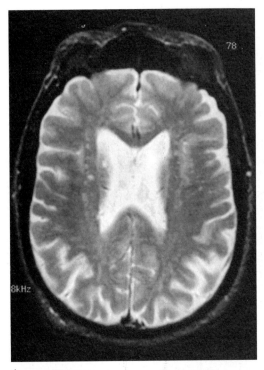

A

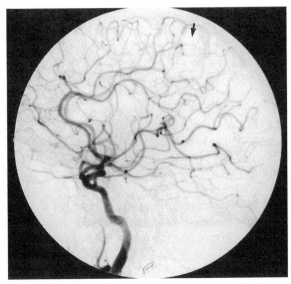

B

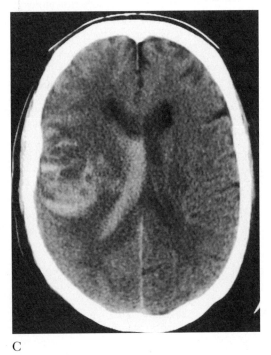

C

Figure 27–2. (*A*) Axial magnetic resonance image revealing foci of right-sided subcortical isch-emia on pre-endarterectomy imaging. (*B*) Cerebral angiography was performed immediately af-ter right carotid endarterectomy when the patient awoke from anesthesia with left-sided hemi-paresis. Imaging revealed a distal middle cerebral artery embolus with pial collateral flow (*arrow*). The patient received anticoagulation therapy with intravenously administered heparin (1000 U/hour) without a bolus. (*C*) Computed tomography scan image showing that 4 hours later, an intracranial hematoma bled into the area of infarction, with intraventricular extension. (From Henderson et al.[33] By permission of the American Association of Neurological Surgeons.)

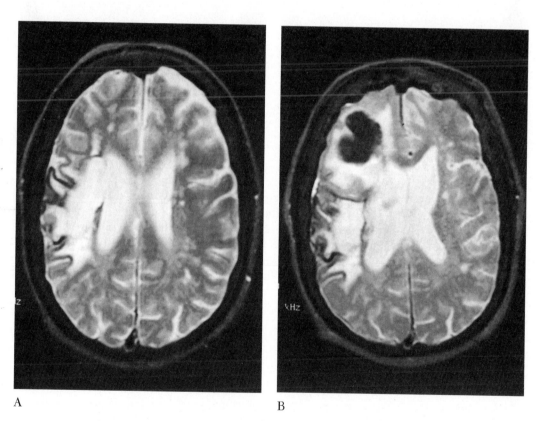

A   B

Figure 27–3. Axial magnetic resonance images. (*A*) Large right-sided middle cerebral artery in-farct was revealed on pre-endarterectomy imaging. (*B*) An intracranial hematoma bled into the area of infarction or surrounding brain tissue within 24 hours of right carotid endarterectomy performed within 1 week of the infarction. During endarterectomy, cerebral blood flow dou-bled. (From Henderson et al.[33] By permission of the American Association of Neurological Sur-geons.)

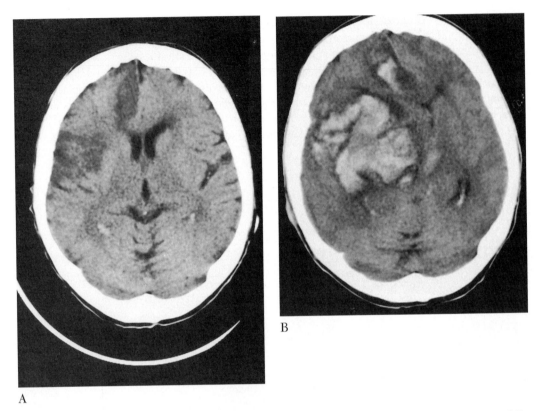

A

B

Figure 27–4. Computed tomography scan images demonstrating (A) a large right-sided middle cerebral artery infarct, (B) with bleeding from the intracranial hematoma into the adjacent right frontal lobe 5 days after right carotid endarterectomy. The patient had postoperative hypertension, was confused, and had a seizure in the 48 hours preceding infarction. (From Henderson et al.[33] By permission of the American Association of Neurological Surgeons.)

each of these cranial nerve deficits are shown in Table 27–4.

A major concern is a lesion of the recurrent laryngeal nerve with vocal cord paralysis. Hoarseness or dysphagia clearly improves within 6 months after carotid endarterectomy. In a few patients, the deficit is permanent.

Ischemic Stroke

The incidence of ischemic stroke after carotid endarterectomy has been estimated to be up to 5%.[22,31,38,75] Not all strokes are ipsilateral to carotid endarterectomy, and some involve the posterior circulation.[3] Moreover, ischemic injury due to manipulation may remain silent.[12,28] A recent study examining postoper-

ative diffusion-weighted imaging found that carotid endarterectomy was associated with a significantly increased risk of small, probably embolic, scattered infarcts in the same territory.[51] The abnormalities were much more prevalent in patients who had carotid endarterectomy with shunting. However, a recent study of 1001 carotid endarterectomies in which electroencephalography was used as a monitoring technique and selected shunting was done revealed a combined stroke and mortality rate of 1% to 3%.[31]

Ischemic stroke may be associated with acute occlusion of the carotid artery in the early postoperative period.[49] Occlusion can also occur during the surgical procedure, probably from embolization of atheromatous debris or

Table 27–3. Incidence of Peripheral Nerve Lesions after Carotid Endarterectomy in Prospective Studies

Author	Publication Year	Number of Patients	INCIDENCE OF PERIPHERAL NERVE DAMAGE (%)							
			VII	IX	X inf	X sup	XII	Aur	CS	Total (%)
Hertzer et al.[34]	1980	240	3		6	2	5			16
Liapis et al.[45]	1981	40	5		27		20	7		59
Evans et al.[23]	1982	128		1	35		11			47
Astor et al.[7]	1983	133			6	1	6			13
Forssell et al.[27]	1985	162	1	1	3		10	7	1	23
Aldoori & Baird[6]	1988	52	6		6		16			28
Forssell et al.[26]	1995	689		0.3	1	0.3	11			12
Schauber et al.[66]	1997	183	1		8		4	1		14
Ballotta et al.[10]	1999	200	1		4	1	5	1		12
Scavée et al.[65]	2001	600	0.2		6		0.5			6

X inf, inferior or recurrent laryngeal nerve; X sup, superior laryngeal nerve; Aur, great auricular nerve; CS, cervical sympathetic chain.

Source: Modified from D'Addato M, Mirelli M: Cranial nerve injury after carotid artery surgery. In Branchereau A, Jacobs M (eds): *Complications in Vascular and Endovascular Surgery. Part I.* Armonk, New York, Futura Publishing Company, 2001, pp 141–149. By permission of the publisher.

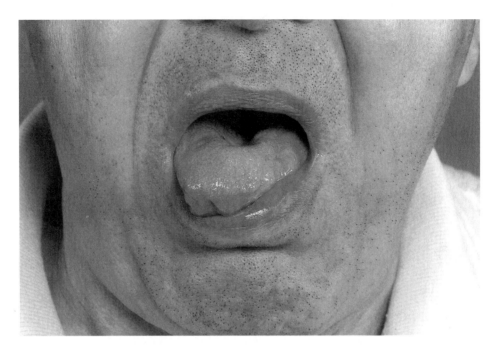

Figure 27–5. Hypoglossal nerve lesion on the right with deviation of the tongue to the right after carotid endarterectomy.

thrombus. In other patients, however, an asymptomatic postoperative interval is followed by an acute severe neurologic deficit that involves hemiparesis of the face, arm, and leg and gaze preference, all indicative of a stroke in a large arterial territory. Prompt surgical re-exploration has been done, but it is unclear whether thrombectomy or repair of the technical defect and patch angioplasty have had any effect on recovery of function.[4] Ischemic stroke

Table 27–4. Clinical Features of Cranial Nerve Deficits after Carotid Endarterectomy

Type	Symptoms	Mechanism	Permanent
Facial nerve (VII)	Mimics central VII Asymmetry of upper lip	Hyperextension Head rotation	Rare
Glossopharyngeal nerve (IX)	Dysphagia Nasal regurgitation Hemiparesis Soft palate Hypertension common (Hering's nerve)	Shunt placement (more retraction) Subluxation of mandible	Up to 5%
Vagus nerve (X)	Hoarseness Reduced coughing Inability to produce high tones	Ligation or transection of superior thyroid artery	Infrequent after 3 months
Accessory nerve (XI)	Drooping shoulder Painful acromioclavicular joint	Retractor injury Electrical trauma	Unclear
Hypoglossal nerve (XII)	Deviation of tongue Dysarthria Chewing difficulties	Short neck after transection of digastric muscle	Infrequent after 6 months

may also occur with acute intraluminal thrombosis that can be documented by selective angiography (Fig. 27–6).

Immediate reexploration was found to be successful in a study from the New York University Medical Center.[62] This study found intraluminal thrombus in 15 of 18 reexplorations (83%), and it was possible to correct any technical defects. After 18 reexplorations in 12 patients, there was complete resolution or significant improvement in neurologic deficit. Reexploration could be tailored toward patients with a severe deficit (National Institutes of Health Stroke Scale score ≥ 8).[25] Signs pertaining to large territory stroke (gaze preference, hemianopia, and flaccid hemiplegia) of the middle cerebral artery warrant early exploration for occlusion of a major vessel. Isolated monoparesis can indicate a branch occlusion of the middle cerebral artery, which is treated by control of blood pressure surges or intravenous administration of dextran (20 mL bolus followed by infusion of dextran 40 at 20 mL/hour), but it may fall short, and many surgeons would still want to proceed. Anecdotal reports of intraoperative infusion of thrombolytics have been published, but the risks of this intervention are unclear.[11,77]

MEDICAL COMPLICATIONS

Medical complications after carotid endarterectomy need attention.[55] A wound hematoma occurs from capillary oozing and, in approximately one-fourth of patients, arterial bleeding. Wound hematoma in the operated neck is uncommon, but severity of airway compromise

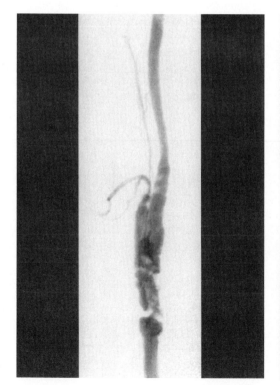
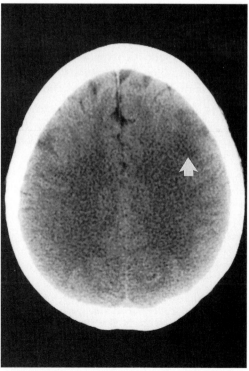

Figure 27–6. Patient with acute postoperative aphasia. *Left,* Angiogram obtained after carotid endarterectomy showing typical rugged-shaped carotid artery but also contrast defects indicating thrombus (confirmed at reexploration). *Right,* Computed tomography scan image showing early development of hypodensity (*arrow*) in cortical branch of middle cerebral artery.

varies. Clinically obvious airway obstruction requiring reintubation is very uncommon, but obstruction may be more prevalent (up to 25%) in patients studied by computed tomography.[18] Major predictors of a wound hematoma are failure to reverse intravenous heparin, intraoperative hypotension (adequate hemostasis during hypotension may prove to be false after blood pressure is increased), and carotid shunt placement.[18] Coughing due to prior chronic obstructive pulmonary disease and brief hypertensive surges may contribute.[42,53] A large wound hematoma requires emergency evacuation, even at the bedside in some instances. Most of the time, compromise by the wound hematoma is transient and self-limiting. Corticosteroids, moist steam inhalers, and nursing care in a sitting position have been successful.[37] Dehiscence of the venous patch, caused by a tear in the middle of the vein graft, is obviously more serious.[68,69,81] Rupture may lead to hypoperfusion and massive cerebral infarction and also respiratory distress. A rupture with venous patching has been described, but the incidence of this serious complication is very low. At the Mayo Clinic, 5 postoperative vein ruptures occurred after 2888 carotid endarterectomies.[81] Reinforcing the vein patch with a synthetic mesh wrap may account for the infrequency of rupture.

Postoperative hypertension is a major concern and requires treatment with antihypertensive agents, as outlined in Chapter 6. Hypertension is a common manifestation of a lesion affecting Hering's nerve, a branch of the glossopharyngeal nerve.[78] Factors that increase the risk of postoperative hypertension are high-grade carotid stenosis, cardiac dysrhythmias, and preoperative hypertension with a systolic blood pressure of more than 160 mm Hg and evidence of renal failure. Postoperative hypertension can be expected in patients with preoperative hypertension, but in 20% of instances, the finding is new. Carotid baroreceptor sensitivity (increased activity of the carotid sinus nerve) in addition to true dysfunction after vagal nerve damage is the proposed mechanism. The same mechanism accounts for bradycardia. Postoperative hypertension (systolic blood pressure of more than 180 mm Hg or 35 mm Hg from baseline) has been linked to cardiac complications, such as angina pectoris, congestive heart failure, myocardial infarction, and arrhythmias.

CONCLUSIONS

- Adequate postoperative blood pressure control and discontinuation of anticoagulation may be justified in patients at high risk for intracerebral hematomas.
- Admission to the NICU is warranted to monitor for wound hematomas, hypertension, and cardiac stress.
- Reexploration may be needed in stroke occurring after carotid endarterectomy.

REFERENCES

1. AbuRahma AF, Choueiri MA: Cranial and cervical nerve injuries after repeat carotid endarterectomy. *J Vasc Surg* 32:649–654, 2000.
2. AbuRahma AF, Lim RY: Management of vagus nerve injury after carotid endarterectomy. *Surgery* 119:245–247, 1996.
3. AbuRahma AF, Robinson P, Holt SM, et al: Perioperative and late stroke rates of carotid endarterectomy contralateral to carotid artery occlusion: results from a randomized trial. *Stroke* 31:1566–1571, 2000.
4. AbuRahma AF, Robinson PA, Short YS: Management options for post carotid endarterectomy stroke. *J Cardiovasc Surg (Torino)* 37:331–336, 1996.
5. Ackerstaff RG, Moons KG, van de Vlasakker CJ, et al: Association of intraoperative transcranial Doppler monitoring variables with stroke from carotid endarterectomy. *Stroke* 31:1817–1823, 2000.
6. Aldoori MI, Baird RN: Local neurological complication during carotid endarterectomy. *J Cardiovasc Surg (Torino)* 29:432–436, 1988.
7. Astor FC, Santilli P, Tucker HM: Incidence of cranial nerve dysfunction following carotid endarterectomy. *Head Neck Surg* 6:660–663, 1983.
8. Ayari R, Ede B, Bartoli M, et al: Neurologic compli-

cations of carotid surgery. In Branchereau A, Jacobs M (eds): *Complications in Vascular and Endovascular Surgery*. Part I. Armonk, NY: Futura Publishing Company, 2001, pp 119–131.

9. Bailes JE: Carotid endarterectomy. *Neurosurgery* 50:1290–1295, 2002.

10. Ballotta E, Da Giau G, Renon L, et al: Cranial and cervical nerve injuries after carotid endarterectomy: a prospective study. *Surgery* 125:85–91, 1999.

11. Barr JD, Horowitz MB, Mathis JM, et al: Intraoperative urokinase infusion for embolic stroke during carotid endarterectomy. *Neurosurgery* 36:606–611, 1995.

12. Barth A, Remonda L, Lovblad KO, et al: Silent cerebral ischemia detected by diffusion-weighted MRI after carotid endarterectomy. *Stroke* 31:1824–1828, 2000.

13. Bowyer MW, Zierold D, Loftus JP, et al: Carotid endarterectomy: a comparison of regional versus general anesthesia in 500 operations. *Ann Vasc Surg* 14:145–151, 2000.

14. Branchereau A, Ondo N'Dong F, Scotti L: Mécanismes des complications neurologiques postopératoires enhancement chirurgie carotidienne. In Kieffer E, Natali J (eds): *Aspects Techniques de la Chirurgie Carotidienne*. Paris: AERCV, 1987, pp 317–331.

15. Breen JC, Caplan LR, DeWitt LD, et al: Brain edema after carotid surgery. *Neurology* 46:175–181, 1996.

16. Brooks WH, McClure RR, Jones MR, et al: Carotid angioplasty and stenting versus carotid endarterectomy: randomized trial in a community hospital. *J Am Coll Cardiol* 38:1589–1595, 2001.

17. Caplan LR, Skillman J, Ojemann R, et al: Intracerebral hemorrhage following carotid endarterectomy: A hypertensive complication? *Stroke* 9:457–460, 1978.

18. Carmichael FJ, McGuire GP, Wong DT, et al: Computed tomographic analysis of airway dimensions after carotid endarterectomy. *Anesth Analg* 83:12–17, 1996.

19. Counsell CE, Salinas R, Naylor R, et al: A systematic review of the randomised trials of carotid patch angioplasty in carotid endarterectomy. *Eur J Vasc Endovasc Surg* 13:345–354, 1997.

20. Curran AJ, Smyth D, Sheehan SJ, et al: Recurrent laryngeal nerve dysfunction following carotid endarterectomy. *J R Coll Surg Edinb* 42:168–170, 1997.

21. Dalman JE, Beenakkers IC, Moll FL, et al: Transcranial Doppler monitoring during carotid endarterectomy helps to identify patients at risk of postoperative hyperperfusion. *Eur J Vasc Endovasc Surg* 18:222–227, 1999.

22. Enevoldsen EM, Torfing T, Kjeldsen MJ, et al: Cerebral infarct following carotid endarterectomy. Frequency, clinical and hemodynamic significance evaluated by MRI and TCD. *Acta Neurol Scand* 100:106–110, 1999.

23. Evans WE, Mendelowitz DS, Liapis C, et al: Motor speech deficit following carotid endarterectomy. *Ann Surg* 196:461–464, 1982.

24. Fearn SJ, Parry AD, Picton AJ, et al: Should heparin be reversed after carotid endarterectomy: a randomised prospective trial. *Eur J Vasc Endovasc Surg* 13:394–397, 1997.

25. Findlay JM, Marchak BE: Reoperation for acute hemispheric stroke after carotid endarterectomy: Is there any value? *Neurosurgery* 50:486–493, 2002.

26. Forssell C, Kitzing P, Bergqvist D: Cranial nerve injuries after carotid artery surgery. A prospective study of 663 operations. *Eur J Vasc Endovasc Surg* 10:445–449, 1995.

27. Forssell C, Takolander R, Bergqvist D, et al: Cranial nerve injuries associated with carotid endarterectomy. A prospective study. *Acta Chir Scand* 151:595–598, 1985.

28. Gaunt M, Naylor AR, Lennard N, et al: Transcranial Doppler detected cerebral microembolism following carotid endarterectomy. *Brain* 121:389–390, 1998.

29. Ghali R, Palazzo EG, Rodriguez DI, et al: Transcranial Doppler intraoperative monitoring during carotid endarterectomy: experience with regional or general anesthesia, with and without shunting. *Ann Vasc Surg* 11:9–13, 1997.

30. Hafner DH, Smith RB III, King OW, et al: Massive intracerebral hemorrhage following carotid endarterectomy. *Arch Surg* 122:305–307, 1987.

31. Hamdan AD, Pomposelli FB Jr, Gibbons GW, et al: Perioperative strokes after 1001 consecutive carotid endarterectomy procedures without an electroencephalogram: incidence, mechanism, and recovery. *Arch Surg* 134:412–415, 1999.

32. Hayes PD, Allroggen H, Steel S, et al: Randomized trial of vein versus Dacron patching during carotid endarterectomy: influence of patch type on postoperative embolization. *J Vasc Surg* 33:994–1000, 2001.

33. Henderson RD, Phan TG, Piepgras DG, et al: Mechanisms of intracerebral hemorrhage after carotid endarterectomy. *J Neurosurg* 95:964–969, 2001.

34. Hertzer NR, Feldman BJ, Beven EG, et al: A prospective study of the incidence of injury to the cranial nerves during carotid endarterectomy. *Surg Gynecol Obstet* 151:781–784, 1980.

35. Ho DS, Wang Y, Chui M, et al: Epileptic seizures attributed to cerebral hyperperfusion after percutaneous transluminal angioplasty and stenting of the internal carotid artery. *Cerebrovasc Dis* 10:374–379, 2000.

36. Hobson RW II: Update on the Carotid Revascularization Endarterectomy versus Stent Trial (CREST) protocol. *J Am Coll Surg* 194:S9–S14, 2002.

37. Hughes R, McGuire G, Montanera W, et al: Upper airway edema after carotid endarterectomy: the effect of steroid administration. *Anesth Analg* 84:475–478, 1997.

38. Jacobowitz GR, Rockman CB, Lamparello PJ, et al: Causes of perioperative stroke after carotid endarterectomy: special considerations in symptomatic patients. *Ann Vasc Surg* 15:19–24, 2001.

39. Jansen C, Sprengers AM, Moll FL, et al: Prediction of intracerebral haemorrhage after carotid endarterec-

tomy by clinical criteria and intraoperative transcranial Doppler monitoring. *Eur J Vasc Surg* 8:303–308, 1994.

40. Jordan WD Jr, Alcocer F, Wirthlin DJ, et al: High-risk carotid endarterectomy: challenges for carotid stent protocols. *J Vasc Surg* 35:16–22, 2002.

41. Kieburtz K, Ricotta JJ, Moxley RT III: Seizures following carotid endarterectomy. *Arch Neurol* 47:568–570, 1990.

42. Kunkel JM, Gomez ER, Spebar MJ, et al: Wound hematomas after carotid endarterectomy. *Am J Surg* 148:844–847, 1984.

43. Lanska DJ, Kryscio RJ: In-hospital mortality following carotid endarterectomy. *Neurology* 51:440–447, 1998.

44. L'AURC, Becquemin JP, Souadka F, et al: Risque opératoire actuel de la chirurgie carotidienne: expérience du groupe vasculaire de l'AURC. In Kieffer E, Bousser MG (eds): *Indications et Résultats de la Chirurgie Carotidienne.* Paris: AERCV, 1988, pp 41–50.

45. Liapis CD, Satiani B, Florance CL, et al: Motor speech malfunction following carotid endarterectomy. *Surgery* 89:56–59, 1981.

46. Manninen PH, Tan TK, Sarjeant RM: Somatosensory evoked potential monitoring during carotid endarterectomy in patients with stroke. *Anesth Analg* 93:39–44, 2001.

47. Maroulis J, Karkanevatos A, Papakostas K, et al: Cranial nerve dysfunction following carotid endarterectomy. *Int Angiol* 19:237–241, 2000.

48. McCrory DC, Goldstein LB, Samsa GP, et al: Predicting complications of carotid endarterectomy. *Stroke* 24:1285–1291, 1993.

49. McKinsey JF, Desai TR, Bassiouny HS, et al: Mechanisms of neurologic deficits and mortality with carotid endarterectomy. *Arch Surg* 131:526–531, 1996.

50. Morasch MD, Hirko MK, Hirasa T, et al: Intensive care after carotid endarterectomy: a prospective evaluation. *J Am Coll Surg* 183:387–392, 1996.

51. Muller M, Reiche W, Langenscheidt P, et al: Ischemia after carotid endarterectomy: comparison between transcranial Doppler sonography and diffusion-weighted MR imaging. *AJNR Am J Neuroradiol* 21:47–54, 2000.

52. O'Neill L, Lanska DJ, Hartz A: Surgeon characteristics associated with mortality and morbidity following carotid endarterectomy. *Neurology* 55:773–781, 2000.

53. O'Sullivan JC, Wells DG, Wells GR: Difficult airway management with neck swelling after carotid endarterectomy. *Anaesth Intensive Care* 14:460–464, 1986.

54. Ouriel K, Shortell CK, Illig KA, et al: Intracerebral hemorrhage after carotid endarterectomy: incidence, contribution to neurologic morbidity, and predictive factors. *J Vasc Surg* 29:82–87, 1999.

55. Paciaroni M, Eliasziw M, Kappelle LJ, et al: Medical complications associated with carotid endarterectomy. North American Symptomatic Carotid Endarterectomy Trial (NASCET). *Stroke* 30:1759–1763, 1999.

56. Piepgras DG, Morgan MK, Sundt TM Jr, et al: Intracerebral hemorrhage after carotid endarterectomy. *J Neurosurg* 68:532–536, 1988.

57. Pomposelli FB, Lamparello PJ, Riles TS, et al: Intracranial hemorrhage after carotid endarterectomy. *J Vasc Surg* 7:248–255, 1988.

58. Radak D, Popovic AD, Radicevic S, et al: Immediate reoperation for perioperative stroke after 2250 carotid endarterectomies: differences between intraoperative and early postoperative stroke. *J Vasc Surg* 30:245–251, 1999.

59. Reigel MM, Hollier LH, Sundt TM Jr, et al: Cerebral hyperperfusion syndrome: a cause of neurologic dysfunction after carotid endarterectomy. *J Vasc Surg* 5:628–634, 1987.

60. Rigdon EE, Monajjem N, Rhodes RS: Criteria for selective utilization of the intensive care unit following carotid endarterectomy. *Ann Vasc Surg* 11:20–27, 1997.

61. Riles TS, Imparato AM, Jacobowitz GR, et al: The cause of perioperative stroke after carotid endarterectomy. *J Vasc Surg* 19:206–214, 1994.

62. Rockman CB, Cappadona C, Riles TS, et al: Causes of the increased stroke rate after carotid endarterectomy in patients with previous strokes. *Ann Vasc Surg* 11:28–34, 1997.

63. Rockman CB, Jacobowitz GR, Lamparello PJ, et al: Immediate reexploration for the perioperative neurologic event after carotid endarterectomy: Is it worthwhile? *J Vasc Surg* 32:1062–1070, 2000.

64. Ross SD, Tribble CG, Parrino PE, et al: Intensive care is cost-effective in carotid endarterectomy. *Cardiovasc Surg* 8:41–46, 2000.

65. Scavée V, Viejo D, Buche M, et al: Six hundred consecutive carotid endarterectomies with temporary shunt and vein patch angioplasty: early and long-term results. *Cardiovasc Surg* 9:463–468, 2001.

66. Schauber MD, Fontenelle LJ, Solomon JW, et al: Cranial/cervical nerve dysfunction after carotid endarterectomy. *J Vasc Surg* 25:481–487, 1997.

67. Schroeder T, Sillesen H, Sorensen O, et al: Cerebral hyperperfusion following carotid endarterectomy. *J Neurosurg* 66:824–829, 1987.

68. Scott EW, Dolson L, Day AL, et al: Carotid endarterectomy complicated by vein patch rupture. *Neurosurgery* 31:373–376, 1992.

69. Self DD, Bryson GL, Sullivan PJ: Risk factors for postcarotid endarterectomy hematoma formation. *Can J Anaesth* 46:635–640, 1999.

70. Shuaib A, Hunter KM, Anderson MA: Multiple intracranial hemorrhages after carotid endarterectomy. *Can J Neurol Sci* 16:345–347, 1989.

71. Solomon RA, Loftus CM, Quest DO, et al: Incidence and etiology of intracerebral hemorrhage following carotid endarterectomy. *J Neurosurg* 64:29–34, 1986.

72. Steed DL, Peitzman AB, Grundy BL, et al: Causes of stroke in carotid endarterectomy. *Surgery* 92:634–641, 1982.

73. Sundt TM Jr, Ebersold MJ, Sharbrough FW, et al: The risk-benefit ratio of intraoperative shunting during carotid endarterectomy. Relevance to operative and postoperative results and complications. *Ann Surg* 203:196–204, 1986.

74. Sundt TM Jr, Sharbrough FW, Piepgras DG, et al: Correlation of cerebral blood flow and electroencephalographic changes during carotid endarterectomy: with results of surgery and hemodynamics of cerebral ischemia. *Mayo Clin Proc* 56:533–543, 1981.

75. Tretter MJ Jr, Hertzer NR, Mascha EJ, et al: Perioperative risk and late outcome of nonelective carotid endarterectomy. *J Vasc Surg* 30:618–631, 1999.

76. van Harten B, van Gool WA, Bienfait HM, et al: Brain edema after carotid endarterectomy. *Neurology* 48:544–545, 1997.

77. Winkelaar GB, Salvian AJ, Fry PD, et al: Intraoperative intraarterial urokinase in early postoperative stroke following carotid endarterectomy: a useful adjunct. *Ann Vasc Surg* 13:566–570, 1999.

78. Wong JH, Findlay JM, Suarez-Almazor ME: Hemodynamic instability after carotid endarterectomy: risk factors and associations with operative complications. *Neurosurgery* 41:35–41, 1997.

79. Woodward G, Venkatesh R: Spinal accessory neuropathy and internal jugular thrombosis after carotid endarterectomy. *J Neurol Neurosurg Psychiatry* 68:111–112, 2000.

80. Yagnik PM, Chong PS: Spinal accessory nerve injury: a complication of carotid endarterectomy. *Muscle Nerve* 19:907–909, 1996.

81. Yamamoto Y, Piepgras DG, Marsh WR, et al: Complications resulting from saphenous vein patch graft after carotid endarterectomy. *Neurosurgery* 39:670–675, 1996.

28

Craniotomy and Biopsy

Both elective and emergency craniotomy are unchallenged indications for admission to a neurologic-neurosurgical intensive care unit. We may have a tendency to overestimate small risks but the probability of a major complication after elective craniotomy is rare, and such a complication is unlikely to contribute to overall morbidity. In many patients with planned craniotomy, stay in the NICU is precautionary and brief.

Tumor surgery is most often the indication for elective craniotomy. Wound infections,[24] brain edema, seizures, and postoperative hemorrhage in any compartment along the track of surgical excision constitute most of the complications. Other equally common complications, discussed in other chapters of this monograph, include increased intracranial pressure (Chapter 9), status epilepticus (Chapter 24), and hyponatremia (Chapter 31). Neurosurgical problems in perioperative care, such as wound infections, pseudomeningocele,[7,41] and cerebrospinal fluid leaks are not discussed here. The organizing principle of this chapter is to provide a brief overview of specific unusual complications. Most of these complications are handled by the neurosurgeon. However, the neurointensivist or any of the attending neurologists may be consulted or asked to comanage postoperative care.

GENERAL CARE AFTER CRANIOTOMY

Airway management remains an important priority after any type of craniotomy. Recovery of consciousness may be prolonged after exten-

sive surgical procedures requiring brain retraction, and this may result in partial collapse of the airway. Reduced activation of the muscles of the upper airway, such as the pharyngeal constrictor muscle and genioglossus, may not keep the pharynx patent. Inability to maintain a normal airway then results in hypoxemia. Airway obstruction due to bilateral vocal cord paralysis after surgery in the posterior fossa that injures the vagal nerves (e.g., ependymoma, acoustic neuroma) may produce stridor. Temporary tracheostomy may be needed if the cords remain fixed in position.

An abundance of seemingly mundane problems may occur after craniotomy. Refractory nausea and vomiting appear more commonly in women and younger patients and after removal of lesions in the posterior fossa.[13] Effective therapeutic agents are ondansetron, 1 to 4 mg intravenously, and promethazine, 12.5 to 25 mg intravenously. Unrest, anxiety, and discomfort are more common than profound agitation (Chapter 4). Patients with these postoperative manifestations have a good response to infusion of dexmedetomidine.[2,10–12] This new drug, an α_2-adrenergic agonist, has a higher affinity for its corresponding receptor than clonidine. Because respiratory depression does not occur, the drug is ideal as an anxiolytic agent in patients who cannot tolerate the endotracheal tube (patients appear asleep but are quickly awakened). However, dexmedetomidine has a very narrow therapeutic range (1 μg/kg intravenously over 10 minutes followed by 0.2 to 0.7 μg/kg per hour intravenously). Hypotension, bradycardia, and nausea remain of concern as side effects. Experience with dexmedetomidine is limited, and it has been approved for use on only the first 2 postoperative days.[10]

Postoperative hiccups can be difficult to manage. Placement of a nasogastric tube alone can be successful, but many drugs have been tried, including baclofen and valproate (Chapter 18). In the postoperative period, success has recently been claimed with nefopam, a non-narcotic analgesic, 10 mg intravenously.[3]

Craniotomy is a major surgical procedure and typically is followed by significant facial swelling, unilateral soft tissue eyelid hematoma, and pain from transient removal of a bone flap. These discomforts subside gradually, but pain may be severe and is traditionally handled with drugs such as codeine, 60 mg intramuscularly. Generally, drugs are avoided that potentially suppress megakaryopoiesis (for example, H_2 blockers and many antibiotics). A typical postcraniotomy order is shown in Table 28–1.

SPECIFIC COMPLICATIONS

Obtaining the frequency of morbidity and mortality after craniotomy is complicated because neurosurgery has proliferated in specialty areas. Specific complications may occur, although a common denominator is cerebrospinal fluid leak, hemorrhage in the surgical bed, or vascular—arterial or venous—injury.[36,43] Series involving craniotomy for glioma have reported mortality of 3% and morbidity approaching 10%.[9,14,39] Worsening of motor weakness and herniation are substantial surgical risks, varying from 10% to 20% in most large series.[9,14,39]

Epilepsy surgery for intractable seizures has been established and proven.[52] The most frequent concerns are infectious complications, including wound infections that require bone flap removal.[1] Injury to the anterior choroidal artery in temporal lobectomy with radical medial resection may cause hemiplegia. Word-finding deficits can be present after left anterior temporal lobectomy.[1,27] An intracerebral hematoma with depth electrode implantation is usually uncommon, but the incidence may reach 3%.[34,49] Patients with early postoperative seizures have a slightly less favorable outcome, particularly if the seizures are similar in type to presurgical seizures. Isolated auras, however, do not predict a poor surgical result.[28]

Pituitary surgery may lead to neurologic, endocrine, and sinonasal complications.[18] Cerebrospinal fluid leaks, hemorrhage in the surgical site, diabetes insipidus, and panhypopituitarism are leading complications. Adrenal, thyroid, and gonadal deficiencies may become noticeable and are often permanent.[18] Evaluation of postoperative hormonal status may show low thyroxine level and low free thyroxine index due to central hypothyroidism. Adrenal insufficiency may be difficult to detect clinically, but a random sample of cortisol less than 5 μg/dL is highly suggestive.

Diabetes insipidus is evident when polyuria occurs with increased serum tonicity, insufficient water intake, and hypotonic urine (Chapter 31).

Transsphenoidal surgery for pituitary adenoma may cause hyponatremia (up to postoperative day 9),[23] and rapid correction can lead to pontine or extrapontine myelinolysis.[4,19,37,48] The type of hyponatremia and hypernatremia associated with transsphenoidal surgery is further discussed in Chapter 31.

Remote Hemorrhages

Postoperative hemorrhages in the surgical bed (see Chapter 13) are more common than hemorrhages at distant sites.[21,46] However, several cases have been described of intracranial hemorrhage occurring at a site remote from the craniotomy. The hemorrhages may occur in the opposite hemisphere and in the cerebellum after surgery on, for example, one of the frontal

Table 28–1. Standard Postoperative Craniotomy Order*

Codeine	60 mg IM, q4h p.r.n.
Cefazolin sodium	500–1000 mg IV, q4h
Dexamethasone	4 mg IV, q4h
Phenytoin	100 mg, q8h
Subcutaneous heparin	5000 U, q12h

*Also includes swallowing precautions, incentive spirometry, crystalloid fluids, and prevention of intracranial pressure surges.

lobes or after drainage of a subdural hematoma. The mechanism for these hemorrhages may be different in each location, the pathophysiology remains unclear, and the clinical significance is not always obvious. Predisposing factors are coagulopathy, preoperative use of mannitol, prior alcohol abuse, use of valproic acid, which could interfere with anticoagulation,[47] and traumatic origin of the hematoma but not postoperative hypertension.[6] These remote hemorrhages have been devastating, causing significant morbidity, but they can be small without contributing much to the overall neurologic condition. The frequency is estimated to be 1 in 300 craniotomies.

Most remote hemorrhages become evident clinically and on CT scan within the first 24 hours. Often, a postoperative CT scan documents remote hemorrhages in a patient who does not awaken from general anesthesia. Postoperative headache may be a warning sign of a remote hemorrhage in the cerebellum. In several case reports in the literature, generalized tonic-clonic seizures signaled a hematoma involving a hemispheric location. Clinical features vary depending on the location. Hemorrhages in the cerebellar peduncles produce a tremor and in the cerebellar hemisphere result in cerebellar ataxia and slurred speech. Nystagmus may change in direction with different positions of gaze (a typical feature of central nystagmus).

In cerebellar hematomas, the CT characteristics of the hemorrhage—much of the blood tracks through the folia—may suggest a venous hemorrhage from tearing of the superior vermian veins or any of their tributaries.[47,53] Some data suggest that postoperative hemorrhage in the cerebellum is more likely with cerebrospinal fluid drainage during surgery, possibly a reflection of a mechanical shift of the cerebellum ("cerebellar sag").[16,53] These factors suggest that acute reduction in intracranial pressure from removal of a supratentorial mass can lead to a critical increase in transmural pressure in veins and venules, culminating in possible hemorrhage. Another hypothesis is that extension and rotation during positioning obstruct the veins of the cerebellum and result in a hemorrhagic infarct. Pterional craniotomy often involves various de-

grees of contralateral rotation and 20° of extension of the neck that may predispose the patient to obstruction of the internal jugular vein. An examination of the biomechanics of this region confirmed that angulation and obstruction of the internal jugular vein at the transverse process of C1 on the same side as the craniotomy may be a contributing cause.[44]

Craniotomy for a traumatic intracranial lesion may be associated with a contralateral extradural hematoma. Failure to awaken after surgery is the most common presenting feature and is striking in some, with fixed, dilated pupils and bilateral extensor posturing.[54] However, remote hemorrhages after craniotomy for traumatic brain injury may be a result of the development of hemorrhagic contusions rather than a consequence of the surgical procedure.[8]

Multiple intracerebral hemorrhages, a contralateral extradural hematoma,[54] and subarachnoid hemorrhage[26] have been described in exceptional cases and may include supratentorial and intratentorial hemorrhages.[32,35] Examples of remote hemorrhages are shown in Figures 28–1, 28–2, and 28–3.

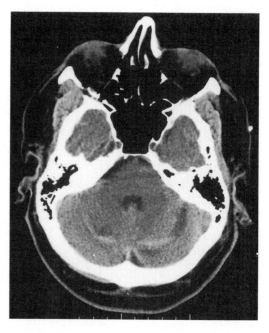

Figure 28–1. Remote cerebellar hematoma. Note tracking along folia suggesting venous hemorrhage.

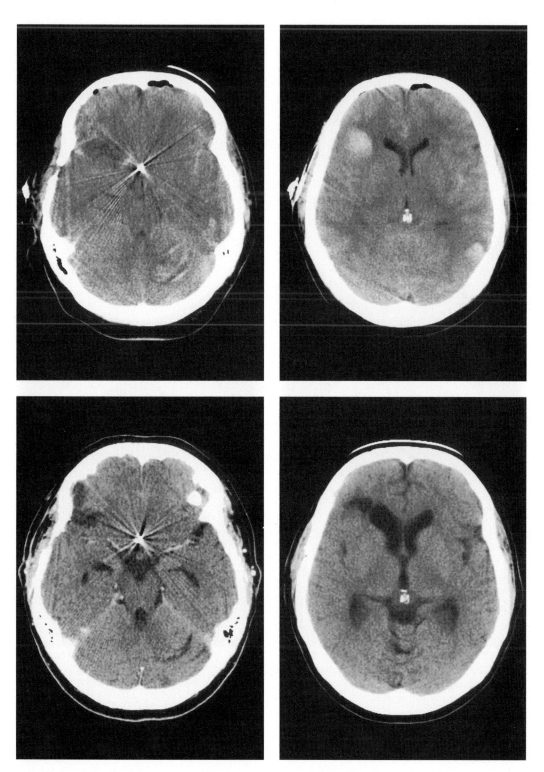

Figure 28–2. Serial computed tomography scans. (*Top row*) Supratentorial and infratentorial remote cerebral hemorrhages and clipping of communicating artery aneurysm. (*Bottom row*) 3 months later, hypodense scars as telltale signs of the postoperative hemorrhages.

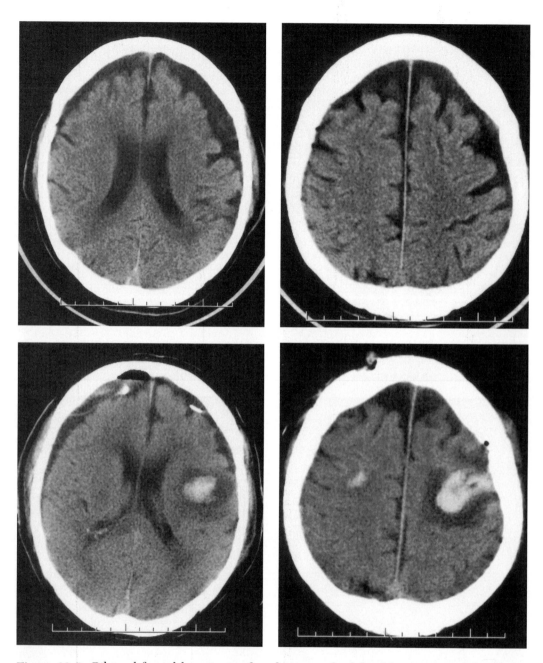

Figure 28–3. Bilateral frontal hematoma after drainage of subdural hygromas with bur holes and placement of a suction drain.

With so few examples, the ideal management is not well established. When the hematoma involves the cerebellum and is causing herniation, surgery is necessary to remove the mass effect. Small hemorrhages in both hemispheres can probably be left alone. Undoubtedly, outcome is determined by the time to recognition, and if a mass effect exists, surgical evacuation is necessary. Many patients who initially fail to awaken have a poor outcome, particularly when the signs involve upward or downward herniation. However, most patients in cases reported in the literature have a predominantly poor outcome, often with serious disability. Prevention of cerebellar hemorrhage may be equally important. It is imperative to focus on drainage only (no suction) and avoid intraoperative use of mannitol and valproic acid.[20]

Postbiopsy Hemorrhage

Biopsy-associated intracerebral hemorrhage occurs in only a small percentage of patients[15,40,51,56] (Table 28–2). A prospective study found delayed neurologic deterioration in only a few patients (0.4%).[25] Silent hemorrhage was more common, occurring in more than half the studied cases. Multivariate analysis documented increased risk with a platelet count below 150,000 cells/mm^3 or a lesion in the pineal gland due to the extreme vascularity of pinealomas and pinealoblastomas. There was increased risk with a higher number of specimens or postoperative hypertension.[15] A recent study of patients who had biopsy for presumed lymphoma after organ transplantation found an unexpectedly high incidence (four of six patients) of postbiopsy hemorrhage.[33] Evacuation of the hematoma is rarely needed and only if mass effect occurs (Fig. 28–4). Intracerebral hematoma may also occur with ventriculostomy but is rarely observed or clinically of much relevance[38] (Fig. 28–5).

Cerebral Infarction

Cerebral infarction is most commonly due to venous occlusion. This complication may occur after resection of a meningioma and is related to prior invasion of the dura and venous sinuses. Convexity, parasagittal, and falcine meningiomas are close to the superior sagittal sinus, causing a particular risk of infarction.[22] In some instances, the neurosurgeon has already attempted to reconstruct the cerebral venous sinus. Hemorrhagic infarction may incorporate the operative bed but also may occur at a distance or involve the deeper cerebral veins, causing bithalamic hemorrhagic infarcts, particularly if the operation is to remove a tumor in the pineal region.

A tentorial meningioma may require sacrifice of the transverse or sigmoid sinus, but if the torcula remains patent, venous cerebellar or supratentorial hemorrhage is less likely. Cerebellar infarction after the suboccipital approach is used to remove an acoustic neuroma is a known complication to neurosurgeons. In some patients, cerebellar softening is already obvious before closure, and the neurosurgeon resects the lateral part of the cerebellum. Postoperative CT scans may not be able initially to distinguish between edema and infarction, and magnetic resonance imaging with magnetic resonance venography may be needed.

Arterial occlusion may occur because of sacrifice of branches of the middle cerebral artery adherent to the sylvian fissure in patients who underwent surgery for a convexity meningioma. Cerebral infarction may be a consequence of complicated repair of an aneurysm despite use

Table 28–2. Literature Review of Hemorrhagic Complications (1990–2000) Detected after Stereotactic Brain Biopsy Procedures

Authors (Year)	No. of Patients	Patients with Hemorrhage (%)
Voges et al., 1993[51]	338	2.4
Sawin et al., 1998[40]	225	3.6
Yu et al., 1998[56]	310	1.6
Field et al., 2001[15]	500	8.0

Source: Modified from Field M, Witham TF, Flickinger JC, et al: Comprehensive assessment of hemorrhage risks and outcomes after stereotactic brain biopsy. *J Neurosurg* 94:545–551, 2001. By permission of the American Association of Neurological Surgeons.

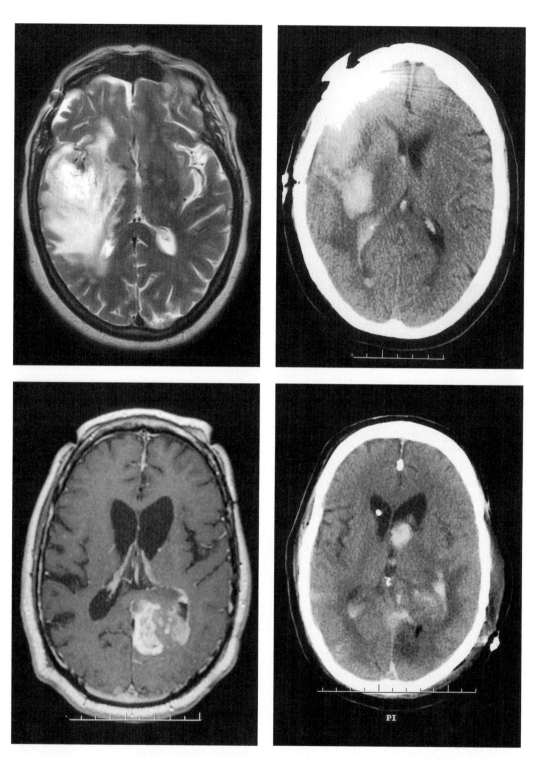

Figure 28–4. Preoperative magnetic resonance image (*top and bottom left*) and postoperative computed tomography scan (*top and bottom right*) in each of two patients with astrocytoma and postbiopsy intracerebral hematoma.

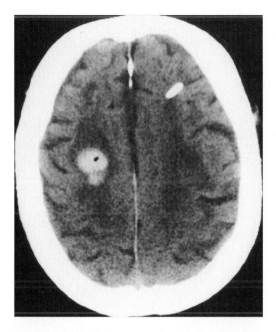

Figure 28–5. Postventriculostomy intracerebral hematoma. Note air in hematoma. The ventriculostomy drain has been moved to the opposite side.

of high-flow saphenous vein grafts. Resection of an arteriovenous malformation may cause retrograde thrombosis of the feeding arteries.[30]

Postoperative Cerebral Edema

Partial resection or stereotactic biopsy is more commonly associated with postoperative cerebral edema than gross total resection (Fig. 28–6). Prolonged retraction in the brain and an anesthetic regimen that increases cerebral blood volume may contribute. Opioids (leading to respiratory depression, high arterial carbon dioxide, and increased cerebral blood flow), isoflurane and nitrous oxide (vasodilators increasing cerebral blood volume), and enflurane and halothane (decreasing cerebral fluid resorption) can increase intracranial pressure from edema.[50]

Dexamethasone (10 to 20 mg intravenously followed by 4 mg every 6 hours) possibly reduces postoperative edema, and its use peri-operatively in craniotomy is universally accepted although not borne out by hard evidence.

Prevention (or treatment) of postoperative cerebral edema includes placement of the patient in a semirecumbent (30° to 40°) position to facilitate venous drainage, restriction of free water, and limitation of fluid intake to 2 L of isotonic saline. The role of blood pressure control is not known, and blood pressure goals in the perioperative period are not well established. Mannitol (Chapter 9) may be used temporarily, but most of the edema subsides spontaneously.

Seizures

Seizures may be due to a precipitous drop in antiepileptic drug level from failure to monitor levels in a patient with previous epileptic episodes or to drug interactions (Chapter 24). In other patients, high-risk situations, such as evacuation of subdural empyema and tumors abutting the primary motor cortex, may predispose to seizures. Use of prophylactic antiepileptic drugs (phenytoin and carbamazepine) in craniotomy is controversial because no effect on prevalence of postoperative seizures has been demonstrated up to 13 weeks after surgery.[45] Focal seizures are most common and may be refractory to treatment. Electroencephalography should document periodic epileptiform discharges. Aggressive management is needed, because some patients have prolonged hemiparesis, and partial status epilepticus lasting several days has been associated with permanent hemiparesis.[5] Control may be achieved with administration of phenobarbital, 20 mg/kg. Intravenous administration of valproate, 15 to 30 mg/kg loading dose over 1 hour, may be successful. Management of status epilepticus has been further discussed in Chapter 24.

Air Embolus

The incidence of air embolization after posterior fossa surgery is difficult to estimate and

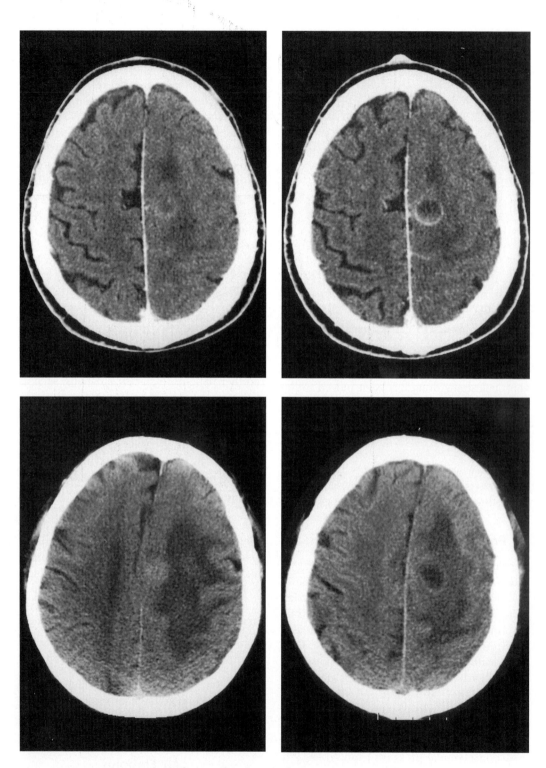

Figure 28–6. Biopsy-associated secondary brain edema presenting with seizure. (*Top row*) preoperative and (*bottom row*) postoperative computed tomography images.

Table 28–3. Air Embolism after Neurosurgical Procedures

Position	Incidence (%)
Sitting	25
Supine	14.6
Prone	10
Lateral	8.3

Source: Modified from Albin MS, Carroll RG, Maroon JC: Clinical considerations concerning detection of venous air embolism. *Neurosurgery* 3:380–384, 1978. By permission of the Congress of Neurological Surgeons.

depends on the detection methods. When Doppler ultrasonography is used for detection, air embolization is very common, particularly in a sitting position. Table 28–3 shows that the incidences are variable and related to neurosurgical positioning. Routine use of 10 cm of positive end-expiratory pressure during neurosurgery in the sitting position has no effect on the incidence of air embolization, although earlier studies suggested its use. Giebler et al.[17] documented significant adverse cardiovascular effects with the use of positive end-expiratory pressure. However, in most patients, the symptoms are not clinically significant.[29,42] The clinical presentation of a paradoxical air embolus is a sudden decrease in arterial PO_2 or saturation (to low 50s) followed by a decrease in end-tidal PCO_2 (from 30s to single digits), almost immediately followed by hypotension and tachycardia. When air enters the coronary arteries, electrocardiographic changes, including widening of the QRS complex and ST segment elevation or depression, can be seen, and cardiac arrest may occur. Air embolus entering the brain may cause a devastating injury. When anesthesiologists suspect air embolization, the surgeon should flood the wound with Ringer's solution and carefully inspect for open venous channels. The cut surfaces of the bone should be waxed and the open veins coagulated with bipolar forceps. In addition, the patient must be carefully moved to the right side to an upward position. Computed tomography scan in patients who have had air embolization may

show gas (black areas within the large arteries that can be seen on CT).

MEDICAL COMPLICATIONS

The available series on the medical complications of craniotomy have reported an incidence of 2% to 8%. This approximation compares with an operative mortality of about 3%. As alluded to, most series involve patients who had craniotomy for brain tumors.[9,14,39] The complications after surgery, seldom specific, include deep venous thrombosis, pulmonary embolus, myocardial ischemia or cardiac arrhythmias, gastrointestinal bleeding, and pneumonia. (Each of these abnormalities is covered extensively in other chapters of this book.) Several observations, however, are noteworthy. Medical complications were more likely to occur in patients who had two or more anatomical areas affected than in patients who had a lesion in only one area. Patients with a Karnofsky score of less than 80 had an increased risk of venous thrombus or pulmonary embolus.[14] Gastrointestinal bleeding after craniotomy was observed in several studies, but the incidence appears to be comparatively low in comparison with incidences from other major surgical procedures. In one study of patients who underwent craniotomy, however, the incidence approached 9%.[31] There was no relationship to age, corticosteroid administration, or casual use of prophylactic medication.

A prospective multicenter study of 2944 patients found that 4% had infections at the surgical site, including wound infections, bone flap infections, osteitis, meningitis, and brain abscesses. Risk factors identified were postoperative cerebrospinal fluid leakage, recurrent surgery, emergency surgery, contaminated surgical fields, and operative time longer than 4 hours. In this study, antibiotic prophylaxis did not appear to decrease the risk of a postoperative wound infection.[24] However, one earlier randomized trial documented that postcraniotomy infections were virtually eliminated.[55]

CONCLUSIONS

- The typical postcraniotomy order should include pain management with codeine, cefazolin, dexamethasone, phenytoin, and subcutaneous heparin; swallowing precautions; adequate fluids with crystalloids; and reduction of free water intake.
- Worsening after craniotomy may be due to hemorrhage in the surgical bed, remote hemorrhage, cerebral edema, or ischemic stroke from sacrifice of a large vein or artery.
- Careful evaluation of the endocrine axis (triiodothyronine, thyrotropin, cortisol, urine osmolarity) after pituitary surgery may detect panhypopituitarism.
- Postoperative seizures may be due to postoperative drug interactions.

REFERENCES

1. Behrens E, Schramm J, Zentner J, et al: Surgical and neurological complications in a series of 708 epilepsy surgery procedures. Neurosurgery 41:1–9, 1997.
2. Bhana N, Goa KL, McClellan KJ: Dexmedetomidine. Drugs 59:263–268, 2000.
3. Bilotta F, Pietropaoli P, Rosa G: Nefopam for refractory postoperative hiccups. Anesth Analg 93:1358–1360, 2001.
4. Boehnert M, Hensen J, Henig A, et al: Severe hyponatremia after transsphenoidal surgery for pituitary adenomas. Kidney Int Suppl 64:S12–S14, 1998.
5. Borchert LD, Labar DR: Permanent hemiparesis due to partial status epilepticus. Neurology 45:187–188, 1995.
6. Brisman MH, Bederson JB, Sen CN, et al: Intracerebral hemorrhage occurring remote from the craniotomy site. Neurosurgery 39:1114–1121, 1996.
7. Brown LJ: Suprasellar tension pneumocyst after transsphenoidal surgery. Case report. J Neurosurg 89:146–148, 1998.
8. Bullock R, Hanemann CO, Murray L, et al: Recurrent hematomas following craniotomy for traumatic intracranial mass. J Neurosurg 72:9–14, 1990.
9. Cabantog AM, Bernstein M: Complications of first craniotomy for intra-axial brain tumour. Can J Neurol Sci 21:213–218, 1994.
10. Coursin DB, Maccioli GA: Dexmedetomidine. Curr Opin Crit Care 7:221–226, 2001.
11. De Wolf AM, Fragen RJ, Avram MJ, et al: The pharmacokinetics of dexmedetomidine in volunteers with severe renal impairment. Anesth Analg 93:1205–1209, 2001.
12. Ebert TJ, Hall JE, Barney JA, et al: The effects of increasing plasma concentrations of dexmedetomidine in humans. Anesthesiology 93:382–394, 2000.
13. Fabling JM, Gan TJ, Guy J, et al: Postoperative nausea and vomiting. A retrospective analysis in patients undergoing elective craniotomy. J Neurosurg Anesthesiol 9:308–312, 1997.
14. Fadul C, Wood J, Thaler H, et al: Morbidity and mortality of craniotomy for excision of supratentorial gliomas. Neurology 38:1374–1379, 1988.
15. Field M, Witham TF, Flickinger JC, et al: Comprehensive assessment of hemorrhage risks and outcomes after stereotactic brain biopsy. J Neurosurg 94:545–551, 2001.
16. Friedman JA, Piepgras DG, Duke DA, et al: Remote cerebellar hemorrhage after supratentorial surgery. Neurosurgery 49:1327–1340, 2001.
17. Giebler R, Kollenberg B, Pohlen G, et al: Effect of positive end-expiratory pressure on the incidence of venous air embolism and on the cardiovascular response to the sitting position during neurosurgery. Br J Anaesth 80:30–35, 1998.
18. Heilman CB, Shucart WA, Rebeiz EE, et al: Endoscopic pituitary surgery. Clin Neurosurg 46:507–514, 2000.
19. Hensen J, Henig A, Fahlbusch R, et al: Prevalence, predictors and patterns of postoperative polyuria and hyponatraemia in the immediate course after transsphenoidal surgery for pituitary adenomas. Clin Endocrinol (Oxf) 50:431–439, 1999.
20. Honegger J, Zentner J, Spreer J, et al: Cerebellar hemorrhage arising postoperatively as a complication of supratentorial surgery: a retrospective study. J Neurosurg 96:248–254, 2002.
21. Kalfas IH, Little JR: Postoperative hemorrhage: a survey of 4992 intracranial procedures. Neurosurgery 23:343–347, 1988.
22. Keiper GL Jr, Sherman JD, Tomsick TA, et al: Dural sinus thrombosis and pseudotumor cerebri: unexpected complications of suboccipital craniotomy and translabyrinthine craniectomy. J Neurosurg 91:192–197, 1999.
23. Kelly DF, Laws ER Jr, Fossett D: Delayed hyponatremia after transsphenoidal surgery for pituitary adenoma. Report of nine cases. J Neurosurg 83:363–367, 1995.
24. Korinek AM: Risk factors for neurosurgical site infections after craniotomy: a prospective multicenter study of 2944 patients. The French Study Group of Neurosurgical Infections, the SEHP, and the C-CLIN Paris-Nord. Service Epidemiologie Hygiene et Prevention. Neurosurgery 41:1073–1079, 1997.
25. Kulkarni AV, Guha A, Lozano A, et al: Incidence of silent hemorrhage and delayed deterioration after stereotactic brain biopsy. J Neurosurg 89:31–35, 1998.

26. Kuroda R, Nakatani J, Akai F, et al: Remote subarachnoid haemorrhage in the posterior fossa following supratentorial surgery. Clinical observation of 6 cases. *Acta Neurochir* 129:158–165, 1994.

27. Langfitt JT, Rausch R: Word-finding deficits persist after left anterotemporal lobectomy. *Arch Neurol* 53:72–76, 1996.

28. Malla BR, O'Brien TJ, Cascino GD, et al: Acute postoperative seizures following anterior temporal lobectomy for intractable partial epilepsy. *J Neurosurg* 89:177–182, 1998.

29. Matjasko J, Petrozza P, Cohen M, et al: Anesthesia and surgery in the seated position: analysis of 554 cases. *Neurosurgery* 17:695–702, 1985.

30. Miyasaka Y, Yada K, Ohwada T, et al: Retrograde thrombosis of feeding arteries after removal of arteriovenous malformations. *J Neurosurg* 72:540–545, 1990.

31. Muller P, Jirsch D, D'Sousa J, et al: Gastrointestinal bleeding after craniotomy: a retrospective review of 518 patients. *Can J Neurol Sci* 15:384–387, 1988.

32. Papanastassiou V, Kerr R, Adams C: Contralateral cerebellar hemorrhagic infarction after pterional craniotomy: report of five cases and review of the literature. *Neurosurgery* 39:841–851, 1996.

33. Phan TG, O'Neill BP, Kurtin PJ: Posttransplant primary CNS lymphoma. *Neuro-oncol* 2:229–238, 2000.

34. Pilcher WH, Roberts DW, Flanigin HF, et al: Complications of epilepsy surgery. In Engel J Jr (ed): *Surgical Treatment of the Epilepsies*. 2nd ed. New York: Raven Press, 1993, pp 565–581.

35. Rapana A, Lamaida E, Pizza V: Multiple postoperative intracerebral haematomas remote from the site of craniotomy. *Br J Neurosurg* 12:364–368, 1998.

36. Raymond J, Hardy J, Czepko R, et al: Arterial injuries in transsphenoidal surgery for pituitary adenoma: the role of angiography and endovascular treatment. *AJNR Am J Neuroradiol* 18:655–665, 1997.

37. Salvesen R: Extrapontine myelinolysis after surgical removal of a pituitary tumour. *Acta Neurol Scand* 98:213–215, 1998.

38. Savitz MH, Bobroff LM: Low incidence of delayed intracerebral hemorrhage secondary to ventriculoperitoneal shunt insertion. *J Neurosurg* 91:32–34, 1999.

39. Sawaya R, Hammoud M, Schoppa D, et al: Neurosurgical outcomes in a modern series of 400 craniotomies for treatment of parenchymal tumors. *Neurosurgery* 42:1044–1055, 1998.

40. Sawin PD, Hitchon PW, Follett KA, et al: Computed imaging-assisted stereotactic brain biopsy: a risk analysis of 225 consecutive cases. *Surg Neurol* 49:640–649, 1998.

41. Sawka AM, Aniszewski JP, Young WF Jr, et al: Tension pneumocranium, a rare complication of transsphenoidal pituitary surgery: Mayo Clinic experience 1976–1998. *J Clin Endocrinol Metab* 84:4731–4734, 1999.

42. Schaffranietz L, Gunther L: The sitting position in neurosurgical operations. Results of a survey. [German.] *Anaesthesist* 46:91–95, 1997.

43. Semple PL, Laws ER Jr: Complications in a contemporary series of patients who underwent transsphenoidal surgery for Cushing's disease. *J Neurosurg* 91:175–179, 1999.

44. Seoane E, Rhoton AL Jr: Compression of the internal jugular vein by the transverse process of the atlas as the cause of cerebellar hemorrhage after supratentorial craniotomy. *Surg Neurol* 51:500–505, 1999.

45. Shaw MD, Foy PM: Epilepsy after craniotomy and the place of prophylactic anticonvulsant drugs: discussion paper. *J R Soc Med* 84:221–223, 1991.

46. Taylor WA, Thomas NW, Wellings JA, et al: Timing of postoperative intracranial hematoma development and implications for the best use of neurosurgical intensive care. *J Neurosurg* 82:48–50, 1995.

47. Toczek MT, Morrell MJ, Silverberg GA, et al: Cerebellar hemorrhage complicating temporal lobectomy. Report of four cases. *J Neurosurg* 85:718–722, 1996.

48. Tosaka M, Kohga H: Extrapontine myelinolysis and behavioral change after transsphenoidal pituitary surgery: case report. *Neurosurgery* 43:933–936, 1998.

49. Van Buren JM: Complications of surgical procedures in the diagnosis and treatment of epilepsy. In Engel J Jr (ed): *Surgical Treatment of the Epilepsies*. New York: Raven Press, 1987, pp 465–475.

50. Vender JR, Black P, Natter HM, et al: Post-anesthesia uncal herniation secondary to a previously unsuspected temporal glioma. *J Forensic Sci* 40:900–902, 1995.

51. Voges J, Schroder R, Treuer H, et al: CT-guided and computer assisted stereotactic biopsy. Technique, results, indications. *Acta Neurochir* 125:142–149, 1993.

52. Wiebe S, Blume WT, Girvin JP, et al: A randomized, controlled trial of surgery for temporal-lobe epilepsy. *N Engl J Med* 345:311–318, 2001.

53. Yacubian EM, de Andrade MM, Jorge CL, et al: Cerebellar hemorrhage after supratentorial surgery for treatment of epilepsy: report of three cases. *Neurosurgery* 45:159–162, 1999.

54. Yague LG, Rodriguez-Sanchez J, Polaina M, et al: Contralateral extradural hematoma following craniotomy for traumatic intracranial lesion. Case report. *J Neurosurg Sci* 35:107–109, 1991.

55. Young RF, Lawner PM: Perioperative antibiotic prophylaxis for prevention of postoperative neurosurgical infections. A randomized clinical trial. *J Neurosurg* 66:701–705, 1987.

56. Yu X, Liu Z, Tian Z, et al: CT-guided stereotactic biopsy of deep brain lesions: report of 310 cases. *Chin Med J (Engl)* 111:361–363, 1998.

PART V

MANAGEMENT OF SYSTEMIC COMPLICATIONS

29

Pulmonary Complications

Acute pulmonary disease is a complicating factor in acutely ill neurologic patients, whereas in other medical intensive care units, exacerbation of long-standing pulmonary disease is often the primary reason for admission. Acute respiratory distress in the NICU can be due to aspiration pneumonia, pulmonary emboli, and nosocomial pneumonia. In fact, outcome from critical neurologic illness may be determined in many patients by whether or not pulmonary complications arise. Better outcomes can be expected with closer attention to prevention, recognition, and management of potentially fatal pulmonary complications. Impaired arousal or defective swallowing mechanism most likely is an important factor in the development of aspiration pneumonia. Pulmonary embolism from immobilization, particularly in patients not protected by intermittent compression devices or subcutaneous heparin, can surprisingly emerge as early as several days after admission.[50]

This chapter describes two important issues: the general pathophysiologic principles of acute respiratory failure and the most significant respiratory complications in patients with acute neurologic catastrophes. The goal in any of these patients is to reduce $PaCO_2$ or improve oxygenation, or both. Brief mechanical ventilation (invasive or noninvasive positive pressure) may be required (Chapter 5).

PATHOPHYSIOLOGY OF ACUTE RESPIRATORY FAILURE

Respiration is often understood in terms of ventilation-perfusion match. The parts of the lung that do not participate in respiration are known as the *physiologic dead space*, the sum of *anatomical dead space* (the part of the airway system not connected with the alveoli, possibly including the tubing between the Y connector and the patient, the pharynx, and the major conduction airways) and *alveolar dead space* (the part of the airway system that does not permit gas exchange, in which inspired gas is similar to exhaled gas). This component of the respiratory system is 20% to 30% of total ventilation. The ratio of dead-space gas volume to tidal gas volume (V_D/V_T) can be measured in two ways. The respiratory therapist may collect expired gas from several tidal volumes exhaled over 5 minutes into a collection bag, and this sample is analyzed together with an arterial sample. Currently, most often an infrared light device can measure mixed expired PCO_2 ($PECO_2$). This simple device is connected to the exhalation hose, and end-tidal carbon dioxide is measured just before the arterial blood gas is obtained. The dead space can then be measured from the following formula:

$$V_D/V_T = \frac{PaCO_2 - PECO_2}{PaCO_2}$$

(Normal range, 0.2 to 0.3.) Increasing dead space over time is an indicator of worsening pulmonary function and mortality (highest when ≥ 0.57).[28]

Another measure of bedside assessment of gas exchange is the alveolar-arterial oxygen difference ("A-a gradient"). The alveolar P_{O_2} (P_{AO_2}) is calculated from the following formula: $P_{AO_2} = F_{IO_2} \times 713 - P_{aCO_2}/0.8$. The difference between P_{AO_2} and P_{aO_2} is 10 to 20 mm Hg. An A-a gradient greater than 20 mm Hg indicates pulmonary dysfunction.

The third important measure is maximum inspiratory pressure (PImax). Maximum inspiratory pressure can be used (together with vital capacity) and maximum expiratory pressure to differentiate a neuromuscular cause from other causes of respiratory failure (Chapter 5).

Measurement of one set of arterial blood gases determines the seriousness of respiratory impairment. It is convenient to divide acute respiratory failure into acute hypoxemia ($P_{O_2} < 50$ mm Hg) and acute hypercapnia ($P_{CO_2} > 50$ mm Hg).

Hypoxemia occurs in conditions causing alveolar hypoventilation or in instances of perfusion directed toward lung areas in which the ratio of alveolar ventilation ($\dot{V}A$) to perfusion ($\dot{Q}$) is less than 1.0. The hallmarks of bedside evaluation of acute hypoxemic respiratory failure are determination of the A-a gradient, whether hypoxemia is corrected by 100% oxygen, and if the PImax has changed from the norm (Table 29–1). The most common clinical disorders in the NICU associated with acute hypoxemic respiratory failure and ventilation-perfusion mismatch are atelectasis, aspiration pneumonitis, pulmonary embolism, and pulmonary edema (cardiac or neurogenic). The clinical features of acute hypoxemia are fairly consistent and include impaired arousal, restlessness, tachypnea, tachycardia, and, sometimes, hypertension and peripheral vasoconstriction.

Similarly, acute hypercapnic respiratory failure is delineated by both the A-a gradient and PImax. Decreased PImax identifies many of the neuromuscular disorders, including those of motor neurons (e.g., amyotrophic lateral sclerosis), neuromuscular junction (e.g., myasthenia gravis, Lambert-Eaton syndrome, botulism, neuromuscular junction blockade by specific paralytic agents), peripheral nerve (e.g., Guillain-Barré syndrome, critical illness polyneuropathy), and muscle (e.g., polymyositis, acid maltase deficiency). When the respiratory muscles fail, alveolar ventilation is insufficient to eliminate carbon dioxide, and the result is increased tidal volume or respiratory rate.[49] A normal PImax often indicates central hypoventilation (e.g., primary brain stem lesion) or increased carbon dioxide production by sepsis or from a flurry of generalized tonic-clonic seizures. A bedside approach to hypoxemia and hypercapnia is shown in Tables 29–1 and 29–2.

ACUTE RESPIRATORY DISTRESS IN MECHANICALLY VENTILATED PATIENTS

Although many patients with an acute brain injury can breathe unassisted, a proportion of patients require support by mechanical ventilation. Agitated patients with an acute central nervous system catastrophe have an increased respiratory drive culminating in large minute volumes and ventilator-patient asynchrony. In

Table 29–1. Initial Bedside Approach to Acute Hypoxemic Respiratory Failure

A-a Gradient	Other Variable	Disorder
Normal	PImax decreased	Neuromuscular cause of hypoventilation
	PImax normal	Central cause of hypoventilation
Increased	Correction with 100% O_2	Ventilation-perfusion mismatch
	No correction with 100% O_2	Right-to-left shunt, intraparenchymal or intracardiac

A-a, alveolar-arterial; PImax, maximum inspiratory pressure.

Table 29–2. Initial Bedside Approach to Acute Hypercapnic Respiratory Failure

A-a Gradient	Other Variable	Disorder
Normal	PImax decreased	Neuromuscular
	PImax normal	
	Increased CO_2 production	Sepsis, seizures
	Normal CO_2 production	Central hypoventilation
Increased		Cardiopulmonary

A-a, alveolar-arterial; PImax, maximum inspiratory pressure.

other mechanically ventilated patients, a quasistable situation is abruptly disturbed by tachypnea, diaphoresis, nasal flaring, and complete arrhythmic breathing, often with use of the accessory respiratory muscles.

Important initial clinical signs in a mechanically ventilated patient with acute respiratory distress and a sudden increase in respiratory rate are hypotension, hypoxemia, and cardiac arrhythmias, all possibly connected with one another. An analytic approach is imperative to resolve the causes of acute critical respiratory distress in mechanically ventilated patients (Fig. 29–1). The first step is to immediately check the patient-ventilator connection by measuring exhaled tidal volume to see if it agrees with that displayed on the ventilator control panel. Marginal exhaled tidal volume or low exhaled inspiratory pressure may indicate a leak in the system connections. The patient is disconnected from the ventilator and connected to a manual bag with 100% oxygen. This bypasses any problem in the machine, and immediate clinical improvement with 100% oxygen unmasks a ven-

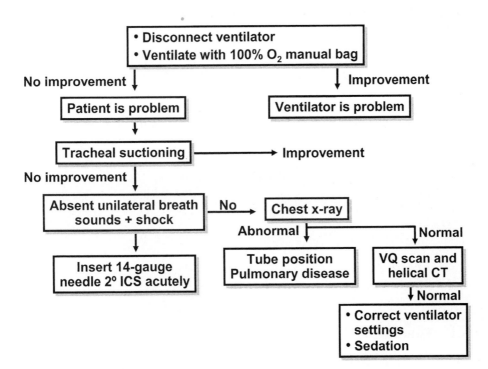

Figure 29–1. Algorithm for initial management of mechanically ventilated patients in acute respiratory distress. 2° ICS, second intercostal space; VQ, ventilation-perfusion.

tilator-related cause. If the pulse oximeter does not indicate immediate improvement in oxygenation, the next step is to check the patency of the airway. If secretions are heard, tracheal suctioning must be performed immediately after preoxygenation with 100% oxygen. In addition, if asymmetrical breath sounds are heard on auscultation of the lungs, main stem intubation or obstruction may be present. One should acknowledge, however, that asymmetrical breath sounds are not specific, and many conditions can produce these findings, including acute pneumothorax, pleural effusions, and atelectasis of large segments.

Nonetheless, pneumothorax is highly probable in patients in shock who have unilateral absence of breath sounds.[7] Pneumothorax in mechanically ventilated patients, fortunately rare (5%), most likely is caused by large tidal volumes (more than 12 mL/kg) and high positive end-expiratory pressure (PEEP) values (more than 15 mm Hg) in patients with known obstructive lung disease. Highly suspicious signs are a sudden increase in peak airway pressure and hypotension. Tension pneumothorax may develop quickly; therefore, a 14-gauge needle must be placed in the second intercostal space at the anterior midclavicular line. Further management includes tube thoracostomy (Fig. 29–2).

Failure to resolve respiratory distress after an attempt at tracheobronchial suctioning is followed by emergency chest radiography to determine the position of the tube and the existence of a primary pulmonary problem (pneumothorax, pulmonary edema) or abdominal distention (gastric distention, bowel perforation), which is suggested by diaphragmatic elevation. Fiber-optic bronchoscopy may follow in patients with diminished bilateral breath sounds to check the endotracheal position and possibly clear excess secretions or remove a foreign body.[48]

Patients with persistent hypoxemia and normal findings on initial chest radiography pose a diagnostic challenge. The differential diagnosis includes pulmonary embolism, acute bronchospasm, and microatelectasis. It is important to consider pulmonary emboli and, when clinical suspicion is high, to perform a ventilation-perfusion scan, helical CT scanning, duplex ultrasound examination of the legs, and D-dimer assay.

If the laboratory findings are normal, the ventilator settings should be corrected. Inappropriate ventilator settings may underlie patient-ventilator asynchrony, a maladaptation of the patient-to-ventilator timing.[36] Patients with reduced respiratory drive may insufficiently trigger the ventilator if the trigger threshold is insensitive. Flow triggering could be different from pressure triggering, and adjustments should be made. A high proportion of mandatory breaths with synchronous intermittent

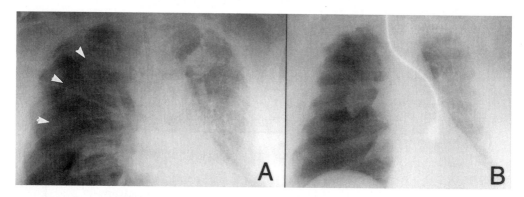

Figure 29–2. Rapidly evolving tension pneumothorax on chest radiographs. (A) *Arrows* point to collapsed lung. (B) Repeat radiograph obtained just before chest tube placement shows displacement.

mandatory ventilation or a high-pressure support level with the pressure-support ventilator may cause problems in these patients. Auto-PEEP, a very important phenomenon, must be evaluated. This condition of air trapping must be considered in patients with a sudden increase in pulmonary artery wedge pressure. Auto-PEEP occurs in patients with obstructed airways, often in those with underlying bronchospastic disease.

Auto-PEEP is the difference between the alveolar pressure and the pressure at the airway opening at end-expiration. Exhalation is incomplete in patients with airway obstruction from whatever cause, and the alveolar pressure remains positive at end-expiration. Auto-PEEP increases mean intrapleural pressure and decreases venous return, and the result may be hypotension. In addition, auto-PEEP increases the threshold at which the ventilator is triggered, and this diminished sensitivity may become particularly distressing for acutely ill neurologic patients with decreased levels of consciousness. In this clinical situation, the typical sequence of events is inability to trigger the ventilator, a controlled breath completely asynchronous with the patient's respiratory pattern, immediate increase in the work of breathing, discomfort, and agitation. When suspicion of auto-PEEP is high—because of otherwise unexplained sudden hypotension, increased pulmonary artery wedge pressures, and increased work of breathing—auto-PEEP can be resolved by increasing the respiratory flow rate to increase the expiratory time, by decreasing the respiratory rate in patients with spontaneous efforts, and by decreasing the tidal volume in assist-control ventilation.[45]

If no obvious cause is found, agitation with markedly increased respiratory drive becomes a strong contender, and sedation must be considered (for pharmacotherapy of agitation, see Chapter 4). It may be difficult to separate pain from agitation, and opioids may be needed in addition. Remifentanil hydrochloride should be considered because of its short half-life and brevity of action[35] (initial dose, 0.5 to 1 μg/kg per minute intravenously; maintenance, 0.05 to 2 μg/kg per minute intravenously). A more extensive list of causes of acute respiratory distress in mechanically ventilated patients is shown in Table 29–3.

Table 29–3. Differential Diagnosis of Acute Respiratory Distress in Mechanically Ventilated Patients

Acute main bronchus obstruction
Inappropriate ventilator setting
Auto-PEEP
Pneumothorax
Atelectasis
Pulmonary embolus
Pulmonary edema
Dislodgment of tracheostomy tube
Endotracheal malposition
Machine dysfunction
Abdominal distention

PEEP, positive end-expiratory pressure.

ASPIRATION PNEUMONIA

Altered level of consciousness alone is a major risk factor for aspiration, but many other factors coincide (Chapter 6). The gastric reservoir, presence of gastroesophageal reflux (common in mechanically ventilated patients), and position may contribute. In a randomized trial, when patients were placed in a semirecumbent position (45°), a 75% reduction in the rate of nosocomial pneumonia and a fourfold reduction in the rate per 1000 ventilator days were found.[9]

Clinical Features and Management

Aspiration is often subclinical, and very rarely a fulminant aspiration syndrome is observed. Overspill of large amounts of gastric acid into the airways may cause acute hypoxemia, wheezing, cyanosis, and shock.[4]

Many patients have no clinical symptoms or transient hypoxemia before a chest radiograph uncovers infiltrates. In others, hypoxemia can be profound, with PaO_2 values in the 40 mm Hg range. Hypoxemia associated with aspiration is explained by a large intrapulmonary shunt, and pulmonary artery pressures may increase because of hypoxemic vasoconstriction.

Pulmonary edema from acid-induced damage to capillaries eventually may lead to a fatal clinical course.

The radiologic features are pivotal in the evaluation because the clinical symptoms can be attenuated. The most consistent findings in adults are right lower lobe infiltrates (the left main stem bronchus has a more angular course) (Fig. 29–3), atelectasis, and air bronchogram in large-segment aspiration. Infiltrates can be bilateral and more diffuse when restricted to the lower lobes, and usually repeat chest radiography demonstrates these abnormalities (Fig. 29–4).

Conservative treatment is indicated in many patients, and the radiographic abnormalities usually subside rapidly. Corticosteroids are of no benefit and are potentially harmful. The emergence of fever may signal aspiration pneumonitis, but antibiotic coverage must await the demonstration of a likely pathogen. Cultures containing anaerobes such as *Bacteroides melaninogenicus*, *Fusobacterium nucleatum*, *Peptostreptococcus*, *Bacteroides fragilis*, and *Streptococcus* species suggest active infection from aspiration.[27] For most patients, an empirical antibiotic regimen includes beta-lactam/beta-lactamase inhibitor or cephalosporin combined with an aminoglycoside or clindamycin for *Bacteroides* species.[32,37] (A more comprehensive discussion of antibiotic management is found in the subsection on nosocomial pneumonia in Chapter 33.) Mechanical ventilation may be indicated if progressive infiltrative abnormalities are demonstrated. Standard modes of mechanical ventilation may not provide adequate ventilatory support, and occasionally the mode of mechanical ventilation must be switched to a more aggressive mode of pressure-support ventilation with, at times, inverse ratio in patients with fulminant aspiration pneumonitis or adult respiratory distress syndrome. As a last resort, a prone (face down) position can be tried. It has been shown to improve oxygenation, regional changes in ventilation, and ventilation-perfusion match. Change in pulmonary mechanics in this position may also account for quick improvement in oxygenation. Accidental extubation in this unusual position was uncommon in a recent study, but facial edema was prevalent.[12]

NEUROGENIC PULMONARY EDEMA

Acute injury to the brain or brain stem may cause massive pulmonary edema, but the true frequency seems very low.[10] Conditions that have traditionally been associated with neurogenic pulmonary edema are aneurysmal subarachnoid hemorrhage, primary medullary hemorrhage,[20] status epilepticus, and severe head injury, and neurogenic pulmonary edema may develop in patients with the clinical diagnosis of brain death.[5,6,8,11,52] In its full presentation, the clinical picture is very specific, almost always appearing soon after the initial impact. The clinical entity may be mistaken for other pulmonary conditions, such as massive aspiration pneumonia or pulmonary contusion. Delayed neurogenic pulmonary edema (much less common, if it exists at all) should be differentiated from more prevalent multiple pulmonary emboli.

Recent observations in subarachnoid hemorrhage have raised provocative questions about the underlying mechanism and challenged the classic explanation that pulmonary edema is of neurogenic origin. Traditionally, neurogenic pulmonary edema is attributed to

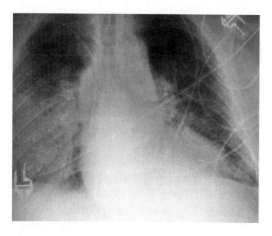

Figure 29–3. Matured aspiration pneumonitis in right lower lobe.

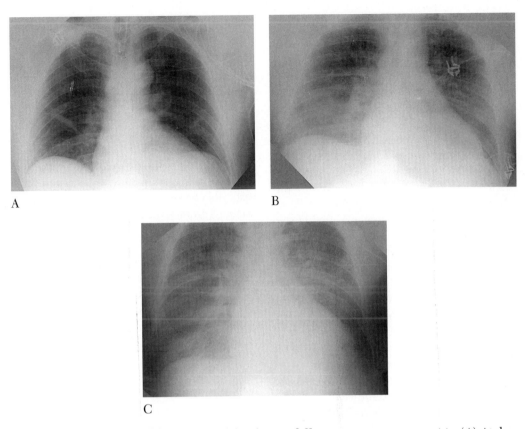

Figure 29–4. Serial chest radiographs of developing diffuse aspiration pneumonitis. (*A*) Atelectasis. (*B* and *C*) Gradual appearance of whiteout-like infiltrates.

a massive sympathetic discharge, probably mediated by the anterior hypothalamus and triggered by an initial overwhelming increase in intracranial pressure during the arterial rupture. The increased sympathetic activity leads to generalized vasoconstriction, hypertension, and direct damage to endothelial cells, which may result in increased permeability ("capillary leak") and subsequent airspace flooding, commonly known as "blast injury."

However, there is increasing evidence that pulmonary edema in subarachnoid hemorrhage may have a cardiogenic origin. Structural damage to the myocardium has been amply documented, and contraction bands and focal and subendocardial myocardial injury are characteristic histologic features. There is sufficient clinical evidence that myocardial dysfunction is common in poor-grade subarachnoid hemorrhage. Hemodynamic measurements demonstrated significant reduction in ventricular performance as measured by left ventricular stroke index, cardiac index, and echocardiogram in patients with subarachnoid hemorrhage who had an increase in the MB fraction of creatine kinase (see Chapter 30). The true incidence in subarachnoid hemorrhage is not known, and we have observed dramatic pulmonary edema without any echocardiographic evidence of ventricular dysfunction. In a recent study that obtained pleural fluid and compared pulmonary edema fluid with plasma protein, hydrostatic edema was found in more than half the patients.[42] This result suggested either myocardial dysfunction with increase in left cardiovascular pressures or, alternatively, profound venoconstriction. Pulmonary venoconstriction may force fluid into the lungs.

Clinical Features and Management

The clinical picture is striking. Excessive sweating, hypertension, tachypnea, and production of frothy sputum are typical. The diagnosis of neurogenic pulmonary edema is supported by the combination of marked hypoxemic respiratory failure (hypoxemia, greatly increased A-a gradient) with normal pulmonary artery wedge pressure (values less than 15 mm Hg), excluding a cardiogenic cause for pulmonary edema. Chest radiography demonstrates diffuse pulmonary infiltrates (Fig. 29–5).

Management of neurogenic pulmonary edema is focused on recruitment of collapsed alveoli with PEEP to correct the marked ventilation-perfusion mismatch. Mechanical ventilation with PEEP nearly always reverses the condition, and definite radiographic improvement is evident within hours.

Positive end-expiratory pressure is titrated by maximizing oxygen delivery at the lowest FIO_2 settings, usually possible at a level of 10 to 15 cm H_2O. Positive end-expiratory pressure ventilation alone should be sufficient to resolve neurogenic pulmonary edema, and weaning can be achieved fairly rapidly in many patients when the effect of the acute impact has subsided. If the origin of pulmonary edema is not clear or is possibly confounded by cardiac stunning, dobutamine (5 to 15 $\mu g/kg$ per minute) to improve ventricular forward flow could be considered.

CHEST TRAUMA

Thoracic injuries may be observed in a significant number of trauma patients admitted to the NICU. Chest wall injuries vary from a single rib fracture without significant impairment to major pulmonary contusion. Fracture of a first rib, however, is indicative of major trauma[34] from involvement of vascular structures. Most instances of chest trauma can be managed nonsurgically. Emergency thoracotomy is indicated for cardiac tamponade, control of air embolization, and shock not responding to aggressive resuscitation.[21] This section does not further consider mediastinal trauma or great vessel injury but focuses on pulmonary lesions.

Pulmonary trauma can be life-threatening if it produces such conditions as pneumothorax, flail chest, and tracheobronchial injury.

Clinical Features and Management

Usually, a consecutive series of ribs is fractured, and in patients with marked flail chest, paradoxical motion of the chest wall occurs with spontaneous breathing (Fig. 29–6) and gas exchange rapidly becomes compromised.

Pulmonary contusion from blunt trauma may not be immediately noticeable but in most patients becomes apparent within hours. Serial chest radiographs or CT scans[46] taken on the same day show evolution of patchy, often ill-defined parenchymal densities that do not coincide with the anatomical division of the lung.[33,40] Post-traumatic pneumatoceles (thin-walled air sacs) develop hours to days later. The differentiation from aspiration pneumonia is that the density is more centrally located in aspiration pneumonia and limited to a bronchial distribution. Treatment of a pulmonary contusion is conservative. Flail chest does not necessarily warrant intubation or mechanical ventilation if gas exchange is within normal limits, and relief of pain suffices.[33,40]

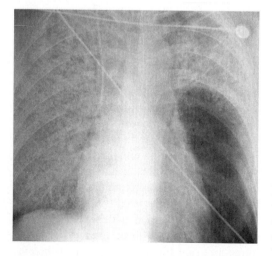

Figure 29–5. Neurogenic pulmonary edema.

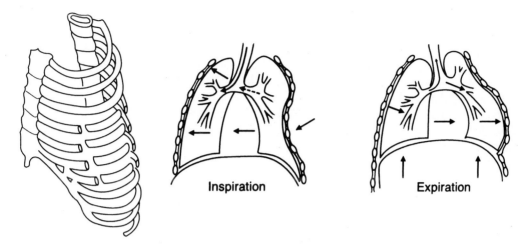

Figure 29–6. Paradoxical movement with flail chest.

Traumatic pneumothorax should be treated with thoracotomy tube drainage, and in patients with progressive deterioration from tension pneumothorax, drainage is preceded by needle decompression. Many patients with tension pneumothorax have hyperresonance, hypotension, distended neck veins, and tracheal deviation on examination.

PULMONARY EMBOLISM

Patients with acute neurologic diseases are susceptible to deep venous thrombosis. Pulmonary emboli may occur in the first week after initial presentation of any acute stroke and are not necessarily the consequence of long-term immobilization.[41,50] Deep venous thrombosis is significantly more common in a paralyzed leg.[47] Large proximal veins in the thigh may clot, and the risk of pulmonary embolization is considerably higher than in patients with calf vein thrombosis alone (40% versus 15%).[23] In addition, one should appreciate that postoperative neurosurgical patients have an incidence of pulmonary embolism similar to that with hip and knee surgery (1% to 3% fatal pulmonary embolism).[15,19] The risk of deep venous thrombosis is probably also increased in patients with previous deep venous thrombosis, skin pigmentation of the legs, and varices.

In these circumstances, the risk of deep venous thrombosis is reduced, but not sufficiently, by use of pneumatic devices.[2,3]

Clinical Features and Management

The clinical presentation of pulmonary embolism is never straightforward, and data from the Prospective Investigation of Pulmonary Embolism Diagnosis (PIOPED) study have confirmed the widely held conception that pulmonary embolism is often silent and difficult to diagnose.[1]

Pulmonary embolism is likely if patients have two or three typical manifestations: low-grade fever, sudden tachypnea (respiratory rate of 20 or more), and pleuritic pain together with hypocapnia from hyperventilation and marginal Po_2 (which may be only positional).[16,17] However, the clinical examination may not be helpful; rales, wheezing, and signs of pleural effusion are absent in many patients. Massive pulmonary embolism is often dramatic and may cause sudden death. When this occurs, pulmonary embolism may superficially resemble rebleeding in subarachnoid hemorrhage. (However, in our patients with subarachnoid hemorrhage, pulmonary emboli occurred after surgical clipping.)

The most startling presentation of pulmonary embolus is right ventricular failure, usually developing only if more than two-thirds of the pulmonary circulation is obstructed.[51] Acute dilatation of the right ventricle causes increased ventricular pressure that is transmitted to the right atrium and clinically detected by pronounced neck veins, right-sided S_3 gallop, and, rarely, parasternal lift.

The clinical features of pulmonary embolism have a low specificity. In one study, the highest specificities were in tachypnea (0.80), hemoptysis (0.76), and pleuritic chest pain (0.64). Laboratory support for the diagnosis of pulmonary embolism is summarized in Table 29–4. Electrocardiographic abnormalities may have some value, but they are often momentary. The most frequently seen abnormalities are T-wave inversions and a nonreciprocal ST depression.

The use of D-dimer values has generated considerable interest. D dimers are fibrin breakdown products that become measurable when the fibrin matrix of fresh emboli fragments. D-dimer assay of whole blood agglutination has a reported sensitivity of 96% but a very low specificity of 48%. D dimers may be increased in the first 30 days after an ischemic stroke involving the cortex,[43] and warfarin may reduce the sensitivity of the assay.[24] Its negative predictive value (values below 500 μg/L) may have some use as an additional test to rule out segmental or massive pulmonary embolism in patients with ventilation-perfusion scans of low probability.[25] If clinical suspicion is low, these findings may preclude invasive pulmonary angiography. A combination of a normal D dimer and normal alveolar dead-space fraction was associated with a probability of less than 1% in a multicenter study.[24]

Bedside echocardiography could be useful in a few instances. The indirect demonstration of increased right ventricular dimension, a dilated right pulmonary artery, and flattening of the intraventricular septum may be more supportive of pulmonary emboli. Demonstration of intraluminal thrombi is not common.

If clinical probability is high (based on a combination of abnormal clinical, electrocardiographic, arterial blood gas, and chest X-ray findings), almost 70% of the patients have confirmation on pulmonary angiograms. If the probability is low, the percentage is reduced to less than 10%. However, in most patients, clinicians are not able to attach a high or low probability to a certain clinical presentation. In this intermediate category, the yield of positive pulmonary angiography is as low as 30%. Therefore, before one proceeds to this invasive study, a ventilation-perfusion scan or helical CT scan is warranted and could reduce the need for pulmonary angiography. Another disappointment is that two-fifths of the scans are not helpful (so-called intermediate probability). A high-probability ventilation-perfusion scan indicates an 80% to 85% probability of pulmonary embolism. Criteria for scintigraphic detection of pulmonary embolism are shown in Table 29–5, and a high-probability ventilation-perfusion scan is shown in Figure 29–7.

An extremely important recent development is the use of helical CT. In a prospective study of 60 patients with 15 angiographically proven pulmonary emboli, sensitivity was 65% and specificity 97%. This imaging study has the advantage of directly demonstrating emboli in areas of ventilation-perfusion shunts[44] (Fig. 29–8) and may image other, confounding pulmonary lesions. Emboli in small subsegmental pulmonary arterial branches may not be visualized. Helical CT scans miss subsegmental emboli with standard 3 mm sections, but detection increases 40% with 1 mm scans. These small peripheral emboli most likely are also

Table 29–4. Laboratory Test Results Supportive of Pulmonary Embolism

Hypocapnia and hypoxemia
Electrocardiographic abnormalities
  T-wave inversion in the right precordial leads, III, and aVF
  ST depression (nonreciprocal)
  T-wave inversion (patients with history of cardiopulmonary disease)
  Sudden atrial fibrillation
  P pulmonale
  Right bundle-branch block
D-dimer increase (> 500 μg/L)
High probability of embolism on ventilation-perfusion scan
Spiral computed tomography documentation of intra-arterial clot
Increased right ventricular dimension or dilated right pulmonary artery on echocardiography

Table 29–5. Diagnostic Criteria for Pulmonary Embolism on Ventilation-Perfusion Scan

Low probability (< 20%)	Small V/Q mismatches
	Perfusion defect substantially smaller than chest X-ray opacity
	Multiple subsegmental V/Q mismatches and normal chest radiograph
	V/Q match less than 50% of one lung filled
Intermediate probability (20%–80%)	Diffuse V/Q mismatch
	Perfusion defect with matched density on chest radiograph
	Abnormality neither "high" nor "low" in probability
High probability (> 80%)	Two or more large V/Q mismatches with normal ventilation and chest radiograph
	Perfusion substantially larger than chest X-ray opacity, which shows some areas of mismatch

V, ventilation; Q, perfusion.

clinically relevant, because they may cause pulmonary hypertension.[38]

Pulmonary angiography remains the standard procedure to confirm the diagnosis of pulmonary emboli (Fig. 29–9). The perceived risk outweighs the actual risk of pulmonary arteriography, and, in fact, the procedure is generally safe. Very occasionally, pulmonary angiography causes ventricular arrhythmias. The procedure, however, is expensive. There have been multiple attempts to scale back diagnostic tests to arrive at a diagnosis, and some have argued that D-dimer assay, helical CT, and leg ultrasonography should provide sufficient information. For example, helical CT scans have

a false-negative rate of 5% in patients with clinically suspected pulmonary embolus, increased D dimer (> 500 μg/L), and normal leg ultrasound findings.[30] In addition, a recent Canadian cost-benefit analysis suggested that helical CT can replace pulmonary angiography when ventilation-perfusion scans and leg ultrasound findings are negative.[29] Definitive studies on safety, sensitivity, and specificity of helical CT for suspected pulmonary embolus are not available, and we and others[31] remain reluctant to withhold anticoagulant therapy on the basis of negative results of a helical CT examination. It is complicated to marshall all these data sets into a workable decision algo-

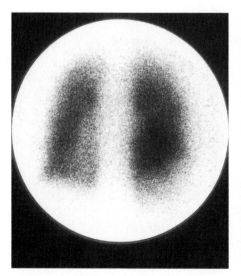
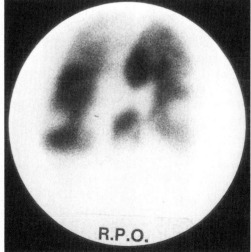

Figure 29–7. High-probability ventilation-perfusion scans. (*Left*) Normal ventilation. (*Right*) Multiple large perfusion defects.

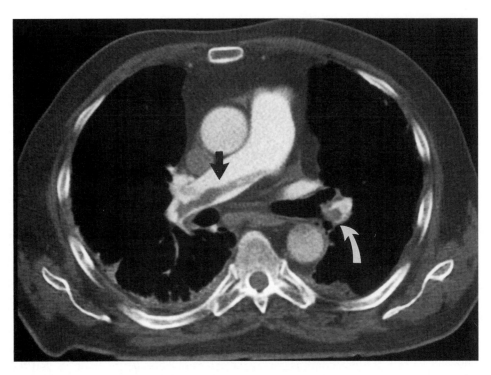

Figure 29–8. Helical computed tomography scan demonstrates thrombus within the right pulmonary artery (*black arrow*) and within the left descending trunk (*white arrow*).

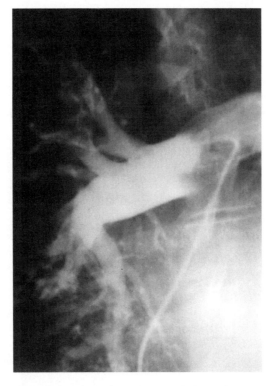

Figure 29–9. Pulmonary embolus demonstrated on angiogram (upper lobe vessels on the right).

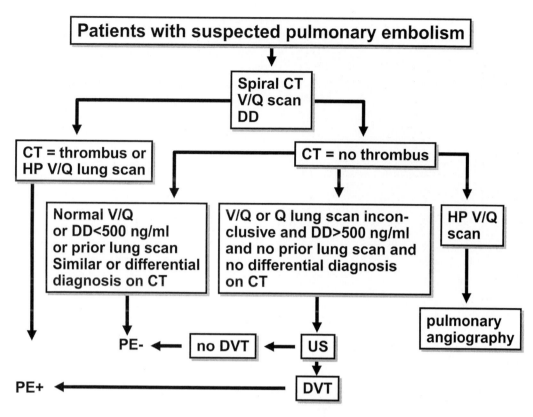

Figure 29–10. Diagnostic algorithm of the likelihood of pulmonary embolism (PE) with various test results. CT, computed tomography; DD, D-dimer; DVT, deep venous thrombosis; HP, high probability; PE, pulmonary embolism; V/Q, ventilation/perfusion; US, ultrasonography. (From Lorut C, Ghossains M, Horellou MH, et al: A noninvasive diagnostic strategy including spiral computed tomography in patients with suspected pulmonary embolism. *Am J Respir Crit Care Med* 162:1413–1418, 2000. By permission of the American Thoracic Society.)

rithm. One recently suggested possible approach is shown in Figure 29–10.

Treatment of pulmonary embolism depends on the size of the embolus. Patients with massive pulmonary embolus most often are in shock from acute cor pulmonale, which justifies aggressive treatment with thrombolytic agents. Studies with thrombolytic agents have indeed shown improvement in hemodynamic variables but no significant effect on mortality.[13] Tissue plasminogen activator, 0.6 mg/kg over 15 minutes, can be administered.[51] A retrospective study from France of patients treated with thrombolysis for massive pulmonary emboli and associated right ventricular dilatation found three patients with intracranial hemorrhage and no benefit over heparin.[14] A recent

trial found no fatal hemorrhages but benefit from alteplase.[26] There is no published experience in patients with an acute ischemic or hemorrhagic stroke, and undoubtedly management may substantially increase the probability of hemorrhage in a recent hemispheric infarct.

Emergency embolectomy may be indicated in patients with no improvement in hemodynamic measurements, but this measure is a last resort.

Supportive treatment therefore remains the mainstay of management in patients with pulmonary emboli. Correcting hypoxemia with FIO_2 of 0.6 to 1.0 is effective. Patients with low cardiac output are best served by norepinephrine in a continuous infusion of 0.1 $\mu g/kg$ per minute in an attempt to improve right ventricular performance. Volume expansion in patients

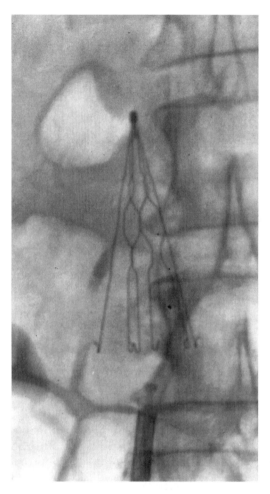

Figure 29–11. Vena cava filter (Greenfield).

in shock from massive pulmonary embolization is indicated only for those who need additional volume to counter the effects of positive pressure ventilation; in many other patients, fluid loading may cause further right ventricular distention and more ventricular strain.

Heparin treatment is initiated immediately. A weight-based nomogram with partial thromboplastin time at two times the normal value is used[18] (see Chapter 8). Heparin treatment should not be adjusted to a lower level for fear of hemorrhagic conversion of ischemic stroke—albeit real—because failure to give a bolus or, worse, failure to provide adequate anticoagulation—particularly in patients with massive consumption of heparin associated with widespread embolization—may increase mortality from pulmonary embolism. Administration of warfarin can begin 48 hours after the start of heparinization. Patients are not mobilized until warfarin is therapeutic, and administration is continued for 6 months.[39] Stable patients with massive pulmonary emboli may benefit from alteplase.[26]

Filter devices (e.g., Greenfield) should be placed in patients with an absolute contraindication to anticoagulation and in patients with recurrent episodes despite adequate anticoagulation (Fig. 29–11). Filters, which may be obstructive and cause leg edema, should be inserted very selectively.[22] Deep venous thrombosis is treated with high-pressure stockings, leg elevation, and rest.

CONCLUSIONS

- The most common cause of acute hypoxemic respiratory failure in the NICU is ventilation-perfusion mismatch from atelectasis, aspiration, pulmonary edema, or pulmonary embolism.
- Sudden respiratory distress in a mechanically ventilated patient should prompt disconnection (excludes machine failure), tracheal suctioning or bronchoscopy (excludes bronchial obstruction), chest radiography (excludes pneumothorax), and ventilation-perfusion scan or spiral CT scan (may exclude large pulmonary emboli). Inappropriate ventilator settings may cause patient-ventilator asynchrony.

REFERENCES

1. Anderson GB: Noninvasive testing in the diagnosis of pulmonary embolism. PIOPED revisited (editorial). *Chest* 109:5–6, 1996.
2. Black PM, Baker MF, Snook CP: Experience with ex-

ternal pneumatic calf compression in neurology and neurosurgery. *Neurosurgery* 18:440–444, 1986.
3. Black PM, Crowell RM, Abbott WM: External pneumatic calf compression reduces deep venous thrombosis in patients with ruptured intracranial aneurysms. *Neurosurgery* 18:25–28, 1986.

4. Bynum LJ, Pierce AK: Pulmonary aspiration of gastric contents. *Am Rev Respir Dis* 114:1129–1136, 1976.

5. Carlson RW, Schaeffer RC Jr, Michaels SG, et al: Pulmonary edema following intracranial hemorrhage. *Chest* 75:731–734, 1979.

6. Chen HI, Sun SC, Chai CY: Pulmonary edema and hemorrhage resulting from cerebral compression. *Am J Physiol* 224:223–229, 1973.

7. Chiles C, Ravin CE: Radiographic recognition of pneumothorax in the intensive care unit. *Crit Care Med* 14:677–680, 1986.

8. Colice GL: Neurogenic pulmonary edema. *Clin Chest Med* 6:473–489, 1985.

9. Drakulovic MB, Torres A, Bauer TT, et al: Supine body position as a risk factor for nosocomial pneumonia in mechanically ventilated patients: a randomised trial. *Lancet* 354:1851–1858, 1999.

10. Fein IA, Rackow EC: Neurogenic pulmonary edema. *Chest* 81:318–320, 1982.

11. Fredberg U, Botker HE, Romer FK: Acute neurogenic pulmonary oedema following generalized tonic clonic seizure. A case report and a review of the literature. *Eur Heart J* 9:933–936, 1988.

12. Gattinoni L, Tognoni G, Pesenti A, et al: Effect of prone positioning on the survival of patients with acute respiratory failure. *N Engl J Med* 345:568–573, 2001.

13. Goldhaber SZ: Thrombolysis in pulmonary embolism: a large-scale clinical trial is overdue. *Circulation* 104:2876–2878, 2001.

14. Hamel E, Pacouret G, Vincentelli D, et al: Thrombolysis or heparin therapy in massive pulmonary embolism with right ventricular dilation: results from a 128-patient monocenter registry. *Chest* 120:120–125, 2001.

15. Hamilton MG, Hull RD, Pineo GF: Venous thromboembolism in neurosurgery and neurology patients: a review. *Neurosurgery* 34:280–296, 1994.

16. Hoellerich VL, Wigton RS: Diagnosing pulmonary embolism using clinical findings. *Arch Intern Med* 146:1699–1704, 1986.

17. Huet Y, Lemaire F, Brun-Buisson C, et al: Hypoxemia in acute pulmonary embolism. *Chest* 88:829–836, 1985.

18. Hull RD, Raskob GE, Rosenbloom D, et al: Optimal therapeutic level of heparin therapy in patients with venous thrombosis. *Arch Intern Med* 152:1589–1595, 1992.

19. Inci S, Erbengi A, Berker M: Pulmonary embolism in neurosurgical patients. *Surg Neurol* 43:123–128, 1995.

20. Inobe JJ, Mori T, Ueyama H, et al: Neurogenic pulmonary edema induced by primary medullary hemorrhage: a case report. *J Neurol Sci* 172:73–76, 2000.

21. Jones NS: An audit of the management of 250 patients with chest trauma in a regional thoracic surgical centre. *Arch Emerg Med* 6:97–106, 1989.

22. Kaufman JA: Filter placement in deep venous thrombosis. *AJR Am J Roentgenol* 166:457–458, 1996.

23. Kelly J, Rudd A, Lewis R, et al: Venous thromboembolism after acute stroke. *Stroke* 32:262–267, 2001.

24. Kline JA, Israel EG, Michelson EA, et al: Diagnostic accuracy of a bedside D-dimer assay and alveolar dead-space measurement for rapid exclusion of pulmonary embolism: a multicenter study. *JAMA* 285:761–768, 2001.

25. Kline JA, Nelson RD, Jackson RE, et al: Criteria for the safe use of D-dimer testing in emergency department patients with suspected pulmonary embolism: a multicenter US study. *Ann Emerg Med* 39:144–152, 2002.

26. Konstantinides S, Geibel A, Heusel G, et al: Heparin plus alteplase compared with heparin alone in patients with submassive pulmonary embolism. *N Engl J Med* 347:1143–1150, 2002.

27. Lorber B, Swenson RM: Bacteriology of aspiration pneumonia. A prospective study of community- and hospital-acquired cases. *Ann Intern Med* 81:329–331, 1974.

28. Nuckton TJ, Alonso JA, Kallet RH, et al: Pulmonary dead-space fraction as a risk factor for death in the acute respiratory distress syndrome. *N Engl J Med* 346:1281–1286, 2002.

29. Paterson DI, Schwartzman K: Strategies incorporating spiral CT for the diagnosis of acute pulmonary embolism: a cost-effectiveness analysis. *Chest* 119:1791–1800, 2001.

30. Perrier A, Howarth N, Didier D, et al: Performance of helical computed tomography in unselected outpatients with suspected pulmonary embolism. *Ann Intern Med* 135:88–97, 2001.

31. Rathbun SW, Raskob GE, Whitsett TL: Sensitivity and specificity of helical computed tomography in the diagnosis of pulmonary embolism: a systematic review. *Ann Intern Med* 132:227–232, 2000.

32. Rebuck JA, Rasmussen JR, Olsen KM: Clinical aspiration-related practice patterns in the intensive care unit: a physician survey. *Crit Care Med* 29:2239–2244, 2001.

33. Richardson JD, Adams L, Flint LM: Selective management of flail chest and pulmonary contusion. *Ann Surg* 196:481–487, 1982.

34. Richardson JD, McElvein RB, Trinkle JK: First rib fracture: a hallmark of severe trauma. *Ann Surg* 181:251–254, 1975.

35. Rosow CE: An overview of remifentanil. *Anesth Analg* 89 (Suppl):S1–S3, 1999.

36. Sassoon CS, Foster GT: Patient-ventilator asynchrony. *Curr Opin Crit Care* 7:28–33, 2001.

37. Scheld WM, Mandell GL: Nosocomial pneumonia: pathogenesis and recent advances in diagnosis and therapy. *Rev Infect Dis* 13 Suppl 9:743–751, 1991.

38. Schoepf UJ, Holzknecht N, Helmberger TK, et al: Subsegmental pulmonary emboli: improved detection with thin-collimation multi-detector row spiral CT. *Radiology* 222:483–490, 2002.

39. Schulman S, Rhedin AS, Lindmarker P, et al: A comparison of six weeks with six months of oral anticoagulant therapy after a first episode of venous thromboembolism. *N Engl J Med* 332:1661–1665, 1995.

40. Shorr RM, Crittenden M, Indeck M, et al: Blunt thoracic trauma. Analysis of 515 patients. *Ann Surg* 206:200–205, 1987.

41. Silver FL, Norris JW, Lewis AJ, et al: Early mortality following stroke: a prospective review. *Stroke* 15:492–496, 1984.

42. Smith WS, Matthay MA: Evidence for a hydrostatic mechanism in human neurogenic pulmonary edema. *Chest* 111:1326–1333, 1997.

43. Takano K, Yamaguchi T, Uchida K: Markers of a hypercoagulable state following acute ischemic stroke. *Stroke* 23:194–198, 1992.

44. Teigen CL, Maus TP, Sheedy PF II, et al: Pulmonary embolism: diagnosis with contrast-enhanced electron-beam CT and comparison with pulmonary angiography. *Radiology* 194:313–319, 1995.

45. Tobin MJ: Respiratory monitoring in the intensive care unit. *Am Rev Respir Dis* 138:1625–1642, 1988.

46. Tocino I, Miller MH: Computed tomography in blunt chest trauma. *J Thorac Imaging* 2:45–59, 1987.

47. Warlow C, Ogston D, Douglas AS: Venous thrombosis following strokes. *Lancet* 1:1305–1306, 1972.

48. Weiss YG, Deutschman CS: The role of fiberoptic bronchoscopy in airway management of the critically ill patient. *Crit Care Clin* 16:445–451, 2000.

49. Wijdicks EFM: Short of breath, short of air, short of mechanics. *Pract Neurol* (In press, 2002).

50. Wijdicks EFM, Scott JP: Pulmonary embolism associated with acute stroke. *Mayo Clin Proc* 72:297–300, 1997.

51. Wood KE: Major pulmonary embolism: review of a pathophysiologic approach to the golden hour of hemodynamically significant pulmonary embolism. *Chest* 121:877–905, 2002.

52. Yabumoto M, Kuriyama T, Iwamoto M, et al: Neurogenic pulmonary edema associated with ruptured intracranial aneurysm: case report. *Neurosurgery* 19:300–304, 1986.

30

Cardiac Complications

The patterns of myocardial injury are diverse in acute disorders of the central nervous system. It can result in cardiac arrhythmias, cardiac failure, and hard-to-manage hemodynamic instability. Cardiac abnormalities can be grouped into three categories. First, left ventricular dysfunction occurs in many patients with terminal acute central nervous system catastrophes and may imply a phenomenon called *stunning.* Second, cardiac arrhythmias are prevalent. The most common causes are underlying structural heart disease, associated drug therapy, left ventricular strain, pulmonary embolism, fever, and anemia. Third, although traumatic injury to the heart is uncommon, traumatic aortic dissection; damage to the right ventricle, septum, and tricuspid valve (susceptible because of proximity to the sternum); and pericardial effusion are all possible considerations in patients with polytrauma. Laceration of the left anterior descending coronary artery and right ventricular wall contusion have been diagnosed in exceptional cases.

It is important to investigate cardiac injury in acute neurologic disease precisely. The presence of acute myocardial ischemia has important repercussions if patients need neurosurgical intervention. In some patients, evolving cardiac failure may result in pulmonary edema that compromises gas exchange. In others, cardiac arrhythmias are life-threatening, and a temporary pacemaker may be indicated. This chapter considers frequently observed cardiac abnormalities and provides practical basic knowledge.

PATHOPHYSIOLOGIC MECHANISMS OF CARDIAC ABNORMALITIES

Cardiac injury and arrhythmias have been linked to a transient *sympathetic storm,* which may result in objective myocardial damage, mostly in the form of dispersed areas of hemorrhages and myocytolysis, myofibrillar degeneration, myocyte eosinophilia, and contraction bands, but not necrosis.[17,22,28,51]

Sympathetic preponderance includes sustained hypertension, dilatation of pupils, fever, profuse sweating, and, at times, peripheral cutaneous vasoconstriction resulting in characteristically cold fingers and toes. The alleged anatomical site associated with sympathetic stimulation is the anterior hypothalamus.[3] Other structures besides the diencephalon possibly involved in sympathetic response are neurons in the ventrolateral medulla oblongata and right-sided insular cortex.[11,36,44] The role of the right insula in sudden death due to tachyarrhythmias has been suggested in clinical studies.[11] Pressure, stretch, or hypoxemia may trigger depolarization of these sensitive neurons, leading to a persistent sympathetic tone.

The effector mechanisms of autonomic function are traditionally divided into sympathetic fibers that accelerate and parasympathetic fibers that slow the sinoatrial node. The system is balanced, but the parasympathetic system predominates in many drowsy patients with an acute central nervous system lesion. In other patients, particularly during the acute first hours, the sympathetic system is charged.

In patients with catastrophic brain lesions, increased systemic levels of catecholamines may result in an extreme increase in peripheral vascular resistance. The inability of the left ventricle to overcome this resistance may result in an acute increase in ventricular wall stress. Ventricular wall stress together with a continuing catecholamine surge may lead to electrical instability, eventually culminating in ventricular tachyarrhythmias. Myofibrillar degeneration may occur, with prominent contraction bands typical of the hypercontracted state.[17]

Another hypothesis suggested that a large increase in norepinephrine from sympathetic nerve terminals opens calcium channels and results in interchange of calcium (influx) and potassium (efflux).[51] Persistently high levels of calcium would explain the hypercontracted state followed by cell membrane destruction. Hyperkalemia would explain the peaked T waves on the electrocardiogram (ECG). However, these so-called "cerebral waves" are quite uncommon in the spectrum of ECG abnormalities associated with acute major brain injury.

Another theoretical possibility is coronary vasospasm incited by catecholamine release. However, a study in mongrel dogs showed no evidence of coronary spasm after cisternal blood injection despite regional wall motion abnormalities and contraction bands in two-thirds of the studied canines.[61]

Cardiac arrhythmias may also occur in acute neuromuscular disorders, particularly Guillain-Barré syndrome (GBS). Life-threatening cardiac arrhythmias in GBS are very uncommon, and the pathologic substrate of cardiac arrhythmias in GBS has not been elucidated. Clinicopathologic studies, however, have demonstrated scattered lymphocytic infiltrates in ganglia and in parasympathetic and sympathetic branches. In GBS, sinus tachycardia is the most common cardiac arrhythmia and may be related to lesions of the afferent baroreceptors.

In general, the cardiac manifestations can be considered to result from triggers of the central or peripheral nervous system, but in some conditions, the pathophysiologic state truly originates from the heart. Animal data cannot be easily extrapolated to the NICU population with a high proclivity for coronary artery disease. Other examples of primary cardiac causes are cardiac contusion in severe head injury, acute myocardial infarction complicated by embolic ischemic stroke, and the occasional situation in which endocarditis is associated with intracranial hematoma from a ruptured infectious aneurysm. Electrolyte disorders or drug toxicity can be implicated in some patients with cardiac arrhythmias, but this situation is uncommon in the NICU. In addition, multifocal atrial tachycardia (often mistaken for atrial fibrillation) may occur in response to a brief hypoxemic event, particularly in patients with pulmonary disease.

CARDIAC MANIFESTATIONS IN SPECIFIC NEUROLOGIC CIRCUMSTANCES

The fascinating link between acute lesions to the brain and the heart has been investigated clinically by both cardiologists and neurologists. It remains largely terra incognita, with major research opportunities.

This section reviews cardiac arrhythmias and the most pertinent ECG abnormalities in acute neurologic disorders.

Aneurysmal Subarachnoid Hemorrhage

The incidence of cardiac arrhythmias in aneurysmal SAH is difficult to estimate. Most likely, differences in monitoring result in varying incidences of ECG abnormalities and arrhythmias. The incidence of cardiac arrhythmias may also be inaccurate because sudden death in SAH (approximately 10% of all patients) is possibly associated with ventricular fibrillation or any other type of immediately life-threatening arrhythmia.

The most common cardiac rhythm disturbances in SAH are sinus bradycardia and sinus tachycardia, but both are nonspecific and can be associated with multiple causes. Possible causes for sinus bradycardia are administration of morphine, increased vagal tone from vomiting, and use of β-blockers. Potential causes of sinus tachycardia are fever, hypovolemia with anemia (a frequently overlooked cause of tachycardia), and sympathomimetic drugs such as dopamine (or other inotropes).

The incidence of life-threatening tachyarrhythmias varies considerably in studies.[2,43] Tachyarrhythmias are observed significantly more often in patients with SAH and massive intraventricular hemorrhage. When Holter monitoring was used within 48 hours of admission in patients with SAH, 41% of the patients had life-threatening arrhythmias, such as torsades de pointes, ventricular flutter, and ventricular fibrillation.[16] This high incidence of potentially life-threatening arrhythmias is unusual and was not found in a series of patients with serial ECG recordings and daily bedside monitoring.[8] Other SAH-associated cardiac arrhythmias are runs of ventricular premature complexes, sustained ventricular tachycardia, and bradyarrhythmias, mostly transient idioventricular rhythm and atrioventricular block.[2,14,16]

Morphologic ECG changes are common in SAH.[8,35] One study suggested that frequencies of ECG abnormalities were higher in patients with blood in the right sylvian fissure and quadrigeminal cistern, a finding that may argue for irritation of the insular cortex.[27] The signif-

Table 30–1. Electrocardiographic Changes in Subarachnoid Hemorrhage*

	No. of Patients
Ischemic ST segment	44
Ischemic T wave	41
Prominent U wave	39
QT$_c$ interval prolongation	34
Flat or isoelectric T wave	24
Short PR interval	14
Long PR interval	13
Transient pathologic Q wave	11
Peaked P wave	10
Tall T wave	10
Broad P wave	4

*Based on findings in 61 patients with serial electrocardiograms.
Source: Modified from Brouwers PJ, Wijdicks EFM, Hasan D, et al: Serial electrocardiographic recording in aneurysmal subarachnoid hemorrhage. *Stroke* 20:1162–1167, 1989. By permission of the American Heart Association.

icance of ECG changes remains unclear; they do not affect overall outcome,[8,60] and studies have not been able to separate out patients with higher risks of cardiac death. The most common ECG changes are shown in Table 30–1. Most frequently, the morphologic abnormalities are related to changes in the QRS complex. Very often, ST-segment sagging appears (leads I, aVL); T waves are deeply inverted, and the QT interval is prolonged (Fig. 30–1). (The QT interval varies with the heart rate, and a corrected QT [QT$_c$] is calculated by dividing the QT interval

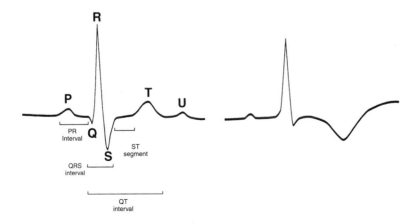

Figure 30–1. Typical morphologic changes in electrocardiographic tracing associated with acute central nervous system event: (*Left*) Normal tracing. (*Right*) ST segment depression, marked T-wave inversion, and QT interval prolongation.

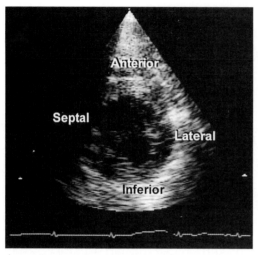
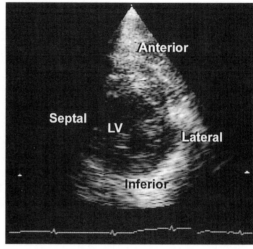

A   B

Figure 30–2. Transthoracic echocardiograms in a patient with aneurysmal subarachnoid hemorrhage. End-diastolic (*A*) and end-systolic (*B*) phases are shown in short-axis views. Note marked electrocardiographic tracing showing the view in relation to the cardiac cycle. Global severe hypokinesis is shown as virtually no change in left chamber size from end-diastole to end-systole. LV, left ventricle.

by the square root of the interval between two R waves; normal is 0.41 second in women and 0.39 second in men.) A recent retrospective study found ST- and T-wave abnormalities, most commonly T-wave inversions and ST elevations, in 27% of patients with ECG readings. None of these abnormalities predicted cardiac mortality.[60] However, echocardiographic studies have repeatedly shown ventricular dysfunction in these patients (Fig. 30–2). One study found corresponding regional wall motion abnormalities in patients with transient ST segment elevation.[47] Another study found that inverted T waves and QT-segment prolongation were significantly correlated with left ventricular function.[38] In patients with poor-grade SAH cardiac dysfunction can be profound (Fig. 30–3). Often, myocardial damage in SAH is subendocardial in the form of small, scattered hemorrhages. In an important study of 72 patients with aneurysmal SAH without prior cardiac disease, abnormal left ventricular wall motion was found in only 9 (13%) and was directly linked to peak creatine kinase MB levels of more than 2%.[39]

Echocardiographic abnormalities could persist for weeks, although spontaneous re-versibility has been described (Fig. 30–4).[57] An echocardiogram may demonstrate significant regional wall motion abnormalities that, unlike acute myocardial infarction, may be reversible as early as 4 days later[24] Serial ECGs and echocardiography are important because "acute myocardial infarction patterns" may dramatically change, even within 1 day.[8,37]

Head Injury

Cardiac arrhythmias have been studied less frequently in head injury.[29] Cardiac arrhythmias have been reported in patients with acute subdural hematoma. In a study of 100 patients, 41% had new rhythm disturbances, half with ventricular arrhythmias.[54] Confounding factors could exist, particularly in patients with multitrauma who may have direct cardiac trauma.[23] Electrocardiographic abnormalities in closed head injury may indicate pericardial effusion, myocardial infarction from laceration of coronary arteries, or ventricular wall motion abnormalities from stunning. If the ECG findings are normal 3 hours after trauma, the chance of later complications is greatly reduced. The diagnosis

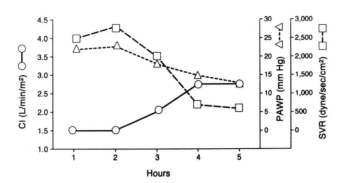

Figure 30–3. Transient ventricular failure (*cardiac stunning*) in a patient with poor-grade subarachnoid hemorrhage. CI, cardiac index; PAWP, pulmonary artery wedge pressure; SVR, systemic vascular resistance. (From Wijdicks EFM: Worst-case scenario: management in poor-grade aneurysmal subarachnoid hemorrhage. *Cerebrovasc Dis* 5:163–169, 1995. By permission of S Karger AG.)

of myocardial contusion is facilitated by echocardiographic findings of regional wall motion abnormalities and, most important, pericardial effusion. Cardiogenic shock is uncommon, and left ventricular ejection fraction usually is not reduced, because the right ventricle is preferentially involved in blunt trauma.[45] Cardiac tamponade is most impressive in its presentation, with hypotension, cyanosis of the upper chest and face, and distended neck veins.

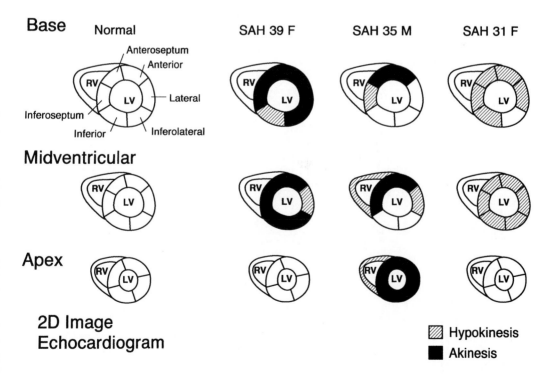

Figure 30–4. Two-dimensional (2-D) echocardiographic drawings showing ventricular hypokinesis and akinesis at different locations in the heart in three patients with subarachnoid hemorrhage (SAH). F, female; LV, left ventricle; M, male; RV, right ventricle.

Acute Ischemic or Hemorrhagic Stroke

Patients with a major stroke in arterial territory often have previous evidence of underlying heart disease. Therefore, in this clinical cate-gory, cardiac arrhythmias may be a cause rather than a result of stroke. In a prospective study by Rokey et al.,[49] asymptomatic coronary artery disease was found in approximately one-third of the patients with stroke. We reported on a patient with a pristine coronary angiogram,

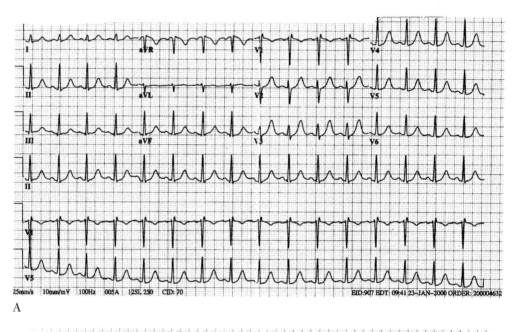

A

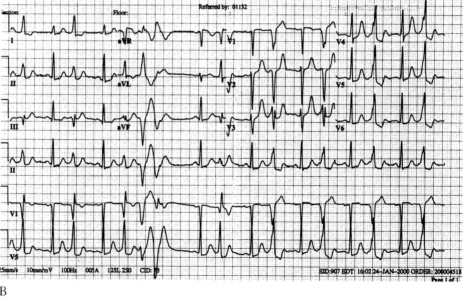

B

Figure 30–5. (*A*) Electrocardiogram (ECG) on admission with minimal ST segment depression and regular sinus rhythm pattern in V_1. (*B*) ECG showing bigeminal rhythm, peaked T waves and mild ST segment depression in inferolateral leads.

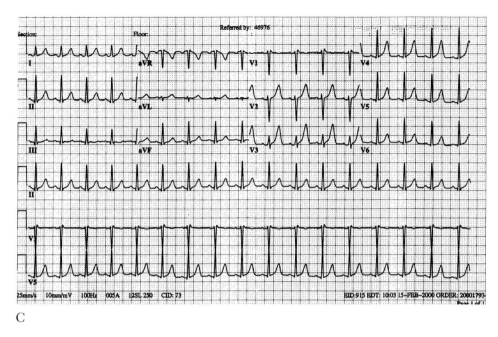

C

Figure 30–5. *(Continued) (C)* Return of ECG to baseline 3 weeks later. (From Rogers et al.[48] By permission of the American Academy of Neurology.)

new regional wall motion abnormalities on echocardiography, and transient ECG abnormalities after a hemorrhage damaging the rostral ventrolateral medulla oblongata[48] (Fig. 30–5).

The prevailing rhythm abnormality in acute ischemic stroke is atrial fibrillation, but sinus tachycardia, premature ventricular complexes, and premature atrial complexes are almost as frequent.[7,15] The Lausanne Stroke Registry Study found "new-onset" atrial fibrillation in 42% of patients, including those with spontaneous intracerebral hematoma and those with parietal-insular and brain stem infarcts.[55] In a retrospective study, only patients with right-sided hemispheric stroke had supraventricular tachycardia, whereas patients with left-sided hemispheric stroke more often had multiform premature ventricular complexes, couplets, and ventricular tachycardia, findings that suggested differences in influence of the hemispheres.[32] Whether aggressive monitoring is indicated in patients with left hemispheric strokes, whose cardiac arrhythmias seem more life-threatening, remains unresolved and doubtful.

Life-threatening arrhythmias in acute stroke are very unusual and should point to other causes, particularly acute myocardial infarction.

Status Epilepticus

Cardiac arrhythmias are possibly more often present in status epilepticus than truly recognized. In our review of patients admitted to the emergency department with status epilepticus, cardiac arrhythmias occurred in 15 of 38 (39%).[58] Sinus tachycardia was found in the vast majority, but two patients had ventricular tachycardia and a brief asystole after sudden bradycardia. No relationship was found with respiratory or metabolic (lactic) acidosis, a common occurrence in this condition.[58] Another study found bradycardia during seizures but only in the context of associated brief apnea.[40] An unresolved question is whether patients with status epilepticus and cardiac arrhythmia need β-blockers for myocardial protection.

Guillain-Barré Syndrome

The whole gamut of cardiac arrhythmias can be seen in GBS, including complete heart block. In the large plasma exchange trials conducted by the GBS study group and the French Cooperative Group, fatal cardiac arrest occurred in 3 of the combined total of 445 patients. Fortunately, pacemaker intervention is very rarely necessary in GBS.[50]

Sinus tachycardia and so-called vagal bradycardia spells are most frequent in patients with GBS. Persistent sinus tachycardia invariably occurs in patients with complete quadriplegia and mechanical ventilation, may appear at any time during the illness, and generally is not associated with hypotension or angina pectoris. Slowing of rate is indicated with signs of myocardial ischemia on ECG.

Vagal spells are brief salvos of bradycardia or sinus arrest, and tracheal suctioning is a common trigger. Vagal spells are usually a feature seen in the plateau phase but may extend into the recovery phase. When these episodes occur, ECG monitoring should continue until the patient becomes ambulant. Recently, bradycardia was associated with reversible myocardial stunning in a young woman with GBS,[5] but this finding remains unexplained.

Morphologic ECG abnormalities are uncommon and nonspecific in GBS, but when they are present, ST-segment abnormalities are frequent.[50] It is uncertain whether they represent myocardial damage.

Brain Death

Cardiac arrhythmias may occur in patients who fulfill the criteria for brain death, and ventricular tachycardia is frequent. It may be associated with severe surges in blood pressure due to increased intracranial pressure.

During apnea testing, cardiac arrhythmia may occur with severe acidosis (pH < 7.0), and it is commonly ventricular tachyarrhythmia. This arrhythmia may be associated with hypotension, which has the potential to jeopardize organ recovery if it is not rapidly corrected. The risk of cardiac arrhythmia is often related to significant hypoxemia during the apnea test. This risk is not increased in patients with known coronary artery disease. Only when acidosis becomes severe and PCO_2 approaches 90 mm Hg can cardiac arrhythmias be expected despite adequate preoxygenation. In general, connection to the ventilator corrects the arrhythmia.

Myocardial dysfunction after catastrophic brain injury leading to brain death is common and often associated with ventricular arrhythmias. Myocardial dysfunction is more severe in patients with traumatic head injury than in those with SAH or intraparenchymal hemorrhage. In our study of 66 patients, myocardial dysfunction in brain death from SAH was more regional and ejection fraction more marginally abnormal and not accompanied by histologic changes in the ventricular myocardium. However, a very significant reduction in ejection fraction and global hypokinesis interspersed with large akinetic segments (average of 25%) was found in patients with head trauma who had progression to brain death.[19] Ventricular arrhythmias occurred in 30% of patients with severe echocardiographic abnormalities and in none with normal echocardiographic findings.

Echocardiography (and also coronary angiography) is routinely used to screen brain-dead donors. Technetium Tc 99m pyrophosphate may have a future role in identifying severe myocardial injury, but no data are yet available in humans.[52] Patients who fulfill the clinical criteria of brain death have an invariate heart rate due to autonomic uncoupling. Cardiac arrest is an inevitable consequence of brain death. Lack of autonomic nervous system input results in a decrease in contractility and coronary perfusion and in terminal cardiac rhythms, such as sinus bradycardia, or isolated atrial activity.[21,25,26,33]

CARDIAC ARRHYTHMIAS

The most commonly observed cardiac arrhythmias in central nervous system catastrophes and their management options are systemati-

Ventricular Tachycardia

Ventricular tachycardia is one of the most frequently observed tachycardias in acute central nervous system injury. Many patients have nonsustained tachycardia.

The diagnostic hallmark of ventricular tachycardia is a wide QRS complex of 140 msec or more. The P waves are mostly obscured within the ST segment and difficult to detect at high rates[10,53] (Fig. 30–6I). This type of tachycardia can be mistaken for supraventricular tachycardia, but intravenous administration of adenosine, which converts reentry supraventricular tachycardia (rarely seen in NICUs), can be used for differentiation. In fact, adenosine gives information similar to that of the vagal maneuver by blocking atrioventricular nodal conduction.

Treatment depends on the level of blood pressure. Cardioversion is indicated in patients with a significant reduction in blood pressure. Lidocaine is indicated in patients with normal blood pressure.

Miscellaneous Cardioarrhythmias

Occasionally, torsades de pointes arrhythmias appear in patients with poor-grade aneurysmal SAH, typically in association with bradyarrhythmia and prolonged QT interval. The wide QRS complexes twist around the baseline, continuously change in shape, are extremely rapid, with rates around 300 beats/minute, and are brief[4] (Fig. 30–6J). Hypokalemia and hypomagnesemia are risk factors, as are many drugs (antipsychotic and antidepressant agents, antibiotics, and many cardiovascular drugs).

Cardiac arrhythmias of no consequence are single premature atrial complex (Fig. 30–6K) and premature ventricular complex (Fig. 30–6L). Management of cardiac arrhythmias is summarized in Table 30–3.

MANAGEMENT OF CARDIAC ABNORMALITIES

Cardiac abnormalities of any sort may signal myocardial injury or dysfunction. Cardiac wall motion abnormalities are frequently found but generally do not pose a particular management

Table 30–3. Guidelines for the Initial Management of Common Cardiac Arrhythmias

Arrhythmia	Therapy
Sinus tachycardia	Esmolol
Sinus bradycardia	Atropine, cardiac pacing
Atrial fibrillation	Verapamil, diltiazem
Atrial flutter	Verapamil, diltiazem
Multifocal atrial tachycardia	Verapamil or metoprolol
Junctional rhythm	Atropine
Atrioventricular block	Cardiac pacing
Venticular tachycardia	Cardioversion
Torsades de pointes	Magnesium sulfate

problem. Their potential to be present in poor-grade SAH and head injury should be recognized, but significant hemodynamic instability is uncommon. Dobutamine (5 μg/kg starting dose) can be helpful if blood pressure decreases and pulmonary edema occurs.

In every patient with cardiac arrhythmia and an ECG abnormality, a full 12-lead ECG and echocardiography are warranted. Management becomes highly complex in patients with new ECG abnormalities suggesting myocardial infarction. In particular, the decision to evaluate these patients with ECG abnormalities for possible coronary artery disease is difficult, as alluded to earlier. Any pattern of myocardial infarction can be observed, but when infarction is truly present, a subendocardial pattern is most common, with large T waves and a major ST segment decrease, often exceeding 2 or 3 mm. ST elevation in the precordial leads (predominantly V_4 through V_6) has been associated with acute brain injury (particularly SAH) without angiographic evidence of coronary artery disease.[30] In addition, acute myocardial infarction causes a major increase in creatine kinase in contrast to the minor increases from cerebral creatine kinase. Creatine kinase MB samples obtained every 8 to 12 hours for at least 24 to 48 hours should generate reliable information. The ratio of myocardial isoenzyme (creatine kinase MB fraction) to total creatine kinase, however, is only marginally increased in patients with nonsignificant ECG abnormalities associated with acute central nervous system disease. Troponin (T or I) is not detectable in healthy persons and is a better marker for cardiac injury because isoforms expressed in skeletal muscle are not detected by current assays. The sensitivity and specificity of cardiac troponin I for myocardial dysfunction, at least in aneurysmal SAH, is much higher than those of creatine kinase MB.[46] The usefulness of this sensitive cardiac assay in acute brain injury warrants more study. Increased troponin I correlates with ECG abnormalities, gallop rhythm, and pulmonary edema, relationships not found with increased MB fraction of creatine kinase. This assay is very sensitive, and only mild increases can be detected after cardioversion[6] or in mimicking disorders such as pulmonary embolism due to acute right ventricular strain, dilation, and injury.[18]

Factors that should influence the decision to further investigate significant coronary artery disease are history of myocardial infarction, angina pectoris, and older age. Emergency cardiology consultation is imperative, certainly when ECGs suggest critical proximal left anterior descending coronary stenosis (ST segment elevation in precordial leads and progressive symmetrical T-wave inversion without pathologic precordial Q waves). In addition, bundle branch block or hemiblock in association with acute myocardial infarction increases the risk of early death. However, despite these discriminating signs, nuclear perfusion imaging should be performed in patients with a high likelihood of acute myocardial infarction, and coronary angiography and possibly angioplasty should also be considered.

A detailed review of the perioperative cardiac risks and guidelines have been published by the American College of Cardiology and American Heart Association task force on practice guidelines.[1,34] Craniotomy should be considered an intermediate surgical risk, with a reported cardiac death and nonfatal myocardial infarction rate of less than 5%.[1,34] However, cardiac complications are up to five times more common in emergency procedures, such as evacuation of a traumatic intracerebral hematoma. This increase most likely reflects the inclusion of patients with significant coronary disease who were not evaluated because of the brief time between ictus and surgery. Generally, the risk of perioperative myocardial infarction in patients with no coronary disease (by ECG, history of angina, or coronary angiogram) is low.

The risk increases significantly in patients with unstable coronary syndromes, decompensated congestive heart failure, arrhythmias, and severe valvular disease. A full cardiologic evaluation, if time allows, is needed, often with noninvasive testing. New wall motion abnormalities within one or two coronary vessel territories on echocardiography or abnormal findings on dobutamine stress echocardiography justify coronary angiography or aggressive medical management. No data on whether preoperative percutaneous transluminal coronary angioplasty or bypass grafting in the event of coronary artery disease reduces the perioperative risk are available in patients with acute neurologic illness, although this benefit seems likely. (The data are also unclear in other types of surgery.)

Perioperative management in patients with suspected myocardial ischemia probably should include more aggressive monitoring during anesthesia (12-lead ECG) and intravenous administration of nitroglycerin intraoperatively or intraoperative administration of diltiazem or oral administration of metoprolol. Clonidine may have potential and seems beneficial, but further evaluation in a prospective trial is needed.[42]

Postoperative ECG studies are needed on the first and second days, and cardiac enzymes are studied only in patients with demonstrated ECG abnormalities.[1]

CONCLUSIONS

- Most cardiac arrhythmias in acute central nervous system disorders are transient and do not require therapeutic intervention.
- Additional evaluation (nuclear scan, coronary angiography) for acute myocardial infarction and coronary artery disease should be considered if persistent ECG and echocardiographic

abnormalities (particularly major ST segment decrease, large T waves) are found in patients with acute central nervous system events, patients with previous myocardial infarction or angina pectoris, and elderly patients.
- The most common morphologic ECG changes in acute central nervous system catastrophes are prolonged QT interval, ST segment sagging, and deeply inverted T waves.
- Echocardiography may be a useful noninvasive tool for early diagnosis of cardiac anatomical or functional abnormalities that may underlie the arrhythmias.
- The risk of cardiac mortality and nonfatal myocardial infarction with craniotomy is less than 5% but increases in patients with unstable angina, congestive heart failure, cardiac arrhythmias, or valvular disease.

REFERENCES

1. ACC/AHA Task Force Report: Guidelines for perioperative cardiovascular evaluation for noncardiac surgery. *J Am Coll Cardiol* 27:910–948, 1996.
2. Andreoli A, di Pasquale G, Pinelli G, et al: Subarachnoid hemorrhage: frequency and severity of cardiac arrhythmias. A survey of 70 cases studied in the acute phase. *Stroke* 18:558–564, 1987.
3. Attar HJ, Gutierrez MT, Bellet S, et al: Effect of stimulation of hypothalamus and reticular activating system on production of cardiac arrhythmia. *Circ Res* 12:14–21, 1963.
4. Ben-David J, Zipes DP: Torsades de pointes and proarrhythmia. *Lancet* 341:1578–1582, 1993.
5. Bernstein R, Mayer SA, Magnano A: Neurogenic stunned myocardium in Guillain-Barré syndrome. *Neurology* 54:759–762, 2000.
6. Boriani G, Biffi M, Cervi V, et al: Evaluation of myocardial injury following repeated internal atrial shocks by monitoring serum cardiac troponin I levels. *Chest* 118:342–347, 2000.
7. Britton M, de Faire U, Helmers C, et al: Arrhythmias in patients with acute cerebrovascular disease. *Acta Med Scand* 205:425–428, 1979.
8. Brouwers PJ, Wijdicks EFM, Hasan D, et al: Serial electrocardiographic recording in aneurysmal subarachnoid hemorrhage. *Stroke* 20:1162–1167, 1989.
9. Brugada P, Gursoy S, Brugada J, et al: Investigation of palpitations. *Lancet* 341:1254–1258, 1993.
10. Campbell RW: Ventricular ectopic beats and non-sustained ventricular tachycardia. *Lancet* 341:1454–1458, 1993.
11. Cheung RTF, Hachinski V: The insula and cerebrogenic sudden death. *Arch Neurol* 57:1685–1688, 2000.
12. Cruickshank JM, Neil-Dwyer G, Degaute JP, et al: Reduction of stress/catecholamine-induced cardiac necrosis by beta 1-selective blockade. *Lancet* 2:585–589, 1987.
13. Cushing H: The blood-pressure reaction of acute cerebral compression, illustrated by cases of intracranial hemorrhage; a sequel to the Mütter lecture for 1901. *Am J Med Sci* 125:1017–1044, 1903.
14. Davies KR, Gelb AW, Manninen PH, et al: Cardiac function in aneurysmal subarachnoid haemorrhage: a study of electrocardiographic and echocardiographic abnormalities. *Br J Anaesth* 67:58–63, 1991.
15. Davis TP, Alexander J, Lesch M: Electrocardiographic changes associated with acute cerebrovascular disease: a clinical review. *Prog Cardiovasc Dis* 36:245–260, 1993.
16. Di Pasquale G, Pinelli G, Andreoli A, et al: Holter detection of cardiac arrhythmias in intracranial subarachnoid hemorrhage. *Am J Cardiol* 59:596–600, 1987.
17. Doshi R, Neil-Dwyer G: Hypothalamic and myocardial lesions after subarachnoid haemorrhage. *J Neurol Neurosurg Psychiatry* 40:821–826, 1977.
18. Douketis JD, Crowther MA, Stanton EB, et al: Elevated cardiac troponin levels in patients with submassive pulmonary embolism. *Arch Intern Med* 162:79–81, 2002.
19. Dujardin KS, McCully RB, Wijdicks EFM, et al: Myocardial dysfunction associated with brain death: clinical, echocardiographic, and pathologic features. *J Heart Lung Transplant* 20:350–357, 2001.
20. Falk RH: Atrial fibrillation. *N Engl J Med* 344:1067–178, 2001.
21. Goldstein B, Toweill D, Lai S, et al: Uncoupling of the autonomic and cardiovascular systems in acute brain injury. *Am J Physiol* 275:R1287–R1292, 1998.
22. Greenhoot JH, Reichenbach DD: Cardiac injury and subarachnoid hemorrhage. A clinical, pathological, and physiological correlation. *J Neurosurg* 30:521–531, 1969.
23. Hackenberry LE, Miner ME, Rea GL, et al: Biochemical evidence of myocardial injury after severe head trauma. *Crit Care Med* 10:641–644, 1982.
24. Handlin LR, Kindred LH, Beauchamp GD, et al: Reversible left ventricular dysfunction after subarachnoid hemorrhage. *Am Heart J* 126:235–240, 1993.
25. Herijgers P, Borgers M, Flameng W: The effect of brain death on cardiovascular function in rats. Part I. Is the heart damaged? *Cardiovasc Res* 38:98–106, 1998.
26. Herijgers P, Flameng W: The effect of brain death on cardiovascular function in rats. Part II. The cause of the in vivo haemodynamic changes. *Cardiovasc Res* 38:107–115, 1998.
27. Hirashima Y, Takashima S, Matsumura N, et al: Right sylvian fissure subarachnoid hemorrhage has electrocardiographic consequences. *Stroke* 32:2278–2281, 2001.

28. Hockman CH, Mauck HP Jr, Hoff EC: ECG changes resulting from cerebral stimulation. II. A spectrum of ventricular arrhythmias of sympathetic origin. *Am Heart J* 71:695–700, 1966.

29. Jacobson SA, Danufsky P: Marked electrocardiographic changes produced by experimental head trauma. *J Neuropathol Exp Neurol* 13:462–466, 1954.

30. Kono T, Morita H, Kuroiwa T, et al: Left ventricular wall motion abnormalities in patients with subarachnoid hemorrhage: neurogenic stunned myocardium. *J Am Coll Cardiol* 24:636–640, 1994.

31. Kuck KH, Schlüter M: Junctional tachycardia and the role of catheter ablation. *Lancet* 341:1386–1391, 1993.

32. Lane RD, Wallace JD, Petrosky PP, et al: Supraventricular tachycardia in patients with right hemisphere strokes. *Stroke* 23:362–366, 1992.

33. Logigian EL, Ropper AH: Terminal electrocardiographic changes in brain-dead patients. *Neurology* 35:915–918, 1985.

34. Mangano DT, Goldman L: Preoperative assessment of patients with known or suspected coronary disease. *N Engl J Med* 333:1750–1756, 1995.

35. Manninen PH, Ayra B, Gelb AW, et al: Association between electrocardiographic abnormalities and intracranial blood in patients following acute subarachnoid hemorrhage. *J Neurosurg Anesthesiol* 7:12–16, 1995.

36. Manning JW, deV Cotten M: Mechanism of cardiac arrhythmias induced by diencephalic stimulation. *Am J Physiol* 203:1120–1124, 1962.

37. Marion DW, Segal R, Thompson ME: Subarachnoid hemorrhage and the heart. *Neurosurgery* 18:101–106, 1986.

38. Mayer SA, LiMandri G, Sherman D, et al: Electrocardiographic markers of abnormal left ventricular wall motion in acute subarachnoid hemorrhage. *J Neurosurg* 83:889–896, 1995.

39. Mayer SA, Lin J, Homma S, et al: Myocardial injury and left ventricular performance after subarachnoid hemorrhage. *Stroke* 30:780–786, 1999.

40. Nashef L, Walker F, Allen P, et al: Apnoea and bradycardia during epileptic seizures: relation to sudden death in epilepsy. *J Neurol Neurosurg Psychiatry* 60:297–300, 1996.

41. Nichol G, McAlister F, Pham B, et al: Meta-analysis of randomised controlled trials of the effectiveness of antiarrhythmic agents at promoting sinus rhythm in patients with atrial fibrillation. *Heart* 87:535–543, 2002.

42. Nishina K, Mikawa K, Uesugi T, et al: Efficacy of clonidine for prevention of perioperative myocardial ischemia: a critical appraisal and meta-analysis of the literature. *Anesthesiology* 96:323–329, 2002.

43. Oppenheimer SM, Cechetto DF, Hachinski VC: Cerebrogenic cardiac arrhythmias. Cerebral electrocardiographic influences and their role in sudden death. *Arch Neurol* 47:513–519, 1990.

44. Oppenheimer SM, Gelb A, Girvin JP, et al: Cardiovascular effects of human insular cortex stimulation. *Neurology* 42:1727–1732, 1992.

45. Orliaguet G, Ferjani M, Riou B: The heart in blunt trauma. *Anesthesiology* 95:544–548, 2001.

46. Parekh N, Venkatesh B, Cross D, et al: Cardiac troponin I predicts myocardial dysfunction in aneurysmal subarachnoid hemorrhage. *J Am Coll Cardiol* 36:1328–1335, 2000.

47. Pollick C, Cujec B, Parker S, et al: Left ventricular wall motion abnormalities in subarachnoid hemorrhage: an echocardiographic study. *J Am Coll Cardiol* 12:600–605, 1988.

48. Rogers ER, Phan TG, Wijdicks EFM: Myocardial injury after hemorrhage into the lateral medulla oblongata. *Neurology* 56:567–568, 2001.

49. Rokey R, Rolak LA, Harati Y, et al: Coronary artery disease in patients with cerebrovascular disease: a prospective study. *Ann Neurol* 16:50–53, 1984.

50. Ropper AH, Wijdicks EFM, Truax BT: *Guillain-Barré Syndrome*. Philadelphia: FA Davis Company, 1991.

51. Samuels MA: Cardiopulmonary aspects of acute neurologic diseases. In Ropper AH (ed): *Neurological and Neurosurgical Intensive Care*. 3rd ed. New York: Raven Press, 1993, pp 103–119.

52. Satur CM, Doyle D, Darracott-Cankovic S, et al: Can technetium 99m pyrophosphate be used to quantify myocardial injury in donor hearts? *Ann Thorac Surg* 68:2225–2230, 1999.

53. Shenasa M, Borggrefe M, Haverkamp W, et al: Ventricular tachycardia. *Lancet* 341:1512–1519, 1993.

54. VanderArk GD: Cardiovascular changes with acute subdural hematoma. *Surg Neurol* 3:305–308, 1975.

55. Vingerhoets F, Bogousslavsky J, Regli F, et al: Atrial fibrillation after acute stroke. *Stroke* 24:26–30, 1993.

56. Waldo AL, Wit AL: Mechanisms of cardiac arrhythmias. *Lancet* 341:1189–1193, 1993.

57. Wells C, Cujec B, Johnson D, et al: Reversibility of severe left ventricular dysfunction in patients with subarachnoid hemorrhage. *Am Heart J* 129:409–412, 1995.

58. Wijdicks EFM, Hubmayr RD: Acute acid-base disorders associated with status epilepticus. *Mayo Clin Proc* 69:1044–1046, 1994.

59. Wood MA, Brown-Mahoney C, Kay GN, et al: Clinical outcomes after ablation and pacing therapy for atrial fibrillation: a meta-analysis. *Circulation* 101:1138–1144, 2000.

60. Zaroff JG, Rordorf GA, Newell JB, et al: Cardiac outcome in patients with subarachnoid hemorrhage and electrocardiographic abnormalities. *Neurosurgery* 44:34–39, 1999.

61. Zaroff JG, Rordorf GA, Titus JS, et al: Regional myocardial perfusion after experimental subarachnoid hemorrhage. *Stroke* 31:1136–1143, 2000.

31

Acid–Base Disorders and Sodium Handling

Although frequent in medical and surgical intensive care units, life-threatening acid–base disorders are uncommon in patients with acute neurologic disorders. When they occur, they are often transient (e.g., metabolic acidosis in status epilepticus) or purposely induced (respiratory alkalosis to treat increased intracranial pressure). Consequently, a persistent acid–base disorder more often indicates a complicating major medical problem.

The most commonly encountered abnormalities in the NICU are hyponatremia and hypernatremia. A number of electrolyte abnormalities are unusual in patients with acute neurologic illnesses. Potassium depletion is most often associated with diuretic agents, vomiting and diarrhea related to gastrointestinal feeding, and use of mineralocorticoids to expand intravascular volume. Calcium and magnesium metabolism is seldom disturbed except in profound alcohol abuse. Hypomagnesemia may contribute to seizures, and hypophosphatemia may be associated with significant muscle weakness, but often renal loss due to use of mannitol can be implicated.[44]

The many other electrolyte abnormalities, far more common in other medical or surgical intensive care units, are described in a companion monograph.[61] A guideline for evaluation and management is included in the Appendix. This chapter presents a foundation of the basic principles, but its use also lies in the interpretation of these derangements.

ACID–BASE ABNORMALITIES

This section explores the mechanisms underlying acidosis and alkalosis. Clinically, these derangements—when deviation from the normal range is severe—are important because the level of consciousness may decrease and major cardiac arrhythmias can result.

Principles of Acid–Base Physiology and Interpretation

The H^+ concentration in body fluids is held constant by buffers. Changes in H^+ concentration and reciprocal pH concentration are important, because vital cellular enzyme systems depend on a constant milieu for functioning. The most important buffer in the extracellular fluid is the HCO_3^-/CO_2 system, although other buffers (H_2PO_4, NH_3) are recruited to maintain the balance.

Changes in the acid–base balance are reflected by changes in arterial P_{CO_2} (respiratory acidosis with an increase, respiratory alkalosis with a decrease) or changes in arterial HCO_3^- concentration (metabolic acidosis with a decrease, metabolic alkalosis with an increase). Changes of this nature result in an appropriate compensatory response. To maintain a constant ratio of arterial P_{CO_2} to arterial HCO_3, a change must be in the same direction: an increase in arterial P_{CO_2}, an increase in arterial HCO_3, and, vice versa, a decrease in arterial P_{CO_2} and a decrease in arterial HCO_3.

Blood gas interpretation remains complex, even for experienced clinicians in critical care. Before an attempt is made to interpret a blood gas, an erroneous result should be excluded. A well-known cause for acidosis is related to heparin used to anticoagulate the sample before transport to the laboratory. This is often recognized by extreme reductions in values, approaching a pH of 6.5, with associated clinical discrepancy. Venous blood sampling may occur and actually is rather common, and it has resulted in inappropriate admission to the intensive care unit of patients with suspected acute neuromuscular failure. Usually, oxygen saturation is in the 70s, and a marked discrepancy with pulse oximetric values is noted. Another helpful method is to compare oxygen content with that of hemoglobin (the oxygen content of arterial blood is greater than that of hemoglobin). Obtaining blood gases from an arterial catheter after the patient has been stabilized in the unit eliminates this error.

Blood gas interpretation is usually guided by changes in arterial pH and arterial P_{CO_2}. A change in pH defines acidosis or alkalosis. Given a decrease in arterial pH, metabolic acidosis is present when the arterial P_{CO_2} is normal or decreased. Metabolic acidosis is then differentiated into metabolic acidosis with a normal or high anion gap (anion gap = $Na^+ - [Cl^- + HCO_3^-]$; 10 to 12 mEq/L). An increased anion gap occurs in lactic acidosis (e.g., status epilepticus), uremic acidosis, diabetic or alcoholic ketoacidosis, and intoxication (ethylene glycol, methanol, and salicylate), situations that are uncommon in critically ill neurologic patients but are occasionally causes for coma of unexplained origin or contribute to impaired arousal. A normal anion gap identifies loss of alkali from the gastrointestinal tract (e.g., diarrhea), which also results in compensatory reciprocal change in chloride and bicarbonate or renal acidosis. Given a decrease in arterial pH, respiratory acidosis is present when arterial P_{CO_2} is increased.

Conversely, given an increase in arterial pH, metabolic alkalosis is present when arterial P_{CO_2} is normal or increased. Respiratory alkalosis is present when arterial P_{CO_2} is decreased. A useful acid–base nomogram is shown in Figure 31–1.

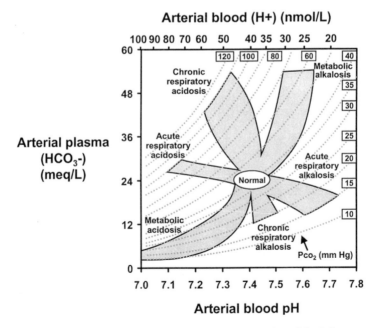

Figure 31–1. Acid–base nomogram. Boxed values are P_{CO_2}. (Modified from DuBose TD Jr: Acid-base disorders. In Brenner BM [ed]: *Brenner & Rector's The Kidney.* 6th ed. Vol 1. Philadelphia: WB Saunders Company, 2000, pp 925–997. By permission of the publisher.)

Treatment of acid–base disorders requires correction of the trigger and, less often, additional active intervention. Metabolic or respiratory acidosis is mostly asymptomatic until the pH reaches 7.2. The systemic effects of metabolic acidosis usually instigate correction. These systemic effects begin with tachycardia, which is replaced by bradycardia when the blood pH approaches 7.1. Ventricular contractility is markedly reduced with these degrees of acidosis. The risk of acute ventricular fibrillation increases significantly at these levels. Patients with previous cardiac disease may be predisposed.

Metabolic Acidosis

The most probable conditions that produce metabolic acidosis in patients with central or peripheral nervous system disorders are shown in Table 31–1. Metabolic acidosis is not frequently observed in acutely ill neurologic patients and must alert neurologists to other, unrelated, conditions. The most common conditions that must be excluded are diabetic ketoacidosis and renal failure. Lactic acidosis from a series of tonic-clonic seizures or status epilepticus, however, is comparatively more common. Ethylene glycol intoxication should be considered in patients with an increased anion gap. These patients may present with status epilepticus and increased anion gap that initially are falsely attributed to lactic acidosis from seizures. However, an osmolar gap (for formula, see the Appendix) should increase the clinical suspicion.

Rhabdomyolysis should be considered in patients with greatly increased creatine kinase values. Although the condition is uncommon, it may be observed after status epilepticus and in patients with a major stroke, in whom it is discovered after days of muscular ischemia

Table 31–1. Common Causes of Metabolic Acidosis in the Neurologic Intensive Care Unit

Lactic acidosis (status epilepticus)
Ketoacidosis (diabetes, alcoholism, malnourishment)
Septic shock
Rhabdomyolysis

Table 31–2. Common Causes of Metabolic Alkalosis in the Neurologic Intensive Care Unit

Gastrointestinal losses
Diuretics (loop or thiazide)
Massive blood transfusion in multitrauma
Severe hypokalemia
Penicillin (high doses)

from prolonged compression of a hemiplegic limb. No treatment of the metabolic acidosis is indicated, because spontaneous correction can be expected after rehydration. Bicarbonate infusion in status epilepticus (up to 90 mEq initially) may be considered when the pH is lower than 7.0. However, when cardiac arrhythmias are absent, bicarbonate supplementation can be postponed. Replenishment may lead to unexpected alkalosis, which lowers the seizure threshold (see Chapter 24). Large fluid volumes are necessary in diabetic ketoacidosis, and bicarbonate is administered cautiously if severe hyperkalemia is present. Hemodialysis is virtually always indicated in patients with methanol or ethylene glycol intoxication.

Metabolic Alkalosis

The causes of metabolic alkalosis are listed in Table 31–2. Most patients with metabolic alkalosis have lost sodium and water from excessive use of diuretic agents (contraction alkalosis), excessive vomiting, or nasogastric suctioning. Typically, urinary chloride concentration is less than 15 mEq/L. Metabolic alkalosis with increased urinary loss of chloride (and potassium) often identifies hyperaldosteronism, which may be causing hypertension. Metabolic alkalosis can cause a significant decrease in level of consciousness and can be a possible reason for clinical deterioration in any patient with an acute central nervous system disorder. Management is directed toward judicious repletion of the volume deficit.

Respiratory Acidosis

Respiratory acidosis remains the most frequent acid–base disorder in patients requiring me-

Table 31–3. Common Causes of Respiratory Acidosis in the Neurologic Intensive Care Unit

Aspiration pneumonitis
Adult respiratory distress syndrome
Acute pulmonary edema
Pneumothorax
Mechanical ventilation
Neuromuscular respiratory failure and imminent arrest

chanical ventilation. In patients with acute respiratory acidosis, there is additional laboratory evidence of hypercapnia and decreased pH, often with associated hypoxemia. The most likely causes of respiratory acidosis in critically ill neurologic patients are summarized in Table 31–3. The obvious first considerations are aspiration and acute pulmonary edema. Particularly in patients with underlying pulmonary disease, a single bout of aspiration or aspiration pneumonitis compromises their condition. Acute pulmonary edema triggered by the central nervous system insult alone (neurogenic pulmonary edema) is uncommon. It most commonly occurs in patients with poor-grade subarachnoid hemorrhage, particularly ruptured basilar artery aneurysm, and in patients who fulfill the clinical criteria for brain death within hours after the insult.

Patients with an acute neuromuscular disorder may have rapid progression to acute hypercapnia if the initial clinical signs of air hunger, tachycardia, brow sweating, and use of accessory muscles (sternocleidomastoid) are not appreciated as signals of imminent danger (see Chapter 5). These patients often are markedly hypoxemic, and in some patients, more often those with long-standing neuromuscular disease, correction with only 1 to 2 L of oxygen may substantially increase PCO_2 (and reduce alertness) without measures to increase alveolar ventilation. In addition, in patients with long-standing carbon dioxide retention and hypoxemia drive, removal of the stimulus with oxygen therapy eliminates the drive, reduces ventilation, and intensifies hypercapnia.

In general, treatment of respiratory acidosis consists of mechanical ventilation and correction of the more relevant life-threatening hypoxemia.

Respiratory Alkalosis

Induced hyperventilation is the most common reason for respiratory alkalosis, and patients typically have an increased ventilatory drive after acute central nervous system catastrophes. The causes are found in Table 31–4. In newly admitted patients with unexplained coma, aspirin poisoning, amphetamines, and cocaine should be considered when appropriate. Hyperventilation in an attempt to overcome hypoxemia must be excluded. Respiratory alkalosis is common in patients with mechanical ventilation because of large tidal volumes and can easily be corrected if necessary. Treatment is directed to the cause and may vary from mild sedation to correction of hypoxemia and its underlying cause.

DISORDERS OF SODIUM AND WATER HOMEOSTASIS

Critically ill neurologic patients are exposed to multiple factors that can perturb sodium and volume homeostasis. Many factors stimulate secretion of the antidiuretic hormone. Mechanical ventilation with positive end-expiratory pressure, overwhelming pain and stress, and medications may all result in abnormal water retention and dilutional hyponatremia. At the other extreme, hypernatremia is less frequent but most commonly due to diabetes insipidus and osmotic diuretics.

Possible routes for additional fluid and electrolyte losses are the skin in patients with high fever and profuse diaphoresis, the lung in patients with induced hyperventilation, and the stomach from gastric suctioning.

Table 31–4. Common Causes of Respiratory Alkalosis in the Neurologic Intensive Care Unit

Induced hyperventilation
 Mechanical ventilation
 Intracranial pressure management
Compensatory response to hypoxemia
Pulmonary embolism
Central neurogenic hyperventilation
Early sepsis

Several general principles must be considered. The absolute value of the electrolyte abnormality is less important than the rate of change. Furthermore, the accompanying change in intravascular status is more relevant than the absolute serum sodium level.

HYPOTONIC AND HYPERTONIC STATES

The most common disorders of tonicity or effective osmolality are hyponatremia and hypernatremia. Plasma sodium values should be monitored daily, sometimes hourly. Management, particularly of hyponatremia, is often difficult, and rapid correction of the abnormalities could prove disastrous.

Evaluation of Hyponatremia

Hyponatremia (serum sodium ≤ 135 mmol/L) is classified on the basis of tonicity (effective osmolality). Hyponatremia may be associated with normal or increased osmolality when additional solutes are present, such as in hyperglycemia or with recent administration of a hypertonic solution such as mannitol. Hyperglycemia reduces plasma sodium because an extracellular shift of water driven by glucose cannot emanate from the extracellular space. A correction factor of a decrease of 2.4 mEq/L in sodium concentration per 100 mg/dL increase in glucose concentration has been recommended.[20]

With recent administration of mannitol, calculation of serum osmolality demonstrates lower serum osmolality (see below).

(Blood urea nitrogen [BUN] and glucose values are expressed as milligrams per deciliter. The calculated value should be at least 10 mOsm/kg lower than the measured value.)

Normal serum osmolality with hyponatremia (pseudohyponatremia) may indicate severe hyperlipemia (e.g., in patients with known brittle diabetes admitted with acute stroke), severe hyperproteinemia (e.g., in patients with multiple myeloma admitted with central nervous system infection), or use of intravenous immunoglobulin.[26] Intravenous administration of immunoglobulin increases the protein-containing nonaqueous phase of plasma. The ion-selective electrodes measure sodium concentration per liter of serum but do not correct for increased protein or lipid concentration. Sodium is present only in the aqueous phase; each unit volume of plasma measured has less sodium-containing water. When measured after infusion of intravenous immunoglobulin, serum protein concentration is increased. However, most hospital laboratories have measures in place to adjust for this abnormality.

Hyponatremia is further divided into three major categories, and each may have clinical attributes. The major categories are hyponatremia associated with volume depletion (relative tachycardia, orthostasis, marginal skin turgor), hyponatremia associated with volume expansion (edema, weight gain), and hyponatremia associated with normal volume (lack of edema, normal blood pressure and pulse).

Hypovolemic hyponatremia may result from extrarenal spills (vomiting, diarrhea, and third-space fluid losses in trauma) or from nephrotic syndrome, cirrhosis, or cardiac failure. A random urine specimen with a urine sodium concentration below 20 mEq/L is useful because it indicates hypovolemia.

Hyponatremia can be generated when water is excessive in relation to sodium. This physiologic state of hypo-osmolality prompts an appropriate response of reduced antidiuretic hormone (ADH) secretion, which results in excess excretion of water, dilution of urine, and decrease in urine osmolality. Conversely, in patients with hypovolemia and hyponatremia, the volume-sensitive carotid sinus baroreceptors stimulate the paraventric-

$$\text{plasma osmolality} = 2 \times [\text{Na}] + \frac{\text{glucose}}{18} + \frac{\text{BUN}}{2.8} = \text{mOsm/kg H}_2\text{O}$$

ular neurons to secrete ADH and cause water to be retained in an attempt to restore the depleted volume (a marked ADH response is seen after blood volume depletion of more than 20%).

Many other nonosmotic stimuli of ADH have been identified. Pain, nausea, and drugs such as morphine (often used in NICUs for pain management; see Chapter 4) and carbamazepine may profoundly stimulate ADH secretion.[25] However, when carefully studied, oxcarbazepine (an analogue of carbamazepine) was not associated with increased ADH, but hyponatremia occurred with failure to excrete a waterload, suggesting an effect on collecting tubules by the drug itself.[50]

Traditionally, syndrome of inappropriate antidiuretic hormone (SIADH) has been a major cause of hyponatremia in patients with central nervous system disease. The diagnostic criteria for SIADH include hyponatremia with hypoosmolar serum, inappropriately concentrated urine, continued sodium excretion (urinary sodium of > 25 mEq/L), and exclusion of renal or endocrine disease (hypothyroidism or hypoadrenalism). There must also be no stimuli that could produce a nonosmotic release of ADH, such as hypovolemia, hypotension, pain, stress, and nausea.[52] It should be noted that increased urine sodium concentration is difficult to interpret. Unfortunately, it is commonly explained as indicative of SIADH, particularly when found in combination with increased urine osmolality. However, increased urinary sodium concentration may also have its origin in cerebral salt wasting or large sodium intake. Increased concentration may also occur in patients with hypovolemia and metabolic alkalosis from profuse vomiting. (The increased load on the renal tubules from sodium bicarbonate produced by the stomach results in increased excretion of sodium to neutralize the HCO_3^- load.)

Other laboratory tests that may be helpful in further determination of hyponatremia are serum uric acid concentration (increased in volume depletion, decreased in volume expansion and euvolemia) and blood urea nitrogen (increased in volume depletion, normal in volume expansion). It now appears that cerebral salt wasting syndrome is more likely in many central nervous system disorders,[8,17,30,43] although some continue to disagree with this concept.[38] The possible causes of hyponatremia in neurologic disease are listed in Table 31–5. The following sections discuss hyponatremia associated with specific clinical neurologic disorders.

Hyponatremia in Aneurysmal Subarachnoid Hemorrhage

Hyponatremia is the most common electrolyte disturbance after aneurysmal SAH. The precise physiologic changes in hyponatremia associated with SAH have yet to be elucidated. Early studies noted that only 10% of patients with SAH had hyponatremia, but later studies showed sodium values below 134 mmol/L in 34% of patients with SAH.[18] Severe hyponatremia (plasma sodium level < 125 mmol/L) is rarely seen in SAH; as a consequence, neurologic deterioration can seldom be attributed to hyponatremia alone. Hyponatremia can usually be expected within the first week after the ini-

Table 31–5. Potential Causes of Hypo-osmolar Hyponatremia in the Neurologic Intensive Care Unit

Hypovolemia	*Normovolemia or Hypervolemia*
Diuretics (thiazide, loop)	SIADH
Addison's disease (acute corticosteroid withdrawal)	Acute renal failure
Gastrointestinal and skin losses	Congestive heart failure
Dietary sodium restriction with excess hypotonic fluid intake	Hepatic failure
Cerebral salt wasting	

SIADH, syndrome of inappropriate antidiuretic hormone.

tial hemorrhage and closely parallels the period of cerebral vasospasm.[67]

For many years, neurosurgeons viewed the development of hyponatremia as a marker for impending cerebral ischemia in SAH, but the relationship had never been systematically studied. In a post hoc analysis of a prospectively acquired series of patients with SAH, cerebral infarction occurred significantly more often in patients with hyponatremia (61%) than in patients with normal serum sodium values (21%).[67]

Initially, hyponatremia in patients with SAH was attributed to SIADH, and it was believed that excessive water retention led to dilutional hyponatremia.[13] Nelson et al.[37] should be credited for initially challenging the concept of SIADH in intracranial disease. Both human and animal studies suggested hypovolemic hyponatremia caused by excessive natriuresis and diuresis rather than hypervolemic or euvolemic hyponatremia from water retention. These studies first suggested that cerebral salt wasting more accurately explained hyponatremia after SAH than SIADH. Later, a prospective study of 21 patients with aneurysmal SAH demonstrated that plasma volume was decreased in most patients with hyponatremia. Hyponatremia was preceded by a negative sodium balance in all instances. Blood ADH levels were increased or normal on admission but had decreased by the time hyponatremia occurred. The ADH levels remained slightly higher than those in controls, but this increase could have been a response to hypovolemia.[68]

Later data in patients with SAH, however, suggested that ADH remains increased despite the prevention of volume contraction.[12] In a prospective study of 19 patients who received hypervolemic therapy, volume contraction was prevented but ADH levels were detectable during a hypo-osmolar state. Whether critically ill patients with recent aneurysmal rupture have an additional disturbance in vasopressin regulation remains to be defined. As alluded to earlier, nonosmolar stimuli to ADH may cause an increase in ADH and may be difficult to ferret out in clinical studies.

Certain computed tomography scan characteristics may predict the development of hyponatremia. The risk of hyponatremia developing after aneurysmal rupture is significantly increased in patients with enlargement of the third ventricle, with or without dilatation of the lateral ventricles, on initial computed tomography scanning.[66] The relationship between enlargement of the third ventricle and hyponatremia suggests that pressure on the hypothalamus produces hyponatremia by release of natriuretic peptides located in the anteroventral region of the third ventricle.

Much of the recent research has concentrated on the role of natriuretic factors. These are digoxin-like immunoreactive substance (endogenous ouabain), natriuretic peptides, and adrenomedullin. In a preliminary study of a digoxin-like substance, enlargement of the third ventricle and the lateral ventricles and, particularly, location of the center of the hemorrhage in the frontal interhemispheric fissure in association with rupture of the anterior communicating artery, increased the detection of this natriuretic substance, but no clear relationship to hyponatremia was detected.[69] Although the source and nature of digitalis-like circulating factors (endogenous ouabain) are largely unknown, these substances inhibit Na^+, K^+-ATPase and cause natriuresis. These factors are very limited in effect, but they may also have a role in maintaining increased blood pressure.[16] In an as yet unconfirmed study, it was found that after the plasma was heated and the sensitivity of a digoxin radioimmunoassay was increased, an endogenous substance that cross-reacted with antibodies to digoxin was identified in 18 of 25 consecutive patients with SAH.[69] Detection of this substance increased in the days after the hemorrhage and was found more often in patients with natriuresis and volume depletion. Its role in SAH remains unclear, and interest has waned.[17,73]

The putative role of another, better characterized natriuretic substance, atrial natriuretic peptide (ANP), in clinical deterioration after SAH has been extensively studied.[11,22,60,63] Several studies, using single daily measurements of ANP, found marked elevation of plasma ANP levels but no association with the development of hyponatremia or the net sodium balance. A study with diurnal measurements of ANP and vasopressin found a second surge of ANP followed by natriuresis and net sodium loss. In addition, ANP peaks were accompanied by a reciprocal decrease in ADH levels, allowing diuresis. All patients with cerebral infarction after SAH had a brief natriuresis associated with an ANP peak in the previous day.[63]

The possible role of other members of the natriuretic peptide family was recently studied in SAH.[22,56,57,62,65] The natriuretic peptide family now consists of ANP, brain natriuretic peptide (BNP), C-type natriuretic peptide (CNP), and dendroaspis natriuretic peptide (DNP). BNP is also markedly increased in SAH, but both BNP and ANP increase after SAH and seem to be regulated differently. The natriuretic properties of CNP are few, if any, and it may be more involved with vasodilatation. It usually is released by endothelial cells. In a preliminary study, a possible vasoregulatory role for CNP was suggested because it was more often increased in patients in whom cerebral vasospasm developed. DNP (discovered in the venom of the green mamba snake) is increased in plasma of patients with congestive heart failure and found in human atrial myocardium. Injected into rat ventricles, it increased renal water excretion.[27] It has not yet been fully characterized to prove its genuine endogenous origin,[47] nor has it been systematically studied in aneurysmal SAH,[28,29,53] but in our pilot study, we found a relative increase, particularly in patients with hyponatremia.[24] A loop similar to that of a comparable amino acid sequence is shared (Fig. 31–2). C-type natriuretic peptide has very little natriuretic activity, and DNP is markedly diuretic; thus, the major differences appear in the tail. The relationship of the natriuretic peptide system with renin-angiotensin and ADH has been carefully delineated. Atrial natriuretic peptide not only causes natriuresis but also reduces ADH and inhibits renin aldosterone release.[23,71] How these natriuretic factors—particularly ANP and BNP, secreted respectively from atrium and ventricle—increase is not known.[71] The time course

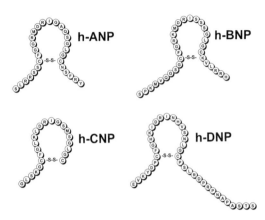

Figure 31–2. Natriuretic peptide system amino acid sequences of human atrial natriuretic peptide (h-ANP), human brain natriuretic peptide (h-BNP), human C-type natriuretic peptide (h-CNP), and human dendroaspis natriuretic peptide (h-DNP). One-letter amino acid code: A, alanine; C, cysteine; D, aspartic acid; F, phenylalanine; G, glycine; H, histidine; I, isoleucine; K, lysine; L, leucine; M, methionine; N, asparagine; P, proline; Q, glutamine; R, arginine; S, serine; T, threonine; V, valine; Y, tyrosine. Note 17-amino acid disulfide ring structure in all types. DNP has the longest C-terminus amino acid "tail."

of these abnormalities in SAH is depicted in Figure 31–3.

Recently, adrenomedullin, an endogenous peptide with both vasodilatory and natriuretic properties, was discovered. Adrenomedullin is structurally related to calcitonin, and thus its main biologic action is vasodilatation. When administered, it decreases peripheral vascular resistance, reduces blood pressure, and vasodilates cerebral arteries. Its biologic actions are shown in Figure 31–4. Its effects seem uncoupled from the natriuretic system effects but significantly correlated with vasospasm, so that it may have a role in countering vasoconstriction and inhibiting vasoconstrictor hormone production.[34,62]

The relevance of these studies into the pathophysiology of cerebral vasospasm remains to be determined. One possible explanation for

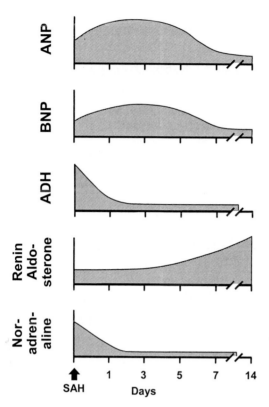

Figure 31–3. Time course of plasma levels of natriuretic peptides, antidiuretic hormone (ADH), and renin-aldosterone after subarachnoid hemorrhage (SAH). ANP, atrial natriuretic peptide; BNP, brain natriuretic peptide.

development into symptomatic vasospasm could be the additional reduction of cerebral perfusion from a simultaneous hypovolemic state due to natriuresis. Current management reflects that concept.

Hyponatremia in Head Injury
Severe traumatic brain injury has also been linked to SIADH, but both its prevalence and its mechanism have been poorly studied. The preliminary impression is that, as in SAH, blood volume is decreased with appropriately increased ADH levels.[42,45] Reports of patients with hyponatremia and natriuresis resistant to fluid restriction have appeared. Hyponatremia could only be corrected after expansion with isotonic saline or an increase in the daily so-

dium load. These patients may also be susceptible to cerebral vasospasm, which may be more common in those with traumatic subarachnoid bleeding. Hyperosmolarity and possible hypernatremia after severe head injury, however, are far more common in clinical practice. Many physicians deliberately induce a hyperosmolar state by administering mannitol to treat increased intracranial pressure.

Hyponatremia in Meningitis
Studies, mainly in children, have found that SIADH is present in bacterial, tuberculous, and aseptic meningitis.[9,14] One study[14] found that 88% of 50 children with *Haemophilus influenzae* meningitis had evidence of increased secretion of ADH. In another large study, 32% of 300 pediatric patients with bacterial meningitis had plasma sodium values between 122 and 133 mmol/L.[59]

Although some reports in children suggest a role for initial water restriction after meningitis, experience in adults is very limited. One study found that ADH in urine was increased during the course of aseptic and bacterial meningitis, but hyponatremia did not develop.[40] This study emphasized that patients with meningitis may be at risk for SIADH. Another study, however, also suggested a possible role for ANP,[36] challenging the concept of SIADH. Plasma levels of ADH have been increased, most likely appropriately so because of dehydration and hypovolemia. Prophylactic restriction of fluid in patients with developing cerebral edema remains controversial, is possibly detrimental, and should not be initiated.[32]

Hyponatremia in Guillain-Barré Syndrome
Hyponatremia occurs in up to 30% of patients with GBS, but severe, symptomatic hyponatremia is rare.[46,49] The risk of hyponatremia developing is much greater in mechanically ventilated patients.

In a prospective series, symptomatic mild hyponatremia appeared at an average of 10 days after intubation (range, 1 to 23 days).[49] Hyponatremia occurred in 42% of ventilated patients and in 19% of nonventilated patients with GBS and responded well to fluid restriction. Hy-

Human Adrenomedullin (ADM)

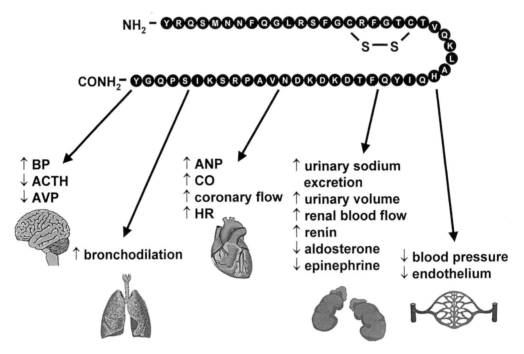

Figure 31–4. Physiologic actions of adrenomedullin. ACTH, adrenocorticotropic hormone; ANP, atrial natriuretic peptide; AVP, arginine vasopressin or ADH; BP, blood pressure; CO, cardiac output; HR, heart rate. (From Wijdicks et al.[62] By permission of the American Association of Neurological Surgeons.)

ponatremia in mechanically ventilated patients with GBS probably results from SIADH. In a study of 12 consecutive patients with GBS, plasma ADH levels were higher (mean, 28 ± 15 pg/mL) than in nonventilated patients (mean, 13 ± 12 pg/mL) and controls (mean, 9 ± 7 pg/mL), although hyponatremia did not occur in any patient. Atrial natriuretic peptide levels were increased only in patients with extreme blood pressure changes from dysautonomia, possibly simply as a reflection of atrial stretch from increased blood volume.[64]

In ventilated patients, secretion of ADH is stimulated by impaired venous return, particularly when positive end-expiratory pressure is applied. Syndrome of inappropriate antidiuretic hormone may also result from abnormalities in afferent nerves of volume receptors, but patients with SIADH and GBS do not invariably have marked dysautonomia. Osmotic resetting due to afferent defect has been suggested but this mechanism has not been carefully studied.[41]

Hyponatremia after Pituitary Surgery

After transsphenoidal surgery, almost 50% of patients have a disorder of water homeostasis within the first 2 postoperative weeks. Several patterns may occur (Fig. 31–5), but early postoperative polyuria is most common. This phenomenon can be attributed to unloading of large amounts of perioperative fluid or to depletion of ADH induced by surgical trauma. More interesting are the biphasic or triphasic patterns of polyuria and hyponatremia[19,39] (Fig. 31–5). Hyponatremia can be severe, with values less than 125 mmol/L. A higher risk of hyponatremia seems more likely in patients operated on for microadenomas. The tentative explanation is possible involvement of the stalk or upward displacement of the posterior lobe outside the

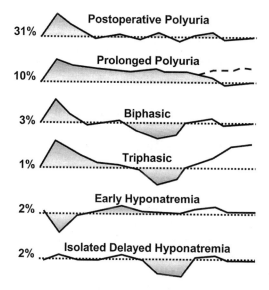

Figure 31–5. Patterns and frequency (%) of postoperative polyuria (> 2500 mL). Hypernatremia, upward movement, and hyponatremia, downward movement, after transsphenoidal surgery in 1571 patients. (From Hensen et al.[19] By permission of Blackwell Science.)

surgical field. Hyponatremia can possibly be linked to cortisol deficiency, a stimulus from one of the natriuretic peptides, unregulated vasopressin secretion from the damaged posterior pituitary body, or prolonged treatment with desmopressin (delayed hyponatremia). Continuous monitoring of plasma sodium is imperative, together with reduction of free water intake.

Miscellaneous Neurologic Disorders Associated with Hyponatremia

Syndrome of inappropriate antidiuretic hormone or any other cause of hyponatremia has been reported after chronic subdural hematoma, stroke, carotid endarterectomy,[31] obstructive hydrocephalus, and fulminant multiple sclerosis.[21] In patients infected with human immunodeficiency virus who have recent encephalitis, hyponatremia could point to cytomegalovirus-induced adrenalitis (see Chapter 21).

Treatment of Hyponatremia

The treatment of hyponatremia is focused on correction of the volume derangement alone;

the absolute serum sodium value has much less clinical relevance. The management of asymptomatic hyponatremia, irrespective of severity, should be conservative. If hyponatremia is associated with contraction of intravascular volume (and secondary release of ADH), treatment should consist of volume replacement with isotonic saline. Once the intravascular volume is normalized, the stimulus to ADH release is eliminated and the patient excretes excess water to correct hyponatremia. If the cause is SIADH, restriction of free water alone slowly corrects hyponatremia. Syndrome of inappropriate antidiuretic hormone is self-limited in neurologic patients; therefore, a brief period of free water restriction may be definitive therapy. In resistant cases, lithium carbonate is an option because it inhibits the renal response to ADH. (The recommended initial dose is 900 to 1200 mg daily.) Demeclocycline hydrochloride also inhibits the renal response to ADH.[10,15] (The recommended initial dose is 1200 mg per day, which should be reduced to the lowest effective dose.) Both agents are very rarely used in neurologic patients with acute hyponatremia and are more often administered in patients with long-standing hyponatremia.

The management of symptomatic hyponatremia is more controversial, and an osmotic demyelination syndrome or central pontine myelinolysis demyelination[1,7,55,58] can occur if hyponatremia is corrected by more than 12 mmol/L in 24 hours or to values greater than the upper limit of normal.[6,35]

Most cases of acute severe symptomatic hyponatremia that require correction result from excessive water; therefore, facilitating the excretion of water is the appropriate therapy.[54] This is best achieved with furosemide-induced diuresis (20 mg) and a hypertonic saline (3%) solution.[4] The diuretic produces renal loss of free water (hypotonic diuresis), and the excreted sodium is returned in a smaller volume with a hypertonic solution.

Conventional formulas calculate the sodium requirement by multiplying total body water by the difference between the desired serum sodium concentration and the current sodium concentration. An elegant approach introduced by Adrogué and Madias[3] uses a formula that proj-

Table 31–6. Treatment of Symptomatic Hyponatremia

Volume Contraction	Volume Dilution
0.9% NaCl (or 1.5%) 3% NaCl Fludrocortisone acetate, 0.4 mg/day	Calculate need to normalize serum sodium by using 3% NaCl (513 mmol/L) in the formula $$\frac{513 - \text{current plasma Na}}{0.5 \times \text{body weight} + 1}$$ to provide total millimoles per liter Rate: raise serum sodium 1 mmol/L per hour

Data from Adrogué HJ, Madias NE: Hyponatremia. *N Engl J Med* 342:1581–1589, 2000. By permission of the Massachusetts Medical Society.

ects the change in serum sodium after infusion and retention of 1 L of a previously chosen infusate, mostly 3% sodium chloride (Table 31–6).

Treatment of hyponatremia in SAH is complex. Again, volume status is more important than hyponatremia per se. Ideally, the volume status should be evaluated by immediate placement of a Swan-Ganz catheter. Volume resuscitation is needed when pulmonary artery wedge pressure is below 10 mm Hg. Volume resuscitation is achieved with normal saline or 5% albumin alone. Oral administration of salt may further increase sodium intake to balance natriuresis. If the fluid balance remains negative or less than 500 mL a day, fludrocortisone, 0.4 mg a day orally, is very effective.[33,70,72] Recommendations are given in Table 31–6. The effect of fludrocortisone is apparent within hours and may last 24 to 48 hours. Often, administration for more than 5 days is without merit because of a "mineralocorticoid escape" phenomenon. (Sodium retention is overcome by renal mechanisms, including increase in plasma ANP and decrease in renin and sympathetic nerve activity, and no further positive sodium balance is observed.) Fludrocortisone remains an important adjunct in the management of resistant hyponatremia and negative fluid balance.

Hypernatremia

Hypernatremia is defined as sodium values exceeding 145 mEq/L. The conditions associated with increased serum sodium concentration are listed in Table 31–7.

Hypernatremia is commonly associated with acute neurologic events, often from dehydration in patients unable to obtain water. The clinical manifestations of acute hypernatremia appear only when serum osmolalities approach 400 mOsm/kg of water and may lead to a decrease in level of consciousness and generalized tonic-clonic seizures. Hypernatremia in the NICU is due commonly to pure water loss and less commonly to an artificially administered large dose of sodium (e.g., hypertonic saline enemas or feeding preparations) causing a gain in hypertonic sodium.[2]

Evaluation of Hypernatremia

Hypernatremia is similarly categorized by the volume of extracellular fluid. Loss of proportionally more water than salt causes hypernatremia in most patients if water is not replenished. Examples of acute severe hypernatremia are correction of lactic acidosis by intravenously administered sodium bicarbonate and massive doses of hypertonic saline to achieve hypervolemic therapy. The combination of hypernatremia, hypovolemia, and hypotonic urine indicates that the patient is not conserving water. In the NICU, the cause of hypernatremia is often defective central release of ADH or induced osmotic diuresis.

Table 31–7. Causes of Hypernatremia in the Neurologic Intensive Care Unit

Hypovolemia	Normovolemia or Hypervolemia
Gastrointestinal loss	Hypertonic sodium solutions
Diuretics (e.g., mannitol)	Corticosteroid excess
Diabetes insipidus	

Table 31–8. Treatment of Symptomatic Hypernatremia

Pure Water Loss or Hypotonic Hypernatremia	*Hypertonic Hypernatremia*
Calculate need to normalize serum sodium by using 5% dextrose in the formula	Furosemide, 40–80 mg IV Switch to electrolyte-free water infusion (5% dextrose)

$$\frac{(0 - \text{current plasma Na})}{0.5 \times \text{body weight} + 1}$$

or

0.45% NaCl in the formula

$$\frac{(77 - \text{current plasma Na})}{0.5 \times \text{body weight} + 1}$$

to provide total millimoles per liter
Rate: reduce serum sodium 10 mmol/L
in 24 hours
Desmopressin, 0.5–2 g IV every 3 hours

Data from Adrogué HJ, Madias NE: Hypernatremia. *N Engl J Med* 342:1493–1499, 2000. By permission of the Massachusetts Medical Society.

Osmotic diuresis is initiated by drugs such as mannitol and glycerol, or it may be due to hyperglycemia when the renal threshold for conserving glucose is exceeded. (Nephrogenic diabetes insipidus is very uncommon but can be acquired through drug toxicity [lithium, demeclocycline, amphotericin B, gentamicin, glyburide, or furosemide]. It can be differentiated from neurogenic diabetes insipidus by lack of response to administration of ADH.)[2,5]

Patients with head injury, massive cerebral edema, or rapid central diencephalic herniation injuring the stalk and certainly patients with the clinical criteria for brain death are at considerable risk for the development of diabetes insipidus.[51] Therefore, fluid balance, urine specific gravity, and serum sodium concentration must be carefully monitored. Obviously, increased urine output has multiple potential causes. In head injury, for example, diuresis may be an appropriate response to fluid administered during resuscitation from trauma, or the output may be a result of osmotic diuresis from administration of mannitol.

Diabetes insipidus is characterized by hypotonic urine (osmolality < 300 mOsm/kg or specific gravity < 1010) and polyuria (> 30 mL/kg per day).[5,48] Clinically significant polyuria does not develop until approximately 75% of the ADH-secreting neurons are destroyed; in most patients, therefore, the impairment of ADH release is incomplete. The disruption of ADH secretion is transient in 50% to 60% of patients with severe head injury. Normal osmoregulation returns in 3 to 5 days.

Treatment of Hypernatremia

Hypernatremic dehydration is best corrected by judicious use of intravenous fluids. In very rare clinical situations of overt shock, colloids are administered. The water deficit can be calculated as shown below. (See also the Appendix.)

The rate of correction is not exactly known, but water deficits are best corrected within 48 hours. If the clinical situation allows, half the water deficit is restored within 24 hours and the rest over 48 hours. Preferably a formula similar to that in hyponatremia can be used,[2] however, typically using hypotonic fluids. Recommendations are given in Table 31–8.

$$\text{water deficit in liters} = 0.6 \times \text{body weight (kg)} \times \left(\frac{\text{serum NA}}{140} - 1\right)$$

In general, patients unable to sense thirst require careful monitoring of fluid balance, urine specific gravity, body weight, and serum sodium concentration. If urine volume is not excessive, replacement of urine output and insensible losses with intravenous fluids may be sufficient. Treatment of acute diabetes insipidus requires meticulous management. Intravenous fluids or aqueous vasopressin may be used if the polyuria and polydipsia are difficult to manage. Hormonal replacement with vasopressin in acute diabetes insipidus should be considered if urine output is more than 300 mL/hour for 2 consecutive hours. Therapy should begin with desmopressin, 0.5 to 2 μg every 3 hours intravenously (see Chapter 34).

CONCLUSIONS

- Most patients with metabolic acidosis in the NICU have transient lactic acidosis after seizures. Correction of metabolic acidosis with bicarbonate is seldom needed. A major systemic illness should be considered in other circumstances.
- Hyponatremia must be viewed against volume status. Cerebral salt wasting (hypovolemic hyponatremia) is more common in certain central nervous system disorders than SIADH (normovolemic hyponatremia). The laboratory criteria are identical. Differentiation from SIADH is possible with serial body weight (decrease), fluid balance (negative), and pulmonary artery wedge pressures (low) and with clinical signs of early dehydration, relative tachycardia, orthostasis, and marginal skin turgor.
- Hypernatremia from dehydration is most common with diabetes insipidus from head injury, at the time of diagnosis of brain death, or with use of osmotic diuretic agents.

REFERENCES

1. Adams RD, Victor M, Mancall EL: Central pontine myelinolysis: a hitherto undescribed disease occurring in alcoholic and malnourished patients. *Arch Neurol Psychiatry* 81:154–172, 1959.
2. Adrogué HJ, Madias NE: Hypernatremia. *N Engl J Med* 342:1493–1499, 2000.
3. Adrogué HJ, Madias NE: Hyponatremia. *N Engl J Med* 342:1581–1589, 2000.
4. Ayus JC, Olivero JJ, Frommer JP: Rapid correction of severe hyponatremia with intravenous hypertonic saline solution. *Am J Med* 72:43–48, 1982.
5. Blevins LS Jr, Wand GS: Diabetes insipidus. *Crit Care Med* 20:69–79, 1992.
6. Brunner JE, Redmond JM, Haggar AM, et al: Central pontine myelinolysis and pontine lesions after rapid correction of hyponatremia: a prospective magnetic resonance imaging study. *Ann Neurol* 27:61–66, 1990.
7. Calakos N, Fischbein N, Baringer JR, et al: Cortical MRI findings associated with rapid correction of hyponatremia. *Neurology* 55:1048–1051, 2000.
8. Cort JH: Cerebral salt wasting. *Lancet* 1:752–754, 1954.
9. Cotton MF, Donald PR, Schoeman JF, et al: Plasma arginine vasopressin and the syndrome of inappropriate antidiuretic hormone secretion in tuberculous meningitis. *Pediatr Infect Dis J* 10:837–842, 1991.
10. De Troyer A: Demeclocycline. Treatment for syndrome of inappropriate antidiuretic hormone secretion. *JAMA* 237:2723–2726, 1977.
11. Diringer M, Ladenson PW, Stern BJ, et al: Plasma atrial natriuretic factor and subarachnoid hemorrhage. *Stroke* 19:1119–1124, 1988.
12. Diringer MN, Wu KC, Verbalis JG, et al: Hypervolemic therapy prevents volume contraction but not hyponatremia following subarachnoid hemorrhage. *Ann Neurol* 31:543–550, 1992.
13. Doczi T, Bende J, Huszka E, et al: Syndrome of inappropriate secretion of antidiuretic hormone after subarachnoid hemorrhage. *Neurosurgery* 9:394–397, 1981.
14. Feigin RD, Stechenberg BW, Chang MJ, et al: Prospective evaluation of treatment of *Haemophilus influenzae* meningitis. *J Pediatr* 88:542–548, 1976.
15. Forrest JN Jr, Cox M, Hong C, et al: Superiority of demeclocycline over lithium in the treatment of chronic syndrome of inappropriate secretion of antidiuretic hormone. *N Engl J Med* 298:173–177, 1978.
16. Hamlyn JM, Hamilton BP, Manunta P: Endogenous ouabain, sodium balance and blood pressure: a review and a hypothesis. *J Hypertens* 14:151–167, 1996.
17. Harrigan MR: Cerebral salt wasting syndrome: a review. *Neurosurgery* 38:152–160, 1996.
18. Hasan D, Lindsay KW, Wijdicks EFM, et al: Effect of fludrocortisone acetate in patients with subarachnoid hemorrhage. *Stroke* 20:1156–1161, 1989.
19. Hensen J, Henig A, Fahlbusch R, et al: Prevalence,

predictors and patterns of postoperative polyuria and hyponatraemia in the immediate course after trans-sphenoidal surgery for pituitary adenomas. *Clin Endocrinol (Oxf)* 50:431–439, 1999.

20. Hillier TA, Abbott RD, Barrett EJ: Hyponatremia: evaluating the correction factor for hyperglycemia. *Am J Med* 106:399–403, 1999.

21. Ishikawa E, Ohgo S, Nakatsuru K, et al: Syndrome of inappropriate secretion of antidiuretic hormone (SIADH) in a patient with multiple sclerosis. *Jpn J Med* 28:75–79, 1989.

22. Isotani E, Suzuki R, Tomita K, et al: Alterations in plasma concentrations of natriuretic peptides and antidiuretic hormone after subarachnoid hemorrhage. *Stroke* 25:2198–2203, 1994.

23. Johnston CI, Phillips PA, Arnolda L, et al: Modulation of the renin-angiotensin system by atrial natriuretic peptide. *J Cardiovasc Pharmacol* 16 Suppl 7:S43–S46, 1990.

24. Khurana GV, Wijdicks EFM, Heublein DM, et al: Dendroaspis natriuretic peptide (DNP) in aneurysmal subarachnoid hemorrhage. Preliminary observations. (Submitted for publication.)

25. Lahr MB: Hyponatremia during carbamazepine therapy. *Clin Pharmacol Ther* 37:693–696, 1985.

26. Lawn N, Wijdicks EFM, Burritt MF: Intravenous immune globulin and pseudohyponatremia (letter to the editor). *N Engl J Med* 339:632, 1998.

27. Lee J, Kim SW: Dendroaspis natriuretic peptide administered intracerebroventricularly increases renal water excretion. *Clin Exp Pharmacol Physiol* 29:195–197, 2002.

28. Lisy O, Jougasaki M, Heublein DM, et al: Renal actions of synthetic dendroaspis natriuretic peptide. *Kidney Int* 56:502–508, 1999.

29. Lisy O, Lainchbury JG, Leskinen H, et al: Therapeutic actions of a new synthetic vasoactive and natriuretic peptide, dendroaspis natriuretic peptide, in experimental severe congestive heart failure. *Hypertension* 37:1089–1094, 2001.

30. Maesaka JK, Gupta S, Fishbane S: Cerebral salt-wasting syndrome: Does it exist? *Nephron* 82:100–109, 1999.

31. Magovern JA, Sieber PR, Thiele BL: The syndrome of inappropriate secretion of antidiuretic hormone following carotid endarterectomy. A case report and review of the literature. *J Cardiovasc Surg (Torino)* 30: 544–546, 1989.

32. Møller K, Larsen FS, Bie P, et al: The syndrome of inappropriate secretion of antidiuretic hormone and fluid restriction in meningitis—how strong is the evidence? *Scand J Infect Dis* 33:13–26, 2001.

33. Mori T, Katayama Y, Kawamata T, et al: Improved efficiency of hypervolemic therapy with inhibition of natriuresis by fludrocortisone in patients with aneurysmal subarachnoid hemorrhage. *J Neurosurg* 91:947–952, 1999.

34. Nagaya N, Nishikimi T, Horio T, et al: Cardiovascular and renal effects of adrenomedullin in rats with heart failure. *Am J Physiol* 276:R213–R218, 1999.

35. Narins RG: Therapy of hyponatremia: Does haste make waste? (Editorial.) *N Engl J Med* 314:1573–1575, 1986.

36. Narotam PK, Kemp M, Buck R, et al: Hyponatremic natriuretic syndrome in tuberculous meningitis: the probable role of atrial natriuretic peptide. *Neurosurgery* 34:982–988, 1994.

37. Nelson PB, Seif SM, Maroon JC, et al: Hyponatremia in intracranial disease: perhaps not the syndrome of inappropriate secretion of antidiuretic hormone (SIADH). *J Neurosurg* 55:938–941, 1981.

38. Oh MS, Carroll HJ: Cerebral salt-wasting syndrome. We need better proof of its existence. *Nephron* 82:110–114, 1999.

39. Olson BR, Gumowski J, Rubino D, et al: Pathophysiology of hyponatremia after transsphenoidal pituitary surgery. *J Neurosurg* 87:499–507, 1997.

40. Padilla G, Ervin MG, Ross MG, et al: Vasopressin levels in infants during the course of aseptic and bacterial meningitis. *Am J Dis Child* 145:991–993, 1991.

41. Penney MD, Murphy D, Walters G: Resetting of osmoreceptor response as cause of hyponatraemia in acute idiopathic polyneuritis. *Br Med J* 2:1474–1476, 1979.

42. Penney MD, Walters G, Wilkins DG: Hyponatraemia in patients with head injury. *Intensive Care Med* 5:23–26, 1979.

43. Peters JP, Welt LG, Sims EAH, et al: A salt-wasting syndrome associated with cerebral disease. *Assoc Am Physicians Trans* 63:57–63, 1950.

44. Polderman KH, Bloemers FW, Peerdeman SM, et al: Hypomagnesemia and hypophosphatemia at admission in patients with severe head injury. *Crit Care Med* 28:2022–2025, 2000.

45. Poon WS, Mendelow AD, Davies DL, et al: Secretion of antidiuretic hormone in neurosurgical patients: appropriate or inappropriate? *Aust N Z J Surg* 59:173–180, 1989.

46. Posner JB, Ertel NH, Kossmann RJ, et al: Hyponatremia in acute polyneuropathy. Four cases with the syndrome of inappropriate secretion of antidiuretic hormone. *Arch Neurol* 17:530–541, 1967.

47. Richards AM, Lainchbury JG, Nicholls MG, et al: Dendroaspis natriuretic peptide: Endogenous or dubious? *Lancet* 359:5–6, 2002.

48. Robertson GL: Differential diagnosis of polyuria. *Annu Rev Med* 39:425–442, 1988.

49. Ropper AH, Wijdicks EFM, Truax BT (eds): *Guillain-Barré Syndrome*. Philadelphia: FA Davis Company, 1991.

50. Sachdeo RC, Wasserstein A, Mesenbrink PJ, et al: Effects of oxcarbazepine on sodium concentration and water handling. *Ann Neurol* 51:613–620, 2002.

51. Sazontseva IE, Kozlov IA, Moisuc YG, et al: Hormonal response to brain death. *Transplant Proc* 23:2467, 1991.

52. Schwartz WB, Bennett W, Curelop S, et al: A syndrome of renal sodium loss and hyponatremia probably resulting from inappropriate secretion of antidiuretic hormone. *Am J Med* 23:529–542, 1957.

53. Schweitz H, Vigne P, Moinier D, et al: A new member of the natriuretic peptide family is present in the venom of the green mamba (*Dendroaspis angusticeps*). *J Biol Chem* 267:13928–13932, 1992.

54. Sterns RH: The management of hyponatremic emergencies. *Crit Care Clin* 7:127–142, 1991.

55. Sterns RH, Riggs JE, Schochet SS Jr: Osmotic demyelination syndrome following correction of hyponatremia. *N Engl J Med* 314:1535–1542, 1986.

56. Sviri GE, Feinsod M, Soustiel JF: Brain natriuretic peptide and cerebral vasospasm in subarachnoid hemorrhage. Clinical and TCD correlations. *Stroke* 31:118–122, 2000.

57. Tomida M, Muraki M, Uemura K, et al: Plasma concentrations of brain natriuretic peptide in patients with subarachnoid hemorrhage. *Stroke* 29:1584–1587, 1998.

58. Tormey WP: Central pontine myelinolysis and changes in serum sodium (letter to the editor). *Lancet* 335:1169, 1990.

59. von Vigier RO, Colombo SM, Stoffel PB, et al: Circulating sodium in acute meningitis. *Am J Nephrol* 21:87–90, 2001.

60. Weinand ME, O'Boynick PL, Goetz KL: A study of serum antidiuretic hormone and atrial natriuretic peptide levels in a series of patients with intracranial disease and hyponatremia. *Neurosurgery* 25:781–785, 1989.

61. Wijdicks EFM: *Neurologic Complications of Critical Illness*. 2nd ed. Oxford: Oxford University Press, 2002.

62. Wijdicks EFM, Heublein DM, Burnett JC Jr: Increase and uncoupling of adrenomedullin from the natriuretic peptide system in aneurysmal subarachnoid hemorrhage. *J Neurosurg* 94:252–256, 2001.

63. Wijdicks EFM, Ropper AH, Hunnicutt EJ, et al: Atrial natriuretic factor and salt wasting after aneurysmal subarachnoid hemorrhage. *Stroke* 22:1519–1524, 1991.

64. Wijdicks EFM, Ropper AH, Nathanson JA: Atrial natriuretic factor and blood pressure fluctuations in Guillain-Barré syndrome (letter to the editor). *Ann Neurol* 27:337–338, 1990.

65. Wijdicks EFM, Schievink WI, Burnett JC Jr: Natriuretic peptide system and endothelin in aneurysmal subarachnoid hemorrhage. *J Neurosurg* 87:275–280, 1997.

66. Wijdicks EFM, VanDongen KJ, VanGijn J, et al: Enlargement of the third ventricle and hyponatraemia in aneurysmal subarachnoid haemorrhage. *J Neurol Neurosurg Psychiatry* 51:516–520, 1988.

67. Wijdicks EFM, Vermeulen M, Hijdra A, et al: Hyponatremia and cerebral infarction in patients with ruptured intracranial aneurysms: Is fluid restriction harmful? *Ann Neurol* 17:137–140, 1985.

68. Wijdicks EFM, Vermeulen M, ten Haaf JA, et al: Volume depletion and natriuresis in patients with a ruptured intracranial aneurysm. *Ann Neurol* 18:211–216, 1985.

69. Wijdicks EFM, Vermeulen M, van Brummelen P, et al: Digoxin-like immunoreactive substance in patients with aneurysmal subarachnoid haemorrhage. *Br Med J (Clin Res)* 294:729–732, 1987.

70. Wijdicks EFM, Vermeulen M, van Brummelen P, et al: The effect of fludrocortisone acetate on plasma volume and natriuresis in patients with aneurysmal subarachnoid hemorrhage. *Clin Neurol Neurosurg* 90:209–214, 1988.

71. Williams TD, Walsh KP, Lightman SL, et al: Atrial natriuretic peptide inhibits postural release of renin and vasopressin in humans. *Am J Physiol* 255:R368–R372, 1988.

72. Woo MH, Kale-Pradhan PB: Fludrocortisone in the treatment of subarachnoid hemorrhage-induced hyponatremia. *Ann Pharmacother* 31:637–639, 1997.

73. Yamada K, Goto N, Nagoshi H, et al: Role of brain ouabainlike compound in central nervous system-mediated natriuresis in rats. *Hypertension* 23:1027–1031, 1994.

32

Gastrointestinal Complications

Gastrointestinal discomfort is not often voiced by patients with acute brain injury. Impaired level of consciousness often precludes an adequate history of abdominal pain, and, in trauma, there may be distracting injuries.[17] Often, only significant laboratory changes, such as a decrease in hematocrit, point to a gastrointestinal complication.

The gastrointestinal disorders in the NICU are not unique but of a different nature. For example, conditions associated with sepsis (acute pancreatitis, acalculous cholecystitis) are observed often in medical or surgical intensive care units and are less prevalent in the NICU. The single most important complication is gastrointestinal bleeding. Although there may be a tendency to underreport gastrointestinal complications, the true incidence after any acute neurologic illness is, in reality, low. In addition, disorders of bowel motility may occur, of which diarrhea is most common in hospitalized patients. Diarrhea associated with enteral nutrition is virtually ubiquitous.

This chapter summarizes the important principles of recognition and management of acute conditions in the gastrointestinal tract complicating acute neurologic illness. Bowel care in spinal cord injury, which is complicated because of neurogenic bowel disorder, receives attention here.

GASTROINTESTINAL BLEEDING

Acute central nervous system disorders may induce lesions in the lining of the gastrointestinal tract, which generally appear at multiple sites. They may be confined to the mucosa (erosions) or extend into the submucosa or beyond (ulcers).[34] Ulcers may be the result of sympathetic overactivity, but the vulnerability of the mucosa may also be increased by substances such as acetylcholine, histamine, and endogenous thyrotropin-releasing hormone.[5,24] Disruption of the mucus gel overlying the gastric epithelium may also be a consequence of bile reflux, uremia, alcohol, aspirin, and nonsteroidal anti-inflammatory drugs.

Gastrointestinal hemorrhages from stress-associated erosions are minor and seldom lead to massive, life-threatening situations or require frequent blood transfusions.[40] In addition, complications of a rapid decline in hematocrit (e.g., acute myocardial infarction) are rare. Nonetheless, a measurable risk remains in patients in the NICU, and this risk is greater in anticoagulated patients, patients with previous use of nonsteroidal anti-inflammatory drugs, and patients with underlying coagulopathies. For patients with red blood in gastric aspirate or red blood from the rectum, mortality may be 30%.[3,32]

Clinical Features and Evaluation

Mucosal lesions in patients with a catastrophic central nervous system event are common and have become more evident since the introduction of endoscopy.[28] Appreciable bleeding, however, occurs in less than 5% of the patients and reaches the clinical stage of shock in a much smaller percentage.[29]

The clinical signs of gastrointestinal bleeding can be dangerously subtle. Feelings of oppression, nausea associated with excessive sweating, relative tachycardia, and pale facial features may soon be followed by oozing of blood or, at times, massive production of blood. Gastrointestinal bleeding can first be signaled by a coffee-ground color in aspirate.

The clinical presenting signs that should be recognized as possible indicators of severe hemorrhage are orthostatic hypotension and, eventually, decrease in hemoglobin and hematocrit concentrations. Clinically, orthostatic hypotension is the most reliable forerunner of hypovolemic shock. After the head of the bed is changed to at least 60° with the patient's legs in a dependent position, sequential measurement of systolic blood pressure and pulse provides a reasonable estimate of the volume of blood loss. New-onset tachycardia without change in systolic blood pressure indicates a fractional loss of blood volume of 15% or less. Tachycardia with a change in systolic blood pressure of 10 mm Hg when position is changed indicates a blood volume depletion of at least 20%, and a spontaneous change in blood pressure to systolic levels below 100 mm Hg indicates a loss of 25% or more.[4] At this juncture, oliguria (urine volume < 15 mL/hour) is invariably present.

With loss of whole blood, the hematocrit does not change, because the percentage of erythrocyte mass to total blood mass remains similar. Decrease in hematocrit lags behind and appears after redistribution of plasma to the intravascular space. Replacement of fluid with saline or volume expanders decreases the hematocrit further, and the decrease should not be misinterpreted as an indicator of continuing gastrointestinal bleeding. In this circumstance, active gastrointestinal bleeding is suggested only when hypotension persists and the hematocrit does not increase after infusion of whole blood or packed cells. Hematemesis or sudden appearance of large fresh clots per anum is also a sign of active bleeding in the gastrointestinal tract but does not indicate whether the site is in the upper or the lower part of the tract.

Gastrointestinal bleeding after acute stroke appears as hematemesis or melena and occasionally with a sudden decrease in hemoglobin value. In our study, orthostatic hypotension and massive hematemesis developed in a minority of patients.[59] Others found more severe gastrointestinal hemorrhages after acute stroke and hypotension or a decrease in hemoglobin in 50% of the patients.[15] Minor (and probably less clinically significant) gastrointestinal hemorrhages may not be noticed, and some patients may have only a transient tinge of blood with nasogastric return, possibly related to mucosal damage from the nasogastric tube alone.

The source of gastrointestinal bleeding should be actively sought. Intuitively, stress ulcers are implicated as a cause of gastrointestinal bleeding, but many other causes should be pursued. Hemorrhage from the nasopharynx should be investigated in any patient with prolonged intubation or tracheostomy. Proper inspection of the mouth may sporadically identify damage to the mucosa of the oral pharynx incurred during placement of the endotrachial tube. Bleeding is common in nasally intubated patients, even occasionally excessive, and may lead to accumulation in the dependent portions of the stomach. Bleeding from a tracheostomy can appear minimal because the blood is swallowed. Massive bleeding at the tracheostomy site from erosion of the brachiocephalic artery is fortunately rare (1% to 5%) but often fatal, appearing much more commonly with hemoptysis.

Mallory-Weiss tears should be considered in patients with profound vomiting. Associated conditions with profound vomiting are acute cerebellar stroke and aneurysmal subarachnoid hemorrhage. Repeated retching and vomiting may cause a circumferential mucosal laceration in the cardia portion of the stomach or longitudinally in the proximal esophagus[23] (Fig. 32–1). However, it can occur in any situation that increases abdominal pressure, such as repeated bucking and coughing with tracheostomy in situ, seizures, and episodic autonomic storms. An important predisposing factor for Mallory-Weiss tears is a history of alcohol or aspirin abuse. Hemorrhage from Mallory-Weiss tears ceases spontaneously, and half the

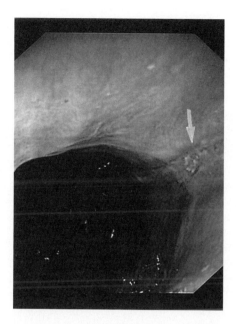

Figure 32–1. Typical linear injury (*arrow*) at gastroesophageal junction (Mallory-Weiss).

patients do not require blood transfusion. An underlying profound gastritis is often confirmed by endoscopy. Definitive treatment with multipolar electrocoagulation is needed in only a few patients with these complications.

Some form of esophagitis occurs in 50% of patients receiving mechanical ventilation. The cause is mechanical irritation from nasogastric tubes or induction of gastroenteric reflux from interference with sphincter function.[45]

In-hospital upper gastrointestinal bleeding usually is associated with peptic ulcers and gastritis. An autopsy study of gastrointestinal bleeding in intracranial disease found significant occurrences of gastric petechiae (50%) and gastric or duodenal ulcers (30%), but some of these lesions may have represented agonal changes.[28] A retrospective review in neurosurgical patients found that 7% of 526 had gastrointestinal bleeding, mostly from superficial mucosal erosions.[10] Comatose patients and patients with acute ulcers at endoscopy were at significantly higher risk for life-threatening complications. Lower gastrointestinal bleeding is much less common in acutely ill neurologic patients and in many is related to local mucosal

trauma. In 14 patients who had gastrointestinal hemorrhage in acute stroke, the most common associated possible causes were long-term use of aspirin, other nonsteroidal anti-inflammatory drugs, and anticoagulation.[59]

These alternative explanations for gastrointestinal bleeding suggest that medication-induced gastrointestinal bleeding, at least in acute stroke, may be underappreciated.[15,59] Other studies found that the risk of gastrointestinal bleeding was increased in patients with a Glasgow coma scale score of less than 9, mechanical ventilation, coagulopathy,[8,13] or sepsis.[9]

Enteral nutrition is insufficient as a measure to prevent stress ulcers.[41] The use of prophylactic medication (antacids or histamine$_2$-blockers) for gastrointestinal bleeding in traumatic brain injury has been addressed in prospective studies. Cimetidine prophylaxis was effective in a single controlled trial.[25] The use of the more expensive drug ranitidine in "high-risk" neurosurgical patients significantly reduced gastrointestinal bleeding.[9] However, alkalization of gastric contents may result in colonization with gram-negative organisms.

Proton pump inhibitors act by selectively inhibiting H^+/K^+ adenosine triphosphatase in the stimulated parietal cells of the stomach and decrease acid secretion. This new class of drugs is considered equally efficacious and less expensive. However, proton pump inhibitors have not been compared with histamine receptor antagonists. Omeprazole (Prilosec) is better and easier to use than ranitidine and is administered through the nasogastric tube. Omeprazole is dissolved in sodium bicarbonate (20 mg dissolved in 10 mL of 8.4% sodium bicarbonate) and administered in the morning,[35,37] but it can be administered intravenously in a 40 mg bolus injection.[36] Pantoprazole (Protonix) has become available in an intravenous formulation, and costs are comparable to, if not less than, those of alternatives. Pantoprazole, 40 mg intravenously once or twice a day, provides good protection and is safe. It has become the preferred agent in our NICU.

The policy of prophylaxis in acutely ill neurologic patients remains to be determined.

One should appreciate the significant hospital charges of stress ulcer prophylaxis. Practice guidelines can reduce inappropriate use of costly drugs[44] but have not been developed for NICU patients. If one extrapolates the results of studies in other intensive care units to NICUs, administration of proton pump inhibitors is reasonable in patients who have used aspirin or other nonsteroidal anti-inflammatory drugs, are taking anticoagulants, have a history of peptic ulcer, or are receiving mechanical ventilation. Specific neurologic conditions associated with a comparatively high risk of gastrointestinal bleeding and for which prophylaxis is indicated are pontine hemorrhage, severe diffuse axonal head injury, poor-grade subarachnoid hemorrhage, and acute spinal cord injury.[22,54,58]

Management of Gastrointestinal Bleeding

The order of priority and the problems in the management of patients with an underlying neurologic disorder and acute gastrointestinal bleeding are different from those in other intensive care populations. The most pertinent differences are a lower threshold for replacement of lost red blood cells to secure adequate oxygen uptake and a need for more stringent control of blood pressure. Immediate stabilization of blood pressure is important in any patient but more so in a patient with an acute brain injury. Blood pressure–dependent areas in the acutely injured brain and a shift in cerebral autoregulation in patients with chronic hypertension imply that hypotension may not be well tolerated (see Chapter 6). Fortunately, most gastrointestinal bleeding in critically ill neurologic patients is minor and stops even before endoscopy is performed.

Volume replacement is the first line of treatment, and pharmacologic support with inotropic agents is usually not indicated.[4,38] At least two short peripheral venous catheters should be inserted. If the primary goal is to improve infusion rate, cannulation of central veins is not recommended and may complicate matters further from its high incidence of iatrogenic complications in an emergency situation.

Replacement fluid usually consists of isotonic saline. Transfusion becomes important when the hematocrit decreases below a critical level of 30%.

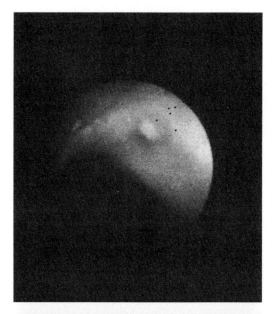

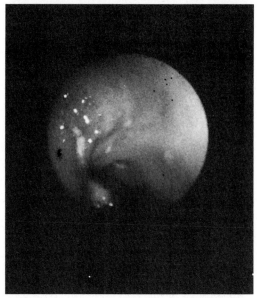

Figure 32–2. (*Top* and *bottom*) Typical endoscopic view of superficial erosion in acute neurologic central nervous system events. (The same ulcer may be seen with use of nonsteroidal anti-inflammatory drugs.)

The blood transfusion principles in patients with neurologic critical illness are similar to those in any other critically ill population. Massive gastrointestinal hemorrhages should be treated with whole blood alone to replace loss of both components of blood volume. When to begin infusion of whole blood or red blood cells depends on the ability of the patient to tolerate acute anemia. Patients with signs of imminent cardiac failure or transient electrocardiographic changes should have blood transfusion immediately. However, with the growing awareness of the risk of virally transmitted diseases, blood transfusions should not be ordered indiscriminately. One unit of fresh frozen plasma after 4 units of packed erythrocytes replaces lost coagulation factors. When gastrointestinal bleeding is associated with a coagulopathy, fresh frozen plasma (2 to 4 units) or platelet infusion (platelet count < 50,000) is needed for correction.

Empirical treatment with a continuous intravenous infusion of histamine$_2$- or proton pump blockers is advised because of tenable evidence of a reduced incidence of recurrent bleeding and, more important, of reduced mortality in randomized trials. Despite its costs, ranitidine infusion at 0.30 mg/kg per hour can be used in gastrointestinal bleeding after a loading dose of 0.5 mg/kg, but proton pump inhibitors are preferred.[61] For example, omeprazole reduced mortality and transfusion requirements in a randomized study (40 mg orally every 12 hours for 5 days).[30]

After initial resuscitation, fiber-optic endoscopy should be considered to localize the bleeding site. Emergency endoscopy localizes the source of bleeding in 95% of patients and, more relevant, determines the activity of the bleeding[14,16,18] (Fig. 32–2). Localization of a bleeding ulcer with a visible vessel (estimated prevalence, 25%) and localization of an ulcer with an adherent clot (estimated prevalence, 10%) have risks of rebleeding of, respectively, 50% and 20%.[12,31,53] At least half the patients with active bleeding, including oozing and spurting, observed during the procedure have rebleeding. A low risk (< 5%) of rebleeding can be expected when a clean base is found containing only old blood or pigments that can be washed away without effort.

Several direct therapeutic approaches can be tried at the time of endoscopy.[19,21] Multipolar electrocoagulation and heater probes are the most common and have reduced the need for early surgery.[33]

After hemodynamic stabilization and identification of the most likely source, specific treatment in most neurologically ill patients is medical. Suggested management tailored to the cause of gastrointestinal hemorrhage is summarized in Table 32–1. Continued bleeding without an identified source after several endoscopic attempts should prompt angiography or colonoscopy.

The decision to surgically intervene in bleeding stress ulcers is not difficult in extreme circumstances, such as failure to control active bleeding endoscopically, shock associated with an endoscopically visible artery, and increasing transfusion needs. Recommendations for surgical management in other clinical situations are more complicated and usually are guided by the age of the patient and the existence of comorbid disease. Before surgery is planned, arteriography for localization, possibly followed by arterial embolization or vasopressin infusion, is often considered.

Table 32–1. Management of Acute Upper Gastrointestinal Bleeding

Mallory-Weiss syndrome	Volume resuscitation
	Endoscopic confirmation
	Observation or electrocoagulation
Peptic ulcer, erosions	Volume resuscitation
	Endoscopic confirmation
	Proton pump inhibitors
	Surgery if at increased risk for bleeding

Lower gastrointestinal tract bleeding is usually associated with angiodysplasia and diverticulitis, very unusual causes of bleeding in the NICU. Localization can be difficult, and radionuclide scanning with technetium-labeled red blood cells may provide essential information[62] (sensitivity of 91% and specificity of 100%) before angiography is performed.[6]

DISORDERED INTESTINAL MOTILITY

Bed rest, medication, and enteral alimentation change bowel movement. Constipation may develop in patients confined to bed, but in many others, diarrhea or frequent loose stools complicate the acute neurologic illness.

Diarrhea

Hospital diarrhea is a serious problem in acutely ill neurologic patients. It is often self-limiting and related to fecal impaction, which in turn is associated with narcotic analgesics, reduced oral intake, and mild dehydration. In patients with GBS, early onset of diarrhea may indicate that *Campylobacter jejuni* infection triggered GBS, certainly if the diarrhea is associated with mucus or blood.

It is important to consider bacterial enteritis from *Clostridium difficile* (for details, see Chapter 33), but in most instances causes are more mundane, and a change in gut flora alone may cause diarrhea.

Most often, clindamycin, penicillins, and cephalosporins are implicated in diarrhea. Theophylline in toxic doses, digoxin, and most central-acting antihypertensive agents can produce diarrhea. Oral intake should be carefully evaluated. Frequent use of apple juice or elixers (e.g., antiepileptic medication) to administer medication can be incriminated in occasional instances.

Initiation of enteral nutrition alone probably is the most common reason for diarrhea (Table 32–2). Most often, sudden exposure of the gut to undiluted enteral formula results in frequent loose stools or diarrhea. High infusion rate (more than 50 mL per hour), certainly when

Table 32–2. Causes of Diarrhea

Hyperosmolar enteral nutrition
Enteral feeding at high infusion rates
Antacids, clindamycin, cephalosporins, histamine$_2$-
   receptor antagonists, angiotensin-converting enzyme
   inhibitors, theophylline
Hypoalbuminemia
Clostridium difficile infection

Source: Benjamin E: Gastrointestinal complications in the intensive care unit. *Clin Chest Med* 20:329–345, 1999.

hyperosmolar enteral formulas are used, is a possible factor. Another possible cause is lactose intolerance. Better adaptation can be achieved by a very gradual increase in the amount and by substitution of lactose-free formulas. Dilution of hyperosmolar solutions reduces diarrhea but dilution of iso-osmolar solutions does not.

In any event, analysis of the stool is warranted, and the examination should include determination of pH, leukocytes, muscle fibers, fat, pathogenic bacteria, osmolality, occult blood, and 24-hour volume. It is useful as well to measure magnesium content, particularly if antacids have been used to prevent stress ulcers.

Adynamic Ileus

Adynamic ileus may be mild or progress to significant cecal distention. It occurs invariably in GBS, after exploratory abdominal surgery in patients with multitrauma, and as a side effect of medication.

The typical presentation is great discomfort but little pain from distention. Vomiting may occur. No visible peristalsis and absolute silence on auscultation are characteristic.

In most patients, conservative management is sufficient. In a few patients, the disorder progresses to life-threatening acute colonic pseudo-obstruction (Ogilvie's syndrome).[46] Pain, distention, and tympany are more likely to be evident on physical examination. Perforation may occur, but in most patients recovery is possible without surgical intervention.

The possible causes of adynamic ileus and

Table 32–3. Possible Causes of Paralytic Ileus and Ogilvie's Syndrome

Neurologic disorders
  Guillain-Barré syndrome
  Meningitis
  Spinal cord injury
Surgical procedures
  Abdominal exploration for blunt trauma and shock
Drugs
  Tricyclic antidepressants
  Phenothiazines
  Opioids

Source: See also Vanek VW, Al-Salti M: Acute pseudo-obstruction of the colon (Ogilvie's syndrome). An analysis of 400 cases. *Dis Colon Rectum* 29:203–210, 1986.

Ogilvie's syndrome are summarized in Table 32–3, and potential triggers should be eliminated. (For a complete overview of causes, see an analysis of 400 cases.[56])

The pathophysiologic explanation remains unclear. In GBS as well as in other etiologic disorders,[57] sympathetic overdrive may be operative as a form of dysautonomia. The incidence in GBS is low (2% to 5%), and cecal perforation is rare, although it was well documented in one patient in the Massachusetts General Hospital series.[50] In our series of patients with severe GBS, ileus developed in 15%, but only a few instances seemed correlated with dysautonomia (Fig. 32–3). Preexisting conditions, such as abdominal surgery and incremental doses of opioids for pain management, were dominant causes.[7]

Abdominal films confirm the diagnosis (Fig. 32–4), usually showing involvement of the cecum and ascending or transverse colon. Air-fluid levels may be present.

Management consists of discontinuing the administration of opioids[20] or any anticholinergic agents, placement of oral and rectal tubes, adequate hydration, no oral intake, and correction of electrolyte abnormalities if they arise.

The recent discovery of the striking effect of neostigmine may result in its acceptance as a first-line agent, particularly since a colonic decompression tube is technically difficult to use. Because neostigmine may slow conduction of the atrioventricular node, it is contraindicated in patients with a heart rate of fewer than 60 beats/minute, systolic blood pressure of less than 90 mm Hg, recent myocardial infarction, previous β-blocker therapy, bronchospasm, or renal failure. Neostigmine increases parasympathetic stimulation, which enhances colonic activity through binding to the motilin receptor.[48] A single intravenous dose of 2 mg of neostigmine has restored colonic function in many patients. The dose may be repeated if necessary. It is prudent to have 1 mg of atropine available should bradycardia occur. An effect can be expected as early as 3 minutes after administration, but 1 hour may be required after a second dose.[1,49,55] Oral pyridostigmine has not been investigated in this condition.

If symptoms persist for more than 2 to 3 days, decompressive colonoscopy may be indicated. Surgical tube cecostomy is considered if cecal distention persists.[46] Perforation is imminent when cecal dilatation reaches 10 cm on plain abdominal films.

Neurogenic Bowel in Spinal Cord Injury

Neurogenic bowel disorder in acute spinal cord injury results in reduced reflex-mediated defecation. The gastrocolic reflex (feeding triggering intestinal peristalsis) may be muted, colon transit time is slowed, and anorectal dyssynergia (anal sphincter contraction with rectal contraction) may occur.[52]

Bowel dysfunction may have different patterns related to the level of spinal injury. Injury above the sacral segments of the spinal cord results in reflexic (upper motor neuron) bowel (defecation cannot be initiated by voluntary relaxation of the external anal sphincter), and injury at the sacral segments or cauda equina results in areflexic (lower motor neuron) bowel (fecal incontinence and hypotonic sphincter). Bowel care is different in each of these types.

Bowel management for reflexic bowel includes insertion of a glycol-based suppository or a small volume of bisacodyl in a saline enema[27] followed by digital stimulation with gentle rolling of a finger while the patient is upright or lying on one side. In contrast, the routine for areflexic bowel is Valsalva's maneuver and manual evacuation of the entire

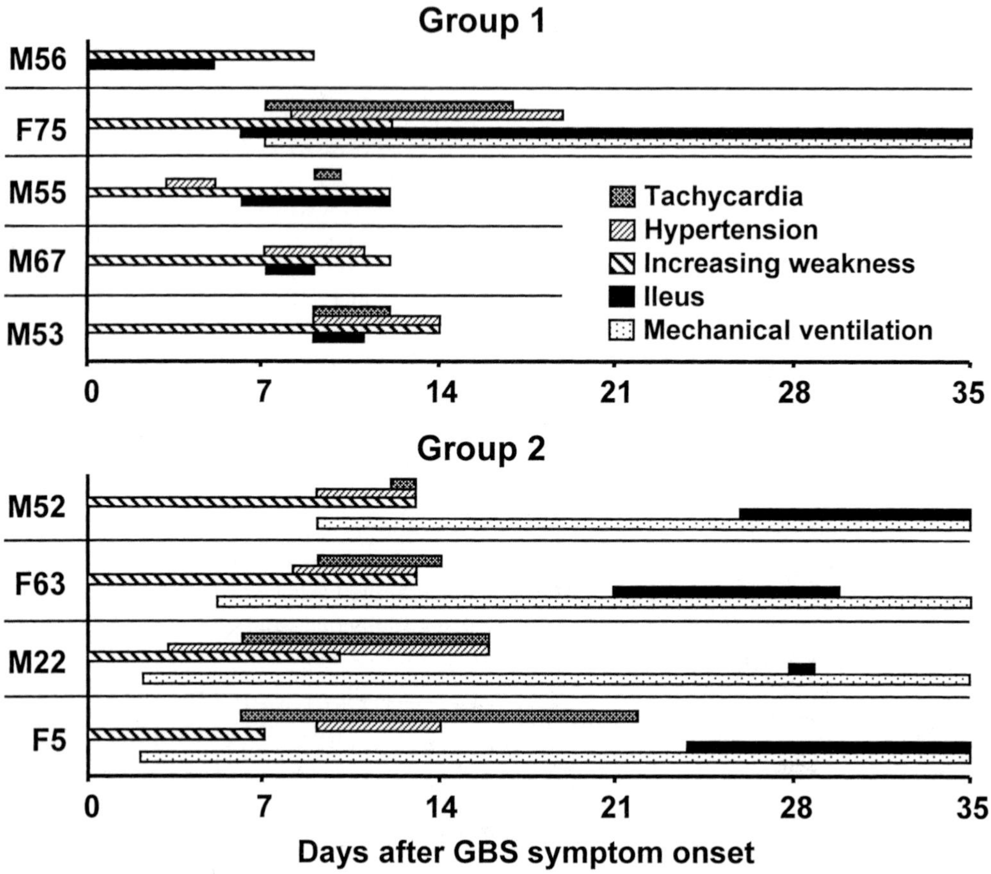

Group 1

Group 2

Figure 32–3. Adynamic ileus in Guillain-Barré syndrome (GBS). Group 1, patients with GBS and worsening strength; group 2, patients with GBS in the phase of improving strength. Note the relation of ileus onset to dysautonomic features. On y-axis: F, female; M, male; age in years. (From Burns et al.[7] By permission of John Wiley & Sons.)

rectum. This technique is preferred for patients in the spinal shock phase.

Major parts of bowel care also include a diet of at least 15 g of fiber daily and an additional 500 mL of fluid to improve stool consistency. Prokinetic agents may cause serious side effects and are generally not effective.[60] Because gastric ulceration is most common in the first month after acute spinal cord injury, dark and tarry stools may indicate gastrointestinal bleeding.[22]

Abdominal Trauma

Patients with closed head injury may have obvious chest (see Chapter 29), urogenital, or ab-

dominal trauma. A detailed discussion is beyond the scope of this book and outside the purview of the neurointensivist. The issues are highly complex, and trauma may involve many intra-abdominal structures. It is mentioned here only to alert attending neurologists to the possibility of its existence.

It is important to consider abdominal trauma in head-injured patients. Abdominal findings on examination could be minimal in patients with profound lesions, such as small bowel perforation, hepatic lacerations, pancreatic transection, and gallbladder injuries.[11,26,51] Abdominal trauma causing extreme changes in blood pressure and a decrease in hematocrit is

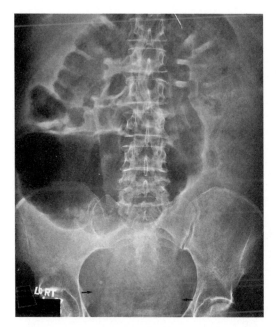

most often identified in the emergency department, and patients are transferred to an operating room for surgical exploration.

Without question, frequent clinical assessment of the abdomen in a recently admitted patient with closed head injury is essential. In many patients with a history of possible intra-abdominal injury, ultrasonography or abdominal CT scanning is needed. Hemodynamically unstable patients require diagnostic peritoneal lavage or laparotomy. In general, increasing abdominal tenderness and a marked decrease in hematocrit without an obvious source of bleeding should prompt exploration. Computed tomography is valuable for detecting free intraperitoneal blood and completely images the intra-abdominal solid organs. Considerable amounts of free fluid but absent solid organ injury on CT still did increase the probability of finding organ injury, and exploratory laparotomy is needed.[47] Contrast medium may be administered, but its additional diagnostic value is uncertain. Administration of a contrast agent may complicate interpretation of CT scans of

Figure 32–4. Abdominal film in a patient with Guillain-Barré syndrome shows striking dilatation of the ascending colon. *Arrows* indicate dilated sigmoid colon and fecal impaction.

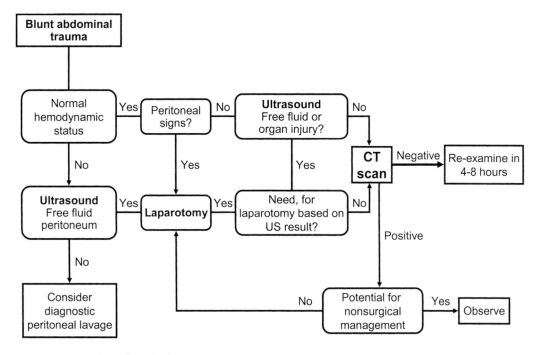

Figure 32–5. Algorithm for blunt trauma. CT, computed tomography; US, ultrasound. (Modified from Amoroso.[2] By permission of WB Saunders Company.)

the brain, because traumatic subarachnoid blood, if present, may not be differentiated from hyperdense contrast material. Ultrasound evaluation is also useful and cost-effective,[43] but the identification of parenchymal injury is more difficult. With multiple views, sensitivity may reach 90% and specificity 98%. Some of the detected findings, such as small hematomas in the liver, may be clinically irrelevant. In addition, a baseline liver function test and determination of serum amylase are warranted.[42] One study suggested that repeat abdominal examination and normal abdominal CT findings beyond the first day sufficiently exclude major injury.[39] An algorithm is shown in Figure 32–5.[2]

Trauma surgeons should be consulted if there is any doubt about whether abdominal injury is present.

CONCLUSIONS

- The severity of gastrointestinal hemorrhage should be assessed immediately. Potentially ominous clinical signs are orthostatic hypotension and tachycardia with change in position. Tachycardia with position change but without change in blood pressure indicates a 15% loss of volume, and decrease in blood pressure to < 100 mm Hg with position change indicates a 25% or greater volume loss.
- Endoscopy is indicated in patients with significant gastrointestinal bleeding, but other sources (oral mucosa, nasal intubation, tracheostomy site) should be excluded.
- Management in gastrointestinal hemorrhage is focused on volume resuscitation and preservation of adequate blood pressure. Proton pump inhibitors should be administered early.
- Diarrhea is most commonly associated with initiation of enteral nutrition and release of fecal impaction related to narcotic analgesics or dehydration.
- Paralytic ileus in GBS usually involves the cecum and ascending colon. Adynamic ileus is treated with oral and rectal tubes, no oral intake, and, if severe dysautonomia is not present, intravenous neostigmine.
- Traumatic abdominal injury may be subtle, and CT scanning and repeat examination for abdominal tenderness are needed within the first day of admission. Laparotomy is required in hemodynamically unstable patients.

REFERENCES

1. Abeyta BJ, Albrecht RM, Schermer CR: Retrospective study of neostigmine for the treatment of acute colonic pseudo-obstruction. *Am Surg* 67:265–268, 2001.
2. Amoroso TA: Evaluation of the patient with blunt abdominal trauma: an evidence based approach. *Emerg Med Clin North Am* 17:63–75, 1999.
3. Beejay U, Wolfe MM: Acute gastrointestinal bleeding in the intensive care unit. The gastroenterologist's perspective. *Gastroenterol Clin North Am* 29:309–336, 2000.
4. Birkett DH: Gastrointestinal tract bleeding. Common dilemmas in management. *Surg Clin North Am* 71:1259–1269, 1991.
5. Bresalier RS: The clinical significance and pathophysiology of stress-related gastric mucosal hemorrhage. *J Clin Gastroenterol* 13 Suppl 2:S35–S43, 1991.
6. Browder W, Cerise EJ, Litwin MS: Impact of emergency angiography in massive lower gastrointestinal bleeding. *Ann Surg* 204:530–536, 1986.
7. Burns TM, Lawn ND, Low PA, et al: Adynamic ileus in severe Guillain-Barré syndrome. *Muscle Nerve* 24:963–965, 2001.
8. Cash BD: Evidence-based medicine as it applies to acid suppression in the hospitalized patient. *Crit Care Med* 30(Suppl): S373–S378, 2002.
9. Chan KH, Lai EC, Tuen H, et al: Prospective double-blind placebo-controlled randomized trial on the use of ranitidine in preventing postoperative gastroduodenal complications in high-risk neurosurgical patients. *J Neurosurg* 82:413–417, 1995.
10. Chan KH, Mann KS, Lai EC, et al: Factors influencing the development of gastrointestinal complications after neurosurgery: results of multivariate analysis. *Neurosurgery* 25:378–382, 1989.
11. Chiang WK: Isolated jejunal perforation from nonpenetrating abdominal trauma. *Am J Emerg Med* 11:473–475, 1993.
12. Clason AE, Macleod DA, Elton RA: Clinical factors in the prediction of further haemorrhage or mortality in

acute upper gastrointestinal haemorrhage. *Br J Surg* 73:985–987, 1986.

13. Cook DJ, Fuller HD, Guyatt GH, et al: Risk factors for gastrointestinal bleeding in critically ill patients. *N Engl J Med* 330:377–381, 1994.

14. Cook DJ, Guyatt GH, Salena BJ, et al: Endoscopic therapy for acute nonvariceal upper gastrointestinal hemorrhage: a meta-analysis. *Gastroenterology* 102:139–148, 1992.

15. Davenport RJ, Dennis MS, Warlow CP: Gastrointestinal hemorrhage after acute stroke. *Stroke* 27:421–424, 1996.

16. Eastwood GL: Endoscopy in gastrointestinal bleeding. Are we beginning to realize the dream? (Editorial.) *J Clin Gastroenterol* 14:187–191, 1992.

17. Ferrera PC, Verdile VP, Bartfield JM, et al: Injuries distracting from intraabdominal injuries after blunt trauma. *Am J Emerg Med* 16:145–149, 1998.

18. Fleischer D: Endoscopic therapy of upper gastrointestinal bleeding in humans. *Gastroenterology* 90:217–234, 1986.

19. Fleischer DE: Endoscopic control of upper gastrointestinal bleeding. *J Clin Gastroenterol* 12 Suppl 2:S41–S47, 1990.

20. Frantzides CT, Cowles V, Salaymeh B, et al: Morphine effects on human colonic myoelectric activity in the postoperative period. *Am J Surg* 163:144–148, 1992.

21. Fromm D: Endoscopic coagulation for gastrointestinal bleeding (editorial). *N Engl J Med* 316:1652–1654, 1987.

22. Gore RM, Mintzer RA, Calenoff L: Gastrointestinal complications of spinal cord injury. *Spine* 6:538–544, 1981.

23. Graham DY, Schwartz JT: The spectrum of the Mallory-Weiss tear. *Medicine (Baltimore)* 57:307–318, 1978.

24. Gudeman SK, Wheeler CB, Miller JD, et al: Gastric secretory and mucosal injury response to severe head trauma. *Neurosurgery* 12:175–179, 1983.

25. Halloran LG, Zfass AM, Gayle WE, et al: Prevention of acute gastrointestinal complications after severe head injury: a controlled trial of cimetidine prophylaxis. *Am J Surg* 139:44–48, 1980.

26. Horst HM, Bivins BA: Pancreatic transection. A concept of evolving injury. *Arch Surg* 124:1093–1095, 1989.

27. House JG, Steins SA: Pharmacologically initiated defecation for persons with spinal cord injury: effectiveness of three agents. *Arch Phys Med Rehabil* 78:1062–1065, 1997.

28. Kamada T, Fusamoto H, Kawano S, et al: Gastrointestinal bleeding following head injury: a clinical study of 433 cases. *J Trauma* 17:44–47, 1977.

29. Karch SB: Upper gastrointestinal bleeding as a complication of intracranial disease. *J Neurosurg* 37:27–29, 1972.

30. Khuroo MS, Yattoo GN, Javid G, et al: A comparison of omeprazole and placebo for bleeding peptic ulcer. *N Engl J Med* 336:1054–1058, 1997.

31. Kohler B, Riemann JF: Upper GI-bleeding—value and consequences of emergency endoscopy and endo-scopic treatment. *Hepatogastroenterology* 38:198–200, 1991.

32. Kupfer Y, Cappell MS, Tessler S: Acute gastrointestinal bleeding in the intensive care unit. The intensivist's perspective. *Gastroenterol Clin North Am* 29:275–307, 2000.

33. Laine L: Multipolar electrocoagulation in the treatment of active upper gastrointestinal tract hemorrhage. A prospective controlled trial. *N Engl J Med* 316:1613–1617, 1987.

34. Laine L, Weinstein WM: Subepithelial hemorrhages and erosions of human stomach. *Dig Dis Sci* 33:490–503, 1988.

35. Lasky MR, Metzler MH, Phillips JO: A prospective study of omeprazole suspension to prevent clinically significant gastrointestinal bleeding from stress ulcers in mechanically ventilated trauma patients. *J Trauma* 44:527–533, 1998.

36. Laterre PF, Horsmans Y: Intravenous omeprazole in critically ill patients: a randomized, crossover study comparing 40 with 80 mg plus 8 mg/hour on intragastric pH. *Crit Care Med* 29:1931–1935, 2001.

37. Levy MJ, Seelig CB, Robinson NJ, et al: Comparison of omeprazole and ranitidine for stress ulcer prophylaxis. *Dig Dis Sci* 42:1255–1259, 1997.

38. Liolios A, Oropello JM, Benjamin E: Gastrointestinal complications in the intensive care unit. *Clin Chest Med* 20:329–345, 1999.

39. Livingstone DH, Lavery RF, Passannante MR, et al: Admission or observation is not necessary after a negative abdominal computed tomographic scan in patients with suspected blunt abdominal trauma: results of a prospective, multi-institutional trial. *J Trauma* 44:273–280, 1998.

40. Lu WY, Rhoney DH, Boling WB, et al: A review of stress ulcer prophylaxis in the neurosurgical intensive care unit. *Neurosurgery* 41:416–425, 1997.

41. MacLaren R, Jarvis CL, Fish DN: Use of enteral nutrition for stress ulcer prophylaxis. *Ann Pharmacother* 35:1614–1623, 2001.

42. McAnena OJ, Moore EE, Marx JA: Initial evaluation of the patient with blunt abdominal trauma. *Surg Clin North Am* 70:495–515, 1990.

43. McKenney MG, McKenney KL, Hong JJ, et al: Evaluating blunt abdominal trauma with sonography: a cost analysis. *Am Surg* 67:930–934, 2001.

44. Mostafa G, Sing RF, Matthews BD, et al: The economic benefit of practice guidelines for stress ulcer prophylaxis. *Am Surg* 68:146–150, 2002.

45. Mutlu GM, Mutlu EA, Factor P: GI complications in patients receiving mechanical ventilation. *Chest* 119:1222–1241, 2001.

46. Nanni G, Garbini A, Luchetti P, et al: Ogilvie's syndrome (acute colonic pseudo-obstruction): review of the literature (October 1948 to March 1980) and report of four additional cases. *Dis Colon Rectum* 25:157–166, 1982.

47. Ng AK, Simons RK, Torreggiani WC, et al: Intra-abdominal free fluid without solid organ injury in blunt

abdominal trauma: an indication for laparotomy. *J Trauma* 52:1134–1140, 2002.

48. Peeters TL: Erythromycin and other macrolides as prokinetic agents. *Gastroenterology* 105:1886–1899, 1993.

49. Ponec RJ, Saunders MD, Kimmey MB: Neostigmine for the treatment of acute colonic pseudo-obstruction. *N Engl J Med* 341:137–141, 1999.

50. Ropper AH, Wijdicks EFM, Truax BT: *Guillain-Barré Syndrome*. Philadelphia: FA Davis Company, 1991.

51. Sharma O: Blunt gallbladder injuries: presentation of twenty-two cases with review of the literature. *J Trauma* 39:576–580, 1995.

52. Stiens SA, Bergman SB, Goetz LL: Neurogenic bowel dysfunction after spinal cord injury: clinical evaluation and rehabilitative management. *Arch Phys Med Rehabil* 78 Suppl:S86–S102, 1997.

53. Swain CP, Storey DW, Bown SG, et al: Nature of the bleeding vessel in recurrently bleeding gastric ulcers. *Gastroenterology* 90:595–608, 1986.

54. Tanaka S, Mori T, Ohara H, et al: Gastrointestinal bleeding in cases of ruptured cerebral aneurysms. *Acta Neurochir (Wien)* 48:223–230, 1979.

55. Turegano-Fuentes F, Muñoz-Jimenez F, Del Valle-Hernandez E, et al: Early resolution of Ogilvie's syndrome with intravenous neostigmine: a simple, effective treatment. *Dis Colon Rectum* 40:1353–1357, 1997.

56. Vanek VW, Al-Salti M: Acute pseudo-obstruction of the colon (Ogilvie's syndrome). An analysis of 400 cases. *Dis Colon Rectum* 29:203–210, 1986.

57. Vantrappen G: Acute colonic pseudo-obstruction. *Lancet* 341:152–153, 1993.

58. Watts CC, Clark K: Gastric acidity in the comatose patient. *J Neurosurg* 30:107–109, 1969.

59. Wijdicks EFM, Fulgham JR, Batts KP: Gastrointestinal bleeding in stroke. *Stroke* 25:2146–2148, 1994.

60. Wysowski DK, Bacsanyi J: Cisapride and fatal arrhythmia. *N Engl J Med* 335:290–291, 1996.

61. Zed PJ, Loewen PS, Slavik RS, et al: Meta-analysis of proton pump inhibitors in treatment of bleeding peptic ulcers. *Ann Pharmacother* 35:1528–1534, 2001.

62. Zuckerman DA, Bocchini TP, Birnbaum EH: Massive hemorrhage in the lower gastrointestinal tract in adults: diagnostic imaging and intervention. *AJR Am J Roentgenol* 161:703–711, 1993.

33

Nosocomial Infections

A nosocomial infection is arbitrarily defined as any infection developing 48 hours after admission. This definition implies that there is no clinical or laboratory evidence of infection in the first 2 days and no infection incubating on admission. An infection manifested earlier is considered community-acquired. Nosocomial infections are much more likely in intensive care units because of the severity of the underlying illness, extremes of age, and multiplicity of devices and instruments. Published epidemiologic surveys have unequivocally shown that hospital-acquired infection contributes greatly to morbidity, mortality, and, often, length of stay in the intensive care unit, with attendant extravagant costs. Cross-contamination from patient to patient by the hands of medical staff ultimately remains the most common and possibly most preventable cause[61,68] (Chapter 3).

Prevalence studies of nosocomial infections in the NICU are few, and it is clear that the results of available prevalence studies in other medical intensive care units cannot be extrapolated to acutely ill neurologic patients.[63] For example, a prospective study in 208 critically ill patients admitted to a medical–surgical intensive care unit in Spain reported a 25% rate of nosocomial pneumonia, mostly from *Staphylococcus aureus*. In contrast, two surveys in a neurosurgery department that included intensive care beds reported crude incidences of 6.7% and 10%, but there was a fivefold increase in nosocomial pneumonia in comatose patients.[52,58] The Centers for Dis-

ease Control National Nosocomial Infections Surveillance system program publishes a semiannual report (www.cdc.gov [search NNIS]) (Table 33–1).

This chapter discusses prophylaxis, recognition, and treatment of nosocomial infection in patients with an acute neurologic disorder. A separate section containing essential information on antibiotics is provided.

EVALUATION OF FEVER

Fever in an acutely ill neurologic patient probably bespeaks infection. Scrupulous attention to asepsis significantly reduces the risk.[44] Bacteremia outbreaks associated with poor handling of propofol (an excellent culture medium) have been described.[2] Other noninfectious causes that can result in increased body temperature must be considered, and generic terms such as "central fever" should be avoided.

A fairly common cause of fever in patients with aneurysmal or traumatic subarachnoid hemorrhage is blood disintegration and resorption. As early as the second day after admission to the unit, a low-grade fever, almost never much higher than 39°C, can arise. A typical feature of fever from blood absorption is relative bradycardia. (One should remain alert to possible early infection when patients are receiving beta-blockade, which blunts tachycardia.) Relative bradycardia as part of an infection may be more common in gram-negative infections.[67]

Table 33–1. Device-Associated Infection Rates by Type of Intensive Care Unit

Type of Unit	No. of Units	Ventilator-associated Pneumonia[*]	Central Line Bloodstream Infection[†]	Urinary Catheter Urinary Tract Infection[‡]
Cardiothoracic	62	9.3 (3.1–18.0)	2.4 (0.4–4.9)	2.3 (0.4–4.8)
Coronary	99	6.9 (0.3–16.9)	4.0 (0.0–7.8)	5.1 (0.9–11.0)
Medical	130	6.5 (2.1–13.6)	5.3 (2.2–9.9)	6.0 (2.5–10.3)
Medical–surgical[§]	113	9.4 (2.8–17.4)	5.0 (2.0–8.2)	5.3 (1.4–10.3)
Neurosurgical	46	11.6 (3.9–22.5)	4.4 (0.0–8.2)	7.0 (2.2–12.1)
Surgical	146	12.1 (5.7–23.3)	4.9 (1.3–9.2)	4.4 (1.4–9.0)
Trauma	24	15.2 (8.7–28.4)	7.8 (1.8–10.9)	6.4 (3.8–10.1)

All numbers are median, 10th percentile, and 90th percentile values.
[*]Number of pneumonia infections per 1000 ventilator days.
[†]Number of infections per 1000 central line days.
[‡]Number of infections per 1000 urinary catheter days.
[§]Major teaching.
Source: *Centers for Disease Control Semiannual Report,* December 2000.

Other major diagnostic categories aside from infectious causes are deep venous thrombosis, drug fever, and atelectasis. An important potential cause for unexplained fever in the intensive care unit is deep venous thrombosis, which may be associated with miliary pulmonary embolism (Chapter 29). Careful examination of patients' calves should be part of a daily routine during rounds (Chapter 3).

Drug fever is commonly associated with tachycardia and chills, typically appears on the 7th to 10th day after continuous administration of a drug, and is often characterized by a stepwise increase in fever after an initial low-grade fever. An accelerated reaction instead of an incremental progression may be seen in patients known to be sensitized to the drug. Fever promptly resolves in 1 to 2 days after the responsible drug is stopped.[16] Virtually any drug can cause fever in a susceptible patient, and in some patients the additional appearance of a skin rash, eosinophilia (only 20% of patients), or abnormal liver function test results is a helpful diagnostic sign.

Postoperative fever has traditionally been linked with atelectasis. Atelectasis may follow early after any type of craniotomy, but attributing fever to atelectasis found on chest radiographs is potentially troublesome, and a careful search for possibly overlooked infections remains important.

The various causes of fever are listed in Table 33–2. Comprehensive laboratory testing for causes of new-onset fever should probably include full hematologic evaluation, including smear and differential count, routine cultures (blood, sputum, urine, stool), chest and sinus radiography, and bronchoscopy, particularly in immunosuppressed patients with pulmonary infiltrates. Cerebrospinal fluid examination (presence of beta$_2$-transferrin) must be strongly considered in any patient with head injury to detect meningitis associated with a possible cerebrospinal fluid leak and in patients with intraventricular catheters and external reservoirs.

NOSOCOMIAL PNEUMONIA

In immunocompetent patients, nosocomial pneumonias are most often caused by bacterial pathogens. In the NICU, bacterial pneumonias are typically caused by gastric and oropharyngeal colonization with aerobic bacteria and repeated small-volume aspiration during sleep, certainly in patients with impaired gag reflexes.[60] The pharynx can be colonized by gram-negative bacilli (*Escherichia coli, Klebsiella, Enterobacter, Proteus, Pseudomonas aeruginosa, Serratia, Acinetobacter, Legionella pneumophila*), gram-positive cocci (*S. aureus, Streptococcus pneumoniae*), and, less often, gram-negative cocci (*Haemophilus influenzae, Branhamella catarrhalis*).[14,15,54,55] Although anaerobic bacteria are frequently isolated in

Table 33–2. Causes of Fever in Acute Neurologic Illness

Cause	Characteristics
Nosocomial pneumonia	Pulmonary infiltrates
	Marginal oxygenation
	Ventilation-perfusion mismatch (increased alveolar-arterial gradient)
Sepsis	Vascular or urinary catheters
	Increase in leukocyte counts with shift to immature polynuclear cells
	Respiratory alkalosis (early sepsis)
Urinary tract infection	100,000 colony-forming units
	White blood cell casts
	Recent "difficult" catheterization
Decubitus ulcer infection	Acute spinal cord injury or severe Guillain-Barré syndrome
Resorption of blood	Subarachnoid hemorrhage
	Head injury
	Traumatic muscle hematomas
Thromboembolism	Persistent tachycardia
	Painful calves, calf edema
	Increased alveolar-arterial gradient
Sinusitis	Nasal intubation
Meningitis	Cerebrospinal fluid leak, hematotympanum
Drug fever	Recent use (≤ 5 days) of new pharmacologic agents (e.g., penicillin, phenytoin, amphotericin B, sulfa preparations)
Propofol contamination	Poor aseptic techniques during preparation
	Postoperative infection
	Staphylococcus aureus in blood cultures

cultures, in critically ill neurologic patients the anaerobic presence in the oropharynx often changes into a predominance of gram-negative rods. *Legionella pneumophila* typically strikes in epidemics and particularly in surgical patients. This very virulent pathogen may hide in humidifiers, nebulizers, ventilation bags, tracheostomy tubes, and tap water.[37,57]

In neurologic patients, the cause of nosocomial pneumonia is often aspiration associated with impaired swallowing mechanism. The distinction between aspiration pneumonia and nosocomial pneumonia, therefore, often is academic. Other risk factors for nosocomial pneumonia are age over 70 years, mechanical ventilation, colonization of the oropharynx, use of histamine$_2$-blockers with or without antacids,[64] daily change of ventilator circuits, underlying chronic lung disease, reintubation,[59] and possibly the procedure of bronchoscopy itself.

A major cause of morbidity in ventilated patients is the development of ventilator-associated pneumonia, which is related to ventilator days[24] (Fig. 33–1). A prospective study of 132 patients with ventilator-associated pneumonia found that tracheostomy, multiple central venous catheter insertions, reintubation, and use of antacids were major contributing factors. *P. aeruginosa* and *S. aureus* were common pathogens. Ventilator-associated pneumonia was frequent within 2 weeks of intubation.[30] Increased mortality has been linked to *P. aeruginosa*, inappropriate antibiotic therapy, and age, but data are derived from medical intensive care units. Prevention of nosocomial pneumonia in mechanically ventilated patients is very important.[22,27] Official guidelines for the prevention of nosocomial pneumonia have been published[8] and summarized in a recent editorial.[31] Selective digestive decontamination has been suggested,[13,35] and indeed gram-negative colonization decreased with a suspension of polymyxin, tobramycin, and amphotericin delivered by nasogastric tube and cefotaxime given intravenously. No difference in incidence of nosocomial pneumonia or mortality was found in one study.[21] Topical antimicrobial prophylaxis with gentamicin-colistin-vancomycin 2% in Orabase every 6 hours significantly reduced oropharyngeal colonization and reduced ventilator-associated pneumonia in a prospective, randomized study.[3] A promising and simple method is continuous aspiration of subglottic se-

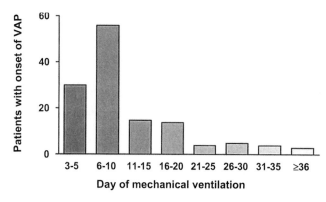

Figure 33–1. Distribution of onset of ventilator-associated pneumonia (VAP). (From Ibrahim et al.[30] By permission of the American College of Chest Physicians.)

cretions, which theoretically may decrease the volume of colonized secretions aspirated into the bronchial tree. A randomized trial in 76 mechanically ventilated patients found a significant reduction in pneumonia and reduction in attributable mortality.[62]

Clinical Features and Evaluation

The clinical diagnosis of nosocomial bronchopneumonia is undisputedly difficult. Fever is a key sign, but the most salient findings remain increased sputum production with a change in its quality to thick, purulent mucus.[11,43] The chest film may be supportive if peripheral infiltrates are demonstrated, but the sensitivity and specificity of radiographic abnormalities are low. *P. aeruginosa* is responsible for many of the ventilator-associated pneumonias, with substantial morbidity from adult respiratory distress syndrome. The radiographic findings are nonspecific, typically consisting of bilateral multifocal and diffuse opacities (Fig. 33–2) with occasional air-space disease cavities, indicating microabscesses. However, although typical for *P. aeruginosa*, microabscesses were found in only 5 of 56 studied patients with ventilator-associated pneumonia.[65] The diagnosis in clinical practice is based on the microbiologic diagnosis of a sample obtained by intratracheal suctioning, but the result is often inaccurate. Because cultures have an overpowering number of gram-nega-

tive bacteria, Gram's stain becomes important. Even if large numbers of single or multiple morphologic types are seen on the sputum Gram stain, only more than 25 polymorphonuclear leukocytes and fewer than 10 contaminating epithelial cells (indicative of the oral cavity rather than the airways) per lower power field suggest nosocomial pneumonia.[40] Alveolar macrophages and elastic fibers suggest that the specimen was obtained from a lung undergoing necrosis. Bronchoalveolar lavage during bronchoscopy in patients on mechanical ventilators may increase detection if the clinical diagnosis is uncertain.[10,45] Both procedures have high sensitivity and specificity. The yield of blood cultures in nosocomial pneumonias is only 5%. Open lung biopsy or transthoracic needle aspiration is a measure of last resort. Routine microbiologic cultures of aspirates before onset of ventilator pneumonia may identify microorganisms that mostly are not involved with later pneumonia and cannot be used to guide antimicrobial agents.[28]

Treatment

The decision to treat pulmonary infiltrates is problematic. Empirical use of antibiotics to avoid missing an infection has unfortunately almost become a "traditional approach." A useful scoring system has been proposed by Pugin et al.[47] (Table 33–3). A score of 6 or less implies a low likelihood for bacterial pneumonia.

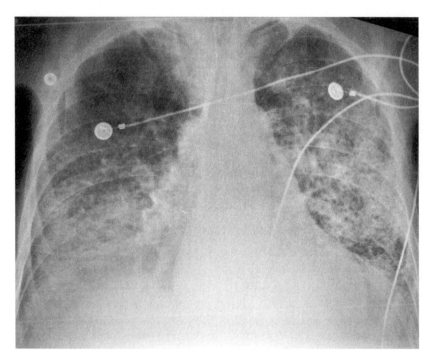

Figure 33–2. *Pseudomonas aeruginosa* pneumonia. Note "patchwork quilt" appearance typical of bronchopneumonia. (The abnormalities may progress to abscesses.)

In most patients, a broad spectrum of empirical treatment is initiated.[1] Most recommended empirical treatment regimens start with a third-generation cephalosporin with an aminoglycoside, but a third- or fourth-generation cephalosporin alone may be sufficient, avoiding the toxicity of many of the aminoglycosides. Cefepime may be preferred in *Pseudomonas aeruginosa*. The broad-spectrum quinolones can be very useful, largely because they penetrate well into secretions. The suggested treatment is summarized in Table 33–4. Vancomycin is the preferred drug if *S. aureus* pneumonia is suspected. The treatment of anaerobic pneumonias is best initiated with the use of clindamycin or imipenem.

INFECTIONS RELATED TO INTRAVENOUS CATHETERS

Transient bacteremias are often related to placement of catheters in intensive care units, including NICUs. Mortality attributed to noso-comial bloodstream infections is high, and a study also found that time in the intensive care unit was significantly prolonged in survivors.[46] The risk of catheter infection seems greater in internal jugular catheters than in subclavian catheters. In addition, an analysis of the potential risk factors in catheter-related infections emphasized that transparent dressings were associated with a significantly higher risk than gauze dressings,[41,48,49] but the link remains controversial. Central venous catheter infections may be prevented if catheter insertion is done with maximal aseptic techniques, topical mupirocin,[29] antibiotic-coated catheters,[32] and obsessional use of cutaneous antiseptics.[38] Recent prospective trials suggested that impregnating catheters with minocycline and rifampin significantly prevents colonization and catheter-related bacteremia,[17,50] with a low likelihood of antibiotic resistance.

Frequent manipulations increase the incidence of catheter-related infections to approximately 10%. Prevention guidelines have diverged on whether to replace the catheter with

Table 33–3. Clinical Pulmonary Infection Score (CPIS) Calculation*

	Score[†]
Temperature, °C	
$\geq$36.5 and $\leq$38.4 = 0 point	0
$\geq$38.5 and $\leq$38.9 = 1 point	1
$\geq$39 and $\leq$36 = 2 points	2
Blood leukocytes, mm³	
$\geq$4000 and $\leq$11,000 = 0 point	0
<4000 or >11,000 = 1 point	1
+ band forms $\geq$50% = add 1 point	2
Tracheal secretions	
Absence of tracheal secretions = 0 point	0
Presence of nonpurulent tracheal secretions = 1 point	1
Presence of purulent tracheal secretions = 2 points	2
Oxygenation: Pa_{O_2}/F_{IO_2}, mm Hg	
>240 or ARDS[‡] = 0 point	0
$\leq$240 and no ARDS = 2 points	2
Pulmonary radiography	
No infiltrate = 0 point	0
Diffuse (or patchy) infiltrate = 1 point	1
Localized infiltrate = 2 points	2
Progression of pulmonary infiltrate	
No radiographic progression = 0 point	0
Radiographic progression (after CHF and ARDS excluded) = 2 points	2
Culture of tracheal aspirate	
Pathogenic bacteria[§] cultured in rare or light quantity or no growth = 0 point	0
Pathogenic bacteria cultured in moderate or heavy quantity = 1 point	1
Same pathogenic bacteria seen on Gram's stain, add 1 point	2

ARDS, adult respiratory distress syndrome; CHF, congestive heart failure; Pa_{O_2}/F_{IO_2}, ratio of arterial oxygen pressure to fraction of inspired oxygen.
*CPIS at baseline was assessed on the basis of five variables, i.e., temperature, blood leukocyte count, tracheal secretions, oxygenation, and character of pulmonary infiltrate. CPIS at 72 hours was calculated on the basis of all seven variables and took into consideration the progression of the infiltrate and culture results of the tracheal aspirate.
[†]The maximum score is 14. A score > 6 at baseline or at 72 hours is considered suggestive of pneumonia.
[‡]ARDS defined as pulmonary arterial wedge pressure $\leq$18 mm Hg and acute bilateral infiltrates.
[§]Predominant organism in the culture.
Source: Modified from Pugin T, Auckenthaler R, Mili N, et al: Diagnosis of ventilator-associated pneumonia by bacteriologic analysis of bronchoscopic and nonbronchoscopic "blind" bronchoalveolar lavage fluid. *Am Rev Respir Dis* 143:1121–1129, 1991. By permission of the American Lung Association.

a new puncture or change the guidewire. Proponents of guidewire change argue that a new puncture only introduces new unnecessary risks of complications and that infection rates between guidewire exchange and new puncture are similar in prospective studies. Indeed, a controlled clinical study found that replacement of central venous catheters every 3 days did not prevent infection but rather, as expected, increased medical complications.[12] Catheter-related sepsis is more common in patients with triple-lumen catheters, which are usually considered when multiple sites for venous access are required. Typically, these catheters are needed in patients with frequent administration of electrolytes, blood products, and parenteral alimentation. The risk of catheter-related infections increases threefold when these types of catheters are used.[53]

Coagulase-negative staphylococci (*Staphylococcus epidermidis* accounts for more than

Table 33–4. Combinations of Antimicrobial Agents for Treatment of Nosocomial Pneumonia

Ceftazidime (Fortaz)	1–2 g q8h IV
Gentamicin (Garamycin)	2–3 mg/kg q8h IV
Aztreonam (Azactam)	2 g q6–8h IV
Clindamycin (Cleocin)	6–12 g q8h IV
Imipenem-cilastatin (Primaxin)	1 g q6–8h IV
Tobramycin (Nebcin)	1–3 mg/kg q8h IV
Ticarcillin (Ticar)	3–4 g q4–6h IV
Tobramycin (Nebcin)	3 mg/kg q8h IV

70%) are most frequently isolated from cultures, followed by *S. aureus*, *Enterococcus* species, *P. aeruginosa*, *Candida* species, *Enterobacter* species, *Acinetobacter* species, and *Serratia* species. *S. aureus* infection is extremely dangerous and can appear fulminantly, with bacteremia terminating in endocarditis and osteomyelitis.

The clinical diagnosis of infection from intravascular catheters usually is based on new-onset fever and colonization of more than 15 colony-forming units in cultures of the catheter tip. Local inflammation may be diagnostic but only in peripheral catheters.

The diagnosis of catheter-related sepsis is based on two positive blood cultures and confirmed by semiquantitative catheter cultures obtained by rolling the catheter tip back and forth across the agar plate. Additional blood cultures (two samples not drawn through the catheter) may be helpful.[9] Treatment is guided by the results of the cultures. For empirical treatment of suspected intravenous line sepsis, vancomycin and a third-generation cephalosporin are advisable (Table 33–5). Amphotericin or fluconazole may be needed if blood cultures are positive for *Candida* infection.

Phlebitis, one of the most common nosocomial infections, has the potential to become serious. Well-recognized causes of phlebitis are antibiotic infusions (e.g., vancomycin) and placement of a peripheral line into the antecubital vein. The risk is also increased when peripheral catheters are inserted in an emergency, because antisepsis could be less guarded. Early phlebitis is suggested by pain, tenderness, erythema, and swelling, later stages by purulence and a palpable cord. Changing the catheter to another site and treating the phlebitis with wet cold compresses

Table 33–5. Antimicrobial Treatment of Catheter-Related Bacteremia or Sepsis

Vancomycin	2 g q12h IV
with cefotaxime	1–2 g q6h IV
or	
Vancomycin	2 g q12h IV
with gentamicin	2–3 mg/kg q8h IV

usually are sufficient. Suppurative peripheral phlebitis, fortunately rare, is a medical emergency, and surgical intervention to remove the infected vein is needed.

NOSOCOMIAL URINARY TRACT INFECTIONS

Of all intensive care unit populations, acutely ill neurologic and neurosurgical patients are at the highest risk for urinary tract infections (Table 33–1). Nosocomial urinary tract infection sharply increases in comatose patients with indwelling catheters. Urinary tract infections may potentially cause sepsis syndrome, but bacteremia is often asymptomatic. However, urinary catheterization should keep the urine sterile in most patients. Bacteriuria takes place when catheters have been inserted for weeks. Urinary catheters impregnated with minocycline and rifampin reduce gram-positive infections but not gram-negative bacteria. Routine use is also discouraged because of cost.[18] More likely, nosocomial urinary tract infections can be reduced if prolonged use of catheters can be avoided, achievable only by constant questioning of the need for catheterization and consideration of alternative methods, such as condom drainage.

Proper separation of infection from colonization is difficult. Suprapubic or flank pain or dysuria has additional diagnostic value but is uncommon in this patient population. The laboratory criteria for urinary tract infection are unclear. Cultures alone may not determine whether significant bacteriuria is present, although 100,000 colony-forming units are at least indicative. New-onset fever and a leukocyte count exceeding 10 cells/mm^3 are highly suggestive of urinary tract infection, and white blood cell casts more strongly indicate involvement of the upper urinary tract.

Urine culture should be repeated if no response is seen in 2 days. Nosocomial urinary tract infections are often caused entirely by *E. coli* and *Proteus mirabilis*, but in patients who earlier received a course of antibiotics, *P. aeruginosa*, *Serratia marcescens*, and *Enterobacter* species are

Table 33–6. Antimicrobial Treatment of Nosocomial Urinary Tract Infection

Gentamicin	2–3 mg/kg q8h
or	
Ceftriaxone	1–2 g q12h IV
or	
Ciprofloxacin	0.2–0.4 g q12h IV
or	
Ampicillin	0.5 g q6h IV
with gentamicin	2–3 mg/kg q8h IV

important contenders, with an occasional disastrous emergence of antibiotic-resistant organisms. Treatment is guided by sensitivity tests or, if the results are not yet available, by the outcome of Gram's stain. Uncomplicated urinary tract infection can be treated with trimethoprim, 100 mg orally twice a day for 7 days, or with oral fluoroquinolones. In uncomplicated catheter-associated sepsis, antibiotics are usually administered for 10 days. In most patients, aminoglycosides are effective (Table 33–6), but in patients with gram-positive cocci, vancomycin is the preferred choice. In immunocompromised patients with neutropenia, an aminoglycoside with ceftazidime or cefepime is recommended.

An unusual occurrence in immunocompromised patients with indwelling catheters is the emergence of candiduria. Topical irrigation of the bladder with infusions of amphotericin B (50 mg/L of sterile distilled water) or miconazole (50 mg/L) at a rate of 40 mL/hour for 5 days should eradicate candidal cystitis.

NOSOCOMIAL GASTROINTESTINAL INFECTIONS

Nosocomial gastroenteritis most often is manifested by diarrhea, but the appearance of diarrhea does not imply an infectious cause (Chapter 32).

Clostridium difficile has been most often implicated. The presenting features of antibiotic-associated colitis can be subtle, with only a minor increase in the number, weight, and liquid content of stools and in fever, but occurrence is also frequently suggested by leukocytosis, severe abdominal cramping, and abdominal

tenderness.[25] Watery diarrhea is much more common than bloody diarrhea. *C. difficile* can be diagnosed from the stool by an assay for its cytotoxin and may be recovered from the stool in 30% to 60% of cultures. Endoscopic confirmation of inflammatory colitis is more specific. However, the prototypical pseudomembranous lesions scattered throughout the bowel mucosa are infrequent, and mild inflammatory changes are more prevalent in antibiotic-related diarrhea.

An important risk factor for nosocomial diarrhea is combination antimicrobial therapy.[6,39] In a survey, exposure to second- and third-generation cephalosporins emerged as the major risk factor for nosocomial diarrhea, more frequent than exposure to clindamycin.[39]

Treatment of nosocomial diarrhea should first focus on mundane causes (Chapter 32). Additional evaluation for *C. difficile*, including endoscopy, cultures, and measurement of toxin assay, should be done. Treatment of nosocomial diarrhea associated with *C. difficile* includes discontinuation of antibiotic therapy, unless it is critical for survival of the patient. The preferred approach is to begin treatment orally with metronidazole; oral vancomycin is reserved for unresponsive infections (Table 33–7). In very mild but persistent cases, cholestyramine (4 g three times a day) is a reasonable approach.

NOSOCOMIAL INFECTIONS IN IMPLANTABLE CENTRAL NERVOUS SYSTEM DEVICES

Patients with a ventriculostomy are at risk for ventriculitis, which has potentially devastating consequences. The incidence of ventriculitis in

Table 33–7. Antimicrobial Treatment of Nosocomial Gastrointestinal Infections*

Discontinuation of previous antibiotics	
and	
Metronidazole[†]	500 mg q.i.d. PO
or	
Vancomycin	250 mg q.i.d. PO

*Virtually always caused by *Clostridium difficile*.
[†]Drug of choice.

the NICU has decreased, most likely because of increased use of fiber-optic parenchymal intracranial pressure monitors,[66] and remains very low. Risk factors for ventriculostomy-associated infections are ventricular catheterization lasting more than 5 days, intracerebral hemorrhage with intraventricular extension, and irrigation of the device.[51] The most frequently isolated bacterial agents in ventriculitis are S. *epidermidis* and *aureus*.

Ventriculitis is typically asymptomatic early in the course and may become evident only with clinical signs of meningeal irritation and fever. Cultures of the cerebrospinal fluid confirm infection, and blood cultures often become positive.

Impregnating the ventricular catheter with rifampin and clindamycin has been suggested to prevent infection, but clinical studies of this procedure are not available. Most neurosurgeons agree that subcutaneous tunneling and prophylactic administration of antibiotics may prevent infections, but firm data are not known. Removal of the catheter after 5 days and meticulous aseptic techniques are probably equally effective. Vancomycin with cefotaxime or vancomycin with gentamicin is preferred (Table 33–8).

ANTIBIOTICS: PREREQUISITES AND USE IN INFECTION CONTROL

Once the bacterial agent is known, many effective antibiotics are available. Preferred choices directed toward specific infections are found in Table 33–9. Dosage adjustment in renal failure is shown in the Appendix. This section describes the most pertinent characteristics of these antibiotics for easy reference.

Cephalosporins

The cephalosporins are divided into classes of generations. The first-generation cephalosporins have a wide spectrum of activity that includes most of the community-acquired infectious organisms, such as S. *pneumoniae*, many E. *coli*, and *Klebsiella* but not the enterococci and not methicillin-resistant *Staphylococcus*.

The prototype of *first-generation cephalosporins* is cefazolin (Ancef, Kefzol).

Dosage
Cefazolin can be used in patients with normal renal function in a dose of 0.5 to 1.0 g every 6 to 8 hours intravenously or intramuscularly. If renal function is impaired, the main adjustment is reducing the frequency of the doses to one or two a day.

Adverse Effects
Allergic rash is probably the most common adverse effect. Commonly, the alkaline phosphatase level is increased. Hemolysis is rare. Other potential side effects are nonspecific diarrhea, abdominal cramps, and nausea.

Indications
First-generation cephalosporins are only very occasionally used in community-acquired respiratory or urinary tract infection. The drug is currently given for perioperative prophylaxis.

Examples of *second-generation cephalosporins* are cefoxitin (Mefoxin), cefamandole (Mandol), and cefotetan (Cefotan).

Dosage
The usual dosages are as follows: cefoxitin, 1 to 2 g every 4 to 6 hours or 3 g every 8 hours intravenously or intramuscularly; cefamandole, 500–1000 mg every 4 to 8 hours intramuscularly or intravenously; and cefotetan, 1 to 2 g every 12 hours intravenously.

Adverse Effects
The second-generation cephalosporins are well known to cause hypoprothrombinemia, which

Table 33–8. Combinations of Antimicrobial Agents for Treatment of Nosocomial Infections Associated with Implantable Central Nervous System Devices

Vancomycin	2 g q12h IV
with cefotaxime	1–2 g q4–6h IV
or	
Vancomycin	2 g q12h IV
with gentamicin	2–3 mg/kg q8h°

°May result in low cerebrospinal fluid levels.

Table 33–9. Drugs of Choice, Arranged by Specific Organisms, for the Treatment of Infection in Critically Ill Patients

Organism	Antimicrobial Agent of Choice	Alternative Agents
Gram-positive cocci (aerobic)		
Staphylococcus aureus		
Non-penicillinase-producing	Penicillin	Vancomycin, cephalosporin
Penicillinase-producing	Nafcillin, oxacillin	Vancomycin, cephalosporin
α-Streptococci (*S. viridans*)	Penicillin	Erythromycin, clindamycin, cephalosporin
β-Streptococci (A, B, C, G)	Penicillin	Cephalosporin, erythromycin
Streptococcus faecalis		
Serious infection	Penicillin or ampicillin + aminoglycoside	Vancomycin + aminoglycoside
Uncomplicated urinary tract infection	Ampicillin	Vancomycin
Streptococcus bovis	Penicillin	Cephalosporin, vancomycin
Streptococcus pneumoniae	Penicillin	Erythromycin, vancomycin, cephalosporin
Gram-positive bacilli (aerobic)		
Corynebacterium, group JK	Vancomycin	
Gram-negative bacilli (aerobic)		
Acinetobacter sp.	Imipenem	Penicillin and gentamicin, aminoglycoside, ceftazidime, trimethoprim-sulfamethoxazole
Campylobacter sp.	Erythromycin or quinolone	Tetracycline, gentamicin
Enterobacter sp.	Imipenem	Cefotaxime, ceftriaxone, ceftazidime, aminoglycoside
Escherichia coli	Third- or fourth-generation cephalosporin	Aminoglycoside, extended-spectrum penicillin
Haemophilus influenzae	Second-, third-, or fourth-generation cephalosporin	Trimethoprim-sulfamethoxazole
Klebsiella pneumoniae	Third- or fourth-generation cephalosporin	Aminoglycoside, aztreonam, extended-spectrum penicillin
Legionella sp.	Erythromycin ± rifampin	Ciprofloxacin
Proteus mirabilis	Ampicillin	Aminoglycoside, cephalosporin
Other *Proteus* sp.	Cefotaxime, ceftriaxone, ceftazidime	Aminoglycoside, aztreonam, imipenem
Providencia sp.	Cefotaxime, ceftriaxone, ceftazidime	Aminoglycoside, imipenem, extended-spectrum penicillin
Pseudomonas aeruginosa	Aminoglycoside + extended-spectrum penicillin	Ceftazidime, aztreonam, imipenem, cefepime
Salmonella sp.	Cefotaxime, ceftriaxone, quinolone	Ampicillin, trimethoprim-sulfamethoxazole
Serratia marcescens	Cefotaxime, ceftriaxone, ceftazidime	Aminoglycoside, imipenem, aztreonam
Shigella sp.	Quinolone	Cefotaxime, ceftriaxone, ceftazidime
Anaerobes		
Anaerobic streptococci	Penicillin	Clindamycin
Bacteroides sp.		
Oropharyngeal strains	Penicillin or clindamycin	Metronidazole
Gastrointestinal strains	Metronidazole	Cefoxitin, clindamycin, imipenem, ticarcillin-clavulanic acid, piperacillin-tazobactam
Clostridium sp. (except *C. difficile*)	Penicillin	Clindamycin, metronidazole, imipenem
Clostridium difficile	Metronidazole	Vancomycin
Other bacteria		
Actinomyces and *Arachnia*	Penicillin G	Tetracycline, clindamycin
Nocardia sp.	Trimethoprim-sulfamethoxazole	Tetracycline, imipenem
Mycobacterium tuberculosis	Isoniazid + rifampin + pyrazinamide + ethambutol	Streptomycin, ciprofloxacin, cycloserine, capreomycin, ethionamide

Source: Modified from Abramowicz M (ed): The choice of antibacterial drugs. *Med Lett Drugs Ther* 38:25–34, 1996. By permission of *The Medical Letter.*

can be prevented by prophylactic administration of vitamin K. Seizures and an acute confusional state may result from high doses.

Indications

These drugs are active against virtually all anaerobic microorganisms, including *Bacteroides fragilis*. Use has been focused on the treatment of purulent pulmonary infections that have evolved into a lung abscess or empyema.

The *third- and fourth-generation cephalosporins* have a major expanded spectrum, and their importance lies in the observation that when they are used against gram-negative infections, toxicity is much lower than that with aminoglycosides. Examples are cefotaxime (Claforan), ceftriaxone (Rocephin), ceftazidime (Fortaz), and cefepime (Maxipime).

Dosage

Cefotaxime is given in a dose of 1 to 2 g every 6 to 8 hours; ceftriaxone, 1 to 4 g every 24 hours; ceftazidime, 0.5 to 2.0 g every 8 hours, and cefepim, 1 to 2 g every 12 hours.

Adverse Effects

The side effects are the same as those with second-generation cephalosporins.

Indications

Because the third- and fourth-generation cephalosporins have an extended spectrum, they are widely used for any potentially serious infection.

Aminoglycosides

This class of antimicrobial agents is typically considered when serious gram-negative infections are present. The main advantage of these drugs over many other antibiotic agents is their superiority in the treatment of *P. aeruginosa* infections. The aminoglycosides may be used in combination with cephalosporins or broad-spectrum penicillins to achieve a synergistic effect. The most frequently used drugs are gentamicin, tobramycin, and amikacin.

Dosage

Gentamicin is given intravenously in a dose of 3 to 6 mg/kg per day divided every 8 hours; to-bramycin intravenously, 3 to 6 mg/kg per day divided every 8 hours; and amikacin, 15 mg/kg per day divided every 12 hours. The desired peak serum level (30 minutes after infusion) for gentamicin and tobramycin is 4 to 6 μg/mL; the desired trough serum level (just before the infusion) is 1 to 2 μg/mL. For amikacin, the peak and trough levels are, respectively, 20 μg/mL and 5 μg/mL.

In patients with renal failure, the interval is adjusted by multiplying the serum creatinine value by 8, which gives the dose interval in hours.

Adverse Effects

The major toxic effects are nephrotoxicity and possible destruction of vestibular or cochlear sensory cells that results in hearing loss, often detectable only with audiometry. The hearing loss may be permanent, whereas the acute tubular necrosis is reversible.

Indications

The use of aminoglycosides in patients is limited to gram-negative infections not susceptible to less toxic drugs. Their use is often reserved for very serious *Pseudomonas* infections and infections in neutropenic patients.

Penicillins

Penicillins continue to be used, particularly because of their favorable safety profile. Penicillins with activity against *Staphylococcus* and *Pseudomonas* have been used frequently. Penicillins typically used in the treatment of nosocomial infection are nafcillin (Unipen), oxacillin (Prostaphlin), piperacillin (Pipracil), mezlocillin (Mezlin), and piperacillin-tazobactam (Zosyn).

Dosage

The doses are nafcillin, 1.5 to 2.0 g every 4 hours; oxacillin, 1.5 to 2.0 g every 4 hours; and piperacillin, 2 to 3 g every 4 hours.

Adverse Effects

Allergic reaction remains the most important limiting factor. In these extended-spectrum penicillins, however, hypokalemia and decreased platelet aggregation may appear, both immediately reversible on discontinuation.

Vancomycin

This drug is widely used in many intensive care units to treat catheter-associated sepsis. It is active against gram-positive microorganisms only.

Dosage

Vancomycin, 1 g every 12 hours, is infused over 1 hour to prevent hypotension, flushing and pruritus ("red man" syndrome), and acute chest pains without demonstrable myocardial ischemia.

Adverse Effects

Prolonged high serum concentrations may produce hearing loss; nephrotoxicity is rare.

Indications

The most important indication is treatment of methicillin-resistant *S. aureus* or *epidermidis* and *Staphylococcus* infections in patients allergic to penicillins. It is also the drug of choice in *C. difficile* colitis.

ANTIBIOTIC RESISTANCE PROBLEM

Strains resistant to antibiotics have become more prevalent in recent years.[23,26,42] Examples are gram-negative bacilli resistant to third-generation cephalosporins or aminoglycosides, pneumococci resistant to penicillins, and, more significantly, enterococci resistant to multiple antibiotics. Important factors are horizontal spread in hospitals, excessive use of antibiotics in intensive care units, and world travel.

Gram-negative bacilli are becoming resistant not only to aminoglycosides but also to third-generation cephalosporins and aztreonam. Treatment with imipenem or ciprofloxacin may be effective. *P. aeruginosa* may therefore be treated with these agents, but tobramycin has been successful as well.

Penicillin-resistant pneumococci, consisting of up to 15% of U.S. strains, may be a major problem in the NICU in patients with pneumonia and meningitis. More comprehensive susceptibility testing is needed. Often, pneumococcal strains have a minimal inhibitory concentration of greater than 2 μg/mL and are resistant to third- and fourth-generation cephalosporins. Management may begin with cefotaxime if the minimal inhibitory concentration is less than 0.25 μg/mL, but in most cases, vancomycin with rifampin, imipenem, or chloramphenicol is required.

Multiple antibiotic-resistant enterococci are less common in NICUs because wound and intra-abdominal infections are less prevalent. Management is highly complex because many strains are resistant to penicillin, ampicillin, aminoglycosides, and vancomycin. The newer antibiotics linezolid and quinupristin-dalfopristin have both been approved for methicillin-resistant *S. aureus* and vancomycin-resistant enterococci. Linezolid (Zyvox) is administered intravenously (600 mg every 12 hours for up to 4 weeks).[19] Headache remains a side effect in 1 of 10 patients and is more common than diarrhea and nausea. The dalfopristin-quinupristin combination (Synercid) is also used for treatment of vancomycin-resistant enterococcus infections (7.5 mg/kg infused intravenously over 1 hour every 8 to 12 hours). Other, yet unproven, strategies are antibiotic cycling (withdrawal for a defined period and reintroduction later), hospital formulary restrictions, use of narrow spectrums and "older," more established antibiotics, and involvement of infectious disease specialists.[7] Several reviews with more detailed discussions are available.[4,5,7,20,33,34,36,56]

CONCLUSIONS

- New-onset fever often indicates infection but may be caused by resorption of blood (relative bradycardia), thromboembolism (persistent tachycardia, painful calves), or drugs (incremental increase in temperature within several days).

- Nosocomial pneumonia is typically recognized by fever, peripheral infiltrates on chest radiographs, change in sputum quality to purulent mucus, and > 25 polymorphonuclear leukocytes on Gram's stain. Empirical treatment consists of intravenous administration of ceftazidime with gentamicin.
- Phlebitis remains the most common catheter-related infection. Changing the catheter site and applying cold wet compresses are often sufficient. Catheter-associated bacteremia is an emergency that should be treated by intravenous administration of vancomycin and a cephalosporin.
- Nosocomial urinary tract infections in catheterized patients are diagnosed by increased leukocyte counts (> 10 cells/mm^3) and cultures. Empirical treatment includes aminoglycosides or vancomycin intravenously. When gram-positive cocci are suspected, vancomycin is preferred.
- Nosocomial gastrointestinal infections are invariably caused by *C. difficile*. Administration of antibiotics is discontinued, and metronidazole is given orally.
- Ventriculitis can be effectively treated with vancomycin and cefotaxime intravenously, assuming that *S. epidermidis* and *aureus* are the causative agents.
- Antibiotic resistance should be considered in patients from countries outside the United States whose condition is worsening and in patients with previous use of multiple antibiotics.

REFERENCES

1. Aoun M, Klastersky J: Drug treatment of pneumonia in the hospital. What are the choices? *Drugs* 42: 962–973, 1991.
2. Bennett SN, McNeil MM, Bland LA, et al: Postoperative infections traced to contamination of an intravenous anesthetic, propofol. *N Engl J Med* 333:147–154, 1995.
3. Bergmans DC, Bonten MJ, Gaillard CA, et al: Prevention of ventilator-associated pneumonia by oral decontamination: a prospective, randomized, double-blind, placebo-controlled study. *Am J Respir Crit Care Med* 164:382–388, 2001.
4. Bergogne-Berezin E: Current guidelines for the treatment and prevention of nosocomial infections. *Drugs* 58:51–67, 1999.
5. Berkowitz FE: Antibiotic resistance in bacteria. *South Med J* 88:797–804, 1995.
6. Brown E, Talbot GH, Axelrod P, et al: Risk factors for *Clostridium difficile* toxin-associated diarrhea. *Infect Control Hosp Epidemiol* 11:283–290, 1990.
7. Byl B, Clevenbergh P, Jacobs F, et al: Impact of infectious diseases specialists and microbiological data on the appropriateness of antimicrobial therapy for bacteremia. *Clin Infect Dis* 29:60–66, 1999.
8. Centers for Disease Control and Prevention: Guidelines for prevention of nosocomial pneumonia. *MMWR Recomm Rep* 46:1–79, 1997.
9. Cercenado E, Ena J, Rodriguez-Creixems M, et al: A conservative procedure for the diagnosis of catheter-related infections. *Arch Intern Med* 150:1417–1420, 1990.
10. Chastre J, Fagon JY: Invasive diagnostic testing should be routinely used to manage ventilated patients with suspected pneumonia. *Am J Respir Crit Care Med* 150:570–574, 1994.
11. Chastre J, Fagon JY, Domart Y, et al: Diagnosis of nosocomial pneumonia in intensive care unit patients. *Eur J Clin Microbiol Infect Dis* 8:35–39, 1989.
12. Cobb DK, High KP, Sawyer RG, et al: A controlled trial of scheduled replacement of central venous and pulmonary-artery catheters. *N Engl J Med* 327:1062–1068, 1992.
13. Cockerill FR III, Muller SR, Anhalt JP, et al: Prevention of infection in critically ill patients by selective decontamination of the digestive tract. *Ann Intern Med* 117:545–553, 1992.
14. Craven DE, Barber TW, Steger KA, et al: Nosocomial pneumonia in the 1990s: update of epidemiology and risk factors. *Semin Respir Infect* 5:157–172, 1990.
15. Craven DE, Steger KA: Nosocomial pneumonia in the intubated patient. New concepts on pathogenesis and prevention. *Infect Dis Clin North Am* 3:843–866, 1989.
16. Cunha BA: Antibiotic side effects. *Med Clin North Am* 85:149–185, 2001.
17. Darouiche RO, Raad II, Heard SO, et al: A comparison of two antimicrobial-impregnated central venous catheters. Catheter Study Group. *N Engl J Med* 340:1–8, 1999.
18. Darouiche RO, Smith JA Jr, Hanna H, et al: Efficacy of antimicrobial-impregnated bladder catheters in reducing catheter-associated bacteriuria: a prospective, randomized, multicenter clinical trial. *Urology* 54:976–981, 1999.
19. Dikema DJ, Jones RN: Oxazolidinone antibiotics. *Lancet* 358:1975–1982, 2001.
20. Felmingham D: Antibiotic resistance. Do we need new therapeutic approaches? *Chest* 108 Suppl 2:70S–78S, 1995.

21. Ferrer M, Torres A, Gonzalez J, et al: Utility of selective digestive decontamination in mechanically ventilated patients. *Ann Intern Med* 120:389–395, 1994.

22. Flaherty JP, Weinstein RA: Infection control and pneumonia prophylaxis strategies in the intensive care unit. *Semin Respir Infect* 5:191–203, 1990.

23. Friedland IR, McCracken GH Jr: Management of infections caused by antibiotic-resistant *Streptococcus pneumoniae*. *N Engl J Med* 331:377–382, 1994.

24. George DL: Epidemiology of nosocomial ventilator-associated pneumonia. *Infect Control Hosp Epidemiol* 14:163–169, 1993.

25. Gerding DN, Olson MM, Peterson LR, et al: *Clostridium difficile*-associated diarrhea and colitis in adults. A prospective case-controlled epidemiologic study. *Arch Intern Med* 146:95–100, 1986.

26. Grayson ML, Eliopoulos GM: Antimicrobial resistance in the intensive care unit. *Semin Respir Infect* 5:204–214, 1990.

27. Hamer DH, Barza M: Prevention of hospital-acquired pneumonia in critically ill patients. *Antimicrob Agents Chemother* 37:931–938, 1993.

28. Hayon J, Figliolini C, Combes A, et al: Role of serial routine microbiologic culture results in the initial management of ventilator-associated pneumonia. *Am J Respir Crit Care Med* 165:41–46, 2002.

29. Hill RL, Fisher AP, Ware RJ, et al: Mupirocin for the reduction of colonization of internal jugular cannulae—a randomized controlled trial. *J Hosp Infect* 15:311–321, 1990.

30. Ibrahim EH, Tracy L, Hill C, et al: The occurrence of ventilator-associated pneumonia in a community hospital: risk factors and clinical outcomes. *Chest* 120:555–561, 2001.

31. Iregui M, Kollef MH: Prevention of ventilator-associated pneumonia: selecting interventions that make a difference. *Chest* 121:679–681, 2002.

32. Kamal GD, Pfaller MA, Rempe LE, et al: Reduced intravascular catheter infection by antibiotic bonding. A prospective, randomized, controlled trial. *JAMA* 265:2364–2368, 1991.

33. Kollef MH: Optimizing antibiotic therapy in the intensive care unit setting. *Crit Care* 5:189–195, 2001.

34. Kollef MH, Fraser VJ: Antibiotic resistance in the intensive care unit. *Ann Intern Med* 134:298–314, 2001.

35. Korinek AM, Laisne MJ, Nicolas MH, et al: Selective decontamination of the digestive tract in neurosurgical intensive care unit patients: a double-blind, randomized, placebo-controlled study. *Crit Care Med* 21:1466–1473, 1993.

36. Kunin CM: Resistance to antimicrobial drugs—a worldwide calamity. *Ann Intern Med* 118:557–561, 1993.

37. Lowry PW, Tompkins LS: Nosocomial legionellosis: a review of pulmonary and extrapulmonary syndromes. *Am J Infect Control* 21:21–27, 1993.

38. Maki DG, Ringer M, Alvarado CJ: Prospective randomised trial of povidone-iodine, alcohol, and chlorhexidine for prevention of infection associated with central venous and arterial catheters. *Lancet* 338:339–343, 1991.

39. McFarland LV, Mulligan ME, Kwok RY, et al: Nosocomial acquisition of *Clostridium difficile* infection. *N Engl J Med* 320:204–210, 1989.

40. Meduri GU: Ventilator-associated pneumonia in patients with respiratory failure. A diagnostic approach. *Chest* 97:1208–1219, 1990.

41. Moro ML, Vigano EF, Cozzi Lepri A: Risk factors for central venous catheter-related infections in surgical and intensive care units. The Central Venous Catheter-Related Infections Study Group. *Infect Control Hosp Epidemiol* 15:253–264, 1994.

42. Murray BE: New aspects of antimicrobial resistance and the resulting therapeutic dilemmas. *J Infect Dis* 163:1184–1194, 1991.

43. Nathens AB, Chu PT, Marshall JC: Nosocomial infection in the surgical intensive care unit. *Infect Dis Clin North Am* 6:657–675, 1992.

44. Nichols RL, Smith JW: Bacterial contamination of an anesthetic agent (editorial). *N Engl J Med* 333:184–185, 1995.

45. Niederman MS, Torres A, Summer W: Invasive diagnostic testing is not needed routinely to manage suspected ventilator-associated pneumonia. *Am J Respir Crit Care Med* 150:565–569, 1994.

46. Pittet D, Tarara D, Wenzel RP: Nosocomial bloodstream infection in critically ill patients. Excess length of stay, extra costs, and attributable mortality. *JAMA* 271:1598–1601, 1994.

47. Pugin J, Auckenthaler R, Mili N, et al: Diagnosis of ventilator-associated pneumonia by bacteriologic analysis of bronchoscopic and nonbronchoscopic "blind" bronchoalveolar lavage fluid. *Am Rev Respir Dis* 143:1121–1129, 1991.

48. Putterman C: Central venous catheter related sepsis: a clinical review. *Resuscitation* 20:1–16, 1990.

49. Raad I, Bodey GP: Infectious complications of indwelling vascular catheters. *Clin Infect Dis* 15:197–208, 1992.

50. Raad I, Darouiche R, Hachem R, et al: The broad-spectrum activity and efficacy of catheters coated with minocycline and rifampin. *J Infect Dis* 173:418–424, 1996.

51. Rebuck JA, Murry KR, Rhoney DH, et al: Infection related to intracranial pressure monitors in adults: analysis of risk factors and antibiotic prophylaxis. *J Neurol Neurosurg Psychiatry* 69:381–384, 2000.

52. Rello J, Ausina V, Ricart M, et al: Nosocomial pneumonia in critically ill comatose patients: need for a differential therapeutic approach. *Eur Respir J* 5:1249–1253, 1992.

53. Richet H, Hubert B, Nitemberg G, et al: Prospective multicenter study of vascular-catheter-related complications and risk factors for positive central-catheter cultures in intensive care unit patients. *J Clin Microbiol* 28:2520–2525, 1990.

54. Rodriguez JL: Hospital-acquired gram-negative pneumonia in critically ill, injured patients. *Am J Surg* 165 Suppl 2A:34S–42S, 1993.

55. Scheld WM, Mandell GL: Nosocomial pneumonia: pathogenesis and recent advances in diagnosis and therapy. *Rev Infect Dis* 13 Suppl 9:743S–751S, 1991.

56. Schentag JJ: Antimicrobial management strategies for gram-positive bacterial resistance in the intensive care unit. *Crit Care Med* 29 Suppl:N100–N107, 2001.

57. Septimus EJ: Nosocomial bacterial pneumonias. *Semin Respir Infect* 4:245–252, 1989.

58. Tay L, Ong PL, Lang L: Nosocomial infections in a neurosurgery department. *Ann Acad Med Singapore* 16:565–570, 1987.

59. Torres A, Gatell JM, Aznar E, et al: Re-intubation increases the risk of nosocomial pneumonia in patients needing mechanical ventilation. *Am J Respir Crit Care Med* 152:137–141, 1995.

60. Tryba M: The gastropulmonary route of infection—fact or fiction? *Am J Med* 91:135S–146S, 1991.

61. Turner J: Hand-washing behavior versus hand-washing guidelines in the ICU. *Heart Lung* 22:275–277, 1993.

62. Valles J, Artigas A, Rello J, et al: Continuous aspiration of subglottic secretions in preventing ventilator-associated pneumonia. *Ann Intern Med* 122:179–186, 1995.

63. Weinstein RA: Epidemiology and control of nosocomial infections in adult intensive care units. *Am J Med* 91:179S–184S, 1991.

64. Weinstein RA: Failure of infection control in intensive care units: Can sucralfate improve the situation? *Am J Med* 91:132S–134S, 1991.

65. Winer-Muram HT, Jennings SG, Wunderink RG, et al: Ventilator-associated *Pseudomonas aeruginosa* pneumonia: radiographic findings. *Radiology* 195:247–252, 1995.

66. Winfield JA, Rosenthal P, Kanter RK, et al: Duration of intracranial pressure monitoring does not predict daily risk of infectious complications. *Neurosurgery* 33:424–430, 1993.

67. Wittesjo B, Bjornham A, Eitrem R: Relative bradycardia in infectious diseases. *J Infect* 39:246–247, 1999.

68. Zimakoff J, Stormark M, Larsen SO: Use of gloves and handwashing behaviour among health care workers in intensive care units. A multicentre investigation in four hospitals in Denmark and Norway. *J Hosp Infect* 24:63–67, 1993.

PART VI

DECISIONS AT THE END OF LIFE AND OTHER RESPONSIBILITIES

34

Brain Death and
Organ Procurement

There are limits beyond which treatment of catastrophic brain injury cannot go, leaving an irrecoverable condition and persistent coma. A clear dividing line exists between severe brain damage and complete loss of brain and brain stem function. *Brain death* is synonymous with total loss of brain function in a nondrugged, normothermic, apneic comatose patient without a major confounding acute systemic or metabolic derangement. We are dead when our brains are dead. Brain death means life has come to an end and the person has passed away. Life support is briefly continued to make organ donation possible. However, regrettably, from time to time essays appear that attempt to portray this state as a steadfast controversy, claiming the clinical diagnosis is an issue that demands serious reconsideration, and some of them even reach a point of arousing unnecessary mistrust.[55] Manipulation of the current carefully constructed law can only harm the 80,000 patients on the waiting list for transplantation.

Brain death in adults is frequently a consequence of severe traumatic brain injury, rerupture in aneurysmal subarachnoid hemorrhage, and intracerebral hemorrhage.[10] It is less common in patients with fulminant encephalitis or bacterial meningitis and after anoxic-ischemic encephalopathy from cardiac resuscitation.

Neurologists with experience in neurologic intensive care and neurosurgeons are commonly involved in the clinical determination of brain death, but physicians on staff of any specialty are potentially allowed to arrive at the same conclusion. This task is highly complicated and includes assessment of the proximate cause, interpretation of neuroimaging findings, recognition of conditions that can mimic brain death, proper execution of the apnea test, knowledge of confirmatory tests and how to interpret results, and management of acute physiologic derangements (e.g., diabetes insipidus) associated with brain death. Early identification of potential organ and tissue donor candidates is very important, but selection of donors can proceed only after the clinical diagnosis of brain death and the consent of family members or a legal representative. The determination of brain death has been reviewed and published as a position paper by the American Academy of Neurology.[72,82] Many other documents exist.[9,10,18,61,62,70,71,81,84,85]

NATIONAL AND INTERNATIONAL CRITERIA

In the United States, legal justification for the determination of death by neurologic criteria is established in the Uniform Determination of Death Act,[80] but neurologists or neurosurgeons should comply with state law and hospital policies and with any other modifications that may be in place.

When a neurologist or neurosurgeon is not involved in care or is unavailable for consultation, staff intensivists or pediatricians typically declare brain death. There is a general consensus that transplant surgeons are not involved in the clinical diagnosis, but this nowadays might be a cliché, and in the United States we have not come across an "aggressive transplant surgeon or representative" interfering with the examination or trying to speed up tests against the physician's will. (Nonetheless, a disturbing account of a pressured neurologist in earlier years has been recorded.[38]) Determination by one physician is sufficient in most states, but independent confirmation by another physician is required in Alabama, California, Connecticut, Florida, Iowa, Kentucky, Louisiana, and Virginia. In Alaska and Georgia, a registered nurse can be the delegated authority to declare death, according to their statutory criteria, but certification by a physician is needed within 24 hours. Other examples of differences in the United States are that only a physician in the neurosciences can make the determination in Virginia and that the right to have a religious exemption is accepted in New Jersey and New York. These amendments in those states require physicians to honor the request to continue medical care in a brain-dead body.

There is a broad acceptance of the concept of brain death throughout the world. However, brain death guidelines are diverse, and some are very complicated.[86] Precise documentation of brain stem reflexes prevails, but apnea testing with $PaCO_2$ confirmation is regulated in approximately two-thirds of the protocols. The number of physicians varies from one to four, and in some countries, only seasoned physicians with at least associate professor status are allowed to make the determination.[86] Equally troubling is the great variation in time of observation. Many countries, without appropriate justification, require a 24-hour interval in patients who become brain dead after cardiac resuscitation. Confirmatory tests are mandatory in approximately one-third of the countries and are skewed toward bedside tests. Several European countries have longer observation periods if anoxia caused brain death.[36] The reason may be that because brain edema develops later, confirmatory tests performed soon after clinical assessment often show residual brain function. This clause is irrelevant if confirmatory tests are not mandated. These differences are undesirable. In the future, consensus on simplified criteria should be obtained.

CLINICAL DIAGNOSIS OF BRAIN DEATH

The clinical diagnosis of brain death is equivalent to irreversible loss of all brain and brain stem function. Loss of consciousness, lack of a coordinated motor response to pain stimuli, absence of brain stem reflexes, and apnea must be documented.

The cause of brain death should be clear from neuroimaging. In most patients, initial cranial CT reveals diffuse cerebral edema, acute mass with profound tissue shift, or multiple hemispheric lesions destroying most of the brain. Obviously, the clinical diagnosis of brain death should be in doubt in patients with normal CT findings. However, this situation occurs in patients with a severe, prolonged anoxic-ischemic insult to the brain (cardiac arrest, asphyxia). In these patients, the clinical diagnosis of brain death should be made only if there is a high degree of certainty about the mechanism that led to brain death. In addition, a CSF examination is warranted to detect infection in patients with initially normal CT scans. In many patients with such a fulminant meningitis or encephalitis, diffuse edema of the brain will appear on CT scans.

Confounding factors that mimic or partly mimic brain death should be excluded. First, hypothermia may blunt brain stem reflexes but only if core temperatures are below 32°C.[23,25] With core temperatures below 27°C, brain stem reflexes most likely become absent. Second, the influence of any drug effect should be excluded. Routine drug screens may be helpful but only when testing is requested for a specific drug or poison. Drug screens may detect alcohol, barbiturates, antiepileptic agents, benzodiazepines, antihistamines, antidepressants, antipsychotic agents, amphetamines, narcotics, and analgesics. The diagnosis of brain death most likely can be made when blood levels of barbiturates are subtherapeutic; however, data are lacking in adults. In brain-dead children with therapeutic levels of barbiturates, no change in isoelectric electroencephalograms was noted during a decrease of barbiturates in the blood to subtherapeutic or undetectable levels.[47] As discussed in Chapter 9, barbiturates also may reduce cerebral blood flow through a mechanism of vasoconstriction, but a more likely explanation for reduced flow is a marked decrease in metabolic demand. The effect of high doses of barbiturates on cerebral blood flow in patients is not known. It is a violation of the protocol to replace a clinical examination confounded by sedative agents such as barbiturates with four-vessel cerebral angiography or another test of blood flow. Third, the clinical diagnosis of brain death is probably not reliable in patients investigated at the time of an acute severe metabolic or endocrine derangement, but clear threshold values are not known. Fourth, alcohol intoxication and head and spine injury are often closely linked. The condition of patients with apnea and quadriplegia due to traumatic cervical spine distraction and alcohol intoxication may superficially mimic brain death if the brain stem reflexes are not carefully examined.[66] Alcohol has a plasma half-life of 10 mL/hour, and the limit for determination of brain death would be similar to the limit for driving, which in most U.S. states is 0.8, or 800 mg/L. (One can argue that if you can drive with this level of alcohol, you can certainly be dead with it.)

In summary, in the United States, the clinical diagnosis of brain death requires that both brain and brain stem function be absent. To overcome the pitfalls of misdiagnosis, the following prerequisites are proposed: (1) definite clinical, neuroimaging, or CSF evidence of an acute central nervous system catastrophe compatible with brain death, (2) lack of complicating medical conditions that may confound clinical assessment (no severe electrolyte, acid-base, or endocrine disturbance), (3) no drug intoxication or poisoning, and (4) core temperature of at least 32°C (90°F). Testing of brain function can proceed only after these requirements have been satisfied.

PRACTICE OF BRAIN DEATH DETERMINATION

The following guidelines have been proposed[82,85] (Fig. 34–1).

Coma or Unresponsiveness

Motor responses of the limbs to painful stimuli should be absent after pressure on the supraorbital nerve, nail-bed pressure stimulus, or simultaneous pressure on both temporomandibular condyles.

One should be aware of several pitfalls. Motor responses (usually brief finger flexion without coordinated responses) of spinal origin may occur spontaneously during apnea testing, often during hypoxic or hypotensive episodes, or during pain stimuli. Sometimes these movements are synchronous with the mechanical ventilator cycle.[57,77] Neuromuscular blocking agents can produce prolonged weakness.[63] If neuromuscular blocking agents have recently been administered, examination with a bedside peripheral nerve stimulator is needed. A train-of-four stimulus should result in four thumb twitches when the neuromuscular blocking agent has been fully washed out.

Absence of Brain Stem Reflexes

Pupils

The response to bright light should be absent in both eyes. Round, oval, or irregular-shaped pupils are compatible with brain death. Most pupils in brain death are in midposition (6 to 7 mm).[51] Dilated pupils are compatible with brain death because intact sympathetic cervical pathways connected with the radially arranged fibers of the dilator muscle may remain intact. Miosis is very uncommon but can occur with massive pontine destruction.

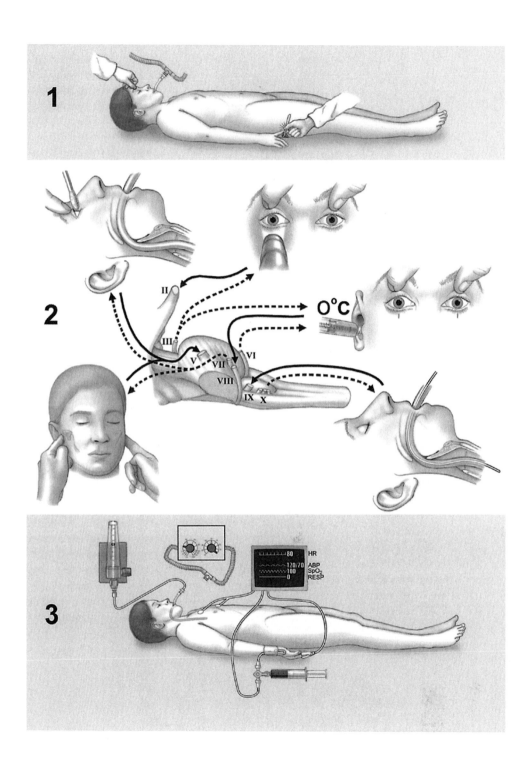

Figure 34–1. Steps in assessing brain death. In step 1, the physician determines that there is no motor response and the eyes do not open when a painful stimulus is applied to the supraorbital nerve or nail bed. In step 2, a clinical assessment of brain stem reflexes is undertaken. The tested cranial nerves are indicated by Roman numerals; the solid arrows represent afferent limbs, and the broken arrows efferent limbs. Depicted are the absence of grimacing or eye opening with deep pressure on both condyles at the level of the temporomandibular joint (afferent nerve V and efferent nerve VII), the absent corneal reflex elicited by touching the edge of the cornea (V and VII), the absent light reflex (II and III), the absent oculovestibular response toward the side of the cold stimulus provided by ice water (pen marks at the level of the pupils can be used as reference) (VIII and III and VI), and the absent cough reflex elicited through the introduction of a suction catheter deep in the trachea (IX and X). In step 3, the apnea test is performed; the disconnection of the ventilator and the use of apneic diffusion oxygenation require precautionary measures. The core temperature should be raised to 36.5°C or higher, the systolic blood pressure should be 90 mm Hg or higher, and the fluid balance should be positive for 6 hours. After preoxygenation (the fraction of inspired oxygen should be 1.0 for 10 minutes), the ventilation rate should be decreased. The ventilator should be disconnected if the partial pressure of arterial oxygen reaches 200 mm Hg or higher and if the partial pressure of arterial carbon dioxide reaches 40 mm Hg or higher. The oxygen catheter should be at the carina (delivering oxygen at a rate of 6 L/minute). The physician should observe the chest and the abdominal wall for respiration for 8 to 10 minutes and should monitor the patient for changes in vital functions. If there is a partial pressure of arterial carbon dioxide of 60 mm Hg or higher or an increase of more than 20 mm Hg from the normal baseline value, apnea is confirmed. ABP, arterial blood pressure; HR, heart rate; RESP, respirations; SpO2, oxygen saturation measured by pulse oximetry. (From Wijdicks.[85] By permission of Mayo Foundation.)

Many drugs can influence pupil size, but light response remains intact. In conventional doses, atropine given intravenously has no marked influence on pupillary response.[27,31] A report of fixed, dilated pupils after extremely high doses of dopamine has not been confirmed.[59] Because nicotine receptors are absent in the iris, neuromuscular blocking drugs do not noticeably influence pupil size.[30] Topical ocular instillation of drugs and trauma to the cornea or bulbus oculi can cause abnormalities in pupil size and produce nonreactive pupils. Preexisting anatomical abnormalities of the iris or effects of previous surgery should be excluded.

Ocular Movements

Ocular movements are absent after head turning and caloric testing with ice water. (Testing is done only when no fractures or instability of the cervical spine is apparent, and in patients with head injury, the cervical spine must be im-

aged to exclude potential fractures or instability, or both.) The oculocephalic reflex, elicited by fast and vigorous turning of the head from middle position to 90° on both sides, normally results in eye deviation to the opposite side of the head turning. Vertical eye movements should be tested with brisk neck flexion. Eyelid opening and vertical and horizontal eye movements must be absent in brain death.

Caloric testing should be done with the head elevated to 30° during irrigation of the tympanum on each side with 50 mL of ice water. Tympanum irrigation can be best accomplished by inserting a small suction catheter into the external auditory canal and connecting it to a 50 mL syringe filled with ice water. One may consider marking the lower eyelid at the level of the pupil with a felt-tip pen to reduce errors in observation. Tonic deviation of the eyes directed to the cold caloric stimulus is absent. The investigator should allow up to 1 minute after injection, and the time between stimulation on each side should be at least 5 minutes.

Drugs that can diminish or completely abolish the caloric response are sedatives, aminoglycosides, tricyclic antidepressants, anticholinergics, antiepileptic drugs, and chemotherapeutic agents. After closed head injury or facial trauma, lid edema and chemosis of the conjunctiva may restrict movement of the globes. Clotted blood or cerumen may diminish the caloric response, and repeat testing is required after otologic inspection. Basal fracture of the petrous bone abolishes the caloric response unilaterally only and may be identified by an ecchymotic mastoid process (Chapter 23).

Facial Sensation and Facial Motor Response

Corneal reflexes should be absent and can be tested by briefly tapping the cornea with a throat swab. The jaw often has drooped. The jaw reflex should be absent. Grimacing to pain can be tested by using standard pain stimuli (Chapter 10).

One should be aware that severe facial trauma may diminish all brain stem reflexes.

Pharyngeal and Tracheal Reflexes

Lack of a cough response to tracheal suctioning (not just placement) should be demonstrated. Usually a suction catheter is advanced to the level of the carina. Movement of the endotracheal tube up and down may not be sufficient to stimulate cough.

Apnea

An important component of the clinical diagnosis of brain death is the demonstration of apnea. Loss of brain stem function produces loss of breathing and vasomotor control that results in apnea and hypotension. Hypotension (from many possible causes) is frequently present at the time of the clinical diagnosis of brain death, but blood pressure can depend on intravascular volume challenged by concomitant diabetes insipidus and on the dose of inotropes. Hypotension is not an absolute criterion for the diagnosis of brain death, but in the vast majority of cases, increasing doses of vasopressors and inotropes are needed.

Apnea is due to destruction of ventrolateral medullary structures. The respiratory neurons are controlled by central chemoreceptors that sense changes in pH of the cerebrospinal fluid, and these accurately reflect changes in arterial PCO_2.[12] There are many other mechanical and chemical stimuli and inhibitory influences to the respiratory neurons of the brain stem.

It is not known at what arterial PCO_2 level the chemoreceptors of the respiratory center are maximally stimulated in hyperoxygenated patients with brain stem destruction. Target arterial PCO_2 of 60 mm Hg is derived from findings in a small number of patients who had respiratory efforts after induction of hypercapnia, but below this value, and who otherwise fulfilled the criteria for the clinical diagnosis of brain death. Lower target levels have been suggested, because one study showed that four patients made effective normal breathing efforts at lower PCO_2 values (range, 30 to 37 mm Hg; mean, 34 mm Hg). At higher arterial PCO_2 values (range, 41 to 51 mm Hg), respiratory-like movements have been observed.[76] These movements are ineffective for ventilation and consist of shoulder elevation and adduction, back arching, and intercostal expansion. These respiratory-like efforts produce negligible tidal volumes and virtually no inspiratory force. In all patients we have seen who otherwise fulfilled the clinical criteria for brain death, breathing also began at a much lower arterial PCO_2 level (approximately 30 to 40 mm Hg). In these patients with a preserved breathing trigger but otherwise completely absent brain stem reflexes, breathing starts within minutes after disconnection from the ventilator, assuming the arterial PCO_2 has been normalized before testing. Repeat testing after no triggering of the ventilator is noted often shows apnea. This may take 24 to 48 hours.

Brain death should be differentiated from an unusual clinical entity, recently pathologically confirmed, of isolated preserved medulla function.[87] Traces of cough response after repeated stimuli, no need for inotropes to support blood pressure, and retained bradycardia after intravenous injection of atropine are salient features of this comatose state ("medulla man"). Technically, the clinical diagnosis of brain death cannot be made, but it is very unlikely that patients survive beyond a vegetative state. In this comatose state, the typical accelerating disintegration of systemic functions leading to cardiac arrest may be absent.[87]

The target arterial P_{CO_2} levels of the apnea tests in brain death determination may be higher in patients with chronic hypercapnia ("CO_2 retainers"). Typically, these patients have severe chronic obstructive pulmonary disease, bronchiectasis, sleep apnea, and morbid obesity. In the absence of metabolic acidosis (e.g., after seizures, sepsis), chronic hypercapnia can be suspected in patients with increased serum concentrations of bicarbonate.[26] If the initial arterial blood gas determination confirms chronic hypercapnia in these patients, the apnea test result could be unreliable, and additional noninvasive confirmatory tests are strongly encouraged.

Hypocapnia can be expected in patients with acute catastrophic structural damage to the central nervous system. In many instances, hypocapnia is caused by high tidal volumes associated with mechanical ventilation, by hyperventilation instituted to decrease intracranial pressure, or by hypothermia. Hypocapnia can be corrected by decreasing either the rate or the tidal volume for several minutes to change the minute volume.

Apnea testing is greatly facilitated by a starting arterial P_{CO_2} value of 40 mm Hg, because the target level of 60 mm Hg is generally reached 6 to 8 minutes after disconnection from the ventilator. (The estimated P_{CO_2} increase is from 3 to 6 mm Hg per minute.[22]) Failure to reach the Pa_{CO_2} target (60 mm Hg, or a 20 mm Hg increase above the normal baseline) may be due to relative hypothermia (32°C to 36°C) and an excessively high flow of oxygen (more than 10 L/min) that washes out rather than provides oxygen.

Cardiac arrhythmias are side effects of severe hypercapnia and respiratory acidosis, occurring mostly in patients with severe hypoxia.[21] Oxygenation may be inadequate, for example, in patients with severe pulmonary disease, acute respiratory distress syndrome, or neurogenic pulmonary edema. The most common abnormalities are premature ventricular

contractions and ventricular tachycardia. Severe hypotension (change in mean arterial blood pressure of more than 15%) has been observed in well-oxygenated patients in whom arterial P_{CO_2} values reached very high levels (average, 90 mm Hg). Respiratory acidosis can be implicated as a cause of myocardial depression.[83] Administration of 100% oxygen through a catheter placed at the level of the carina secures adequate oxygenation during apnea testing. A study of 70 apnea tests found no significant hypoxemia after previous oxygenation and placement of a catheter inside the endotracheal tube.[41] We found that lack of preoxygenation increased the chance of hypotension.[29] Use of high-flow oxygen (10 to 15 L/minute) has been linked to pneumothorax, but the causality is doubtful.[90] Pneumothorax may be seen more often in patients with progression to brain death who had cardiopulmonary resuscitation or polytrauma.

The literature does not provide evidence to favor one method over another.[5,8,20,56,76] Apnea testing by carbon dioxide augmentation was studied in 34 patients. After preoxygenation, carbon dioxide was insufflated at 1 L/minute; at 1 and 2 minutes later, Pa_{CO_2} was checked, followed by disconnection for respiratory movements. The main advantage is that respiratory movements can be observed when Pa_{CO_2} is at a target level rather than after waiting for the Pa_{CO_2} value to increase during continuous observation of the patient for 8 to 10 minutes. The main objections are that the equipment is not readily available in most units and that, most importantly, there is a danger of overcompensation to hypercapnia and acidosis, potentially leading to hypotension and cardiac arrhythmias. In Lang's study,[49] P_{CO_2} values ranged from 60 to 80 mm Hg after 1 minute and from 70 to 95 mm Hg after 2 minutes of insufflation.

Another method of apnea testing is hypoventilation. This method involves a sudden decrease in minute ventilation to 1 L/minute through a decrease in the rate-tidal volume (500 mL) and the ventilator rate (2 breaths/minute) with end-tidal P_{CO_2} monitoring. This method undoubtedly has value, but end-tidal

Pco_2 may not reflect $Paco_2$ in patients with neurogenic pulmonary edema, and the method is more time-consuming (more than 15 minutes may be required to reach target Pco_2 values). Determination of apnea by reliance on the ventilator alarm may be misleading, and we and others have noted "breathing efforts" recorded on the ventilator display in apneic patients purely as a result of positive pressure insufflation.[88]

The apnea test using the apneic oxygen diffusion method is usually safe when performed with a strict protocol. Moderate respiratory acidosis has no significant effect on left ventricular function.[60] Severe respiratory acidosis (pH ≤ 7.0 mm Hg) and severe hypoxemia ($Po_2 < 60$ mm Hg), however, can induce significant cardiac arrhythmias, including ventricular fibrillation.

Important changes in vital signs (e.g., marked hypotension, severe cardiac arrhythmias) during the apnea test may be related to inadequate precautions, although they may occur spontaneously during increasing acidosis. Therefore, the following prerequisites are suggested: (1) core temperature ≥ 36°C (97°F) (4°C higher than the required 32°C for clinical diagnosis of brain death), (2) systolic blood pressure ≥ 90 mm Hg, (3) positive fluid balance in the past 6 hours, (4) arterial Pco_2 ≥ 40 mm Hg, and (5) arterial Po_2 ≥ 200 mm Hg.

One should look closely for respiratory movements. Respiration is defined as abdominal or chest excursions that produce adequate tidal volumes. If present, respiration can be expected early in the apnea test. When respiratory-like movements occur, they can be expected at the end of the apnea test, often when oxygenation may have become marginal. Figure 34–1 illustrates the procedure for the apnea test.

Clinical Observations Compatible with the Diagnosis of Brain Death

Respiratory acidosis, hypoxia, or brisk neck flexion may generate spinal cord responses.[46] Spontaneous movements of the limbs from spinal mechanisms can occur and are more frequent in young adults.[43,44,74] These spinal reflexes include rapid flexion in arms, raising of all limbs or one limb off the bed ("Lazarus sign"), grasping movements, spontaneous jerking of one leg, and walking-like movements. Much more common, if any movements occur, are finger flexion or brief adducting movements of the fingers. Multifocal vigorous myoclonus in the shoulders is occasionally seen in young patients, and its spinal origin is confirmed by an isoelectric electroencephalogram. Stepping movements in the legs (an exaggerated alternating triple-flexion response) may occur just before all brain stem function disappears.

Respiratory-like movements are typical agonal breathing patterns. They are characterized by shoulder elevation and adduction, back arching, and intercostal expansion without any significant measurable tidal volume.

Other, much less common, responses are profuse sweating, blushing, tachycardia, and sudden increases in blood pressure.[15] These hemodynamic responses can sometimes be elicited by neck flexion, and they can be eliminated by ganglionic blockers (e.g., trimethaphan). Muscle stretch reflexes, superficial abdominal reflexes, and Babinski's signs are of spinal origin and thus do not invalidate a diagnosis of brain death. Patients may have initial plantar flexion of the great toe followed by sequential brief plantar flexion of the second, third, fourth, and fifth toes after snapping of one of the toes ("undulating toe flexion sign").

CONFIRMATORY LABORATORY TESTS

Brain death is a clinical diagnosis. A repeat clinical evaluation 6 hours later is advised, but a firm recommendation cannot be given and the interval is very arbitrary. Some hospitals adopt their own guidelines, which may include the opinions of two independent observers. In adults, a confirmatory test is not mandated in the United States, the United Kingdom, and many European countries. In the United States, a confirmatory test could be used for patients in whom some specific components of clinical testing cannot be reliably evaluated, but it should not replace neurologic examination if major confounders are present. Clinical experience with confirmatory tests other than electroencephalography, transcranial Doppler ultrasonography, and conventional angiography is limited. Studies reporting the results of confirmatory tests did not use blind assessment of the results, did not assess interobserver variation, and generally did not perform tests in control subjects with catastrophic central nervous system lesions but not brain death. In addition, many tests require costly equipment and well-trained technicians. Unfortunately, some physicians may supplement a clinical examination with a confirmatory test and then agonize over why the results are conflicting. At least in adults, when a methodically precise clinical examination has been performed, confirmatory tests should be ordered sparingly.

Confirmatory tests that are generally accepted as standards are electroencephalography and conventional cerebral angiography. Consensus criteria have been reported for electroencephalography and transcranial Doppler ultrasonography.[19]

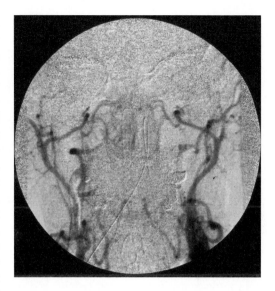

Figure 34–2. Carotid angiogram showing lack of intracranial flow.

Conventional Angiography

Technique
Four-vessel angiography with arch injection is done in the radiology suite. Iodinated contrast medium is injected under high pressure in both the anterior and the posterior circulations. The procedure takes a few hours.[11,13,32,37,50]

Result
Intracerebral filling is absent when arteries enter the dura (Fig. 34–2). The external carotid circulation is patent and fills rapidly. At times delayed filling of the superior longitudinal sinus is seen.

Validity
Interobserver studies have not been published. The procedure has the potential to yield conflicting results because no guidelines for interpretation have been developed.

Disadvantage
Repeated contrast injections may increase the risk of nephrotoxicity and theoretically decrease the acceptance rate in organ recipients.

Electroencephalography

Technique
Usually, a 16- or 18-channel instrument is used with guidelines developed by the American Electroencephalographic Society for recording brain death.[1,7,17,39,45]

Result
No electrical activity occurs above 2 μV at a sensitivity of 2 μV/mm with filter setting at 0.1 or 0.3 second and 70 Hz. Recording should continue for at least 30 minutes (see Chapter 11).

Validity
Most patients meeting the clinical criteria for brain death have isoelectric electroencephalograms. Nevertheless, in a consecutive series of 56 patients fulfilling the clinical diagnosis of brain death, 20% had residual electroencephalographic activity that lasted up to 168 hours.[33]

Disadvantage

Considerable artifacts (intravenous pumps, mechanical ventilator) due to high-gain settings in the intensive care unit may limit interpretation.

Nuclear Brain Scan

Technique

The procedure can be performed at the bedside and takes approximately 15 minutes. The isotope technetium 99m hexamethylpropyleneamine oxime (^{99m}Tc-HMPAO) should be injected within 30 minutes of reconstitution.[24,52,89] A portable gamma camera produces planar views within 5 to 10 minutes. Correct intravenous injection can be checked by taking additional chest and abdominal images.

Result

No uptake occurs in the brain parenchyma ("hollow skull" or "empty light bulb" sign) (see Chapter 11).

Validity

Experience with this technique in adults is limited, but increasing sensitivity has been reported to be as low as 94%, with a specificity of 100%. Reproducibility has been tested in only a few patients. The correlation between cerebral angiography and ^{99m}Tc-HMPAO scintigraphy was excellent.[24]

Disadvantages

The costs are currently high and the technique is not widely available; expertise is limited.

Transcranial Doppler Ultrasonography

Technique

A portable 2-MHz pulsed Doppler instrument can be used at the bedside. Two intracranial arteries should be insonated (middle cerebral artery through the temporal bone above the zygomatic arch and the vertebral or basilar arteries through the suboccipital transcranial window). The transorbital window and the middle cerebral artery may be used and may increase detection of typical flow patterns.[34,35,48,65,68,75]

Result

Transcranial Doppler signals that have been reported in brain death are described in Chapter 11. Lack of transcranial Doppler signals cannot be interpreted as confirmatory of brain death, because 10% of patients may not have temporal insonation windows. Possibly an exception can be made in patients who had transcranial Doppler signals during admission that disappeared at the time of brain death.

Validity

There is a comparatively large experience with transcranial Doppler ultrasonography in the confirmation of brain death. The sensitivity and specificity of the procedure are 91% and 100%, respectively. Occasionally, transcranial Doppler ultrasonography demonstrates "brain death patterns" in patients who are clinically brain dead but have electroencephalographic activity. Small systolic peaks and increased diastolic flow may occur as transient phenomena in patients with aneurysmal rerupture. Transcranial Doppler signals can be normal in patients with primary infratentorial lesions that lead to brain stem death and in patients with anoxic-ischemic brain damage after cardiac arrest, both conditions without increased ICP.

Disadvantages

Transcranial Doppler velocities can be affected by marked changes in arterial P_{CO_2}, hematocrit, and cardiac output. Transcranial Doppler ultrasonography requires considerable practice and skill.

Somatosensory Evoked Potentials

Technique

A portable instrument can be used at the bedside. Median nerve stimulation is performed on both sides.[2,6,14,78]

Result

N20–P22 response is bilaterally absent.

Validity

Somatosensory evoked potentials and auditory brain stem responses were tested in patients with brain death, and most were found to have no responses. One study claimed that both absent brain stem auditory evoked potential and absence of somatosensory evoked potential beyond Erb's point were unique in patients with brain death and not found in comatose patients who still had preserved brain stem function. This study has not been confirmed or refuted.[28]

Miscellaneous Tests

Many of these tests have been done in only small series of patients and are not widely adopted as confirmatory tests.

Computed tomography scanning in brain dead patients often shows the devastating lesion that led to progression to brain death. In patients with anoxic-ischemic damage, brain CT scanning may show diffuse cerebral edema with disappearance of sulci and white-gray differentiation (Fig. 34–3). Contrast CT scanning does not visualize intracranial vessels.[3,69] A good correlation with cerebral angiography has been demonstrated in a few anecdotal reports.

Magnetic resonance imaging and magnetic resonance spectroscopy may be promising, but neither the techniques nor the standards for interpretation are readily available.

Many other confirmatory tests are variants or modifications. Experience is limited, or these tests produce similar results in patients with neurologic catastrophes who do not fulfill the clinical criteria for brain death.

DETERMINATION OF BRAIN DEATH IN CHILDREN

The current guidelines in children were developed by a task force of the American Academy of Pediatrics but have not been recently

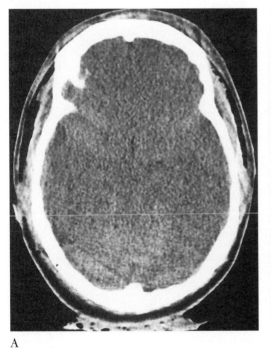
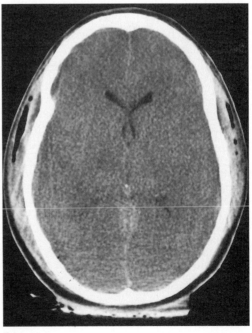

A   B

Figure 34–3. Typical "brain death" computed tomography scans of diffuse cerebral edema showing absence of sulci and gray-white matter differentiation.

Table 34–1. Clinical Criteria for Brain Death in Adults and Children

Coma
Absence of motor responses
Absence of pupillary responses to light and pupils at
    midposition with respect to dilatation
Absence of corneal reflexes
Absence of caloric responses
Absence of gag reflex
Absence of coughing in response to tracheal suctioning
Absence of sucking and rooting reflexes
Absence of respiratory drive at a $PaCO_2$ that is 60 mm
    Hg or 20 mm Hg above normal baseline values
Interval between two evaluations, according to patient's
    age
    Term to 2 months old, 48 hours
    > 2 months to 1 years old, 24 hours
    > 1 years to < 18 years old, 12 hours
    ≥ 18 years old, interval optional
Confirmatory tests
    Term to 2 months old, 2 confirmatory tests
    > 2 months to 1 year old, 1 confirmatory test
    > 1 year to < 18 years old, optional
    ≥ 18 years old, optional

$PaCO_2$, partial pressure of arterial carbon dioxide.
Source: Wijdicks EFM: The diagnosis of brain death. *N Engl J Med* 344:1215–1221, 2001. By permission of the Massachusetts Medical Society.

updated.[4,54,73] These guidelines are summarized in Table 34–1 for easy reference but are not discussed further and are beyond the scope of this monograph.

A study of 93 brain death determinations in children found significant variations in practices.[58] In 25% of patients, the apnea test was not performed, and lack of clear documentation was frequently observed. A task force is needed to revisit the current recommenda-

tions on observation interval and confirmatory tests.

MANAGEMENT OF THE BRAIN-DEAD DONOR

After consent has been obtained (see Chapter 3), serologic tests are done (Table 34–2), and the laboratory tests listed in Table 34–3 are needed to evaluate organ suitability.

Support of the potential organ and tissue donor is complex.[16,42,53] Many physiologic changes occur during the development of brain death, and appropriate management guarantees successful procurement. The criteria for

Table 34–3. Laboratory Tests for Evaluation of Multiorgan Donors

General (needed for all organ donors)
    Electrolytes (Na, K, Cl, CO_2)
    Blood urea nitrogen
    Creatinine
    Glucose
    Complete blood cell count
    Calcium
    Magnesium
    Phosphorus
    Blood cultures (two sets from separate sites; not from
        arterial or central venous lines)
    Diffuse intravascular coagulation panel (if suspected)
Liver
    Aspartate transaminase
    Alanine transaminase
    Total and direct bilirubin
    γ-Glutamyltransferase
    Alkaline phosphatase
    Lactate dehydrogenase
    Prothrombin time
    Partial thromboplastin time
Kidneys
    Urinalysis
    Urine culture
Heart
    Creatine kinase with MB band
    Troponin
Pancreas
    Amylase
    Lipase
Lungs
    Arterial blood gases
    Sputum
    Gram's stain

Source: From Emery SF, Robertson KM: Organ procurement and preparation for transplantation. In Wijdicks EFM (ed): *Brain Death.* Philadelphia: Lippincott Williams & Wilkins, 2001, pp 189–208. By permission of the publisher.

Table 34–2. Serology Tests for All Organ Donors

Human T-lymphotropic viruses 1 and 2
Hepatitis C virus
Hepatitis B surface antigen
Antibody to hepatitis B core antigen
Cytomegalovirus
Rapid plasma reagin, serologic test for syphilis
Antibody to hepatitis B surface antigen
Human immunodeficiency virus, p24 antigen
Epstein-Barr virus (optional)

Source: Emery SF, Robertson KM: Organ procurement and preparation for transplantation. In Wijdicks EFM (ed): *Brain Death.* Philadelphia: Lippincott Williams & Wilkins, 2001, pp 189–208. By permission of the publisher.

becoming a potential organ donor are at the discretion of the organ harvest teams and change frequently. Organ or tissue donation is contraindicated in patients with a possible or demonstrated transmittable disease. This includes patients at high risk for exposure to human immunodeficiency virus (e.g., related to homosexual practice, prostitution, hemophilia, recent skin-piercing treatment) or who recently had treatment with human pituitary extracts.

The most significant initial management problems pertain to hypotension or diabetes insipidus, or both.[67]

Hypotension has many potential causes. These include decreased left ventricular function, loss of systemic vascular resistance, and rewarming of a hypothermic patient with resultant vasodilatation, but hypotension is frequently related to hypovolemia. Hypovolemia can be a result of insufficient fluid resuscitation in patients with diabetes insipidus or a lingering effect of aggressive osmotic diuresis in an attempt to reverse cerebral edema. Hypovolemia can be reversed with isotonic saline or colloids. Administration of dopamine or other inotropic drugs must be postponed, if possible. However, dopamine is indicated if blood pressure cannot be controlled by fluid resuscitation alone; preferably, dosage is low ($< 10 \mu g/kg$ per minute). Alternatively, if ventricular dysfunction is severe by echocardiography, dobutamine can be considered (5 to 10 $\mu g/kg$ per minute). Not uncommonly, blood pressure is extremely dependent on inotropic agents, and

even switching the lining for a new bag by the nursing staff results in a marked drop in blood pressure. Diabetes insipidus can be expected in many patients and can be countered by intravenous desmopressin, 0.5 to 2 μg every 3 hours. Its use can be gauged by urine output (e.g., more than 300 mL/hour for 2 successive hours).[64]

Cardiac arrhythmias are most troublesome in patients with brain death. Hypocalcemia, hypomagnesemia, hypokalemia, hypothermia, use of inotropes, and severe hypoxemia all may contribute. Brain death leads to autonomic uncoupling but also to marked coronary perfusion pressure possibly due to direct endothelial damage.[79] Terminal rhythms include complete heart block, ventricular tachycardia, and sinus bradycardia progressing to asystole. Ventricular arrhythmias predict significant ventricular dysfunction on echocardiograms (Chapter 30). Altered thyroid function has been found in brain dead patients, but it is unclear whether triiodothyronine replacement therapy improves myocardial function, although some studies have found improved ejection fraction after administration of the hormone.[40] Whether this may decrease inotropic therapy is not known. Minute ventilation is usually changed, because hyperventilation may compromise organ function from peripheral vasoconstriction. Organ donation should proceed quickly, because gas exchange rapidly becomes difficult from lung edema, and diffuse intravascular coagulation may damage other vital organs.

CONCLUSIONS

- Brain death can be determined accurately with a neurologic examination but only after hypothermia, drug effects, and acute metabolic derangement have been excluded.
- Apnea testing requires an apneic oxygenation method aiming at PCO_2 of 60 mm Hg or an increase of 20 mm Hg above baseline. With an estimated increase of 3 to 6 mm Hg per minute, 8 minutes is required to reach the target.
- Preoxygenation, increasing temperature to normothermia, and adequate fluid status reduce complications during apnea testing.
- Donor procurement is complex, and, in the hands of organ procurement nurses. Diabetes insipidus and hypotension can be very difficult to manage.

REFERENCES

1. Anonymous: Guideline three: minimum technical standards for EEG recording in suspected cerebral death. American Electroencephalographic Society. *J Clin Neurophysiol* 11:10–13, 1994.
2. Anziska BJ, Cracco RQ: Short latency somatosensory evoked potentials in brain dead patients. *Arch Neurol* 37:222–225, 1980.
3. Arnold H, Kühne D, Rohr W, et al: Contrast bolus technique with rapid CT scanning. A reliable diagnostic tool for the determination of brain death. *Neuroradiology* 22:129–132, 1981.
4. Ashwal S: Brain death in the newborn. Current perspectives. *Clin Perinatol* 24:859–882, 1997.
5. Belsh JM, Blatt R, Schiffman PL: Apnea testing in brain death. *Arch Intern Med* 146:2385–2388, 1986.
6. Belsh JM, Chokroverty S: Short-latency somatosensory evoked potentials in brain-dead patients. *Electroencephalogr Clin Neurophysiol* 68:75–78, 1987.
7. Bennett DR: The EEG in determination of brain death. *Ann N Y Acad Sci* 315:110–120, 1978.
8. Benzel EC, Mashburn JP, Conrad S, et al: Apnea testing for the determination of brain death: a modified protocol. Technical note. *J Neurosurg* 76:1029–1031, 1992.
9. Bernat JL: How much of the brain must die in brain death? *J Clin Ethics* 3:21–26, 1992.
10. Black PM: Brain death (parts 1 and 2). *N Engl J Med* 299:338–344; 393–401, 1978.
11. Bradac GB, Simon RS: Angiography in brain death. *Neuroradiology* 7:25–28, 1974.
12. Bruce EN, Cherniack NS: Central chemoreceptors. *J Appl Physiol* 62:389–402, 1987.
13. Cantu RC: Brain death as determined by cerebral arteriography. *Lancet* 1:1391–1392, 1973.
14. Chancellor AM, Frith RW, Shaw NA: Somatosensory evoked potentials following severe head injury: loss of the thalamic potential with brain death. *J Neurol Sci* 87:255–263, 1988.
15. Conci F, Procaccio F, Arosio M, et al: Viscero-somatic and viscero-visceral reflexes in brain death. *J Neurol Neurosurg Psychiatry* 49:695–698, 1986.
16. Darby JM, Stein K, Grenvik A, et al: Approach to management of the heartbeating "brain dead" organ donor. *JAMA* 261:2222–2228, 1989.
17. Deliyannakis E, Ioannou F, Davaroukas A: Brain stem death with persistence of bioelectric activity of the cerebral hemispheres. *Clin Electroencephalogr* 6:75–79, 1975.
18. Dobb GJ, Weekes JW: Clinical confirmation of brain death. *Anaesth Intensive Care* 23:37–43, 1995.
19. Ducrocq X, Hassler W, Moritake K, et al: Consensus opinion on diagnosis of cerebral circulatory arrest using Doppler-sonography: Task Force Group on Cerebral Death of the Neurosonology Research Group of the World Federation of Neurology. *J Neurol Sci* 159:145–150, 1998.
20. Earnest MP, Beresford HR, McIntyre HB: Testing for apnea in suspected brain death: methods used by 129 clinicians. *Neurology* 36:542–544, 1986.
21. Ebata T, Watanabe Y, Amaha K, et al: Haemodynamic changes during the apnoea test for diagnosis of brain death. *Can J Anaesth* 38:436–440, 1991.
22. Eger EI, Severinghaus JW: The rate of rise of $PaCO_2$ in the apneic anesthetized patient. *Anesthesiology* 22:419–425, 1961.
23. Fischbeck KH, Simon RP: Neurological manifestations of accidental hypothermia. *Ann Neurol* 10:384–387, 1981.
24. George MS: Establishing brain death: the potential role of nuclear medicine in the search for a reliable confirmatory test (editorial). *Eur J Nucl Med* 18:75–77, 1991.
25. Gilbert M, Busund R, Skagseth A, et al: Resuscitation from accidental hypothermia of 13.7 degrees C with circulatory arrest. *Lancet* 355:375–376, 2000.
26. Glauser FL, Fairman RP, Bechard D: The causes and evaluation of chronic hypercapnea. *Chest* 91:755–759, 1987.
27. Goetting MG, Contreras E: Systemic atropine administration during cardiac arrest does not cause fixed and dilated pupils. *Ann Emerg Med* 20:55–57, 1991.
28. Goldie WD, Chiappa KH, Young RR, et al: Brainstem auditory and short-latency somatosensory evoked responses in brain death. *Neurology* 31:248–256, 1981.
29. Goudreau JL, Wijdicks EFM, Emery SF: Complications during apnea testing in the determination of brain death: predisposing factors. *Neurology* 55:1045–1048, 2000.
30. Gray AT, Krejci ST, Larson MD: Neuromuscular blocking drugs do not alter the pupillary light reflex of anesthetized humans. *Arch Neurol* 54:579–584, 1997.
31. Greenan J, Prasad J: Comparison of the ocular effects of atropine or glycopyrrolate with two I.V. induction agents. *Br J Anaesth* 57:180–183, 1985.
32. Greitz T, Gordon E, Kolmodin G, et al: Aortocranial and carotid angiography in determination of brain death. *Neuroradiology* 5:13–19, 1973.
33. Grigg MM, Kelly MA, Celesia GG, et al: Electroencephalographic activity after brain death. *Arch Neurol* 44:948–954, 1987.
34. Hadani M, Bruk B, Ram Z, et al: Application of transcranial Doppler ultrasonography for the diagnosis of brain death. *Intensive Care Med* 25:822–828, 1999.
35. Hassler W, Steinmetz H, Gawlowski J: Transcranial Doppler ultrasonography in raised intracranial pressure and in intracranial circulatory arrest. *J Neurosurg* 68:745–751, 1988.
36. Haupt WF, Rudolf J: European brain death codes: a comparison of national guidelines. *J Neurol* 246:432–437, 1999.
37. Hazratji SM, Singh BM, Strobos RJ: Angiography in brain death. *N Y State J Med* 81:82–83, 1981.
38. Hoffenberg R: Christiaan Barnard: his first transplants and their impact on concepts of death. *BMJ* 323:1478–1480, 2001.

39. Hughes JR: Limitations of the EEG in coma and brain death. *Ann N Y Acad Sci* 315:121–136, 1978.

40. Jeevanandam V, Todd B, Regillo T, et al: Reversal of donor myocardial dysfunction by triiodothyronine replacement therapy. *J Heart Lung Transplant* 13:681–687, 1994.

41. Jeret JS, Benjamin JL: Risk of hypotension during apnea testing. *Arch Neurol* 51:595–599, 1994.

42. Jordan CA, Snyder JV: Intensive care and intraoperative management of the brain-dead organ donor. *Transplant Proc* 19 Suppl 3:21–25, 1987.

43. Jordan JE, Dyess E, Cliett J: Unusual spontaneous movements in brain-dead patients (letter to the editor). *Neurology* 35:1082, 1985.

44. Jørgensen EO: Spinal man after brain death. The unilateral extension-pronation reflex of the upper limb as an indication of brain death. *Acta Neurochir (Wien)* 28:259–273, 1973.

45. Korein J, Maccario M: A prospective study on the diagnosis of cerebral death (abstract). *Electroencephalogr Clin Neurophysiol* 31:103–104, 1971.

46. Kuwagata Y, Sugimoto H, Yoshioka T, et al: Hemodynamic response with passive neck flexion in brain death. *Neurosurgery* 29:239–241, 1991.

47. LaMancusa J, Cooper R, Vieth R, et al: The effects of the falling therapeutic and subtherapeutic barbiturate blood levels on electrocerebral silence in clinically brain-dead children. *Clin Electroencephalogr* 22:112–117, 1991.

48. Lampl Y, Gilad R, Eschel Y, et al: Diagnosing brain death using the transcranial Doppler with a transorbital approach. *Arch Neurol* 59:58–60, 2002.

49. Lang CJG: Apnea testing by artificial CO_2 augmentation. *Neurology* 45:966–969, 1995.

50. Langfitt TW, Kassell NF: Non-filling of cerebral vessels during angiography: correlation with intracranial pressure. *Acta Neurochir (Wien)* 14:96–104, 1966.

51. Larson MD, Muhiudeen I: Pupillometric analysis of the 'absent light reflex.' *Arch Neurol* 52:369–372, 1995.

52. Laurin NR, Driedger AA, Hurwitz GA, et al: Cerebral perfusion imaging with technetium-99m HM-PAO in brain death and severe central nervous system injury. *J Nucl Med* 30:1627–1635, 1989.

53. Lindop MJ: Basic principles of donor management for multiorgan removal. *Transplant Proc* 23:2463–2464, 1991.

54. Lynch J, Eldadah MK: Brain-death criteria currently used by pediatric intensivists. *Clin Pediatr (Phila)* 31:457–460, 1992.

55. Lock MM: *Twice Dead: Organ Transplants and the Reinvention of Death.* Berkeley: University of California Press, 2002.

56. Marks SJ, Zisfein J: Apneic oxygenation in apnea tests for brain death. A controlled trial. *Arch Neurol* 47:1066–1068, 1990.

57. Marti-Fabregas J, Lopez-Navidad A, Caballero F, et al: Decerebrate-like posturing with mechanical ventilation in brain death. *Neurology* 54:224–227, 2000.

58. Mejia RE, Pollack MM: Variability in brain death determination practices in children. *JAMA* 274:550–553, 1995.

59. Ong GL, Bruning HA: Dilated fixed pupils due to administration of high doses of dopamine hydrochloride. *Crit Care Med* 9:658–659, 1981.

60. Orliaguet GA, Catoire P, Liu N, et al: Transesophageal echocardiographic assessment of left ventricular function during apnea testing for brain death. *Transplantation* 58:655–658, 1994.

61. Pallis C: ABC of brain stem death. The position in the USA and elsewhere. *Br Med J* 286:209–210, 1983.

62. Pallis C: Brainstem death. In Vinken PJ, Bruyn GW, Klawans HL (eds): *Handbook of Clinical Neurology.* Vol 57; Revised Series 13. Amsterdam: Elsevier Science Publishers, 1990, pp 441–496.

63. Partridge BL, Abrams JH, Bazemore C, et al: Prolonged neuromuscular blockade after long-term infusion of vecuronium bromide in the intensive care unit. *Crit Care Med* 18:1177–1179, 1990.

64. Pennefather SH, Bullock RE, Mantle D, et al: Use of low dose arginine vasopressin to support brain-dead organ donors. *Transplantation* 59:58–62, 1995.

65. Petty GW, Mohr JP, Pedley TA, et al: The role of transcranial Doppler in confirming brain death: sensitivity, specificity, and suggestions for performance and interpretation. *Neurology* 40:300–303, 1990.

66. Plotkin SR, Ning MM: Traumatic cervical spine disruption. *N Engl J Med* 345:1134–1135, 2001.

67. Power BM, Van Heerden PV: The physiological changes associated with brain death—current concepts and implications for treatment of the brain dead organ donor. *Anaesth Intensive Care* 23:26–36, 1995.

68. Powers AD, Graeber MC, Smith RR: Transcranial Doppler ultrasonography in the determination of brain death. *Neurosurgery* 24:884–889, 1989.

69. Rappaport ZH, Brinker RA, Rovit RL: Evaluation of brain death by contrast-enhanced computerized cranial tomography. *Neurosurgery* 2:230–232, 1978.

70. Report of the Ad Hoc Committee of the Harvard Medical School to Examine the Definition of Brain Death: A definition of irreversible coma. *JAMA* 205:337–340, 1968.

71. Report of the medical consultants on the diagnosis of death to the President's Commission for the Study of Ethical Problems in Medicine and Biomedical and Behavioral Research: Guidelines for the determination of death. *JAMA* 246:2184–2186, 1981.

72. Report of the Quality Standards Subcommittee of the American Academy of Neurology: Practice parameters for determining brain death in adults (summary statement). *Neurology* 45:1012–1014, 1995.

73. Report of Special Task Force: Guidelines for the determination of brain death in children. *Pediatrics* 80:298–300, 1987.

74. Ropper AH: Unusual spontaneous movements in brain-dead patients. *Neurology* 34:1089–1092, 1984.

75. Ropper AH, Kehne SM, Wechsler L: Transcranial Doppler in brain death. *Neurology* 37:1733–1735, 1987.

76. Ropper AH, Kennedy SK, Russell L: Apnea testing in the diagnosis of brain death. Clinical and physiological observations. *J Neurosurg* 55:942–946, 1981.

77. Saposnik G, Bueri JA, Maurino J, et al: Spontaneous and reflex movements in brain death. *Neurology* 54:221–223, 2000.

78. Stöhr M, Riffel B, Trost E, et al: Short-latency somatosensory evoked potentials in brain death. *J Neurol* 234:211–214, 1987.

79. Szabó G, Buhmann V, Bahrle S, et al: Brain death impairs coronary endothelial function. *Transplantation* 73:1846–1848, 2002.

80. Uniform Determination of Death Act, 12 Uniform Laws Annotated (U.L.A.) 589 (West 1993 and West Suppl. 1997).

81. Walker AE: *Cerebral Death*. 2nd ed. Baltimore: Urban & Schwarzenberg, 1981.

82. Wijdicks EFM: Determining brain death in adults. *Neurology* 45:1003–1011, 1995.

83. Wijdicks EFM: In search of a safe apnea test in brain death: Is the procedure really more dangerous than we think? (Letter to the editor.) *Arch Neurol* 52:338–339, 1995.

84. Wijdicks EFM (ed): *Brain Death*. Philadelphia, Lippincott Williams & Wilkins, 2001.

85. Wijdicks EFM: The diagnosis of brain death. *N Engl J Med* 344:1215–1221, 2001.

86. Wijdicks EFM: Brain death worldwide: accepted fact but no global consensus in diagnostic criteria. *Neurology* 58:20–25, 2002.

87. Wijdicks EFM, Atkinson JL, Okazaki H: Isolated medulla oblongata function after severe traumatic brain injury. *J Neurol Neurosurg Psychiatry* 70:127–129, 2001.

88. Willatts SM, Drummond G: Brainstem death and ventilator trigger settings. *Anaesthesia* 55:676–677, 2000.

89. Yatim A, Mercatello A, Coronel B, et al: ^{99m}Tc-HMPAO cerebral scintigraphy in the diagnosis of brain death. *Transplant Proc* 23:2491, 1991.

90. Zisfein J, Marks SJ: Tension pneumothorax and apnea tests (letter to the editor). *Anesthesiology* 91:326, 1999.

35

Ethical and Legal Matters

We can assume, ipso facto, that the neurointensivist or any attending neurologist will be confronted with ethical quandaries and legal challenges. Decisions that are ethically strained commonly involve the futility of care. Because of the profoundly altered consciousness of the patient—more often so than in other intensive care units—resigned acceptance of a devastating neurologic condition is transferred to the family. However, the patient, if consciously involved in decisions, may hold different views. Any of these judgments should give full weight to a person's right to live.

Unlike the situation in medical wards, we should not be surprised to be vulnerable, as such is the nature of the profession. The legal matters particularly focus on risk avoidance, the neurointensivist as expert witness, and some other basic issues. This closing chapter is an attempt to explain a very difficult and dense subject matter but does not pretend to go to all lengths. Conflicting views and illustrative case examples are presented.

ETHICAL CONTROVERSIES

The most controversial topics within the NICU are considered here. Not all of these matters are addressed by the law, and some we opt out of (e.g., active euthanasia).

Futility and Its Consequences

Futility: "a useless act or gesture."[40] From Latin futilis, "leaky." In classic mythology, futility is the condemnation of the 50 daughters of Danaus, who killed their husbands on their wedding night, forever to carry water from the river in leaky jars.

Neurologists have no ethical duty to provide futile interventions. But many neurologists reaffirm that something about the definition of futility of care is still unconvincing. Not many physicians argue that futility is a simple commonsense notion.[51,52] Helft et al.[29] noted that "the illusion of futility is the mistaken assumption that it is an objective entity." Dunphy[18] eloquently summarized the problem: "The incoherence of futility stems, no doubt, from different people at the same time, and the same people at different times, using the word to mean many things."

In a more pragmatic sense, futility most of the time is best characterized as a clear appreciation of a hopeless situation and obvious disparity between the prediction of fatal outcome and aggressiveness of care in the NICU. The term can be used to denote that a certain goal is not worth pursuing, that intervention has no pathophysiologic rationale, that prior therapies have already failed, and that the outcome is not meaningful. It is no longer well-judged to continue support of critical body functions such as respiration and hemodynamic status. Attempts to define futility in percentages of treatment success (e.g., less than 1%) arrive at a loose definition, and the thresholds may look arbitrary to family members. Moreover, a study surveying families 1 year after end-of-life treatment discussions suggested that conflict sometimes arises between family members and medical staff over communication and unprofessional staff behavior.[1] A unilateral decision on futility of care is complex because it can be construed as polarizing, and a second opinion from a colleague may be warranted.

As physicians, we judge some things correctly and some incorrectly. We unconsciously tack on our own skewed experiences. We may underestimate how much some patients and relatives consider life worth living.[14] We should not make a judgment that goes beyond the evidence. We continue to make mistakes in prognostication because hard data on outcome are lacking and accumulation of sedative agents is underappreciated. In fact, only a few neurologic injuries to the brain or spinal cord exist in which the chance of recovery is infinitesimal.

The decisions are more difficult to make when patients are younger. In one such patient (Fig. 35–1), aggressive care was continued at the family's request, but the outcome cannot be easily judged. The patient seems happy with his state of being. Others would tend to deprecate such existence. In Figure 35–2, a major discrepancy between CT scan findings and clinical outcome is evident, pointing to the potential fallacy of too much trust in neuroimaging studies. The examples are not shown here to document that prognostication is an illusion, but it underlines failures.

The main principles of compassionate end-of-life care in the intensive care unit have recently been published.[35] The judicial determinations of withholding and withdrawing life-sustaining treatment are discussed in review

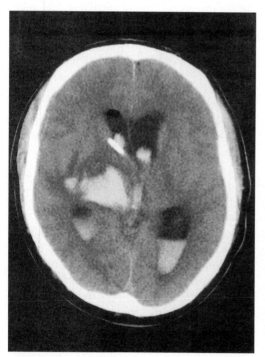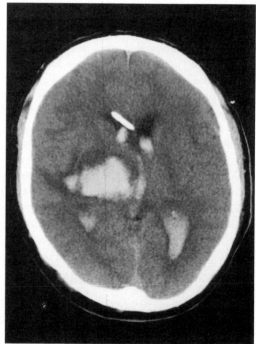

Figure 35–1. Outcome in a 30-year-old man with devastating thalamic hemorrhage. Hospital course: thalamic hemorrhage from arteriovenous malformation; extensor posturing, downward gaze, stupor; tracheotomy, percutaneous endoscopic gastrostomy, ventriculoperitoneal shunt. Seven weeks: awakening. Three months: walking with assistance, hemiplegic, "communicative"; dull, does not laugh much. Two years: adult foster care; independent in self-care; not involved in regular job; quite happy with his situation; spends most of the day in front of a television set.

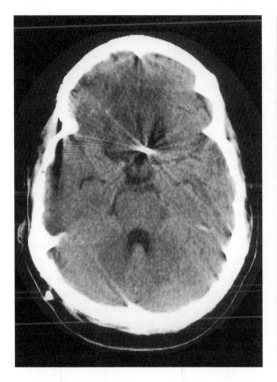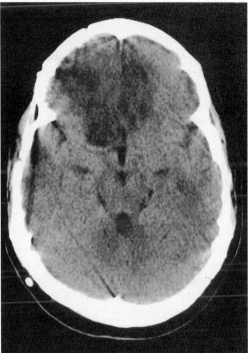

Figure 35–2. Outcome in a 38-year-old woman with multiple cerebral infarcts after subarachnoid hemorrhage. Hospital course: sudden loss of consciousness after acute headache, remained in stupor, anterior communicating aneurysm clipped; pulmonary edema associated with cardiac stunning; marked abulia, dense hemiplegia, severe diffuse vasospasm treated with hemodynamic augmentation; multiple cerebral infarcts emerged. One month: gradually improving transfers and communication. Six months: spastic hemiparesis and some neglect, fully independent and productive; normal cognitive function shown by extensive neuropsychologic tests.

articles and are not considered further in this chapter.[5,10,12,27] Withdrawal and withholding of life support are considered ethically equivalent.[5] The practice is prevalent in many intensive care units around the world but not all (e.g., U.K. and Japan).[22,32,46,58] The prevailing judicial opinion in court decisions in the U.S. is that artificial feedings are similar to other medical interventions.[39]

The circumstances of withdrawal of support in the NICU have only recently been reported.[38] In 43% of patients (excluding patients with brain death), terminal extubation was done; median survival was 7 hours, and almost 70% died within 24 hours. Opioids were needed to relieve agonal or labored breathing in this study.[38] More recently, studies emerged

that scrutinized the reasons and justifications for withdrawal of support in patients admitted to the NICU. Withdrawal of mechanical ventilation was less likely in patients of African-American ethnicity and more likely in patients with lower Glasgow coma scale scores or a diagnosis of subarachnoid hemorrhage or ischemic stroke.[16]

An important retrospective study on withdrawal of support in patients with cerebral supratentorial hemorrhage found a bias toward elderly patients and dominant hemisphere, and withdrawal was less likely when craniotomy was performed. This study, albeit with very small numbers, suggested that despite intracranial hematomas of large volume and low Glasgow coma scores, functional independence was possible when care was continued. Characteristics in some of these patients were not different from those in whom care was withdrawn.[6] The authors expressed concern about a possible self-fulfilling prophecy by family members or physicians, but retrospective comparisons may leave room for error and may not catch important differences.

In our NICU, the suggestion of withdrawal of support is invariably first entertained by family members. Failure to awaken after surgery and absent upper brain stem reflexes, intercurrent infection or sepsis, and progression to herniation with previously expressed wishes not to remain in a severely handicapped state were all reasons to withdraw mechanical ventilation. Care was withdrawn rarely in patients less than 70 years old and only when end-stage herniation occurred. In many instances, failure to improve in level of consciousness after 7 to 10 days of maximal support prompted a radical change in care.

When a final decision is made that treatment or support is not needed at an aggressive level, withdrawal of medication, nutrition, and hydration is discussed. A number of court cases and a number of states have accepted nutrition and hydration as medical interventions. Generally, withdrawal of support should be compassionate, with utmost attention to relief of discomfort and symptoms.[7,8,36] Withdrawal of nutrition and hydration does not lead to starvation, because loss of appetite is common in critically ill patients and some degree of starvation is invariably present. Apart from dryness of the mouth and changes in facial features (decrease in swelling), withdrawal of feeding and hydration leads to a peaceful death in all patients within 2 weeks. Ice chips, sips of liquid, and swabbing of the mouth provide sufficient comfort.

It is probably reasonable not to extubate when further progression will lead to death. However, intubation and maintaining an unobstructed airway should be considered a medical intervention that may prolong dying. Some argue that removal of the tube takes away life, but in fact the brain lesion does. Extubation of a comatose patient results in death within hours to days, usually without respiratory dis-

comfort or overt stridor. In general, breathing may become slightly more rapid, with associated snoring, and evolves into irregular breathing, inspiratory gasps, and, finally, apnea without distress. (It is particularly comforting for family members to know this evolution of the breathing pattern.) The time to apnea depends on the degree of brain stem involvement either from compression associated with herniation or displacement or from direct ischemic or hemorrhagic destruction. The timing of extubation is left to the discretion of the family. Predicting apnea without formal testing can be difficult. Failure to trigger the ventilator is unreliable, often also because of posthyperventilation apnea. Thus, a brief disconnection may not provide reliable information about lack of respiratory drive. This information could be important, because some families expect absent breathing after disconnection and become understandably anxious if breathing continues.

Dyspnea remains the most distressing symptom after extubation. It can be managed by elevation of the head and torso; a humidifier; an intravenous bolus of morphine sulfate, 1 to 2 mg every 10 minutes until dyspnea is relieved. When intravenous access has been removed, opioids (fentanyl, 50 to 100 μg by nebulization; morphine sulfate, 5 mg in 2 mL of sterile water) provide relief and comfort.[21] Anticholinergic agents may be used to reduce secretions (e.g., transdermal scopolamine, one patch every 3 days). Vomiting may be reduced with intramuscular administration of promethazine, 25 mg every 4 hours, and intractable hiccups with nefopam, valproic acid, and baclofen. Recurrence of seizures can be treated with fosphenytoin (300 to 600 mg) given intramuscularly.

Orders Not to Resuscitate

Patients are resuscitated unless it is explicitly directed otherwise. A do-not-resuscitate (DNR) directive is justified when quality of life is very poor or absent, such as in a persistent vegetative state, when upper brain stem reflexes are lost after emergency surgery for herniation, with persistent locked-in syndrome in basilar artery occlusion, after the clinical diagnosis of brain death, and in other catastrophic conditions when a severely disabled state is anticipated.[13] A DNR order may have been determined before admission in an advance directive (Chapter 3), but often the DNR order is written during the hospital stay.[49] Most hospitalized patients would want to discuss DNR orders with their physicians, but data are unknown for the NICU.[49] Other surveys suggest few would want resuscitation in elderly debilitated patients.[37] The DNR order implies withholding cardiopulmonary resuscitation, but all other treatment continues. Concerns that DNR orders may lead to suboptimal management are real but difficult to demonstrate or prove. When DNR is discussed, family members and the patient should understand that cardiopulmonary resuscitation implies placement of a mechanical ventilator, is a complicated procedure (unlike jump-starting a car), and is successful in only 20% of patients, maybe even fewer. Cardiopulmonary resuscitation, despite known questionable long-term outcome,[42,50] is more successful in the intensive care unit. In the NICU, an additional anoxic-ischemic injury to an already impaired brain can occur, and outcome can be worse in this population.

Limited DNR orders (no intubation or defibrillation), or so-called slow codes[26,28,41] (delay in calling; deliberately ineffective attempt), are troublesome, deceiving, and truly unacceptable.[43]

DONORS WITHOUT A HEARTBEAT

In an attempt to reduce a major shortage of organs, protocols have been designed for timely obtaining of organs from patients who died of cardiac arrest. An early estimate of the effect of widespread implementation of so-called non-heart-beating protocols is a 30% increase in the donor pool.[3]

The Uniform Determination of Death Act (UDDA) defines death as (1) irreversible cessation of circulatory and respiratory functions or (2) irreversible cessation of the entire brain. It would seem odd if medicine now were confronted with creation of a new reliable medical standard for death. In brain death, the burden of proof has been with the neurologist, but now the definition of death would again be with the cardiologist or anesthesiologist.[15,30,34,44]

The definition of cardiopulmonary arrest has become a matter of debate, echoing the concerns during the introduction of proposals to determine death by neurologic criteria. However, major differences exist between the evolution of brain death criteria and the evolution of non-heart-beating criteria. A reliable set of criteria for brain death, beginning as early as 1950, was needed to stop futile care.[17] In contrast, criteria for non-heart-beating donors are specifically devised to promote organ donation.

A wide range of opinions has emerged, from use of the protocol in the field ("donors from the streets") to use in the hospital.[2,10] A serious sticking point was best voiced by Lears:[34] "Are we manipulating the death of some person to benefit others?" Proponents of this protocol, used in many countries throughout the world and in U.S. medical centers (Mayo Clinic has not yet decided to participate), have argued that a major source of organs is lost while the disparity between demand and supply is increasing.[24] On the other hand, conflict of interest and lack of informed consent for intra-aortic infusion of cold preservative solution may remain major objections. Some countries have laws allowing presumed consent, which could facilitate the workings of these protocols. Transplant surgeons continue to argue that the function of organs, including pancreas and lung, is very satisfactory.[44] Longer delay would produce so-called warm ischemia that could potentially damage the donor organs. A recent study in Switzerland found delayed graft function but good survival when organs were retrieved 10 minutes after arrest.[56]

To epitomize: This alternative way of increasing the donor pool merits a great deal of thought. One could argue that the complexity of this protocol should be an incentive to search for other creative solutions to this pressing problem of donor shortage. Difficulty in properly dealing with the definition of irreversible cardiac death is real. The proposed interval varies much and has no strong support in data. The Pittsburgh Protocol, introduced in 1992, allows death to be certified on the basis of exclusively cardiopulmonary criteria requiring asystole for 2 minutes before procurement proceeds. A conference at Maastricht, the Netherlands, identified four categories that could provide non-heart-beating donors: I, dead on arrival; II, unsuccessful resuscitation; III, awaiting cardiac death; and IV, cardiac death in a brain-dead donor.[24] This protocol required 10 minutes of cardiopulmonary arrest. The Institute of Medicine outlined recommendations in 1997 that promoted "public openness" and supported these protocols as a means of providing a possible source of organs. It remains unclear whether extension to 5 minutes ("determination of death in controlled non-heart-beating donors by cessation of cardiopulmonary function for at least 5 minutes by electrocardiographic and arterial pressure monitoring") truly is satisfying the skeptics and removing the possible mistrust of the public.[19]

In one of the most recent experiences with these protocols, spanning 15 years, the number of patients with cardiac arrest before diagnosis of brain death was only 9 of 122 donors (7%).[56] Use of this protocol in patients with end-stage herniation may thus seem a possibility, although uncommon. The troubling question is how to make this determination and according to what standards.

Modifications of protocols to have patients with terminal illness but not brain death (e.g., amyotrophic lateral sclerosis) taken off life suport in the operating room before organ recovery verges on active euthanasia.

Active Euthanasia

In active euthanasia, or physician-assisted suicide, a physician commits an act specifically directed to take a patient's life through lethal injection or provision of an orally administered drug with specific directions for an overdose. Both the American College of Physicians and the American Academy of Neurology have issued position papers against this practice.[4,53]

The U.S. Supreme Court ruled that there is no constitutional right to assisted suicide but left open the possibility that individual states (e.g., Oregon) can legalize it.[55] It remains a criminal offense. The U.S. Attorney General recently issued a directive to take punitive action against physicians who hasten death by using medication.[54] This included the possibility of revoking prescription-writing privileges. Recently, a federal judge ruled that the Attorney General went beyond his authority. An appeal is expected. Some continue to argue that legalizing physician-assisted suicide is an act of compassion, a personal and private decision that harms no one else and respects the patient's choice, particularly when suffering cannot be relieved.

In their monograph, Foley and Hendin[23] argue against euthanasia. In a series of convincing essays, a compelling thesis against this practice is developed. Arguments provided include an abominable lack of knowledge and education on palliative care (including side effects of palliative drugs) and failed experiments in the state of Oregon and the Netherlands (lack of informed consent, danger of casualness, unacceptably high rates, and the scope for abuse). Philosophically, there is the potential for disintegration of trust in the patient-physician relationship when the physician can be allowed to inject lethal doses of medicine. The definition of "terrible suffering" is not a problem-free area, and effective palliation is possible in many, if not all, patients.[23] Other scholars argue that active euthanasia demeans the sacredness of human life. The main argument is that it is a direct violation of a moral prohibition against killing human beings.[20,45] In addition, it has been argued that requests of patients are not truly autonomous and are clouded by underlying, potentially treatable depression.[7,8,11] Gradually decreasing attention to providing palliative care, which truly can relieve suffering in many patients, is another concern.

In the United States and most other countries, the neurologist must insistently deny euthanasia to any competent or incompetent person when requested. One should not blur the line between active euthanasia (physician intent to cause death) and aggressive pharmaceutical treatment to provide comfort (physician's intent to relieve perceived suffering).

LEGAL MATTERS

A general assumption, albeit with little substantive information, is that because intensive care units are "high-risk places," they may invite malpractice suits.[9] At the extreme, intensivists' fear of litigation may hamper entry into this subspecialty or facilitate early departure. This section outlines some of the principles and tangible goals of risk-behavior avoidance.

Liability

Medical errors in the NICU could be technical (e.g., misplacement of catheter, tube, or device; continuation of drug despite adverse drug reaction), judgmental (e.g., misdiagnosis of subarachnoid hemorrhage, spinal cord compression, brain tumor; failure to monitor; inappropriate treatment), or normative (e.g., deception, nondisclosure of risk, breach of confidentiality). Motives for filing malpractice claims in the intensive care unit may involve perception of negligence, such as perceived treatment error or delay, missed or delayed diagnosis, equipment misuse, and pharmacologic mishaps. In an NICU, technical–surgical mishaps are prevalent. Negligence or error is ultimately a jury determination and quite loaded. Clearly, some errors could be considered an associated risk of the surgical procedure.

Crippling deficits may be due to failure to uphold reasonable standards of practice (e.g., early antibiotics in meningitis, CT scan in thunderclap headache), but a causal connection between the assumed error and the patient's handicap or death needs to be established. Injury may be difficult to prove because of the critical illness of the patient and the lack of certain customary standards.

One of the first potential problems is when to admit patients to or transfer them out of the NICU.[48] Potential negligence may be claimed by the plaintiff if other intensivists testify that nonadmission to the NICU was a deviation from practice. Examples are failure to admit patients with rapidly worsening Guillain-Barré syndrome or myasthenic crisis for monitoring of respiratory failure, patients with severe head trauma but minimal initial CT scan abnormalities, and patients with an acute mass in the posterior fossa. More complex sources of legal risk are the type of equipment in the unit, failure to consult with related specialists, and the skill, experience, and training of other health care providers, such as nurses and respiratory care practitioners. Claims have also been filed on use of physical restraint, disclosing evidence of battery (unconsented-to, harmful invasion of a patient's bodily integrity).[31]

Disclosure of Mistakes

Serious mistakes could occur in the NICU and may cause permanent morbidity or premature death. Disclosure of mistakes may be deferred because of fear of a negligence suit, punitive responses by colleagues, or a damaged career, but failure to accept responsibility ("no proof whatsoever") or blaming it all on someone else can also be the reason. Disclosure of overt mistakes to those involved does not appear to increase lawsuits,[33,59] but failure to do so will cause patients and family to feel betrayed. In fact, concealing mistakes or negligence may increase liability.[25] In addition, some claims are due to critical remarks by another physician. Disclosure may not be warranted or appropriate if failure to respond to a certain problem did not do any harm (e.g., failure to reverse anticoagulation in a patient already with loss of virtually all brain stem reflexes). In other instances, mistakes may be known complications that have been explained to the patient as causing poor outcome but that cannot truly be considered mistakes (e.g., intracerebral hematoma with thrombolytic agents).

Self-serving interpretations by physicians are of concern, and uncertainties about a possible cause and effect should be expressed to the patient's family. Often honesty is acknowledged.[57] Explicit acknowledgment of thoughtlessness, its consequences, and therapeutic measures to reduce further harm should be discussed in a separate meeting with the family. Judiciousness and skill are required. If the system is at fault (laboratory errors, pharmacist feedback), more systematic research is needed.

Risk Prevention

There is no recipe for prevention of a negligence suit. Important measures are knowledge of the scope of practice and adequate documentation. The medical record remains the central focus for determining whether the physician met the standard of care. Entries should be factual and accurate, timely, and legible. If the physician is candid, is genuinely good and decent, has a sense of fairness, is open to outside concerns, is willing to listen, and can explain an adverse outcome ("fiduciary relationship"), a persistent desire for malpractice action is reduced. Anyone could argue that open display of pharisaical behavior, unavailability, or egotism and cunning could invite filing a suit.

Expert Witness

Neurologic intensive care involves few physicians who are closely knit. Opposition testimony, however, may be obtained from any physician involved in hospital care (so-called hospitalists) that is closely related to the practice.

Proctor[47] summarized the most important questions asked of expert witnesses: "Was it reasonable to have known at such and such a time that a particular substance or procedure was hazardous? And did the people responsible for causing the injury in question act responsibly, given the scientific and ethical standards of the time?"

The court specifically scrutinizes the opinion of the expert for facts, qualification, and personal experience. Discrediting the qualifications and experience of the expert and pointing out areas of vulnerability are common ploys of cross-examining attorneys. The practices of neurointensivists who see acute neurologic disorders differ substantially. Some may have more expertise in trauma, others in acute stroke and neuromuscular disease.

Whether opinions are voiced in depositions or in the courtroom, testimony carries substantial weight and may influence the legal process (settlement or trial) and jury verdict. Potential expert witnesses may remain credible despite selection bias (chosen because of impressive performance or because of clinical brilliance of the expert witness) and financial bias ($100 to $500 per hour).

CONCLUSIONS

- DNR orders should be actively discussed.
- No one has the duty to provide active euthanasia.
- Withdrawal of support when care is deemed futile is an act of compassion, but the patient's autonomy must be respected.
- Non-heart-beating protocols remain highly controversial.
- Adequate documentation, disclosure, and candor should be part of standard care and could reduce the chance of a suit.

REFERENCES

1. Abbott KH, Sago JG, Breen CM, et al: Families looking back: one year after discussion of withdrawal or withholding of life-sustaining support. *Crit Care Med* 29:197–201, 2001.
2. Alvarez J, del Barrio R, Arias J, et al: Non-heart-beating donors from the streets: an increasing donor pool source. *Transplantation* 70:314–317, 2000.
3. Alvarez J, del Barrio R, Arias J, et al: Non-heart-beating donors: estimated actual potential. *Transplant Proc* 33:1101–1103, 2001.
4. The American Academy of Neurology Ethics and Humanities Subcommittee: Palliative care in neurology. *Neurology* 46:870–872, 1996.
5. Anonymous: Withholding and withdrawing life-sustaining therapy. This Official Statement of the American Thoracic Society was adopted by the ATS Board

of Directors, March 1991. *Am Rev Respir Dis* 144:726–731, 1991.

6. Becker KJ, Baxter AB, Cohen WA, et al: Withdrawal of support in intracerebral hemorrhage may lead to self-fulfilling prophecies. *Neurology* 56:766–772, 2001.

7. Block SD: Assessing and managing depression in the terminally ill patient. ACP-ASIM End-of-Life Care Consensus Panel. American College of Physicians–American Society of Internal Medicine. *Ann Intern Med* 132:209–218, 2000.

8. Block SD: Perspectives on care at the close of life. Psychological considerations, growth, and transcendence at the end of life: the art of the possible. *JAMA* 285:2898–2905, 2001.

9. Brennan TA, Leape LL, Laird NM, et al: Incidence of adverse events and negligence in hospitalized patients. Results of the Harvard Medical Practice Study I. *N Engl J Med* 324:370–376, 1991.

10. Clayton HA, Swift SM, Turner JM, et al: Non-heart-beating organ donors: a potential source of islets for transplantation? *Transplantation* 69:2094–2098, 2000.

11. Conwell Y, Caine ED: Rational suicide and the right to die. Reality and myth. *N Engl J Med* 325:1100–1103, 1991.

12. Council on Ethical and Judicial Affairs: Medical futility in end-of-life care: report of the Council on Ethical and Judicial Affairs. *JAMA* 281:937–941, 1999.

13. Curtis JR, Park DR, Krone MR, et al: Use of the medical futility rationale in do-not-attempt-resuscitation orders. *JAMA* 273:124–128, 1995.

14. Danis M, Patrick DL, Southerland LI, et al: Patients' and families' preferences for medical intensive care. *JAMA* 260:797–802, 1988.

15. DeVita MA: The death watch: certifying death using cardiac criteria. *Prog Transplant* 11:58–66, 2001.

16. Diringer MN, Edwards DF, Aiyagari V, et al: Factors associated with withdrawal of mechanical ventilation in a neurology/neurosurgery intensive care unit. *Crit Care Med* 29:1792–1797, 2001.

17. Diringer MN, Wijdicks EFM: Brain death in historical perspective. In Wijdicks EFM (ed): *Brain Death*. Philadelphia: Lippincott Williams & Wilkins, 2001, pp 5–27.

18. Dunphy K: Futilitarianism: knowing how much is enough in end-of-life health care. *Palliat Med* 14:313–322, 2000.

19. Elliott MJ, Mallory G Jr, Khagani A: Transplantation from non-heart-beating donors. *Lancet* 357:819–820, 2001.

20. Emanuel EJ: Euthanasia and physician-assisted suicide: a review of the empirical data from the United States. *Arch Intern Med* 162:142–152, 2002.

21. Farncombe M, Chater S: Clinical application of nebulized opioids for treatment of dyspnoea in patients with malignant disease. *Support Care Cancer* 2:184–187, 1994.

22. Ferrand E, Robert R, Ingrand P, et al: Withholding and withdrawal of life support in intensive-care units in France. A prospective survey. French LATAREA Group. *Lancet* 357:9–14, 2001.

23. Foley K, Hendin H: *The Case Against Assisted Suicide: For the Right to End-of-Life Care.* Baltimore: Johns Hopkins University Press, 2002.

24. Fung JJ: Use of non-heart-beating donors. *Transplant Proc* 32:1510–1511, 2000.

25. Furrow BR, Johnson SH, Jost TS, et al: *Health Law: Cases, Materials, and Problems.* 3rd ed. St Paul: West Publishing Company, 1997, pp 385–388.

26. Gazelle G: The slow code—should anyone rush to its defense? *N Engl J Med* 338:467–469, 1998.

27. Gostin LO: Deciding life and death in the courtroom. From Quinlan to Cruzan, Glucksberg, and Vacco—a brief history and analysis of constitutional protection of the 'right to die.' *JAMA* 278:1523–1528, 1997.

28. Heffner JE, Barbieri C: Compliance with do-not-resuscitate orders for hospitalized patients transported to radiology departments. *Ann Intern Med* 129:801–805, 1998.

29. Helft PR, Siegler M, Lantos J: The rise and fall of the futility movement. *N Engl J Med* 343:293–296, 2000.

30. Herdman R, Potts JT: *Non-Heart-Beating Organ Transplantation: Medical and Ethical Issues in Procurement.* Division of Health Care Services, Institute of Medicine. Washington, DC: National Academy Press, 1997.

31. Kapp MB: Physical restraint use in critical care: legal issues. *AACN Clinical Issues: Adv Pract Acute Crit Care* 7:579–584, 1996.

32. Keenen SP, Busche KD, Chen LM, et al: A retrospective review of a large cohort of patients undergoing the process of withholding or withdrawal of life support. *Crit Care Med* 25:1324–1331, 1997.

33. Kraman SS, Hamm G: Risk management: extreme honesty may be the best policy. *Ann Intern Med* 131:963–967, 1999.

34. Lears L: Obtaining organs from non-heart-beating cadavers. *Health Care Ethics USA* 4:6–7, 1996.

35. Levy MM: End-of-life care in the intensive care unit: Can we do better? *Crit Care Med* 29 Suppl:N56–N61, 2001.

36. Lo B, Snyder L: Care at the end of life: guiding practice where there are no easy answers. *Ann Intern Med* 130:772–774, 1999.

37. Marco CA, Schears RM: Societal opinions regarding CPR. *Am J Emerg Med* 20:207–211, 2002.

38. Mayer SA, Kossoff SB: Withdrawal of life support in the neurological intensive care unit. *Neurology* 52:1602–1609, 1999.

39. Meisel A (ed): *The Right to Die.* 2nd ed. New York: Wiley Law Publications, 1995, pp 592–608.

40. Merriam-Webster's Collegiate Dictionary, 10th ed. 1993, p 475.

41. Muller JH: Shades of blue: the negotiation of limited codes by medical residents. *Soc Sci Med* 34:885–898, 1992.

42. Murphy DJ, Burrows D, Santilli S, et al: The influence of the probability of survival on patients' preferences regarding cardiopulmonary resuscitation. *N Engl J Med* 330:545–549, 1994.

43. Novack DH, Detering BJ, Arnold R, et al: Physicians' attitudes toward using deception to resolve difficult ethical problems. *JAMA* 261:2980–2985, 1989.

44. Orr RD, Gundry SR, Bailey LL: Reanimation: overcoming objections and obstacles to organ retrieval from non-heart-beating cadaver donors. *J Med Ethics* 23:7–11, 1997.

45. Pellegrino ED: Doctors must not kill. *J Clin Ethics* 3:95–102, 1992.

46. Prendergast TJ, Luce JM: Increasing incidence of withholding and withdrawal of life support from the critically ill. *Am J Respir Crit Care Med* 155:15–20, 1997.

47. Proctor RN: Expert witnesses take the stand. *Nature* 407:15–16, 2000.

48. Puffer LB Jr: Legal problems of the intensive care unit. *Med Clin North Am* 55:1365–1374, 1971.

49. Reilly BM, Magnussen CR, Ross J, et al: Can we talk? Inpatient discussions about advance directives in a community hospital. Attending physicians' attitudes, their inpatients' wishes, and reported experience. *Arch Intern Med* 154:2299–2308, 1994.

50. Robinson EM: An ethical analysis of cardiopulmonary resuscitation for elders in acute care. *AACN Clin Issues* 13:132–144, 2002.

51. Rubin SB (ed): *When Doctors Say No: the Battleground of Medical Futility.* Bloomington: Indiana University Press, 1998.

52. Schneiderman LJ, Jecker NS, Jonsen AR: Medical futility: its meaning and ethical implications. *Ann Intern Med* 112:949–954, 1990.

53. Snyder L, Sulmasy DP: Physician-assisted suicide. *Ann Intern Med* 135:209–216, 2001.

54. Steinbrook R: Physician-assisted suicide in Oregon—an uncertain future. *N Engl J Med* 346:460–464, 2002.

55. Washington vs. Glucksberg, 117 S. Ct. 2258, 1997.

56. Weber M, Dindo D, Demartines N, et al: Kidney transplantation from donors without a heartbeat. *N Engl J Med* 347:248–255, 2002.

57. Witman AB, Park DM, Hardin SB: How do patients want physicians to handle mistakes? A survey of internal medicine patients in an academic setting. *Arch Intern Med* 156:2565–2569, 1996.

58. Wood GG, Martin E: Withholding and withdrawing life-sustaining therapy in a Canadian intensive care unit. *Can J Anaesth* 42:186–191, 1995.

59. Wu AW, Folkman S, McPhee SJ, et al: Do house officers learn from their mistakes? *JAMA* 265:2089–2094, 1991.

Appendix

FORMULAS AND TABLES FOR TITRATING THERAPY

The therapeutic options in neurologic intensive care are much greater than those in any other subspecialty in neurology. Pharmaceutical intervention remains a major component, and frequent adjustments are needed. Many patients are on mechanical ventilators and have Swan-Ganz catheters providing data that may prompt adjustment in management. This appendix provides common formulas and nomograms for calculations needed in the daily care of critically ill neurologic patients. The focus is on patients with an acute neurologic disorder. Standard critical care textbooks and pharmaceutical textbooks in critical care can be consulted as well and ideally should be available in every neurologic intensive care unit.

Hemodynamic Equations

Body surface area (BSA) = $(\text{height})^{0.725} \times (\text{weight})^{0.425} \times 71.84 \times 10^{-4}$

Mean arterial pressure (MAP) = $\dfrac{\text{systolic blood pressure} + 2(\text{diastolic blood pressure})}{3}$

$= 70\text{--}105$ mm Hg

Cerebral perfusion pressure (CPP) = MAP − intracranial pressure (ICP)
Stroke volume (SV) = cardiac output (CO)/heart rate (HR) = 32–58 mL/beat
Cardiac index (CI) = CO/BSA = 2.5–4.0 L/min
Cardiac output = SV × HR
Stroke volume index = SV/BSA = 30–65 mL/beat per m^2
Central venous pressure (CVP) = 0–8 mm Hg
Right atrial pressure (RAP) = 0–8 mm Hg
Right ventricular pressure (RVP) = 25/5 mm Hg
Pulmonary artery pressure (PAP)
  Diastolic = 5–12 mm Hg
  Systolic = 15–30 mm Hg
  Mean (PA) = 5–10 mm Hg
Pulmonary capillary wedge pressure (PCWP) = 5–12 mm Hg [pulmonary artery occlusion pressure (PAOP)]

Pulmonary vascular resistance (PVR) = $\dfrac{(\text{PAP} - \text{PCWP})80}{\text{CO}}$ = 150–250 dyne/second per cm^{-5}

Systemic vascular resistance (SVR) $= \dfrac{(\text{MAP} - \text{CVP})80}{\text{CO}} = 800\text{–}1{,}200$ dyne/second per cm^{-5}

Gas Exchange Calculation

FIO_2 Fraction of inspired oxygen: 0.21–1.0
PB Barometric pressure at sea level: 760 mm Hg
PH_2O Partial pressure of H_2O: 47 mm Hg (at 37°C)
RQ $\dfrac{\text{VCO}_2}{\text{VO}_2} = \text{normal} = 0.8$

Calculation for alveolar-arterial (A-a) PO_2 gradient

$$1.\ \text{PAO}_2 = \text{FIO}_2 \,(\text{PB} - \text{PH}_2\text{O}) - \left(\dfrac{\text{PACO}_2}{\text{RQ}}\right)$$

$$= \text{FIO}_2\,(713) - \dfrac{\text{PACO}_2}{0.8}$$

   2. Measure PO_2 from blood gas
      $\text{PAO}_2 - \text{PO}_2 = 10\text{–}20$ mm Hg

$$\text{AVDO}_2 = \dfrac{1.3\ \text{g}(\text{SaO}_2 - \text{SvO}_2)}{\text{hemoglobin}} = 5\text{–}8.3 \text{ volume percent}$$

   $>8.3 =$ oligemic cerebral hypoxemia or low flow
    $<5 =$ hyperemia

Water Deficit

Total body water deficit $= 0.6 \times$ body weight (kg) $\times \left(\dfrac{\text{serum Na}}{140 - 1}\right)$ (e.g., free water deficit for a

70 kg adult with a plasma sodium value of 160 mEq/L $= \dfrac{0.6 \times 70 \times 160}{140 - 1} = 6$ L)

Osmolar Gap

Calculated plasma osmolarity $= 2 \times (\text{Na}) + \dfrac{(\text{glucose})}{18} + \dfrac{(\text{BUN})}{2.8} = \text{mOsm/kg}$

Measured plasma osmolarity $= 275\text{–}295$ mOsm/kg
Osmolar gap $=$ measured Posm $=$ Pcalc $= \leq 10$ mEq/L

Anion Gap

Anion gap $=$ unmeasured anions $-$ unmeasured cations
          $= \text{Na}^+ - (\text{Cl}^- + \text{HCO}_3^-)$
          $= 12$ mEq/L

Table App-1. Adult Enteral Nutrition Formulary

Formula (Brand)	kcal/mL	Protein (g/L)	Osmolality (mOsm/kg)	Volume to meet U.S. RDA	Indications for Use
Osmolite HN	1.06	44	300	1320	Standard formula
Promote	1.0	62.5	340	1000	Stressed patients with higher protein requirements and intact hepatic and renal function
Osmolite	1.06	37	300	1887	Patients with lower protein requirements or protein restriction
Peptamen	1.0	40	270 (unflavored) 380 (flavored)	1500	Patients with severe gastrointestinal disease or pancreatic insufficiency
Sustacal Plus	1.52	61	670	1184	Hypercaloric oral supplement
Nutren 1.5	1.5	60	410 (unflavored)	1000	Hypercaloric tube feeding formula

RDA, recommended dietary allowance.
Note: propofol provides 1 kcal/mL.

Table App-2. Dosage of Hemodynamic Drugs*

	PATIENT'S WEIGHT (kg)						
	40	50	60	70	80	90	100
Dobutamine†	2/5	2/6	2/7	2/8	2/10	2/11	2/12
	4/10	4/12	4/14	4/17	4/19	4/22	4/24
	6/14	6/18	6/22	6/25	6/29	6/32	6/36
	8/19	8/24	8/29	8/34	8/38	8/43	8/48
	10/24	10/30	10/36	10/42	10/48	10/54	10/60
Dopamine†	2/3	2/4	2/5	2/5	2/6	2/7	2/8
	5/8	5/9	5/11	5/13	5/15	5/17	5/19
	10/15	10/19	10/23	10/26	10/30	10/34	10/38
	20/30	20/38	20/45	20/52	20/60	20/68	20/75

*Assumes 60 gtt/mL.
†First number, μg/kg per minute; second number, mL/hour.
Modified from Koch SM: The critical care catalog. In Civetta JM, Taylor RW, Kirby RR (ed): *Critical Care*. 2nd ed. Philadelphia: JB Lippincott Company, 1992, p 1941. By permission of the publisher.

Table App-3. Dosage Adjustment in Renal Failure*

	GLOMERULAR FILTRATION RATE (mL/minute)		
	> 50	10–50	< 10
Aminoglycosides			
Gentamicin	8–12	12	24
Tobramycin	8–12	12	24
Antifungal agents			
Amphotericin B	24	24	24–36
Flucytosine	6	12–24	24–48
Antiviral agents			
Acyclovir	8	24	48
Amantadine	12–24	48–72	168
Cephalosporins			
Cefamandole	6	6–8	8
Cefazolin	6	12	24–48
Cefotaxime	6–8	8–12	12–24
Cefoxitin	8	8–12	24–48
Cephalothin	6	6	8–12
Antibiotics			
Clindamycin	None	None	None
Erythromycin	None	None	None
Metronidazole	8	8–12	12–24
Penicillins			
Amoxicillin	6	6–12	12–16
Ampicillin	6	6–12	12–16
Carbenicillin	8–12	12–24	24–48
Dicloxacillin	None	None	None
Nafcillin	None	None	None
Penicillin G	6–8	8–12	12–16
Piperacillin	4–6	6–8	8
Ticarcillin	8–12	12–24	24–28
Sulfas/trimethoprim			
Sulfamethoxazole	12	18	24
Trimethoprim	12	18	24
Tetracyclines			
Doxycycline	12	12–18	18–24
Minocycline	None	None	None
Vancomycin	24–72	72–240	240

*Interval extension in hours.
Modified from Bennett WM, Aronoff GR, Golper TA, et al: *Drug Prescribing in Renal Failure*. Philadelphia: American College of Physicians, 1987. By permission of the publisher.

Table App–4. Drugs That Alter Antiepileptic Drug (AED) Concentrations

Mechanism of Drug Interaction	Carbamazepine	Phenobarbital	Phenytoin	Valproic Acid
Changes in AED absorption			Antacids	
			Enteral feedings	
Protein-binding displacement			Salicylates	Salicylates
			Sulfas	
			Valproic acid	
Enzyme inhibition of AED	Cimetidine	Chloramphenicol	Amiodarone	
	Danazol	Cimetidine	Chloramphenicol	
	Diltiazem	Isoniazid	Cimetidine	
	Erythromycin	Valproic acid	Ciprofloxacin	
	Fluoxetine		Disulfiram	
	Isoniazid		Isoniazid	
	Propoxyphene		Omeprazole	
	Valproic acid		Phenylbutazone	
	Verapamil		Propoxyphene	
Enzyme induction of AED	Phenobarbital	Carbamazepine	Carbamazepine	Carbamazepine
	Phenytoin	Ethanol	Ethanol	Phenobarbital
	Primidone	Phenytoin	Phenobarbital	Phenytoin
				Primidone
AED effect on other drugs				
Enzyme induction	Clonazepam	Carbamazepine	Carbamazepine	
	Doxycycline	Chlorpromazine	Corticosteroids	
	Ethosuximide	Corticosteroids	Doxycycline	
	Theophylline	Doxycycline	Folic acid	
	Valproic acid	Oral contraceptives	Oral contraceptives	
	Warfarin	Phenytoin	Primidone	
		Quinidine	Pyridoxine	
		Tricyclic antidepressants	Quinidine	
		Warfarin	Vitamin D	
			Warfarin	
Enzyme inhibition				Ethosuximide
				Phenobarbital
				Phenytoin
				Primidone

Table App–5. Major Electrolyte Abnormalities

Electrolyte Abnormality	Cause	Consequence	Treatment°
Hypomagnesemia	GI and renal loss, drug interaction	Cardiac arrhythmias, muscle weakness	1–2 g of magnesium sulfate in 20 mL of normal saline over 2 minutes
Hypermagnesemia	Renal failure, antacids, enemas	Muscle weakness, hypotension, asystole	10% calcium gluconate, 10–20 mL IV over 10 minutes
Hypercalcemia	Diabetes insipidus, malignancy, hyper-parathyroidism	Seizures, coma, cardiac arrhythmias	Hydration, 0.9% NaCl, 500 mL/hour
Hypocalcemia	Critical illness, hypoparathyroidism, fat-deficient diet	Cardiac arrhythmias, tetanus, seizures, laryngospasm	1–2 g of calcium gluconate IV over 10 minutes; then 6 g of calcium gluconate in 500 mL D5W by infusion for 4–6 hours
Hypophosphatemia	Parenteral nutrition, preexisting alcoholism, renal failure	Congestive cardiomyopathy, respiratory failure, rhabdomyolysis	Potassium phosphate, 0.08 mmol/kg IV in 500 mL of 0.45% saline over 6 hours
Hyperphosphatemia	Rare	Similar to those with hypocalcemia	Phosphate binders, 1 g of calcium p.o. t.i.d.
Hypokalemia	Vomiting, prolonged starvation, GI loss	Ventricular fibrillation, quadriplegia	40 mmol of KCl/L IV at 20 mmol/hour
Hyperkalemia	Crush injury, hemolysis, renal failure	Cardiac arrest	Calcium gluconate 10%, 10 mL IV over 3 minutes

GI, gastrointestinal; IV, intravenously.
°When markedly abnormal.
Data from Singer GG: Fluid and electrolyte management. In Ahya SN, Flood K, Paranjothi S (eds): *Washington Manual of Medical Therapeutics*. 30th ed. Philadelphia: Lippincott Williams & Wilkins, 2001, pp 43–75.

Table App–6. Modified National Institutes of Health Stroke Scale*

Item Number	*Item Name*	*Score*
1B	Level of consciousness questions	0 = answers both correctly 1 = answers one correctly 2 = answers neither correctly
1C	Level of consciousness commands	0 = performs both tasks correctly 1 = performs one task correctly 2 = performs neither task
2	Gaze	0 = normal 1 = partial gaze palsy 2 = total gaze palsy
3	Visual fields	0 = no visual loss 1 = partial hemianopsia 2 = complete hemianopsia 3 = bilateral hemianopsia
5a	Left arm	0 = no drift 1 = drift before 10 seconds 2 = falls before 10 seconds 3 = no effort against gravity 4 = no movement
5b	Right arm	0 = no drift 1 = drift before 10 seconds 2 = falls before 10 seconds 3 = no effort against gravity 4 = no movement
6a	Left leg	0 = no drift 1 = drift before 5 seconds 2 = falls before 5 seconds 3 = no effort against gravity 4 = no movement
6b	Right leg	0 = no drift 1 = drift before 5 seconds 2 = falls before 5 seconds 3 = no effort against gravity 4 = no movement
8	Sensory	0 = normal 1 = abnormal
9	Language	0 = normal 1 = mild aphasia 2 = severe aphasia 3 = mute or global aphasia
11	Neglect	0 = normal 1 = mild 2 = severe

*The item numbers correspond to the numbering in the original scale to allow easy identification of the changes. From Lyden PD, Lu M, Levine SR, Brott TG, Broderick J: A modified National Institutes of Health Stroke Scale for use in stroke clinical trials: preliminary reliability and validity. *Stroke* 32:1310–1317, 2001. By permission of the American Heart Association.

Index